REVISED EDITION

Pharmacotherapeutics

FOR ADVANCED NURSING PRACTICE

Edited by

Tammie Lee Demler, PharmD, BS Pharm, RPh, BCGP, BCPP

Clinical Associate Professor

The State University of New York at Buffalo School of Pharmacy and Pharmaceutical Sciences
The State University of New York at Buffalo School of Medicine
Department of Psychiatry

Clinical Assistant Professor

D'Youville College School of Pharmacy
University of Florida College of Pharmacy

Clinical Pharmacist and Pharmacy Practice Residency Program Director

New York State Office of Mental Health
Buffalo, New York

Jacqueline Rhoads, PhD, ACNP-BC, ANP-C, PMHNP-BE, FAANP

Professor

School of Tropical Medicine
Tulane University
New Orleans, Louisiana

Clinical Professor

School of Nursing
University of North Carolina at Charlotte
Charlotte, North Carolina

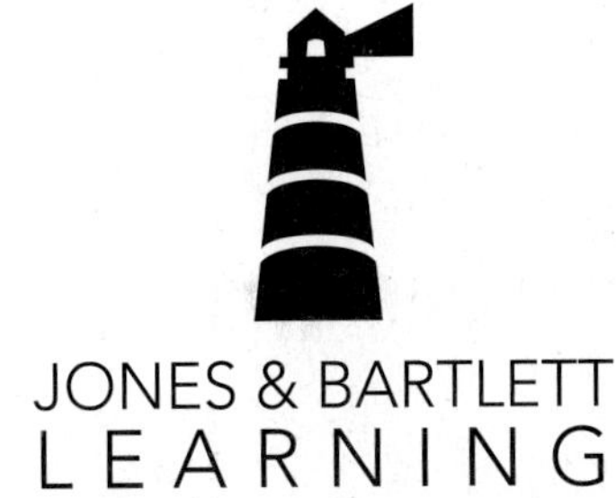

World Headquarters
Jones & Bartlett Learning
5 Wall Street
Burlington, MA 01803
978-443-5000
info@jblearning.com
www.jblearning.com

Jones & Bartlett Learning books and products are available through most bookstores and online booksellers. To contact Jones & Bartlett Learning directly, call 800-832-0034, fax 978-443-8000, or visit our website, www.jblearning.com.

Substantial discounts on bulk quantities of Jones & Bartlett Learning publications are available to corporations, professional associations, and other qualified organizations. For details and specific discount information, contact the special sales department at Jones & Bartlett Learning via the above contact information or send an email to specialsales@jblearning.com.

11056-2

Production Credits
VP, Product Management: Amanda Martin
Director of Product Management: Matthew Kane
Product Manager: Tina Chen
Product Specialist: Christina Freitas
Project Manager: Kristen Rogers
Senior Project Specialist: Vanessa Richards
Senior Marketing Manager: Jennifer Scherzay
Product Fulfillment Manager: Wendy Kilborn
Composition: S4Carlisle Publishing Services
Cover Design: Michael O'Donnell
Rights & Media Specialist: Wes DeShano
Cover Image: © Anatoly Tiplyashin/Shutterstock
Printing and Binding: LSC Communications
Cover Printing: LSC Communications

To order this product, use ISBN: 978-1-284-15429-0

The Library of Congress has cataloged the first printing as follows:

Library of Congress Cataloging-in-Publication Data
Names: Demler, Tammie Lee, editor. | Rhoads, Jacqueline, 1948- editor.
Title: Pharmacotherapeutics for advanced nursing practice / edited by Tammie Lee Demler, Jacqueline Rhoads.
Description: Burlington, Massachusetts : Jones & Bartlett Learning, [2018] | Includes bibliographical references and index.
Identifiers: LCCN 2016038360 | ISBN 9781284110401 (hardcover)
Subjects: | MESH: Drug Therapy--nursing | Advanced Practice Nursing--methods | Examination Questions
Classification: LCC RS97 | NLM WY 18.2 | DDC 615.1076--dc23
LC record available at https://lccn.loc.gov/2016038360

6048

Printed in the United States of America
23 22 21 20 19 10 9 8 7 6 5 4 3 2 1

Contents

Chapter 3

Chapter 4

Chapter 5

Chapter 8

Chapter 9

Chapter 10

Chapter 11

Chapter 12

Chapter 13

Chapter 14

How to Use Our Text

We hope that you find this text to be a helpful, quick and reliable resource for "at-a-glance" and "need-to-know" drug information as well as for therapeutic guidance on general medication management for the majority of drugs currently available on the U.S. market. We understand that at times you need only specific information about a certain drug, and at other times you need information about an entire class of agents or drugs associated with the treatment of medical conditions, as well as prescribing considerations that must be included in the overall treatment plan. To meet these differing needs, we have structured this text to allow you to easily access the information you need. While we are confident that you will find this material to be educational and easy to use, we remind readers that clinical practice and prescribing decisions must be made with real-time resources and clinical judgment that looks past narrative didactic instruction.

We have selected the American Hospital Formulary Service's (AHFS) therapeutic drug classification because it is widely accepted as a primary drug categorization system in both the United States and Canada under which many health system formularies are organized. The AHFS systematic approach used to categorize drugs is based on grouping drugs together that share similar pharmacologic, therapeutic, and /or chemical characteristics. Due to the potential for one drug to be used in more than one therapeutic category, we provide an indexed alphabetical listing with reference to **its primary body system** chapter. For drugs used in more than one body system, a symbol will guide the reader to the additional sections (body systems) that may provide specific and significant detailed information for use in other conditions and therapeutic indications.

Each chapter includes an overview of the body system represented, with a specific focus on the drug classes associated with treatment of medical conditions in that therapeutic area. We have enlisted experts from across the United States to develop the didactic content, including brief narrative overviews of specific categories of drug, and have paired this information with companion drug grids that offer the most significant alerts, warnings, and clinical "pearls" for the busy clinician who needs to extract "the most critical facts" efficiently. These drug precautions, pearls, and "universal prescribing alerts" are based on those emphasized by the drug manufacturers and may not comprehensively reflect the varying degrees of risk for class-related effects. To reduce the risk of information overload (and congestion), we have provided "illustrative" dosing for drugs that have multiple indications for use, with varying dose schedules based on those different indications. This illustrative (usual) dose should be used merely as a benchmark for further exploration if other indications for use are under consideration.

Brand names are provided for those products still available on the U.S. market. Due to ever-changing product availability, you should refer to Food and Drug Administration (FDA) resources to confirm the actual brands available.

This drug summary is intended for educational purposes only. Prescribing decisions should be based on real-time comprehensive drug databases that are updated on a regular basis.

Tips from the Field

Dr. Demler and Dr. Rhoads are practicing clinicians and educators with decades of experience, and they share their experiences to guide your own learning. Thus, this text includes a wealth of tips to enhance your didactic journey and your exploration of clinical pharmacology. Some of the global or universal prescribing alerts are provided at the beginning of the companion drug grids and others are incorporated within the narrative sections of this text.

Case studies are provided to allow the reader to apply didactic knowledge to real-world clinical situations. Conclusions are provided to help the reader apply "lessons learned"; they describe the rationale for the correct answers to the case study questions and explain why other options are not appropriate. To answer the case study questions, readers should refer to both the narrative chapter overviews and the companion drug grids.

Special Populations

Advanced or Early Age Alerts

Of note, we have included only FDA-approved indications for use; however, we recognize that there is considerable non-FDA-approved (i.e., "off-label") use of some drugs in special populations including, but not limited to, older adults (geriatrics) and children (pediatrics). We have included specific symbols that will alert readers to drugs that have specific FDA-approved dosing for these age groups.

In most cases, drugs approved for adult use also are approved for older adults; however, when FDA-approved dosing is different, the (GD) symbol will guide the reader to consult additional resources for specific dose recommendations. Doses listed are for usual adult dosage ranges only. "Geriatric doses" are assumed to be the same as adult doses unless otherwise noted with a symbol. Refer to real-time prescribing references for geriatric doses. Our text does provide a Beers list alert (BL) for all medications that had been identified as meeting criteria of "geriatric risk" at the time of this publication. Even drugs without a Beers list warning may require caution when they are prescribed for older adults (especially first doses and changes to current regimens) and not all Beers criteria list drugs listed in this book may appear on the most current published Beers list. Clinicians must be constantly vigilant when treating this special population.

Additional age-specific caution must be extended to "younger populations" as well. When pediatric use is FDA-approved and age-specific (non-adult) dosing is available, the (PD) symbol will guide the reader to additional prescribing references. Pediatric specialists are often faced with the clinical dilemma of whether to choose to use a medication for children as an "off-label" treatment when adequate studies have not been performed in the pediatric population. These decisions are complicated and require experts in the field to provide guidance in order to deliver the best care. When identifying a medication of interest for use in a pediatric patient, further exploration of the literature should be initiated to determine if studies have been conducted to demonstrate safety and efficacy, even in cases where the FDA has not officially approved its use. In our text, we have included a pediatric symbol when the drug is FDA approved for pediatric use and carries specific pediatric (non-adult) dosing. The lack of a pediatric symbol does not necessarily mean it is not approved for pediatric use.

Altered Organ Function Alerts

Often, the "geriatric doses" are based on the organ function decline expected with advancing age. However, even younger adults with reduced organ function may require a dose adjustment of medications. In our reference, we provide symbols to alert the clinician that there are specific FDA-recommended dose adjustments for patients with hepatic compromise ■ or renal function compromise ▲. When a symbol indicates that specific altered-organ dose adjustment is needed, the clinician should refer to primary real-time dosing references to ensure safe use of that drug in the specific patient. Often manufacturers recommend dose adjustments based on clinical judgment, even when the FDA has not provided specific dosing recommendations.

When significant comorbidities are present, these deficits may impact the pharmacokinetics of drugs more significantly and may alter the safety and efficacy of these drugs in diverse populations. In such circumstances, cautious use of the specific agent is warranted.

All drugs pose a risk of potential allergic reaction. In addition, unpredictable first-dose effects may include, and are not limited to, dizziness, drowsiness, vertigo, or fatigue, and impairment of the patient's ability to perform tasks requiring mental alertness. Caution is always recommended when using any new drug for the first time, when the dose is changed, and with continued use of known offending agents. Prescribers must also be aware that patients may be allergic or intolerant to the inert (non-active) ingredients in medication, thus verification of allergy prior to prescribing, selecting, and administering is essential.

Pregnancy and Lactation

This text is not intended to be a pregnancy and lactation guide. In some chapters, authors may provide a specific caution about use of certain drugs during pregnancy; however, clinicians should not interpret these intermittent cautions to mean that agents in other chapters are "safer" to use during pregnancy. In fact, the FDA recently published changes to the pregnancy-related labeling of prescription drugs that went into effect on June 30, 2015. This policy has been termed the "Content and Format of Labeling for Human Prescription Drug and Biological Products: Requirements for Pregnancy and Lactation Labeling," more succinctly referred to as the "Pregnancy and Lactation Labeling Rule" (PLLR or "final rule"). These content and format changes for information presented in the Physician Labeling Rule (PLR) format were intended to provide more robust information upon which to base risk-versus-benefit decisions when providing care and counseling to pregnant women and nursing mothers who need to take medication. Thus, these women can make informed and educated decisions for themselves and their children. The previously used pregnancy letter categories (i.e., A, B, C, D, and X) are now obsolete; labeling must be updated when information becomes outdated.

Drugs approved by the FDA after June 30, 2015, must use the new format immediately. Labeling for prescription drugs approved on or after June 30, 2001, and prior to June 20, 2015, will be phased in gradually, so we can expect to see both labeling versions for a while. This transition continues during the development of this text. Thus, we recommend that, when identifying any medication of interest for use during pregnancy, clinicians undertake further exploration of data sources to determine the overall safety and efficacy of the agent in pregnancy.

Additional changes we can expect to see with the new PLLR labeling requirement include information on a pregnancy exposure registry for a drug when one is available. Information related to a drug's effects on the reproductive potential of both males and females now must include the need for pregnancy testing, contraception recommendations, and information about infertility as it relates to the drug.

Clinicians should continue to provide education about the reproductive risks of medication use and offer risk-reduction strategies (including contraceptive options when indicated) to women of childbearing age. Many medications—including, but not limited to, anti-infective agents—may decrease the effectiveness of oral contraceptives and intrinsically require counseling in advance about potential pregnancy risks of agents used. These reproductive risks may also extend to males and may preclude sperm donation.

Black Box Warnings

The FDA requires the drug manufacturer to prominently display the most serious and severe warnings at the top of a drug's package insert. One type of warning—commonly referred to as a "black box warning"—appears on a prescription drug's label and is designed to call attention to serious or life-threatening risk; it appears within a box and is considered the highest level of alert to medication safety. The FDA has developed guidelines for manufacturers outlining the structure and content of these boxed warnings; these guidelines are only strongly encouraged, however, and are not legally enforceable. For this reason, there can be confusion over which drugs actually have boxed warnings, the degree of risk these boxed warnings signify, and the reliability of online real-time resources in adequately identifying the boxed warnings issued for each agent.

In our text, we provide the ■ symbol to indicate that the drug listed was associated with a black box warning (BBW) at the time of our publication. Some drugs carry multiple boxed warnings. Thus, when a BBW symbol is present, we encourage the prescriber to seek more detailed information from the package insert about the number and nature of the BBWs associated with the drug.

There are many types of boxed warnings:

- Potential for adverse reaction that is life threatening, permanently disabling, or even fatal
- Potential for serious adverse reaction that may be prevented or reduced in severity by using the drug appropriately
- Restrictions to ensure safe use
- Highlighted warning information that is important for the prescriber to know
- Risk-benefit considerations that are unique to a drug within its drug class

Boxed warnings may be established during clinical trials or during postmarketing surveillance. If human data are not available, the BBW may be based on animal data indicating the drug resulted in serious animal toxicities or adverse events. Drugs with similar properties to the primary offending drug may inherit that drug's boxed warning based on theoretical risk.

Both inconsistency and variability are inherent in the BBW system, and no set requirements or criteria for inclusion of a boxed warning have been established. For this reason, FDA guidelines and professional judgment must guide a clinician's use of, or hesitancy to use, a specific drug. Of note, some contraindications or warnings/precautions become boxed warnings for some medications but not for others. Therefore, absence of a BBW does not make a drug safer, and the precautions noted in the package insert should be considered across the entire risk-benefit drug therapy continuum.

There is no official comprehensive list of BBWs available from the FDA. MedWatch notifications containing boxed warnings are available on the FDA website but are difficult to search by drug name. These notices are archived based on date of release. Drug information resources, such as this text or real-time online databases, are not uniform or comprehensive, either.

How should clinicians use boxed warnings? Review the package insert for BBWs before prescribing, and do not rely solely on the presence or absence of a BBW to alert you to serious precautions or contraindications. Although BBWs are still considered the highest level of alert, not every serious alert will be represented by a BBW. If a drug does not have BBW, it may still have very serious side effects. Always use your best clinical judgment in prescribing, selecting, dispensing, and administering medication and always consider using more than one resource to evaluate potential risks.

Drug Interactions

All drugs are subject to metabolic drug interactions. Drug interactions can be serious, complicated, and difficult to predict. In this text, we specifically identify only those drugs that require dose adjustment according to their manufacturers; however, when prescribing more than one drug, always confirm potential drug interactions prior to the use of a new multiple-drug regimen and when investigating potential adverse effects that may be a result of drug interactions. Consider drug interactions at every point of prescribing, dispensing, or administering medications and on an ongoing basis when monitoring the regimen you have implemented.

Drugs metabolized by the hepatic cytochrome P450 enzymes are subject to either induction or inhibition by other drugs (some are the perpetrating substance), which may result in a decrease or increase in substrate drug plasma concentrations. Patients who have a genetic predisposition to rapid or slow metabolism may be at higher risk of drug-induced side effects and/or subtherapeutic effects of medications administered at the "usual doses."

Potential sources of pharmacokinetic drug interactions are numerous, can be overwhelming, and are often confusing for those clinicians who are not pharmacokineticists. Our text alerts clinicians when manufacturers have provided prescribing recommendations that advise when dose adjustments may be warranted, or when certain drug combinations should be avoided. Although we do not provide a specific symbol indicating the existence of this kind of general risk, all regimens should be continually evaluated in light of potential drug interactions, as the risk of interaction becomes nearly unavoidable with increasing pharmacologic burdens. Drug interactions are a common therapeutic challenge; however, determining the potential risk or outcome and making clinical decisions about how to mitigate, avoid, or monitor such effects are necessary.

One specific drug-related adverse effect that is cumulative, is additive, and can be considered a pharmacodynamic consequence of a pharmacokinetic interaction is prolongation of the heart's QTc interval. The QTc interval is highly individualized and subject to fluctuations throughout the day based on one's level of activity. Even patients without heart complications are at risk of torsades de pointes (malignant heart arrhythmia) if placed on a drug with significant QTc risk. For this reason, we have included a QT symbol if a drug has been associated with a change in the QTc interval. The absence of this symbol should not be considered an indication that a drug carries no risk of QTc prolongation or torsades de pointes. Many medicines have not been tested for this risk in patients, especially those patients with congenital long QT syndrome. Because these safety data are constantly changing and emerging, clinicians are encouraged to identify a real-time resource that they can readily use to evaluate potential QTc risks on an ongoing basis, thereby ensuring that the available evidence supports their continued caution about certain drugs. Because data change regularly regarding these risks, we recommend always checking for the most up-to-date information.

The risk of QTc prolongation is increased in susceptible individuals, including patients with cardiac disease or other conditions that may increase the risk of QTc prolongation including cardiac arrhythmias, congenital long QT syndrome, heart failure, bradycardia, myocardial infarction, hypertension, coronary artery disease, hypomagnesemia, hypokalemia, and hypocalcemia, and patients receiving medications known to prolong the QTc interval or cause electrolyte imbalances. Female patients, geriatric patients, and patients with diabetes, thyroid disease, malnutrition, alcoholism, or hepatic dysfunction may also be at increased risk for QTc prolongation. Patients receiving these medications who have cardiac disease or arrhythmias should be monitored closely, electrocardiography (ECG) should be performed during and after their therapy, and in some cases the clinical decision should be made to avoid the agent entirely if the risk is too great. When evaluating QTc risk, the following risk categories, which are based on the CredibleMeds, should be considered in your overall risk ranking:

- **Drugs to avoid in congenital long QT syndrome.** Substantial evidence supports the conclusion that these drugs pose a risk of torsades de pointes for patients with congenital long QT syndrome. Drugs on this list include those in the three next-higher risk categories and other drugs that do not prolong the QTc interval per se but have a theoretical risk of causing arrhythmia based on their known stimulant actions on the heart.
- **Known risk of torsades de pointes.** Substantial evidence supports the conclusion that these drugs prolong the QTc interval *and* are clearly associated with a risk of torsades de pointes, even when taken as directed in the official labeling.
- **Possible risk of torsades de pointes.** Substantial evidence supports the conclusion that these drugs can cause QTc prolongation, *but* there is insufficient evidence at this time that these drugs, when used as directed in the official labeling, are associated with a risk of causing torsades de pointes.
- **Conditional risk of torsades de pointes.** Substantial evidence supports the conclusion that these drugs are associated with a risk of torsades de pointes *but* only under certain conditions (e.g., excessive dose, hypokalemia, congenital long QT syndrome, or by causing a drug–drug interaction that results in excessive QTc interval prolongation)

Disclaimer

The information presented in this text is intended solely for the purpose of providing general information about health-related matters. It is not intended for any other purpose, including but not limited to medical advice or treatment, nor is it intended to substitute for the users' relationships with their own healthcare providers. To that extent, by use of this text and the information it contains, the user affirms the understanding of the purpose of this text and releases us from any claims arising from the user's comprehension and application of the general information provided in this text.

Additional Resources

American Society of Health-System Pharmacists: http://www.ashp.org

Beers List: https://www.guideline.gov/summaries/summary/49933

Clinical Pharmacology (online database). Tampa, FL: Gold Standard, Inc; 2013.

CredibleMeds: http://www.CredibleMeds.org

FDA Black Box Warnings: http://www.fda.gov/downloads/ForConsumers/ConsumerUpdates/UCM107976.pdf

FDA Pregnancy Label Changes: http://www.fda.gov/Drugs/DevelopmentApprovalProcess/DevelopmentResources/Labeling/ucm093307.htm

About the Editors

Tammie Lee Demler, PharmD, BS Pharm, MBA, RPh, BCGP, BCPP

Dr. Tammie Lee Demler received her Doctor of Pharmacy, Master of Business Administration, and Bachelor of Science degrees at the State University of New York (SUNY) at Buffalo. Dr. Demler is dually Board certified in both geriatrics and psychiatric pharmacy practice, and is currently the Director of Pharmacy Services and Pharmacy residency training at the New York State Office of Mental Health (OMH) at the Buffalo Psychiatric Center. She holds numerous adjunct academic appointments, including Clinical Associate Professor for the State University of New York (SUNY) at Buffalo School of Pharmacy and Pharmaceutical Sciences, Department of Pharmacy Practice and SUNY School of Medicine, Department of Psychiatry, Clinical Assistant Professor at D'Youville College School of Pharmacy, University of Florida School of Pharmacy, and Clinical Instructor for the Erie County Community College Pharmacy Technician Certification Program. Dr. Demler collaborates with both the National Association of the Boards of Pharmacy (NABP) and the Board of Pharmaceutical Specialties (BPS) to develop board examinations that establish the minimum competencies expected for new practitioners for practice in an ever-changing clinical environment. Prior to embarking on her academic and institutional career, Dr. Demler's clinical practice focused on ambulatory care in community pharmacy.

Dr. Demler has authored and co-authored numerous original research articles and expert reviews for print media. She is a member of the editorial board of advisors and regular contributor to *U.S. Pharmacist* and reviewer for *Pharmacist's Letter*. Prior to launching *Pharmacotherapeutics for Advanced Nursing Practice*, Dr. Demler authored a chapter on insomnia in the American College of Clinical Pharmacy's (ACCP's) *Ambulatory Care Self-Assessment*. She also has provided expert pharmacotherapeutic consultation for other books such as the *Side Effects of Drugs: Annual Volume 36* and *Clinical Consult to Psychiatric Nursing for Advanced Practice*. She has presented medication continuing education programs internationally and nationally, and is an Academic Educator for the New York State Medicaid Prescriber Education program sponsored by the New York Department of Health. Dr. Demler served as President of both the Pharmacists Society of the State of New York and the Pharmacists Association of Western New York.

Dr. Demler is also a local media personality, hosting her own weekly TV talk show as well as a weekly community affairs radio segment. She has won a number of prestigious national, state, and local awards acknowledging both her professional and community-based contributions.

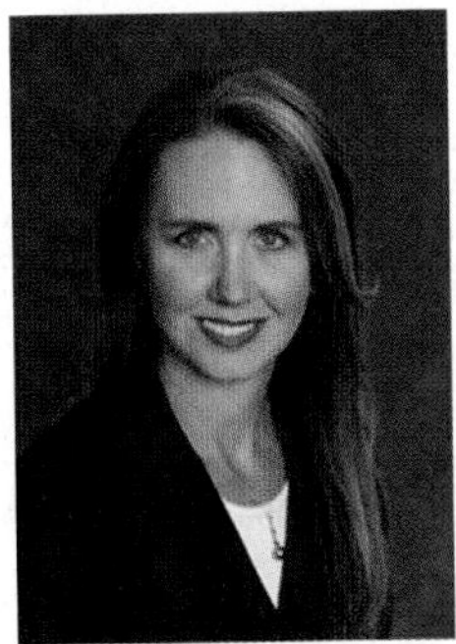

This book is dedicated to my loving family: my husband Tom, my mother Barbara, and my sons Michael and Matthew Carter. Words cannot express my appreciation for your continuous encouragement, love, and support. I acknowledge also my heavenly Father, who continues to bless me abundantly in countless, amazing ways.

—Tammie Lee

Jacqueline Rhoads, PhD, ACNP-BC, ANP-C, PMHNP-BE, FAANP

Dr. Jacqueline Rhoads has held three positions as program director at three major academic institutions. When not in the classroom, she has a history of caring for underserved populations as an adult nurse practitioner at various hospitals and clinics in Texas, Louisiana, and Georgia. Dr. Rhoads has been an acute and primary care nurse practitioner with the U.S. Army Reserves for almost 30 years. Her research focuses on post-traumatic stress disorder (PTSD) in active-duty service personnel, women in the military, medical personnel, post-Vietnam War veterans, and post-Desert Storm PTSD effects.

Dr. Rhoads has written numerous articles on clinical and professional issues for both acute and primary care nursing. She is a frequent speaker and member of several professional organizations. She is also co-author of the American Association of Critical-Care Nurses' ACNP Standards for Practice (2006); she was an expert participant in the American Nurses Credentialing Center's Role Delineation Study.

Dr. Rhoads has been awarded more than 10 Excellence in Teaching awards and has been inducted into the Fellows of the American Academy of Nurse Practitioners. Her professional experience includes 23 years of teaching experience in primary and critical care nursing; 11 years as a nurse practitioner in acute and primary care; 18 years of experience as a clinical nurse specialist (CNS); and 30 years of experience in the Army Nurse Corps, including during the Vietnam War and Desert Storm. Her numerous publications include six books, two of which won the American Nurses Association's book of the year awards in 2011 and 2012. She has written more than 29 articles in refereed and non-refereed journals and newsletters. Her research has involved 4 non-funded state grants and 20 funded grants (federal, state, and local awards). She has also given more than 100 formal presentations in the United States, Europe, and the Middle East.

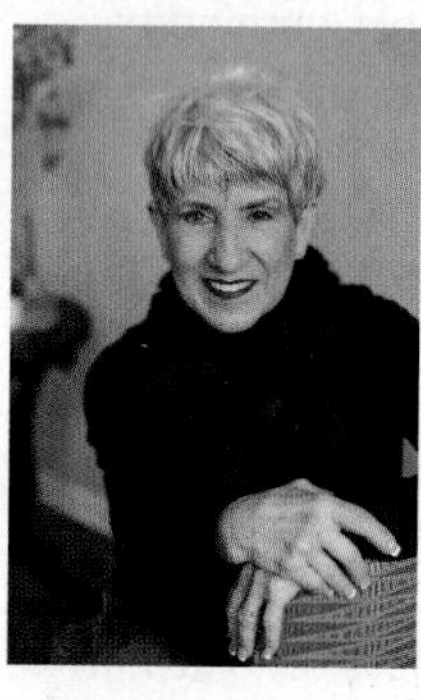

Contributors

Lauren Adams, PharmD, BCPS
Clinical Pharmacist
Hendrick Medical Center
Abilene, Texas

Joseph Bellavia, PharmD
Independent Pharmacist
Compounding Pharmacist
Buffalo, New York

Kirsten Butterfoss, PharmD, CGP
Clinical Assistant Professor
D'Youville College School of Pharmacy
Buffalo, New York

Tammie Lee Demler, PharmD, BS Pharm, MBA, RPh, BCGP, BCPP
Clinical Associate Professor
University at Buffalo School of Pharmacy and Pharmaceutical Sciences
Clinical Assistant Professor
University at Buffalo School of Medicine, Department of Psychiatry
D'Youville College School of Pharmacy
University of Florida College of Pharmacy
Clinical Pharmacist and Pharmacy Practice Residency Program Director
New York State Office of Mental Health
Buffalo, New York

Krystal L. Edwards, PharmD, FCCP, BCPS
Associate Professor, Department of Pharmacy Practice
Ambulatory Care Division
Associate Dean for Career Development, Office of Professional Affairs
Department of Pharmacy Practice
Texas Tech University Health Sciences Center
School of Pharmacy
Dallas, Texas

Katherine Frachetti, MD
Department of Endocrinology and Internal Medicine
Mercy Hospital
Buffalo, New York

Shannon Gowen, PharmD
Post-doctoral Research Fellow
Translational Pharmacology Research Core
NYS Center of Excellence in Bioinformatics and Life Sciences
University at Buffalo
Buffalo, New York

Wayne H. Grant, PharmD, MBA
Clinical Assistant Professor, Adjunct
University of Florida School of Pharmacy
Clinical Pharmacist, Hospice of the Western Reserve
Cleveland, Ohio

Carolyn Hempel, PharmD, BCPS
Clinical Assistant Professor
University at Buffalo School of Pharmacy and Pharmaceutical Sciences
Buffalo, New York

Margaret A. Huwer, PharmD
Director of Pharmacy Services
Riverside Methodist and Dublin Methodist Hospitals
Columbus, Ohio

Stephy Kuriakose, PharmD, BCPS
Clinical Pharmacist
Methodist Medical Center
Dallas, Texas

Claudia Lee, RPh, MD
Clinical Preceptor
University at Buffalo School of Medicine
University at Buffalo School of Pharmacy and Pharmaceutical Sciences
D'Youville College, Department of Health Sciences, Physician Assistant Program
Medical Specialist, New York State Office of Mental Health, Buffalo Psychiatric Center
Buffalo, New York

Michelle Lewis, PharmD, MHA
Clinical Assistant Professor
D'Youville College School of Pharmacy
Buffalo, New York

Jeffrey Lombardo, PharmD, BCOP
Research Assistant Professor
Medication Management Research Network
Associate Director, Empire State Patient Safety Assurance Network
Research Assistant Professor
NYS Center of Excellence in Bioinformatics and Life Sciences
Translational Pharmacology Research Core
Buffalo, New York

Michael S. Mac Evoy, PharmD, BCPS, CDE
Director of Experiential Education
Clinical Assistant Professor
D'Youville College School of Pharmacy
Buffalo, New York

Beatriz Manzor Mitrzyk, PharmD, BCPS, BCACP
Clinical Assistant Professor
Regional Director, Clinical Practice Assessments WPPD program
University of Florida College of Pharmacy
Gainesville, Florida

Gene D. Morse, PharmD, FCCP, BCPS
SUNY Distinguished Professor—Pharmacy Practice (Medicine, Pediatrics)
Co-director, SUNY Global Health Institute
Director, UB Center for Integrated Global Biomedical Sciences
Director, Translational Pharmacology Research Core
NYS Center of Excellence in Bioinformatics and Life Sciences
University at Buffalo
Buffalo, New York

Kimberly Mulcahy, PharmD, BCPS
Clinical Assistant Professor, Adjunct
University at Buffalo School of Pharmacy and Pharmaceutical Sciences
Clinical Pharmacist, New York State Office of Mental Health, Buffalo Psychiatric Center
Buffalo, New York

Charlene Meyer, PharmD
Behavioral Health Pharmacist, Fidelis Care
Clinical Pharmacist, Sisters of Charity Hospital
Buffalo, New York

Steven E. Pass, PharmD, FCCM, FCCP, FASHP, BCPS
Professor and Vice Chair for Residency Programs
Department of Pharmacy Practice
Texas Tech University Health Sciences Center
School of Pharmacy
Dallas, Texas

Gina Prescott, PharmD, BCPS
Clinical Associate Professor
University at Buffalo School of Pharmacy and Pharmaceutical Sciences
Global Health Community Chair
Buffalo, New York

Laura Rumschik, PharmD
Clinical Pharmacist, Ambulatory Care
Buffalo, New York

Christopher Thomas, PharmD, BCPP, BCPS, CGP
Clinical Assistant Professor of Pharmacology
Ohio University Heritage College of Osteopathic Medication
Residency Program Director for PGY-1 and PGY-2 Psychiatry Specialty
Clinical Pharmacy Specialist in Psychiatry
Chillicothe Veterans Affairs Medical Center (VAMC)
Chillicothe, Ohio

Susan D. Thompson DNP, ACNS-BC
Assistant Professor & Graduate Clinical Coordinator
University of St. Francis
Joliet, Illinois

Rebecca Waite, PharmD, BCPP
Clinical Assistant Professor
D'Youville College School of Pharmacy
Buffalo, New York

Amy L. Wojciechowski, PharmD, BCPS-AQ ID, BCCCP
Clinical Assistant Professor
D'Youville College, Department of Pharmacy Practice
Clinical Pharmacist, Niagara Falls Memorial Medical Center
Niagara Falls, New York

The editors would like to acknowledge Kimberly Mulcahy, PharmD, BCPS, and Emily Leppien, PharmD, who are current and past pharmacy residents of Dr. Demler and who have provided additional editing and reviewing of the drug information found in this text.

The editors would like to also acknowledge the work of those who assisted with the drug grid and manuscript content (and additional project support*):

Amanda Conenna, PharmD

Valerie Cooper, PharmD

Anna Gach, PharmD

Haneesha Goli, PharmD

Jessica Isaac, PharmD

Sera Kim, PharmD candidate

Young Ji Amy Lee, PharmD

Tera Mcilwain, PharmD*

Ishita Mehta, PharmD/MBA candidate*

Charlene Meyer, PharmD*

George K. Nimako, PharmD, MS

Michael Rudzinski, PharmD

Laura Rumschik, PharmD*

Finda Sankoh, PharmD

Saundra M. Seep, PharmD*

Christina Shaffer, PharmD

Megan Skelly, PharmD candidate*

Alex Smith, PharmD candidate

Ting You, PharmD/MBA candidate*

Kaitlyn Victor, PharmD candidate*

Kristin Q. Yin, PharmD candidate

Eric Zapalowski, PharmD

Lindsey Zawierucha, PharmD

Reviewers

Cathryn J. Baack, PhD, APRN, FNP-C
Assistant Professor and Program Director, FNP Track of DNP
Marian University Leighton School of Nursing
Indianapolis, Indiana

Kellie Bruce, PhD, RN, FNP-BC
Associate Professor
FNP Program Director
Texas Tech University Health Sciences Center
Lubbock, Texas

Rachel W. Cozort, PhD, MSN, RN, CNE
Assistant Professor of Nursing
Pfeiffer University
Misenheimer, North Carolina

Ann Hallock, DNP, APRN, ANP-C, CNN

Maria Irrera Newcomb, MSN, CRNP, FNP-BC
Assistant Professor
College of Nursing and Health Professions
Drexel University
Philadelphia, Pennsylvania

Catherine Jennings, DNP, MSN, APN
Associate Professor
Felician University
Rutherford, New Jersey

Dr. Kara Jones DNP, CNE, RN-BC, CMSRN
Clinical Assistant Professor
The University of Texas at Tyler School of Nursing
Tyler, Texas

Linda J. Keilman, DNP, MSN, GNP-BC
Assistant Professor, Health Programs
College of Nursing
Michigan State University
East Lansing, Michigan

Christy McDonald Lenahan, DNP, FNP-BC, ENP-C, CNE
University of Louisiana at Lafayette
Lafayette, Louisiana

Debbie Mahoney, PhD, APRN, FNP-BC

Mary Jane Miskovsky, DNP, CRNP, NP
Assistant Professor
DNP Program
Clinical Concentration Coordinator
Adult Gerontology Primary Care Nurse Practitioner Program
Wilkes University
Wilkes-Barre, Pennsylvania

Shelly Noe, DNP, PMHNP-BC
Assistant Professor
New Mexico State University
Las Cruces, New Mexico

Maria Luisa Ramira, DNP, APRN, FNP-BC, CEN
Director and Professor
MSN-FNP Program
United States University
Nurse Practitioner
Emergency Services
Sharp HealthCare
San Diego, California

Patricia A. Rouen, PhD, FNP-BC, RN
Associate Professor
College of Health Professions
University of Detroit Mercy
Detroit, Michigan

Diane Fuller Switzer, DNP, RN, ARNP, FNP/ENP-BC, ENP-C, CCRN, CEN, FAEN
Assistant Clinical Professor
Seattle University College of Nursing
Seattle, Washington

Marjorie A. Vogt, PhD, DNP, CNP, FAANP
Clinical Professor and Associate Director
School of Nursing
Ohio University
Dublin, Ohio

Kathryn W. White, DNP, MA, BS
Associate Clinical Professor and Program Director
University of Minnesota
Minneapolis, Minnesota

Lisa M. Young, DNP, APRN
Assistant Professor, Director of the DNP program
Ashland University
Ashland, Ohio

Introductory Foundations Chapter

Legal and Regulatory Aspects of Prescribing

Author: **Susan D. Thompson, DNP, ACNS-BC**

Editor: **Tammie Lee Demler, PharmD, BS Pharm, MBA, RPh, BCGP, BCPP**

Learning Objectives

- Discuss the various levels of prescriptive authority for the advanced practice nurse.
- Explain the prescribing responsibilities for the advanced practice nurse.
- Synthesize the elements of a well-written prescription.
- Analyze the ethical issues related to prescriptive practice.

Key Terms: regulation, prescribing, controlled substance, scope of practice

Overview of the Legal Aspects of Prescribing

F1.1 Review the Scope of Practice and Regulation of APNs

The scopes of practice and licensing for advanced practice nurses (APNs) are defined by the nurse practice act of each state. The governing body for APN practice is the board of nursing (BON). In some instances, both the BON and the board of medicine govern APN practice. In other instances, the board of midwifery governs the practice of certified nurse–midwives (CNMs).

The term "advanced practice nurse" includes four roles: certified clinical nurse specialist (CNS), certified nurse–midwife (CNM), certified registered nurse anesthetist, and certified nurse practitioner (NP). In addition, several specialty roles fall under the APN category—for example, family nurse practitioner (FNP), psychiatric mental health nurse practitioner (PMHNP), and adult gerontology clinical nurse specialist (AG CNS). Not all four roles are recognized as being part of advanced nursing practice in each state. Consider these examples (National Council of State Boards of Nursing [NCSBN], 2018):

- Connecticut does not recognize CNMs.
- In Florida, CNSs are not recognized as APNs.
- Indiana does not recognize certified registered nurse anesthetists (CRNAs).
- The state of New York only gives recognition to NPs.
- Pennsylvania only recognizes NPs and CNSs.

Additionally, the level of autonomy for each advanced practice role varies by state. In some states, APNs are granted autonomous or full practice authority, meaning that they can practice independently without physician collaboration, attestation, or a collaborative practice agreement. Some states grant full practice to APNs after a period of supervision that is determined by state law. Other states require APNs to practice with physician supervision and/or under a collaborative practice agreement. Additionally, each state may require APNs to meet continuing education requirements to maintain licensure. Refer to your state nurse practice act or BON for full details.

Definition of Prescriptive Authority

Prescriptive authority is granted by each state and gives the APN the legal right to prescribe drugs. Prescriptive authority may or may not fall under the scope of practice. The BON governs prescriptive authority in states that do allow APNs to prescribe medications. However, in some states, the APN's prescriptive authority is governed jointly by the BON and the board of medicine (BOM), or jointly by the BON and the board of pharmacy (BOP).

The level of prescriptive authority is also defined by each state. Some states grant independent prescriptive authority to APNs, whereas other states delineate the parameters of prescriptive authority. For example, independent prescriptive authority allows the APN to prescribe medications without supervision. However, there are exceptions to independent prescriptive authority in some states. For example, the ability to write prescriptions for controlled substances may be limited. Prescriptive authority is delegated by the primary provider through collaborative practice agreements (CPAs) or supervisory agreements in some states, meaning that APNs do not have independent prescriptive authority. In these types of agreements, the APN can prescribe medications according to a written protocol or formulary. Other prescribing restrictions may include limiting prescribing to a specific patient population and/or a specified number of refills.

The laws and regulations surrounding APNs' prescriptive authority vary widely across the states. In January of each year, *The Nurse Practitioner Journal* (*TNPJ*) provides a yearly update of current laws and regulation surrounding APN scope of practice, including prescriptive authority. Other resources include the specific state's nurse practice act, the National Council of State Board of Nursing (NCSBN), and the American Medical Association's (AMA) state law chart. Ultimately, however, the APN is always responsible for practicing within the scope of practice defined by the state of residence and/or license to practice.

Controlled Substances

The federal laws and regulations surrounding controlled substances are created and enforced by the Drug Enforcement Agency (DEA). The Controlled Substance Act regulates the manufacture and distribution of controlled drugs and categorizes these drugs based on their potential for abuse and therapeutic benefit (**Table 1**). Each APN must become familiar with these laws and regulations associated with controlled substance prescribing. All APNs who prescribe controlled

Table 1 Classification of Controlled Substances

Schedule I: Drugs that have a high potential for abuse and no currently accepted medical use in the United States, and that lack accepted safety for use under medical supervision.	Examples: Heroin, LSD, MDMA
Schedule II: Drugs that have a high potential for abuse, which may lead to psychological and physical dependence, but that do have a currently accepted medical use in treatment in the United States.	Examples: Morphine, fentanyl, hydrocodone, methadone, amphetamines
Schedule III: Drugs with a potential for abuse less than substances in Schedules I or II, and whose abuse may lead to moderate or low physical dependence or high psychological dependence.	Examples: Acetaminophen with codeine, buprenorphine, testosterone (Androgel)
Schedule IV: Drugs that have a low potential for abuse relative to substances in Schedule III.	Examples: Alprazolam, zolpidem, phenobarbital
Schedule V: Drugs that have low potential for abuse relative to substances listed in Schedule IV, and that consist primarily of preparations containing limited quantities of certain narcotics.	Examples: Opiate-based antitussives and antidiarrheals

Data from Drug Enforcement Administration (2018). Controlled Substance Schedules. Retrieved from https://www.deadiversion.usdoj.gov/schedules/#define.

substances must obtain a federal DEA number; the application for a DEA number can be obtained from the DEA website or a regional DEA office. In addition to a DEA number (and the advance practice license), some states require APNs to hold a mid-level prescriber license, a controlled substance license, or a prescribing number or certificate.

Many states also require providers who possess a controlled substance license to register with the Prescription Drug Monitoring Program (PDMP). The PDMP is an electronic database that collects information on the prescribing of controlled substances. This state-level mechanism is designed to improve and monitor controlled substance prescribing practices. It is also used to prevent and identify controlled substance abuse. Some states, including Alaska, Illinois, Kentucky, Mississippi, and New York, require APNs who prescribe controlled substances to complete continuing education for prescribing specific controlled substances (such as opiates) (Buppert, 2018).

F1.2 Prescribing Responsibilities for the Advanced Practice Nurse

Prior to prescribing a medication, the APN should perform a physical examination of the patient and obtain a thorough medical history. Prescribing a medication can then be initiated after a diagnosis has been made and a treatment plan has been determined. Before a medication is selected, the APN must consider the risks and benefits for each medication under consideration. Prescribing medications requires a thorough understanding of disease pathology and the medications used to treat the disease. To be a competent and safe prescriber, the APN must possess a solid foundation and understanding of the pharmacokinetics, pharmacodynamics, mechanism of action, adverse drug reactions (ADRs), interactions, routes of administration, efficacy, and cost of medications.

When prescribing, it is important for the APN to follow clinical practice guidelines or protocols. Many such guidelines for prescribing medications have been developed. For example, the Centers for Disease Control and Prevention (CDC) has established guidelines for chronic pain prescribing. Guidelines may be released by different organizations and may vary substantially. For example, the American College of Cardiology (ACC) and the American Heart Association (AHA) task force have recently published guidelines for the treatment of hypertension that differ from the Eighth Joint National Committee (JNC 8); the ACC/AHA guidelines lower the threshold of blood pressure values required to make a diagnosis of hypertension. Although the various guidelines resources are evidence based and should be used to guide medication selection, clinical judgment must always be applied while considering patient-specific factors to individualize treatment.

The APN should have an established provider–patient relationship with the person for whom the nurse is prescribing a medication. The APN should not prescribe medications for friends or relatives.

The APN should ask the patient several questions before prescribing a medication: Are you allergic to any medications? What have you tried to relieve your symptoms? Which other medication and over-the-counter products are you currently taking? Refer to **Table 2** for a more complete list of questions to ask the patient and oneself prior to prescribing.

Table 2 Questions to Ask Before Prescribing a Medication

Ask the Patient	Ask Yourself
Do you have any allergies or sensitivities to medications?	Is there a need for medication to treat the condition?
Which medications are you currently taking?	Is this the most appropriate medication?
Patients who are of childbearing age: • Are you pregnant? • Are you breastfeeding?	Are there any contraindications to prescribing this medication for this patient?
Have you taken this medication in the past? Did it work? Did you experience any side effects?	Is this the correct dosage for this condition? Is this the correct duration?
Do you have any liver or kidney problems?	Is this the most appropriate route?
	What is the cost of the medication?
	Does the patient have a prescription insurance plan?

Patient education is a critical part of the APN's responsibility when prescribing. Elements of patient education include the purpose of the medication, administration instructions, dosing regimen, duration of therapy, possible side effects, management of adverse reactions, food or drug interactions, storage, and laboratory testing. Education should be tailored to each patient. It should be provided verbally, along with instructions written in plain language (fifth-grade reading level) in the patient's primary spoken language.

F1.3 Prescribing Process

Utilizing a consistent prescribing process is imperative for safe prescribing. The World Health Organization (WHO) outlines a six-step model for rational prescribing that can be used as a guideline for decision making. The algorithm for this model is provided later in this chapter (Figure 2). The first step in this model involves identification of the patient's problem by completing a thorough history and performing a physical assessment. After completing the assessment, the APN can formulate a diagnosis and determine whether medication therapy is warranted. The therapeutic objective is then defined. The following question will assist the APN in defining the therapeutic objective: Is the purpose of the medication to cure, reduce symptoms, or replace deficiencies? Establishing goals will allow the APN to further define therapy outcomes, and a review of current practice guidelines will help to identify first-line medication choices. Always consider all patient variables and customize the medication selection for the patient (**Table 3**).

The APN must educate the patient regarding the medication and evaluate the patient's response to the medication therapy. The medication can be continued for the treatment duration if it is effective. However, the APN should monitor appropriate laboratory values and follow prescribing principles. If the treatment is not effective, the APN can change the medication to a second-line therapy and then evaluate the effectiveness of the new medication. Additional prescribing considerations are described in the "Principles of Pharmacology and Rational Drug Selection" section within this *Foundations* chapter.

Although most prescriptions will be submitted to the pharmacy electronically, sometimes a written prescription is necessary. For example, a written prescription may be needed in case of a computer or electrical failure. Additionally, some states may require a written prescription for controlled substances. Patients may also request a written prescription. However, some states accept only electronic prescriptions unless there is an established waiver or in the case of emergencies as described previously.

A written prescription is a legal document that provides direction to both the patient and the pharmacist. Key elements of a prescription should be addressed on all prescriptions (electronic and written) to ensure clarity and avoid miscommunication of information (**Table 4** and **Figure 1**). Included also is the Modified World Health Organization Model of Prescribing for your use and consideration (**Figure 2**).

Table 3 Variables Influencing Prescribing

Age
Sex
Race/ethnicity/culture
Weight
Allergies
Pharmacogenomics
Medical history
Current medications (prescription, over-the-counter, alternative)
Previous medication therapy
Socioeconomic (insurance, income, living environment, daily schedule, support)
Health beliefs

Table 4 Elements of a Well-Written Prescription

Elements of a Well-Written Prescription
Prescriber name and contact information
Prescriber DEA number, if applicable
Patient name and date of birth
Patient allergies
Name of medication
Indication of medication (e.g., enalapril for hypertension)
Form and route of administration
Dosage of medication (e.g., 10 mg once daily)
Duration
Number of refills
Allowable substitutions (generic versus brand)
Signature
Date
The Institute for Safe Medication Practices (ISMP) suggestions to reduce error: do not use abbreviations, do not include a trailing zero (i.e., 2.0)

Susan Harvey, FNP-BC
Family Practice Health Clinic
100 Family Practice Lane
Anytown, USA

Name: Joe Smith Date: 3/8/2018

Address: 3456 Willow St.
Jackson, IL 60608 DOB: 11/25/1948

Enalapril (Vasotec) 10 mg
Take one tablet by mouth daily for high blood pressure for one month, then follow up with our office to assess the need for additional refills

Dispense 30 tablets

Number of refills: 0

Substitution: Yes ☒ No ☐

Signature: Susan Harvey, FNP-BC

DEA Number (if required)

NPI: 1043213698

Figure 1 Prescription Example

Algorithm for Prescribing

1. Define the patient's problem: (History and physical examination)
2. Diagnose: Specify the therapeutic objective
3. Choose the treatment: Based on current practice guidelines—first line therapy
4. Educate the patient
5. Monitor effectiveness
6. Treatment effective?
   a. If YES: Maintain or continue for duration of therapy
   b. If NO: Re-evaluate and change to second line therapy AND monitor effectiveness AND restart process

Figure 2 Modified World Health Organization Model of Prescribing
Data from World Health Organization Model of Prescribing.

F1.4 Ethical Issues

One of the most challenging ethical issues faced by APNs is the absence of a clinical indication for prescribing a medication. Often, patients will be seen by the APN and request a specific medication. The APN must ensure that the medication prescribed is medically necessary. For example, a child with viral cold symptoms does not require antibiotics. In such a case, the APN should spend time with the parent explaining the risks of prescribing antibiotics inappropriately.

Informed consent is another ethical issue. When making medication therapy recommendations, the APN should assess the level of the patient's competence and provide the patient with the information needed to make a decision. The patient must then communicate agreement with the recommended therapy. In some instances, such as when prescribing controlled substances, a medication agreement may be initiated; this can serve as informed consent.

Medications should be prescribed only after a history and physical assessment have been completed. In some instances, patients may call the office for a prescription, or family members or friends may ask for a prescription. Prescriptions should be written only after performing and documenting an examination to prevent harm to the patient as well as to avoid legal ramifications for the APN. Professional practice designations, as well as scope recognitions (ranging from fully independent to those with no practice authority), established by specific Regulatory Agencies are summarized below in **Table 5**. Additional prescribing references have been listed for your review and consideration in **Table 6**.

F1.5 Resources

Table 5 State and Regulatory Agency Professional Practice Designations

State/Regulating Body	Clinical Nurse Specialists	Certified Registered Nurse Anesthetists	Certified Nurse–Midwife	Certified Nurse Practitioner
Alabama: BON/ Board of Medical Examiners	**NPA**	**NPA**	NI	NI
Alaska: BON	**I**	**I**	**I**	**I**
Arizona: BON	NI	**I**	**I**	**I**
Arkansas: BON	NI	NI	NI	NI
California: BON	**NPA**	**NPA**	NI	NI

State/Regulating Body	Clinical Nurse Specialists	Certified Registered Nurse Anesthetists	Certified Nurse–Midwife	Certified Nurse Practitioner
Colorado: BON	I	I	I	I
Connecticut: State Board of Examiners for Nursing	I	I	I	I
Delaware: BON	NI	I	NI	I
Florida: BON/BOM	**NPA**	NI	NI	NI
Georgia: BON	NI	NI	NI	NI
Hawaii: BON	I	I	I	I
Idaho: BON	I	I	I	I
Illinois: BON	NI	NI	NI	NI
Indiana: BON	NI	NI	NI	NI
Iowa: BON	I	I	I	I
Kansas: BON	NI	I	NI	NI
Kentucky: BON	NI	NI	NI	NI
Louisiana: BON	NI	NI	NI	NI
Maine: BON	**NPA**	**NPA**	I	I
Maryland: BON	**NPA**	**NPA**	NI	NI
Massachusetts: Board of Registration in Nursing Board of Registration in Medicine	NI	NI	I	NI
Michigan: BON	NI	**NPA**	NI	NI
Minnesota: BON	I	I	I	I
Mississippi: BON	NR	**NPA**	NI	NI
Missouri: BON	NI	NI	NI	NI
Montana: BON	I: psychiatric/mental health only	I	I	I
Nebraska: BON	**NPA**	I	NI	I
Nevada: BON	I	I	I	I

(*continues*)

Table 5 State and Regulatory Agency Professional Practice Designations *(Continued)*

State/Regulating Body	Clinical Nurse Specialists	Certified Registered Nurse Anesthetists	Certified Nurse–Midwife	Certified Nurse Practitioner
New Hampshire: BON	NR	**I**	**I**	**I**
New Jersey: BON	**NI**	**NPA**	**NI**	**NI**
New Mexico: BON	**I**	**I**	**I**	**I**
New York: BON	NR	NR	**NI**: Board of midwifery	**NI**
North Carolina: BON/BOM	**NPA**	**NPA**	**NI**	**NI**
North Dakota: BON	**I**	**I**	**I**	**I**
Ohio: BON	**NI**	**NI**	I	**NI**
Oklahoma: BON	**NI**	**NI**	**NI**	**NI**
Oregon: BON	**I**	**I**	**I**	**I**
Pennsylvania: BON	**NPA**	NR	**NI**	**NI**
Rhode Island: BON	**NI**	**I**	**I**	**I**
South Carolina: BON	**NI**	**NI**	**NI**	**NI**
South Dakota: BON/Board of Medical and Osteopathic Examiners	**NPA**	**NPA**	**I**	**I**
Tennessee: BON	**NI**	**NI**	**NI**	**NI**
Texas: BON	**NI**	**NI**	**NI**	**NI**
Utah: BON	**I**	**I**	**I**	**I**
Vermont: BON	**I***	**I***	**I**	**I**
Virginia: BON/BOM	**NPA**	**I**	**NI**	**NI**
Washington: Nursing Commission	**I**	**I**	**I**	**I**
West Virginia: Board of examiners for RNs	**I**	**I**	**I**	**NI**
Wisconsin: BON	**NI**	**NI**	**NI**	**NI**
Wyoming: BON	**I**	**I**	**I**	**I**

Abbreviations: BOM: board of medicine; BON: board of nursing; **I**: Independent; **NI**: Not independent; **NPA**: No practice authority; NR: not recognized as APN; RN: registered nurse.

*Check with State regulations to verify current status

Table 6 Prescribing Resources

The Nurse Practitioner Journal	https://journals.lww.com/tnpj/pages/default.aspx
Nurse Practice Act	https://www.ncsbn.org/npa.htm
National Council of State Board of Nursing	https://www.ncsbn.org/5397.htm
Prescription Drug Monitoring Program	https://www.cdc.gov/drugoverdose/pdmp/states.html
Epocrates	http://www.epocrates.com/
LexiComp	http://online.lexi.com/action/home
Pepid	http://www.pepid.com/
Prescribers' Digital Reference (PDR)	http://www.pdr.net/
UptoDate	http://www.uptodate.com/contents/search
DEA	https://www.dea.gov/registration-practitiioners-msg-page.shtml
Family Practice Notebook	https://fpnotebook.com/
Monthly Prescribing Reference	http://www.empr.com/download-empr/section/753/
Clinical Advisor	http://www.clinicaladvisor.com/clinical-advisor-app-download /section/2952/

References

Buppert, C. (2018). *Nurse practitioner's business practice and legal guide.* (6th ed.). Burlington, MA: Jones & Bartlett Learning.

National Council of State Boards of Nursing. (2018). Boards and regulation. Retrieved from https://www.ncsbn.org/boards.htm

Principles of Pharmacology and Rational Drug Selection

Author: **Tammie Lee Demler, PharmD, BS Pharm, MBA, RPh, BCGP, BCPP**

Editors: **Claudia Lee, RPh, MD, and Susan D. Thompson DNP, ACNS-BC**

Learning Objectives

- Identify challenges and opportunities to recommend individualized medication therapy, to increase adherence, and to reduce the risk of potential adverse drug reactions.
- Recommend optimal pharmacologic interventions and recognize vulnerabilities in the current medication use system.
- Provide appropriate patient-specific counseling points to optimize overall medication management.

Key Terms: pharmacotherapy, polypharmacy, drug safety, efficacy, risk, benefit, allergy, contraindication, body system, anaphylaxis, hypersensitivity, contraindication, monotherapy, polypharmacy

Overview of Pharmacology and Rational Drug Selection

This section of the *Foundations* chapter focuses on the practitioner making rational drug selections when prescribing. Primary considerations include keeping in mind the well-documented decline in medication adherence associated with increased pill burden and regimen complexity, and the notable risk of drug interactions and subsequent adverse drug reactions associated with polypharmacy.

A single drug that is indicated for use in a specific primary body system may also demonstrate efficacy in treating conditions in other (secondary) body systems. For a manufacturer to officially promote a drug for additional uses beyond the original indication for which it was initially brought to market, the manufacturer must file an application with the Food and Drug Administration (FDA) and receive FDA approval for the additional use(s). In some cases, a medication may be used "off label" when no other more appropriate agent is available to treat or prevent disease.

Prior to the 1962 U.S. Kefauver-Harris Amendment (the "Drug Efficacy Amendment") to the Federal Food, Drug, and Cosmetic Act, manufacturers were only required to demonstrate that there was no harm associated with the use. Once the amendment was formalized, however, the sponsor also had to demonstrate that the drug both has confirmed efficacy and does not cause harm or present any intolerable risks.

As part of rational drug selection, the use of a single drug for more than one approved indication or condition (thereby targeting illness in more than one body system) is the preferred prescribing practice. An example of this kind of rational pharmacotherapy would be using divalproex for both seizure control and migraine prophylaxis. Conversely, except in cases where no alternative exists, it is best to avoid polypharmacy (taking more than one drug at a time) and to explore opportunities to maximize monotherapy (taking only one drug at a time).

Sometimes a primary essential medication without any appropriate alternative contributes to a side effect that can be managed. In such a case, adding a supplemental secondary medication to manage side effects can allow continued use of the primary medication. However, in cases where acceptable alternatives exist, prescribing a single new primary medication without side effects may prevent the unnecessary prescribing of additional medications, thereby preventing a "prescribing cascade."

When prescribing, dispensing, and administering drug therapy, some recommended "universal alerts" should always be employed. These "universal alerts" are the prescribing equivalent of the reminder to buckle up before driving in a car. We have included some suggested "universal alerts" in our companion drug grids for each therapeutic chapter.

F2.1 Allergies

Known, serious hypersensitivity to the specific drug selected or to any other component of product or formulation selected is a contraindication for use. Allergic reactions have a highly variable presentation pattern. Most clinicians would recognize anaphylaxis as a life-threatening reaction that requires emergency intervention. Typically, this reaction manifests with significant physical distress and may impair the ability to swallow and to breathe. Since drug class allergy considerations may arise with drugs that share similar chemical profiles, avoiding prescribing of a "chemical cousin" in cases with a risk of cross-allergy is warranted.

In other cases, a drug allergy may have a more subtle appearance and be so mild as to be barely noticeable. The development of skin rash and/or hives and generalized itching should, however, prompt further investigation. In some cases, patients with a drug allergy may be treated through desensitization procedures to reduce the degree of reaction upon future exposure.

Drug allergy can occur upon first dose or can emerge later, after repeated exposure to the drug. For this reason, a practitioner should remind the patient to report anything unusual so the incident can be evaluated by a trained clinician. If a true drug allergy is confirmed, removal of the offending agent and careful documentation of the details of the reaction should be made (including symptoms, severity, and date of occurrence) to guide future prescribers in making patient-centered drug selections and to avoid prescribing a drug to a patient who is allergic and could suffer significant harm and even death with a subsequent exposure to that same agent.

F2.2 Adverse Drug Reactions (ADRs)

Adverse reactions associated with the use of some agents include dizziness, drowsiness, vertigo, and fatigue. ADRs such as these may also impair the ability to perform tasks requiring mental alertness. Caution should always be recommended when using any new drug for the first time, when the dose changes, and with continued use of known offending agents.

When the FDA reviews an application for a drug that is intended for commercial use, the side effects reported during clinical trials become an important part of the sponsor's new drug application (NDA). These side effects are reported in terms of the reported percentage of occurrence. They are also benchmarked against a "placebo," so that the true effect of the drug versus potential perceived effects can be more reliably evaluated. Once a product is released to market, these side-effect occurrences are documented in the package insert (i.e., the product package label), along with other FDA required safety and efficacy information.

Since medications are generally studied under "ideal" conditions, patients with specific diseases or lifestyle behaviors (e.g., smoking, heavy alcohol consumption) may be excluded from clinical trials. This process of providing data that does not reflect the general population can potentially result in skewed data. Subsequently, unexpected and unpredictable new adverse reactions may emerge once use of the medication widens to include patients more reflective of the general population.

The FDA's postmarketing notification system, MedWatch, is a critical real-time tool that is intended to collect safety information on drugs that are currently available on the U.S. market for future updated product labeling. In addition to the occurrence of new and/or unexpected adverse effects, patients may experience a range of the predictable adverse effects mentioned at the beginning of this section. For example, some medications, such as selective serotonin-reuptake inhibitor (SSRI) antidepressants, are often reported to boost energy, therefore causing insomnia in many users if taken too late in the day. In contrast, other patients describe sedation with their use. Thus, these sedating effects should be disclosed to patients as a "possibility" when prescribing such medications. Good practice would support educating patients regarding the more common side effects and encouraging patients to report anything they experience that differs from these common side effects.

Any new drug exposure should occur for the first time in a controlled environment (e.g., on a weekend when home and not forced to drive, concentrate, or otherwise). This same precaution should be taken for patients who have been on a drug for a long time, but who are undergoing a dose change, are experiencing a change in their baseline health, or who are reaching advanced age. The Beers Criteria highlight medications that are best avoided in older adults for several reasons. In addition, the Screening Tool of Older People's Prescriptions (STOPP) can detect potential prescribing errors associated with an increase in ADRs in the elderly, and can assist the healthcare team in avoiding the development of ADRs in the older adult population.

F2.3 Brand Versus Generic Drug Names

Brand names are commonly used for agents still available on the U.S. market. However, due to ever-changing product availability, clinicians should refer to FDA resources to confirm the actual brands available. The use of the generic drug name along with its proprietary brand name is an additional safety measure. Often, brand-name drugs may be considered sound-a-like, look-a-like drugs; thus, even when an indication for their use is included in the prescription, they may be subject to misinterpretation or medication errors. Further, after a brand-name drug's patent expires, the generic drug name will be the recognized entity. Consequently, it is beneficial to develop a prescribing habit of using generic (chemical) names whenever possible and, at a minimum, to include an indication for use whenever documenting medication management details on a prescription or in the medical record.

With the transition to electronic prescribing, fields may be provided in the computer application that enable the prescriber to include an instruction to dispense the specific brand-name drug or to substitute for it with a generic equivalent. Examples of computer codes for brand/generic dispensing include the following:

- No product selection indicated
- Substitution not allowed by prescriber
- Substitution allowed: patient requested that brand product be dispensed
- Substitution allowed: pharmacist selected product dispensed
- Substitution allowed: generic drug not in stock
- Substitution allowed: brand drug dispensed as generic
- Substitution not allowed: brand drug mandated by law
- Substitution allowed: generic drug not available in marketplace
- Override
- Other

Insurance plans, including but not limited to Medicare Part D, generally require pharmacies to use the least costly version of the drug prescribed. Sometimes, however, a prescriber may intend for the beneficiary to receive the drug exactly as it is written on the prescription (e.g., to get the brand-name version of a drug). When the prescriber wishes to issue this kind of specific instruction, he/she must use the appropriate action code when initiating an electronic prescription. FDA-approved therapeutically equivalent generics can be found in the FDA's online reference, the Orange Book (https://www.accessdata.fda.gov/scripts/cder/ob/).

The FDA has also published a Purple Book to guide healthcare providers in prescribing "biosimilar and interchangeable biological products" just as they would prescribe other medications. Biological products include a wide range of products, such as gene therapy, vaccines, recombinant therapeutic proteins, blood and blood components, and other tissues that are isolated from a variety of natural sources. According to the FDA, a biosimilar product cannot be substituted for a reference product at the pharmacy level and must be dispensed specifically as prescribed by the healthcare provider. Conversely, a product designated as "interchangeable" may be substituted for the reference product without the intervention of the healthcare provider who prescribed the reference product.

F2.4 Use of Pharmacologic Agents to Achieve Therapeutic Goals

Prescribing decisions should be based on real-time comprehensive drug databases that are updated on a regular basis. Use of pharmacotherapeutic agents should continue until a specific target is achieved, the patient is no longer responsive to treatment, or unacceptable toxicity occurs. Although our text covers the essential and most critical at-a-glance details for most of the drugs available on the market, we acknowledge that guidelines, which are developed and updated frequently by expert consensus, are better referenced via real-time online references and resources that can immediately be updated. That said, understanding the drug-specific details is critical, as the guidelines frequently do not remind prescribers of contraindications, black box warnings, and other more basic drug information that ensures safe and effective use of the medications available.

When drug therapy is initiated, the clinician should begin with the end therapeutic goal in mind. Although this recommendation likely sounds unrealistic, there should always be an intended goal to which we strive; if that goal is not achieved, reconsidering the appropriateness of continuing a drug is essential. Every medication carries some degree of risk, and the decision to continue the use of a drug must always include an evaluation of the risk-versus-benefit balance. The use of real-time databases is essential to ensure that the most updated information is available; however, there may be significant differences in the information available across databases, so it is recommended that a clinician select several resources for reference and comparison.

Pharmacokinetics, Pharmacodynamics, and Pharmacogenomics

Author: **Tammie Lee Demler, PharmD, BS Pharm, MBA, RPh, BCGP, BCPP**

Editors: **Claudia Lee, RPh, MD and Susan D. Thompson DNP, ACNS-BC**

Reviewer: **Joseph Balthasar, PhD**

Learning Objectives

- Identify different pharmacokinetics (PK), pharmacodynamics (PD), and pharmacogenomics (PG) affecting patients' responses to pharmacotherapy.
- Recommend optimal interventions to address pharmacologic complications that may arise from patient-specific determinants of PK-PD-PG.
- Provide appropriate patient-specific counseling points to optimize overall medication management.

Key Terms: Pharmacokinetic, pharmacodynamic, pharmacogenomic, absorption, distribution, metabolism, excretion, elimination, cumulative effects

Overview of Pharmacokinetics, Pharmacodynamics, and Pharmacogenomics

Pharmacokinetics (PK) involves the effects of drug absorption, distribution, metabolism, and excretion (ADME)—processes that may be collectively described as "how the body affects a drug." For a drug to exert an effect, the agent must be first absorbed by the body, then distributed to tissues that are associated with drug action. The efficiency of drug elimination and excretion determines the half-life and overall time-course of drug persistence in the body.

Pharmacodynamics (PD) refers to the relationships between drug concentrations and drug effects; it may be considered to be "how the drug affects the body." The kinetics of unintended or undesirable effect(s) of drugs is described as toxicodynamics, referring to the processes that affect the uptake of, metabolism by, damage to, and disposal of a toxin; these effects are described as adverse drug reactions in a later section of this *Foundations* chapter. The patient's unique set of genes and the functions of those genes serve as prime determinants of drug PK and PD.

Pharmacogenomics (PG) is a relatively new field of study that explores an individual's response, or lack thereof, to a medication and offers potential solutions in providing safe and effective medication interventions that are personalized to meet a patient's specific PG profile. As more information in this area becomes available and as tests become increasingly more accessible, clinicians are beginning to recognize the important role that PG plays in achieving successful medication management outcomes.

F3.1 Pharmacokinetics

Absorption

For a medication to achieve the goal of having the intended therapeutic effects, the drug must be absorbed into the body tissues. Even external (topical) medications must be absorbed into the skin or epithelial tissues to exert influence within the body. A drug must first be absorbed so that it can be distributed through the circulatory system and reach the target organs; the speed with which this absorption occurs varies based on the route by which the drug is administered, the dosage form selected, and patient-specific characteristics. Absorption can occur through the lungs if the medication is inhaled, through the gut if it is swallowed, and through mucosal membranes of the nose, eyes, and rectum if administered via those routes.

Regardless of the absorption pathway, the amount of drug that reaches the circulation and ultimately the end-target tissue or organ, relative to the dose given, is called the "bioavailability" of the medication. Different dose forms may result in different peak concentrations, such that these forms are not equally interchangeable. As an example, the time-course of absorption differs between divalproex extended-release (ER) versus delayed-release (DR) tablets. Dose forms that facilitate a quicker passage through the gut also tend to achieve their target concentrations faster. Generally, liquids are absorbed more quickly than tablets, and chewable (or dissolvable) tablets are absorbed more quickly—sometimes even twice as fast—compared to regular-release oral tablets swallowed whole.

In addition to the specific dosage form, the presence of food may decrease the maximum concentration (C_{max}) and may delay or extend the time required to achieve peak concentrations (T_{max}). Another factor to consider when evaluating the absorption rate of a medication is the lipophilicity (a word of Greek origin, meaning the tendency to "love fat"), referring to the ability for the chemical to dissolve in or pass through lipid membranes. Rapid absorption may be associated with not only more intense therapeutic effects, but also some negative collateral consequences. Valium (diazepam), for example, is a more lipophilic benzodiazepine that, compared to a more hydrophilic ("water loving") agent such as lorazepam, is more quickly absorbed. This rapid absorption of diazepam may explain, in part, the higher abuse potential of this drug, due to the euphoria that results from the "quick absorption rush" of the medication.

The effects of drug transport proteins, such as permeability glycoproteins (P-gp), are also becoming better understood in terms of their role in absorption. The ability of P-gp to actively pump (efflux) drugs and other foreign chemicals out of cells plays a significant role in the kinetics of drug absorption and distribution by limiting passage across the gut mucosa and into the gut and organs such as the brain. Overall, the impact of P-gp may be considered most significant for drugs with a narrow therapeutic index (defined as a characteristically small window between toxic and therapeutic serum concentrations), when using very small doses of a specific drug (thus limiting the degree of saturation of P-gp transport), and for drugs with slow dissolution rates, which also limits the degree of P-gp saturation. P-gp can be both inhibited and induced by certain drugs; however, not all drugs involve P-gp. There appears to be some overlap between drugs that are substrates for P-gp and CYP450 3A4 (a metabolizing enzyme commonly seen in the

Table 7 Pharmacokinetics Terms Associated with Absorption

Term	Definition
Bioavailability	The amount of drug available to elicit pharmacodynamic action at the destination (or target) site in the body after absorption.
Dose form	The chosen vehicle for drug delivery, which may be limited by the drug's physical/chemical characteristics. Dosage form options may be limited for specific drugs (i.e., nitroglycerin must be administered sublingualy and not swallowed).
Chemical form (salts)	The final stable form of the drug that is manufactured (e.g., $CaCO_3$).
Administration rate	Generally considered to be the measure of time recorded for a drug to be administered, but more accurately refers to the desired rate at which a drug should be administered to achieve a steady state of a fixed dose that is therapeutically effective.
Extraction ratio	The fraction of drug available systemically once the drug is absorbed and distributed compared to the original amount of drug administered.
Sustained-, extended-, or controlled-release formulations	A specific vehicle for drug delivery that is developed to release the drug slowly and more evenly (decreased peak and trough) than is possible with the immediate-release formulation. Use of these formulations often allows for a regimen with less frequent dosing.

liver that will be discussed in greater detail in the context of metabolism), such that drug interactions may be complicated by the involvement of both systems. **Table 7** summarizes some of the terms associated with absorption.

Distribution

Distribution of a drug describes the migration of a drug into various body tissues and "compartments" including, but not limited to, the blood, interstitial fluids, cerebrospinal fluid, muscle, and fatty adipose tissue. In most cases, the "central compartment" represents the blood and highly perfused organs, such as the heart, lungs, liver, and kidneys. Peripheral compartments often involve tissues associated with slower rates of drug distribution (e.g., fat and muscle).

Because of these drug distribution differences, the plasma sampling times for laboratory blood draws are often quite specific. For some drugs, there is only a narrow window between the minimum drug concentration considered to be in the therapeutic concentration range (C_{min}) and the maximum concentration allowable to avoid toxicity (C_{max}). Drugs with this kind of small range are referred to as having a narrow therapeutic index. Lithium, one such drug with a narrow therapeutic index, is associated with specific timing recommendations for blood draws, with the lowest expected blood concentration (trough) being seen just prior to the "next dose." These associated recommendations are outlined in the package insert for lithium. To correctly account for the therapeutic index, clinicians should consult references prior to developing a clinical pharmacokinetic drug monitoring plan.

Drug concentration monitoring is most clinically meaningful once a drug has reached steady state—that is, the balance between absorption and elimination that results from a consistent maintenance dose that provides an ongoing optimal therapeutic drug concentration. The use of loading doses and bolus doses may influence the time to achieve steady state due to the variability in these administration options.

The distribution characteristics of a drug can be summarized by the volume of distribution (V_d), which is a parameter used to relate the amount of drug in the body and the plasma concentration achieved. Low plasma concentrations relative to the amount of drug in the body indicate extensive drug distribution to the tissues and a large V_d. The degree to which any one drug is bound to proteins in the blood may also influence the amount of free drug that is available to become distributed to tissues and mediate effects. A small V_d may also indicate a drug is associated with high plasma protein binding, inhibiting the distribution of the drug from the plasma. The V_d also influences other PK metrics, including the drug half-life ($T_{1/2}$) which is defined as the amount of time for half the drug to be eliminated from the body. The extent of drug bound to proteins in the plasma is dependent on the binding affinity of drug for these proteins, which can further vary based on the patient's individual supply of plasma proteins (considered an interpatient variability factor in drug disposition and drug response). Many patients have reduced plasma proteins, so that the increased free fraction of drug available may result in exaggerated side effects of the drug (refer to the special populations section in this *Foundations* chapter for additional detail). **Table 8** summarizes some of the terms associated with distribution.

Table 8 Pharmacokinetics Terms Associated with Distribution

Term	Definition
Drug half-life ($T_{1/2}$)	The time required for the amount of drug in the body to decrease by half.
Therapeutic concentration range	The range of drug serum concentration in the target tissue or blood that is minimally required to elicit the desired pharmacologic response and maximally allowable to avoid toxicity.
Narrow therapeutic index	A drug with a small window of tolerance between the therapeutic drug concentration and the toxic drug concentration.
Interpatient variability in drug disposition and drug response	The unique differences seen in drug pharmacokinetics (ADME) and pharmacodynamics (drug response) in different individuals.
Clinical pharmacokinetic drug monitoring	The routine or intermittent evaluation of the end result/final outcome of ADME, which is often accomplished by evaluating drug concentration in the blood, plasma, or other tissues in the body.
C_{max}	The maximum serum concentration that a drug can achieve in a specified area of the body (or compartment) after the drug has been administered and before the administration of a second dose.
C_{min}	The minimum serum concentration of the drug in the body.
Plasma protein binding	The ability of any drug to bind to protein in the plasma, which varies from person to person based on the amount of protein in the blood and the affinity of any given drug to bind to protein. Human blood proteins to which drugs commonly bind include, but are not limited to, serum albumin, lipoprotein, glycoprotein, and a variety of globulins.
Plasma protein monitoring of free or bound drug	Drugs bound to protein are not available to elicit pharmacologic action, so the "free" unbound portion of the drug is what is "active" and excreted. Pharmacologic monitoring of these binding states (degree of free/bound) is necessary for drugs with a narrow therapeutic index and drugs subject to drug–drug interactions resulting in displacement from proteins.
Binding affinity	The propensity of any drug to bind to plasma proteins. Each drug has a varying degree of protein binding affinity.
Volume of distribution (V_d)	The maximum extent of a drug's ability to migrate into tissues and fluids in the body. The V_d varies with the PK/PD of the drug and the physiologic characteristics of the patient (e.g., obesity, age, gender).
Loading dose	The amount of drug to be administered as the first (initial) dose to achieve the fastest therapeutic serum concentration while attempting to avoid toxicity.
Steady state	The optimal plateau serum concentration achieved after five half-lives of the drug have elapsed, where the amount absorbed equals the amount eliminated.

(*continues*)

Table 8 Pharmacokinetics Terms Associated with Distribution *(Continued)*

Term	Definition
Maintenance dose	The amount of drug required to be administered on an ongoing basis to achieve a steady state of medication that promotes efficacy and avoids toxicity.
Loading versus bolus dose	A loading dose is a higher dose of a drug administered for purposes of achieving a steady-state serum concentration, which will then be decreased to continue as a maintenance dose. A bolus dose is a large amount of any given drug administered all at once or over a short period (e.g., intravenous injection administered over a period of 3–5 minutes).
Plasma sampling time	For certain drugs, samples must be drawn and evaluated at specific times. For example, lithium requires a "trough" concentration, which is the lowest serum concentration just prior to receiving the next dose.

Abbreviations: ADME: absorption, distribution, metabolism, and excretion.

Metabolism

The term *metabolism* is derived from a Greek word meaning "change"; it is applied in the description of a variety of biological processes. For example, food can be "metabolized" or "converted" into energy or building blocks of protein for cellular processes. In the context of pharmacokinetics, metabolism refers to the biotransformation of a drug by chemical reactions (e.g., oxidation, deamidation, conjugation) to form entities (drug metabolites) that are chemically distinct from the parent drug. As such, drug metabolism is a mechanism of drug elimination, and it serves as a key determinant of systemic drug exposure following drug dosing.

Metabolism of drugs may occur in many tissues, including the kidney, lung, and gastrointestinal tract. More generally, however, the liver is the primary organ involved in drug metabolism. When a drug is administered by mouth (oral), it is transported via the portal vein to the liver, where it is metabolized after being absorbed through the gut. Some medications are more likely than others to experience a significant hepatic extraction, a process known as the "first-pass effect"; in such a case, only a small proportion of the active drug reaches the systemic circulation and its intended target tissue. When a drug is known to have a high first-pass effect, oral administration is avoided and other administration options such as parenteral, topical, or sublingual formulations can be used to achieve the desired effect.

Organ function changes over time with advancing age and increased occurrence of comorbid medical illness, often influencing the rate and efficiency of drug clearance by metabolism. A number of demographic variables are associated with differences in drug metabolism:

- Males metabolize drugs more efficiently than females.
- Older adults metabolize drugs less efficiently than younger adults.
- Genetic differences translate into individual differences such as being an extensive metabolizer versus a poor metabolizer (poor metabolizers may experience exaggerated side effects, whereas extensive metabolizers may experience poor/suboptimal drug responses to "usual doses" of the agent prescribed).

The chemistry of metabolism is generally accomplished through "pathways" that facilitate the transformation of a medication via a series of sequential reactions, often allowing the drug substance to be more efficiently excreted from the body. Drugs can either inhibit, induce, or be a substrate (e.g., the target of the change caused by CYP450 inhibitors or inducers) of drug-metabolizing enzymes. In fact, a specific drug may play any of these roles when the right conditions are present. Enzymes target the "substrate" drugs that use these specific pathways: Some drugs have multiple enzymes targeting their metabolism, whereas others experience little, if any, metabolism and are eliminated unchanged in the urine. Drugs and substances that inhibit a specific enzyme (e.g., cytochrome P450 oxidases [CYP450] 1A) are able to decrease the metabolism other drugs that rely on the same enzyme pathway. The drugs that are vulnerable to the impact of inhibitors and/or inducers are called substrates. Drug metabolism is divided into two phases: Phase I (oxidation) and Phase II (conjugation).

Metabolism occurs primarily in the liver, although enzymes located in the kidney, lung, central nervous system, intestine and gastric mucosa, spleen, and circulation (red blood cells [RBCs], lymphocytes) may also be involved. These metabolizing enzymes are themselves subject to the influence of the parent drug(s), in that they can be inhibited (thereby preventing them from breaking down the "substrate" drug).

Numerous CYP enzymes have been identified that account for varying percentages of the overall hepatic enzyme volume and associated contribution to drug metabolism. Patient-specific factors that can influence CYP450 activity include genetic polymorphisms, drug or disease-induced impairment, and altered hepatic metabolism caused by dietary consumption and/or smoking induced hepatic effects (**Table 9**). Drugs with a wide array of CYP450 activity may play a role in numerous enzyme pathways. Notably, evidence suggests that CYP2D6 is not very susceptible to enzyme induction; thus, the person's genetics, rather than drug therapy, accounts for most ultrarapid CYP2D6 metabolism.

Table 10 summarizes some of the terms associated with metabolism.

Table 9 Common Isoforms of Human Cytochrome P450

CYP	Substrate	Inducer	Inhibitor
1A2	Caffeine	Cigarette smoke	Fluvoxamine
2C9	Warfarin	Rifampin	Valproic acid
2C19	Fluoxetine	Rifampin	Isoniazid
2D6	Paroxetine	Genetics	Fluoxetine
2E1	Acetaminophen	Nicotine	Nifedipine
3A4	Diazepam	Phenobarbital	Grapefruit

This table provides only a selection of illustrative examples.

Table 10 Pharmacokinetics Terms Associated with Metabolism

Term	Definition
First-pass effect	The "first pass" of a drug through the body includes its potential extraction after absorption through the gut and before it enters the systemic circulation. Extensive first-pass effects translate into less drug available once it reaches the systemic circulation. As patients age, their first-pass effect is decreased, often resulting in higher drug concentrations compared to the same drug and dose administered to patients of a younger age.
Phase I oxidation	A process of metabolism in which chemical reactions via CYP450 transform chemical agents (i.e., medications) into metabolites that consist of more hydrophilic polar molecules to allow for more efficient excretion. Phase I metabolism also involves chemical reactions of reduction and hydrolysis.
Phase II conjugation	A process of metabolism that converts a parent drug into more hydrophilic polar molecule to allow for more efficient excretion. Drugs metabolized via phase II reactions are renally excreted and may or may not have been previously involved in phase I metabolism. Phase II enzymes (ST, GST, UGT) are responsible for this conjugation process.

(continues)

Table 10 Pharmacokinetics Terms Associated with Metabolism (*Continued*)

Term	Definition
CYP450 inhibitor	A CYP450 metabolism inhibitor can diminish the activity of one or more CYP450 enzymes. Each inhibitor varies in its magnitude of effect based on factors such as the ability to bind to the enzyme and the concentration of the drug available to elicit the action. The resulting inhibition is generally immediate, just like a key opening a lock, resulting in an increased substrate drug concentration.
CYP450 inducer	A CYP450 metabolism inducer that stimulates increased activity of one or more CYP450 enzymes. Each inducer varies in its magnitude of effect based on factors such as the ability to bind to the enzyme and the concentration of the drug available to elicit the action. The resulting induction is generally slow and gradual, because it requires protein synthesis and DNA replication to increase the volume of the targeted substrate CYP enzyme, resulting in the need for higher doses of the substrate drug to accommodate for the accelerated metabolism.
Genetic polymorphisms	A genetic variation that can lead to abnormal expression of a gene or the creation of an abnormal protein that may result in a disease or altered function of the body.
Smoking-induced hepatic effects	Smoking alters hepatic metabolism by inducing the CYP450 1A enzyme. While such effects are most notably recognized as a consequence of cigarette smoking, marijuana has also been reported to lead to this same outcome. The enzyme induction is caused by the polycyclic aromatic hydrocarbons (PAH) that result from the combustion of certain materials, rather than the nicotine itself. Induction caused by smoking is not immediate; instead, it can take up to a week of heavy smoking to elicit enzymatic changes. After cessation of smoking, the individual experiences a gradual return to baseline CYP1A2 activity. Most drug labels do not include recommendations for proactive dose reductions; however, a clinician may want to consider this factor in the overall cessation plan. Toxicity may result when the person stops smoking and serum drug concentrations rise despite the patient continuing on the same dose. Nicotine replacement does not prevent these metabolic changes from occuring during smoking cessation. Conversely, a person who begins to smoke will likely need a dose increase to account for the smoking-induced changes if the drug is a CYP1A2 substrate.
Disease-induced impairment	Although drug metabolism may occur in different areas of the body, hepatic impairment that results from disease can translate into excessive drug concentrations for medications that are extensively metabolized by the liver.
Parent drug	The original form of the drug before it is metabolized.

Excretion

In addition to elimination via metabolism, drugs may be eliminated by excretion into the urine or bile. Excretion of drugs into the urine by the kidneys depends on three processes: glomerular filtration, tubular excretion, and tubular reabsorption. Free drug in the plasma must pass through the glomerular membrane into the renal tubule, allowing for subsequent urinary excretion. Additional augmentation by transporter systems in the tubular membrane can promote further passage of drugs from the plasma into the tubule, and lipophilic drugs may be reabsorbed by passive diffusion from the tubule back into the blood further in later stages at the distal part of the renal tubule.

The glomerular filtration rate (GFR) is often used to assess renal function. GFR is measured in milliliters per minute (mL/min), with a GFR less than 60 mL/min being considered sufficiently reduced (indicating compromised kidney function) to consider drug dose adjustments.

Clinicians continue to debate what is the best method of estimating kidney function in patients with chronic kidney disease (CKD) and acute kidney injury (AKI). Some studies have suggested that the Modification of Diet in

Renal Disease (MDRD) measure for estimated GFR is an acceptable substitute for estimated or measured creatinine clearance (CrCl) as an index for adjusting drug doses in these patients. However, concerns have been raised that this substitution could result in medication dosing errors and possible toxicity, especially for drugs with narrow therapeutic indices. Patients who are likely to be in greatest need for dose adjustments may have their creatinine clearance overestimated if the estimated GFR values are used. Creatinine is a by-product of skeletal muscle breakdown and is derived from dietary meat ingested. It is released into the circulation at a relatively constant rate and has a stable plasma concentration. Creatinine is recognized as an ideal marker for kidney function because it is freely filtered across the glomerulus and is neither reabsorbed nor metabolized by the kidney. There can, however, be progressive overestimation of the GFR with more severe disease. The *Cockcroft-Gault* formula (CG) has been generally recognized as one of the most widely accepted approaches to estimating renal function due to its use and reference in FDA approved product labeling.

Following are some key points related to drug elimination:

- The CG equation is still the best approach for adjusting medication doses based on renal concerns.
- Obese patients will need additional considerations taken into account relative to elimination.
- Older adults should not have their serum creatinine rounded up to 1 mg/dL. However, in non-elderly patients, rounding the creatinine clearance and GFR will make calculations easier to use and the imprecision of these estimates ultimately make the small rounding factor clinically insignificant.
- MDRD is not an appropriate estimation method for patients with a GFR greater than 60 mL/min/1.73 m^2.
- Creatinine clearance and GFR are different measurements and are not interchangeable.

Table 11 summarizes some of the terms associated with elimination.

Table 11 Pharmacokinetics Terms Associated with Elimination

Term	Definition
Renal clearance	The ability and rate at which wastes (i.e., drug metabolites) are excreted through the kidneys and into the urine.
Elimination rate constant (drug elimination, *K* or *Ke*)	The pharmacokinetic measure of the rate by which a drug is eliminated from the body.
Creatinine clearance (CrCl)	The pharmacokinetic measure of the rate by which creatinine, a by-product of muscle metabolism, is excreted through the kidneys and into the urine. Serum creatinine concentrations are reduced in older adults due to the overall decrease in lean muscle mass associated with advancing age, so they may not be an accurate reflection of kidney function for this population.
Glomerular filtration rates (GFR)	The pharmacokinetic measure of the rate by which blood passes through the glomeruli, the small filters found in the kidney.
Dialysis of drugs	The process by which medications, wastes, and/or drug metabolites are removed from the body when the kidneys are not able to carry out this otherwise normal function. Hemodialysis is performed by filtering the blood through a dialysis machine external to the body, whereas peritoneal dialysis is performed within the peritoneal cavity.
Renal function	The pharmacokinetic measure that establishes the health of the organs and the effectiveness to perform the necessary function of the kidneys.

Adverse Drug Reactions and Drug Interactions

Author: **Tammie Lee Demler, PharmD, BS Pharm, MBA, RPh, BCGP, BCPP**

Editors: **Claudia Lee, RPh, MD, and Susan D. Thompson, DNP, ACNS-BC**

Learning Objectives

- Define adverse drug reactions and drug interactions.
- Identify different types of drug warnings and develop plans to reduce the opportunity for harm.
- Understand the challenges in preventing adverse drug reactions and drug interactions, and develop a plan to address these issues when using medication therapy.

Key Terms: Adverse drug reaction, adverse drug event, drug interaction, medication error, Naranjo algorithm, pharmacodynamics, pharmacokinetics, QTc prolongation, seizures, blood dyscrasia, cutaneous reactions, Stevens–Johnson syndrome (SJS), toxic epidermal necrolysis (TEN).

Overview of Adverse Drug Reactions and Drug Interactions

F4.1 Adverse Drug Reactions

An adverse drug reaction (ADR) is an unwanted, and in some cases harmful, reaction following the administration of a drug or a combination of drugs under normal conditions. The unintended or undesirable effect(s) of drugs are often related to the pharmacokinetics (PK) of the drug but result in pharmacodynamic (PD) consequences. This PK/PD relationship is described in greater detail in the PK/PD/PG section of the *Foundations* chapter. Once an ADR is identified and the reaction is thought to be related to the drug, the suspected drug may require dose reduction or discontinuation; the dose reduction; or where the suspected drug is deemed essential and thus required for continued use, alternative interventions must be considered. Since the clinical presentation alone may not confirm a suspect drug is involved or whether the reaction is even due to a drug, assessment tools have been developed to assist clinicians in determining the "likelihood" of an adverse drug event. An example of one such tool is the naranjo rating scale (algorithm), which can determine the likelihood that an ADR is due to a specific drug and not to other factors (Naranjo et al., 1981).

The types of questions shown in **Table 12** (adapted from the Naranjo algorithm) can help the ANP determine the likelihood that an adverse experience is drug induced:

Table 12 Illustrative sample of questions to determine ADR based on modifications of original Naranjo

1. Are there previous definitive reports associating this drug to this reaction?
2. Did the adverse event only occur when the suspected drug was administered?
3. Was an effort made to discontinue the drug and if so, did the adverse reaction improve or resolve when the drug was discontinued?
4. Was a specific antagonist administered and if so, did it reverse or abate the adverse reaction?
5. Was an effort made to rechallenge and if so, did the reaction reoccur upon readministration?

An ADR can occur with the use of any medication in any setting; however, ADRs are reported to occur more frequently in special populations, such as pediatrics or geriatrics. The likelihood of an ADR increases with the use of polypharmacy, which is associated with subsequent secondary drug interactions. It has been reported that approximately 5% of all inpatient admissions are due to ADRs, and approximately 10% to 20% of hospitalized patients will develop an ADR at some point during their hospitalization. These hospital-based ADRs cause significant morbidity, mortality, and increased healthcare costs. Among the ADR-related hospital admissions in the elderly, as many as 88% are reported to be preventable. Efforts are continually made to better understand, and when possible predict, the occurrences of ADRs.

Currently, the most widely recognized categories of events are Type A events, which are defined as predictable and dose-dependent reactions, such as stomach upset with ibuprofen, and Type B events, which are defined as unpredictable and rare reactions. Additional categories have been developed to better describe these events: Type C ADRs (chronic), which relate to the dose and time; Type D ADRs, delayed reactions; Type E ADRs, withdrawal; and Type F, unexpected failure of therapy.

An adverse event—a term that may be confused with adverse drug reaction—is defined as harm that occurs while a patient is taking a drug, regardless of whether the drug is suspected to be the cause. In addition to ADRs, medication errors are considered to be adverse events. A more general description that can be used when communicating with patients to describe ADRs is a drug side effect. However, some might debate the value of describing an ADR as a drug side effect as an effect that is less harmful, is predictable, and may not even require discontinuation of therapy. ADRs due to toxicity can be screened for by using the Naranjo algorithm and/or through clinical interpretation of the laboratory data available.

As mentioned earlier, both older and younger populations are more vulnerable and more likely to experience ADRs. For older adults, the increased risk of ADRs is frequently attributed to the use of polypharmacy to treat comorbid illnesses coupled with the physiologic changes associated with advanced age. An additional challenge in addressing ADRs in the older adult is ensuring that the drug-induced effect is not misdiagnosed as a symptom of another disorder, which might result in the unnecessary prescribing of additional medications, producing a prescribing cascade resulting from the original ADR.

In addition to PK/PD considerations, the Beers criteria highlight medications that are best avoided in older adults and are updated on a regular basis to capture emerging safety information. Use of the Screening Tool of Older People's Prescriptions (STOPP) further assists in detecting potential prescribing errors associated with an increased risk of ADRs in the elderly, and can assist the healthcare team in avoiding the development of ADRs in this population.

F4.2 Drug Interactions

As described in the pharmacokinetics and pharmacokinetics section of this *Foundations* chapter, medications can be subject to an altered journey through the body at almost every point along the absorption, distribution, metabolism, and elimination (ADME) pathway. In addition to the more prominent, and well-recognized, competition through the liver (CYP450) that results in either increased or decreased serum concentration of the affected substrate drug, there are various less-recognized, and less-understood, drug combinations that can lead to alterations in a drug's expected effects. Some medication combinations require dose adjustments of one or both drugs in the regimen. Often, the need for dose adjustment is based on metabolic consequences that cannot be avoided through other means. In some cases, these irreconcilable drug issues can be used purposefully to achieve a "new normal." For example, ritonavir, an HIV medication, is an extremely efficient "inhibitor" of other medications; in other words, ritonavir prevents the expected metabolism and results in an extremely elevated concentration of the other "substrate" drug. This "boosted" concentration may have therapeutic value if the substrate drug otherwise could not achieve the necessary serum concentration without the boosting effects of the inhibitor.

Severe drug interactions may represent imminent danger to the patient and/or potentially significant negative outcomes. Moderate drug interactions may create a significant clinical concern depending on case-specific factors. In such cases, clinicians should consider alternative therapy and/or monitor therapy more closely to ensure safe medication use.

F4.3 Pharmacodynamic Consequences

QTc Prolongation

A prolonged QTc interval can cause irregular heartbeat, which then may result in torsades de pointes (TdP). TdP is a polymorphic ventricular tachycardia (a malignant arrhythmia) that features a change in amplitude and twisting of the QRS complex, and is associated with an increased risk of occurance with a QTc of greater than 500 ms or an increase in the QTc interval to greater than 60 ms. While there is no clear link between the threshold of QTc prolongation and the incidence of TdP, clinicians should evaluate emerging safety information related to this clinical issue and be vigilant when using more than one drug that has the potential to contribute to a prolonged QTc. Because the resulting potential degree or extent of prolongation is not entirely predictable when combining drugs, it is best to avoid pharmacodynamic escalation of this cumulative burden whenever possible. It is also advisable to be familiar with "at-risk patients" and to use extra care to avoid QTc-prolonging drug combinations in these patients.

Examples of high risk patients

- Females
- Older adults
- Patients with electrolyte imbalances
- Patients on QTc-prolonging agents with increased risk and with a cumulative burden of concomitant medications sharing the QTc risk
- Patients with structural heart disease, left ventricular dysfunction, or renal/hepatic disease

Other Pharmacodynamic Issues Resulting from Drug Interactions

Blood Dyscrasias

Medications with varying degree of hemopoietic influence can have additive effects on various blood components. Whether the drug-induced effect targets the platelets (may increase or decrease total platelet counts), red blood cells, or white blood cells, the function of the body's coagulation system and immune system can be altered, resulting in adverse consequences. For example, clozapine, a second-generation antipsychotic, can lower absolute neutrophil counts (ANCs) and may require discontinuation if the FDA established trough threshold count is reached. However, it is important to recognize other factors that are associated with changes to blood components. For instance, clozapine is now more widely available to people with benign ethnic neutropenia, a genetic condition in which the baseline ANC is naturally lower than in the general population; in the past, these patients would have been unable to receive the medication due to their lower normal ANC level.

Seizures

Seizure threshold is a term that describes a person's individual susceptibility to experiencing a seizure. The balance between excitatory and inhibitory processes in the brain can be altered with medications, alcohol consumption, and some physiologic processes associated with illness, such as fever. Drugs that decrease the seizure threshold will increase a person's likelihood of having a seizure; concomitant medications that share this same risk will magnify the potential of inducing a seizure.

Anticholinergic Intoxication

Anticholinergic syndrome (ACS) is induced by drugs that inhibit cholinergic neurotransmission at muscarinic receptor sites. Symptoms of excessive anticholinergic effects include skin flushing, dry skin and mucous membranes, mydriasis, altered mental status, and urinary retention, among other things. Anticholinergic burden scales are available as tools for clinicians to use to predict the potential cumulative burden that taking multiple drugs (polypharmacy) may cause.

Other Serious, But Less Known, Pharmacodynamic Issues

Several psychiatric–neurologic medications, such as lamotrigine, and other aromatic antiepileptic drugs (AEDs), including phenytoin and carbamazepine, may cause severe adverse cutaneous reactions, including Stevens–Johnson Syndrome (SJS) and toxic epidermal necrolysis (TEN). These skin reactions are thought to arise from a disorder of the immune system, and certain medications and genetic predispositions pose varying degrees of risk to patients. In the case of drug interactions, for example, the unintended dose escalation of lamotrigine when taken in combination with another AED, valproate, poses a significant and dangerous risk. Another drug-induced hypersensitivity reaction associated with some second-generation antipsychotic agents (SGAs) is known as "drug reaction with eosinophilia and systemic symptoms" (DRESS). DRESS also initially manifests as a skin reaction, but if not recognized or if left unaddressed, it may progress to a potentially life-threatening condition that includes hematologic abnormalities (eosinophilia, atypical lymphocytosis), lymphadenopathy, and internal organ involvement.

F4.4 Drug Interactions and Alert Fatigue

Among the notable topics covered in the recent medication safety literature is the risk of prescribers becoming overwhelmed with "too much" information—a phenomenon known as "alert fatigue." In this current environment of ever intensifying and evolving technology, electronic warnings that signal less serious alerts may be ignored (passive dismissal) by the prescriber, increasing the risk of significant harm to the patient.

F4.5 Black Box Warnings

The FDA requires black box warnings (BBWs) to be included in the labeling of prescription drugs that have shown potentially serious evidence of harm with use. Often these BBWs will be issued based on data evaluated during clinical trials. Some drugs are released to market with these warnings; for other drugs, the warnings are issued years after their initial launch into the market due to emerging safety data that are recognized during the postmarketing period. While most BBWs are associated with single-agent entities, others may be implicated in class-related BBWs that are formalized by extrapolation of available data under specific circumstances.

In addition, some medications may be contraindicated for use in specific situations in which they may be harmful. Two types of contraindications are possible: relative contraindications (acceptable to use the medication if the benefits outweigh the risks, or the warning only applies under a specific condition such as pregnancy) and absolute contraindications (absolute avoidance recommended such as in patients with a documented primary allergy to the medication due to potential life-threatening outcomes if used). It is important to recognize that not all BBWs are absolute contraindications, and that not all contraindications are BBWs.

References

Naranjo, C. A., Busto, U., Sellers, E. M., Sandor, P., Ruiz, I., Roberts, E. A., . . . Greenblatt, D. J. (1981). A method for estimating the probability of adverse drug reactions. *Clinical Pharmacology & Therapeutics, 30*(2), 239–245.

Special Populations: General Concepts to Address the Medication Needs of Pediatric and Geriatric Patients, Pregnant and Nursing Mothers

Author: **Tammie Lee Demler, PharmD, BS Pharm, MBA, RPh, BCGP, BCPP**

Editors: **Claudia Lee, RPh, MD, and Susan D. Thompson, DNP, ACNS-BC**

Learning Objectives

- Identify challenges and opportunities to recommend individualized recommendations for special populations.
- Recommend optimal pharmacologic interventions based on patient-specific characteristics.
- Provide appropriate patient-specific counseling points and optimal overall medication management.

Key Terms: Geriatric, older, aging, pediatric, neonate, child, adolescent, younger, youth, pregnant, pregnancy, nursing, lactation, breastfeeding, mother, absorption, distribution, metabolism, elimination, protein binding, volume of distribution (V_d)

Overview of Medication Management Within Special Populations

Most FDA drug monographs express adult doses in "usual adult" ranges only and have rarely offered uniquely identified geriatric doses, although this is becoming more common. Because older adults are significantly underrepresented in drug studies, and therefore available data are lacking for decision-making purposes, the safety and efficacy of medications are often extrapolated and assumed to be the same in older patients as in the adult population studied in clinical trials. The lack of specific geriatric dosing does not mean a drug cannot be used in the older adult, nor would such a use be considered "off label use" in this population. Nevertheless, the Beers list has been established as a critical resource to evaluate the use of drugs in older adults and to identify certain medications with known risks in this population.

In the case of pediatric patients, the opposite is true. To prescribe, dispense, and administer medications with FDA approval for use in pediatric patients, the FDA-approved label must expressly designate "pediatric doses" and indications for use. Further complicating this picture, the FDA divides the pediatric population into many different subpopulations. Specifically, the FDA guidance from 1998 breaks down this population into the following groups: neonates (birth to 1 month), infants (1 month to 2 years), developing children (2–12 years), and adolescents (12–16 years). Like the geriatric population, pediatric patients do not have significant representation in studies that would support FDA approval for pediatric use for most of the products available on the market. Due to this gap in FDA approval, coupled with the increasing incidence of pediatric medical and psychiatric illnesses that are also found in the adult population, a significant amount of "off label" prescribing occurs, often with only case reports to support this use. Because the FDA approval process is ongoing and a formal extension of the approved adult indication to pediatric populations can only be considered with a new drug application (NDA) submitted by drug manufacturers, clinicians involved in the medication management process should always refer to prescribing references for age-specific doses.

F5.1 Geriatric Patients

Physiologic Changes

With advanced age comes changes to all areas of the body, but some changes result in more significant pharmacokinetic impacts than others. Increased fat and reduced body water and muscle mass are only two of the major factors that can influence the action of a medication as it journeys through the aging body. Additional factors include decreased small-bowel surface area, slowed gastric emptying, and an increase in gastric pH. Serum protein changes also play a role, with the level of α1-acid glycoprotein increasing with age and the serum albumin decreasing with age (albumin levels may also serve as a biomarker predicting potential morbidity and mortality).

The FDA defines the term "geriatric" as meaning patients 65 years of age or older. However, organizations such as the American Association of Geriatric Psychiatry (AAGP) have criticized this age threshold, noting that the enrollment of healthier elderly subjects in the 65–74 age range allows the pharmaceutical industry to continue to exclude old-old (ages 75–84) and oldest-old (ages 85 and older) from clinical trials, even though these groups of frail patients are most vulnerable to the adverse effects of medications. The AAGP has openly endorsed a new definition of "elderly" that begins at age 70, at least, and perhaps even at age 75, with frailty being recognized as the real issue, rather than chronologic age.

Studies have found decreased levels of P-gp (half the maximal adult levels) in older individuals (67–85 years); however, the clinical importance of such changes in P-gp levels has not been confirmed (refer to earlier text for additional descriptions of P-gp). The efficiency of the cytochrome P-450 enzyme system decreases with age, and these changes become evident far earlier than might be expected. Significant changes are seen as early as 40 years of age, with first-pass metabolism decreasing by about 1% annually after age 40. Renal function also declines with age, although patients with comorbid illness and other clinical factors may experience a steeper and quicker decline.

Creatinine clearance decreases, on average, 8 mL/min/1.73 m^2 per decade; however, the age-related decrease varies substantially from person to person. Serum creatinine levels often remain within normal limits despite a decrease in GFR because the elderly generally have less muscle mass and are generally less physically active than younger adults, which translates into decreased creatinine production. Maintenance of normal serum creatinine levels can mislead clinicians who assume those levels reflect normal kidney function. Decreases in tubular function with age parallel those changes in glomerular function.

Older patients are more likely to experience several concurrent disorders that require medications. They are also likely to have more chronic conditions that can compromise organ function, such as decreased cardiac perfusion (i.e., congestive heart failure, peripheral vascular disease).

F5.2 Medication Management: Examples of Possible Geriatric Implications

Absorption
• *Age-related changes in drug absorption* tend to be clinically insignificant for most drugs. One exception is calcium carbonate, which requires an acidic environment for optimal absorption. • *Age-related increases in gastric pH* decrease calcium (Ca) absorption and increase the risk of constipation. Thus, elderly patients should use a calcium salt (e.g., calcium citrate) that dissolves more easily in a less acidic environment. Another example of altered absorption is an undesireable early release of enteric-coated dosage forms (such as aspirin) with increased gastric pH.
Distribution
• *Increased fat increases* the volume of distribution for highly lipophilic drugs (e.g., diazepam, chlordiazepoxide) and may also increase their elimination half-lives. • *Glycoprotein level increases with age*, but the clinical effect of this change on serum drug binding is unclear. In patients with an acute illness or malnutrition, rapid reductions in serum albumin may enhance drug effects because serum levels of unbound (free) drug may increase (only unbound drug has a pharmacologic effect). Phenytoin and warfarin are drugs with a high risk of toxic effects when serum albumin level decreases.
Metabolism
• *The metabolism and excretion of many drugs decrease.* Clearance due to hepatic metabolism typically decreases roughly 40% in geriatric patients. Theoretically, maintenance drug doses should be decreased by this percentage; however, the rate of drug metabolism varies greatly from person to person, and individual dose adjustment is required. • *Phase I reactions (oxidation, reduction, hydrolysis) are more likely to be prolonged in the elderly.* Usually, age does not greatly affect clearance of drugs that are metabolized by conjugation (phase II reactions). • *First-pass metabolism is reduced.* Thus, for a given oral dose, the elderly patient may have higher circulating drug levels and may experience exaggerated adverse drug effects and/or toxicity.
Elimination
• *Doses of some drugs should be adjusted.* One of the most important pharmacokinetic changes associated with aging is decreased renal elimination of drugs. • *Changes begin to occur after age 30.* Toxicity may develop slowly because levels of chronically used drugs increase for five to six half-lives, until a steady state is achieved.

F5.3 Pediatric Patients

Physiologic Changes

The rapid changes in size, body composition, and organ function that occur during the first year of life notably alter the ADME of medications in the infant's body. Proportions of body water, fat, and protein continuously change during infancy and childhood, and major organ systems mature in size as well as function over this period. Growth and development occur particularly rapidly during the first two years of life, with body weight typically doubling by 6 months of age and tripling by the first year of life. Body surface area (BSA) doubles during the first year of life. Additionally, the pathophysiology of some diseases and pharmacologic receptor functions change during infancy and childhood, and differ from their corresponding mature forms found in adults. Studies of adolescents reveal additional complexities in drug metabolism between the sexes. The FDA classifies the pediatric age spectrum as follows: neonate (birth to 1 month), infant (1 month to 2 years), children (2 to 12 years), and adolescent (12 to less than 16 years).

Absorption

Gastric pH and stomach emptying time have been studied in the pediatric population, just as in the adult and elderly populations. Gastric pH is neutral at birth but becomes more acidic, with a measured pH 1–3 occurring within 24 to 48 hours after birth. The pH then gradually returns to neutral again by the first week of life. This higher (less acidic) pH in neonates and young infants slowly decreases again after that point, becoming more acidic and eventually reaching the adult value at approximately 2 years of age. Gastric emptying time during the neonatal period is prolonged, owing to a reduced intestinal absorption surface area and shorter gut transit time relative to those of the adult.

Metabolic processes are often immature at birth, and later in childhood may be unpredictable. They may be accelerated for certain medications (e.g., codeine), leading to toxic and potentially fatal metabolite formation that is different than what would be expected for adults. Additionally, age-dependent changes observed in pancreatic enzymes and biliary function can compromise the ability to solubilize and subsequently absorb some lipophilic drugs. Developmental changes observed in the activity of drug-metabolizing enzymes and transporters found in the intestine are theorized to potentially alter the bioavailability of drugs as well. However, these potential alterations have not been completely characterized, as few clinical studies have addressed this issue.

P-glycoprotein (P-gp) efflux transporters also play a role in intestinal absorption. An analysis of P-gp expression in human intestinal tissue found relatively low levels in the neonatal group. This expression increased with age to reach maximum levels in young adults (15–38 years).

The skin of pediatric patients, especially newborns, is exposed to greater circulation perfusing the subcutaneous and epidermal tissues. The skin is also generally more hydrated as compared to adult skin. This fact, coupled with the larger ratio of total BSA to body mass in children as compared to adults, can result in an unexpected and undesirable systemic absorption of medications applied to the skin. Reduced blood flow to skeletal muscles has been observed and reported in neonates; however, this is not always the case and estimations may be largely unpredictable at best.

Distribution

Total body water decreases with age, from approximately 80% in newborns to 60% by 1 year of age. Conversely, body fat increases with age, from 1% to 2% in a preterm neonate to 10% to 15% in a term neonate and 20% to 25% in a 1-year-old. The impact of these differences on the volume of distribution (V_d) depends on the physiochemical characteristics of the drug. The reduced amount of plasma proteins, coupled with a diminished binding affinity of those proteins, results in overall decreased plasma protein binding of drugs in neonates and infants. Because the unbound concentration (free drug) is the pharmacologically active critical component, differences seen in pediatric protein binding can complicate the interpretation of measured drug plasma concentrations, which generally reflect the total plasma concentration of a drug. This interpretation is particularly challenging when analyzing drugs that are both highly protein bound and have a narrow therapeutic range.

Hepatic metabolism is altered in infants, primarily due to the immature intestinal cytochrome P450 enzyme system, which results in decreased phase I metabolism. Studies have also suggested that pediatric patients may experience an enhanced first-pass intestinal metabolism. Studies over the last decade evaluating age-dependent development of the drug-metabolizing enzymes have found that each enzyme system has its own unique pattern of development, with activity of these enzymes increasing over time but not in a linear manner with age. However, all the isoenzyme activities are reported to reach a level of function equivalent to that of adults once the child is 1 to 2 years of age.

Renal Elimination

As discussed in the PK/PD section, excretion of drugs by the kidneys depends on three processes: glomerular filtration, tubular excretion, and tubular reabsorption. The glomerular filtration rate is often used to assess renal function, but the efficiency of this process changes over time based on age. In the pediatric population, a full-term newborn has a GFR of 10–20 mL/min/m^2 at birth; this rate then rapidly increases to approximately 20–30 mL/min/m^2 during the first weeks of life, though it varies based on the exact postnatal age of the infant. The GFR generally reaches adult values (approximately 70 mL/min/m^2) by 3 to 5 months of age. Studies suggest that initial dose adjustments can be made in pediatric patients by either decreasing the dose or increasing the dosing interval for drugs that are mainly excreted by glomerular filtration.

Compared to glomerular filtration, tubular excretion and reabsorption seem to mature much more slowly. Tubular secretion has been reported to be approximately 20% to 30% of adult capacity at birth, with maturation occurring by 15 months of age. The roles of factors involved in this process—such as the maturing of renal uptake transporters such as organic cation transporters (OCT) and organic anion transporting polypeptides (OATP)—remain unknown. The last renal function to mature is tubular reabsorption, which does not reach adult capacity until roughly the age of 2 years. The immaturity of this function can result in variable effects on the clearance of drugs that require tubular secretion or reabsorption.

Generally, for drugs principally eliminated by the kidney, immature renal clearance processes result in the inefficient elimination of drugs, prolongation of their half-lives, and potential unexpected toxicity for pediatric patients. In turn, these outcomes require care when prescribing medications to children.

F5.4 Medication Management: Examples of Possible Pediatric Implications

Absorption Changes

Gastrointestinal

- *Prolonged stomach emptying time:* Gastric emptying time during the neonatal period is prolonged relative to that of the adult (delayed absorption).
- *Variable gastric pH:* Less acidic pH for neonates. These pH levels may have a protective effect on acid-labile drugs. They may also result in higher bioavailability of certain medications (e.g., beta-lactam antibiotics) and lower bioavailability of acidic drugs (e.g., phenytoin and acetaminophen) that require acidic conditions for appropriate ionization (increased ionization occurs under achlorhydric conditions).
- *Pancreatic and biliary function:* Reduced absorption of some lipophilic drugs (e.g., prodrug esters such as erythromycin) may occur in children.
- *Reduced intestinal absorption surface area and shorter gut transit time:* These factors may be responsible for the delayed absorption observed in neonates.

Topical

- *Absorption of drugs through skin:* Absorption of topical agents may be high in newborns and infants owing to their more hydrated epidermis, the greater circulation perfusing the subcutaneous layer, and the larger ratio of total BSA to body mass compared to adults. This can result in unexpected and undesirable systemic absorption and potential toxicity.

Parenteral

- *Absorption of parenteral intramuscularly administered drugs:* Absorption of these drugs may be delayed in neonates. Reduced blood flow to skeletal muscles has been observed in neonates; however, this is not always the case and may be largely unpredictable.

Distribution

- *Highly water-soluble drugs:* These drugs have larger volumes of distribution in neonates compared to adults. Therefore, they may require larger loading doses to achieve desired therapeutic concentrations.
- *Lipophilic drugs:* These drugs tend to have smaller volumes of distribution in infants than in older children and adults.
- *Plasma protein binding:* Binding of drugs tends to be reduced in neonates and infants because of reduction of the total amount of plasma proteins and diminished binding affinity.
  - Reduced protein binding may result in an increased distribution of drugs from the plasma to the rest of the body, which may be associated with an increased V_d.
  - Reduced protein binding can result in highly bound acidic drugs (such as sulfonamides) displacing bilirubin via competitive binding processes when plasma albumin level is low. This leads to increased blood levels of unconjugated bilirubin and increased risk of kernicterus or bilirubin encephalopathy in neonates.

Metabolism

- *Immature intestinal cytochrome P450 3A4 (CYP3A4) enzyme system:* This factor may result in reduced clearance and a prolonged half-life for those drugs that are primarily metabolized. Some drugs that are subject to a potentially enhanced first-pass effect may experience reduced bioavailability in young children.

Elimination

- *Immature renal clearance processes:* This factor may result in the inefficient elimination of drugs, prolongation of their half-lives, and potential unexpected toxicity for pediatric patients.
- *Reduced renal excretion:* Renal excretion is also reduced in neonates due to immature glomerular filtration, tubular secretion, and reabsorption.

F5.5 Pregnancy and Female Patients of Childbearing Age

Physiologic Changes

The physiologic changes that occur in the maternal–placental–fetal unit during pregnancy are highly dynamic and influence the pharmacokinetic processes. Pregnancy-induced maternal physiologic changes may affect gastrointestinal function and, therefore, drug absorption rates. Pulmonary changes may influence the absorption of inhaled drugs. As the glomerular filtration rate usually increases during pregnancy, renal drug elimination is generally enhanced, whereas hepatic drug metabolism may increase, decrease, or remain unchanged.

A mean increase of 8 L in total body water during pregnancy alters drug distribution and results in decreased peak serum concentrations of many drugs. Plasma volume increases progressively throughout normal pregnancy, resulting in a 50% total increase in the volume occurring by 34 weeks' gestation; this increase is proportional to the birth weight of the baby. Because the expansion in plasma volume is greater than the increase in red blood cell mass, there is a decline in the hemoglobin concentration, hematocrit, and red blood cell count. The platelet count tends to fall progressively during normal pregnancy, although it usually remains within normal limits. Changes in the coagulation system during pregnancy generally produce a physiologic hypercoagulable state.

Decreased steady-state concentrations have been documented for many agents because of their increased clearance during pregnancy. Pregnancy-related hypoalbuminemia, leading to decreased protein binding, results in increased free drug fraction. However, as more free drug is available for either hepatic biotransformation or renal excretion, the overall net effect is an unaltered free drug concentration. Since the free drug concentration is responsible for drug effects, the previously mentioned changes are probably of no clinical relevance. The placental and fetal capacity to metabolize drugs, together with physiologic factors, such as differences in acid–base equilibrium of the mother versus the fetus, determine the fetal exposure to the drugs taken by the mother.

Use of medication in pregnancy must be based on careful assessment of the clinical benefit versus risk to the patient, including review of specific safety concerns reported in the package labeling. Regardless of the perceived risk of the drug being recommended for use, clinicians should provide education about the reproductive risks of any medication both prior to its administration and on an ongoing basis once the medication is in use.

In addition, clinicians should be prepared to offer risk-reduction strategies for medications associated with reproductive risks, which may include contraceptive use, to women of childbearing age; they should also understand that these reproductive risks may extend to men. Other medications may decrease the effectiveness of oral contraceptives, so, when necessary, an alternative means of birth control should be explored to prevent unplanned pregnancy.

The FDA has provided guidance in establishing risk-versus-benefit analyses. In 1979, the FDA proposed the A, B, C, D, and X codes as quick, at-a-glance sliding-scale risk scores. Although A and B appeared to be safer pregnancy designation code within this system, they more often signaled a lack of information or studies available on which to make an assessment.

In 2015, the FDA's Pregnancy and Lactation Labeling (Drugs) Final Rule (PLLR) went into effect. It required changes to the content and format of the drug labeling for prescription drugs and biologic products submitted after June 30, 2015, and for those approved on or after June 30, 2001, to be phased in gradually. Labeling for over-the-counter (OTC) medications was not included in the PLLR, so OTC medication use in pregnancy continues to be challenging for those involved in assessing this risk. The intended purpose of the FDA's changes to the risk-labeling system was to improve benefit-versus-risk assessments by allowing patients to be better informed and to share in decision making with their healthcare provider.

In addition to eliminating the letter categories (i.e., A, B, C, D, and X), the PLLR requires the drug label to be updated when information becomes outdated. Moreover, the "Pregnancy" subsection (8.1) must now include information about the pregnancy exposure registry, if one is available. These exposure registries allow for the collection of data so more information will be available in the future, and because traditional FDA-required prospective testing excludes pregnant patients due to ethical concerns about potential harms to the unborn. Because the risk of teratogenicity generally declines with the progression of pregnancy to later trimesters, the risk evaluation should be longitudinal over time. Additional information found in this subsection of the PLLR includes a risk summary, clinical considerations, and data and information formerly found in the "Labor and Delivery" subsection but now included in the "Pregnancy" subsection. There is also a new "Females and Males of Reproductive Potential" subsection (8.3) that, when necessary, includes information about the contraception recommendations, the need for pregnancy testing, and information about infertility as it relates to the specific drug.

The A, B, C, D, and X risk categories have been replaced with the following narrative sections and subsections:

Pregnancy (includes Labor and Delivery)

- Pregnancy Exposure Registry
- Risk Summary
- Clinical Considerations
- Data

Lactation (includes Nursing Mothers)

- Risk Summary
- Clinical Considerations
- Data

Females and Males of Reproductive Potential

- Pregnancy Testing
- Contraception
- Infertility

F5.6 Nursing Patients

Physiologic Changes

Because medication is excreted in human breast milk to varying degrees, studies evaluating the amount of drug and the potential effects on the nursing infant are significant factors when making prescribing decisions. In the absence of human studies, animal data may be used to extrapolate the expected excretion into human breast milk. Some medications may reach concentration levels in breast milk like those seen in plasma.

The FDA's 2015 PLLR renamed the "Nursing Mothers" section as the "Lactation" subsection (8.2), and provides information about using the drug while breastfeeding, such as the amount of drug in breast milk and potential effects on the breastfed infant. When manufacturers recommend that a decision should be made either to discontinue breastfeeding or to discontinue the drug so as to continue breastfeeding, the prescriber and the patient are expected to interpret the results of these studies to ensure a shared, informed decision is made and have the opportunity for a comprehensive risk-versus-benefit analysis for each mother and her infant.

Medications that are safe for use directly in an infant that is the same age as the nursing infant's age are generally considered safe for use by the nursing mother. In contrast, medications that are considered safe during pregnancy are not necessarily safe during breastfeeding, because the nursing infant must independently metabolize and excrete the medication. In the first few early weeks postpartum, many medications can pass into breast milk that may not be able to enter mature milk due to temporary gaps in mammary alveolar cells. Some medications are not present in detectable levels in the breast milk in lactating women when their dose times are adjusted appropriately and the medications selected have an optimal PK/PD profile. Medications that are highly protein bound, that have large molecular weights, or that are poorly lipid-soluble tend not to enter the breast milk in clinically important quantities. The transfer of medications into breast milk is largely determined by the maternal serum drug concentration and depends on a concentration gradient that allows passive diffusion of non-ionized, non-protein-bound (free fraction) drugs.

The infant's medication exposure can be limited by prescribing medications to the breastfeeding mother that are poorly absorbed orally, by avoiding breastfeeding during times when the maternal serum drug concentration is at its peak, and by prescribing topical therapy when possible. Maternal serum concentrations tend to be lower with medications that have large volumes of distribution and fluctuate more with medications that have short half-lives. Because drugs are excreted into the milk by passive diffusion, the drug concentration in milk is directly proportional to the corresponding concentration in maternal plasma. The milk to plasma (M:P) ratio, which compares milk with maternal plasma drug concentrations, serves as an index of the extent of drug excretion in the milk. For most drugs, the amount ingested by the infant rarely attains therapeutic levels.

In addition to avoiding drug therapy in breastfeeding women when possible, clinicians should use reliable real-time updated references for obtaining information on medications in breast milk. Although such studies are not commonly available, choosing medications that have been investigated in infants offers the greatest guarantee of safe medication use in the pregnant and nursing mother.

Medication Management for Pregnant Patients and Nursing Mothers

Absorption
• Use topical therapy when possible; use techniques to minimize systemic absorption. • Choose medications with the poorest oral absorption. Breastfeed the infant immediately before taking the medication dose when multiple daily doses are needed. • Administer single daily-dose medications just before the longest sleep interval for the infant, usually after the bedtime feeding.
Distribution
• Choose medications with the lowest lipid solubility. • Choose medications with the highest protein-binding ability.
Metabolism
• Choose medications with the shortest half-life and highest protein-binding ability.

Resources

Merck Manual: https://www.merckmanuals.com/professional/geriatrics/drug-therapy-in-the-elderly/pharmacokinetics-in-the-elderly#v1132340

Pregnancy and Lactation Labeling (Drugs) Final Rule: https://www.fda.gov/Drugs/DevelopmentApprovalProcess/DevelopmentResources/Labeling/ucm093307.htm

Developmental pharmacokinetics in pediatric populations: https://www.ncbi.nlm.nih.gov/pmc/articles/PMC4341411/

General clinical pharmacology considerations for pediatric studies for drugs and biological products: https://www.fda.gov/downloads/drugs/guidances/ucm425885.pdf

Medications in the breastfeeding mother: https://www.aafp.org/afp/2001/0701/p119.html

Pharmacokinetic changes during pregnancy and their clinical relevance: https://www.ncbi.nlm.nih.gov/pubmed/9391746

Chapter 1

Antihistamine Agents

Author: **Kimberly Mulcahy, PharmD, BCPS**

Editor: **Claudia Lee, RPh, MD**

Learning Objectives

- Identify current pharmacologic agents that are appropriate for each condition/diagnosis.
- Recommend optimal pharmacologic interventions based on patient-specific characteristics.
- Provide appropriate patient-specific counseling points and optimal overall medication management.

Key Terms: antihistamine agents, histamine, first-generation antihistamine agents (ethanolamine derivatives, ethylenediamine derivatives, phenothiazine derivatives, piperazine derivatives, propylamine derivatives, miscellaneous), second-generation antihistamine agents, allergy, anaphylaxis, antibody, anticholinergic, antigen, anxiolytic, central nervous system, congestion, conjunctivitis, dermatoses, drowsiness, gastric acid, hay fever, insomnia, motion sickness, nausea, rhinitis, rhinorrhea, sedating, somnolence, urticaria, vomiting

Overview of Antihistamine Agents

Antihistamines are commonly utilized, predominantly over-the-counter (OTC) medications for treatment of allergic conditions. Histamine is found throughout the body, including within the vesicles of mast cells or basophils, and is abundant in the mast cells in areas particularly susceptible to tissue injury, such as the nose, mouth, feet, internal body surfaces, and blood vessels. While intracellular histamine is inert, it is released and becomes activated when a noxious antigen is detected by sensitized antibodies. Histamine that is not found within mast cells functions as a neurotransmitter in the brain and is involved with neuroendocrine control, cardiovascular functions, thermal and weight regulation, and sleep and arousal balance. The enterochromaffin-like (ECL) cells of the stomach release histamine, which is one of the main factors that stimulates the stomach mucosal parietal cells to produce gastric acid for digestion.

Four different histamine receptors have been identified. Each of these receptors is distributed in a different area of the body and elicits a different response to histamine agonism or antagonism. H_1 receptors are found on smooth muscle cells, the endothelium, and the brain; H_2 receptors are distributed in the gastric mucosa, cardiac muscle, mast cells, and the brain; H_3 receptors are located in the brain; and H_4 receptors are predominantly found on eosinophils, neutrophils, and T cells. When histamine stimulates the H_1 receptor, the reaction produces the allergic response commonly observed with insect stings and contact with other allergens, including symptoms such as bronchoconstriction, pain, and itching. H_2 receptors, when exposed to histamine, cause the contraction of gastrointestinal smooth muscles and the release of gastric acid. H_3 receptors in the brain are responsible for the release of many neurotransmitters and may also have an effect on satiety. H_4 receptors on blood cells produce inflammation and other allergic responses when histamine is present. Currently available antihistamine agents affect the H_1 and H_2 receptors; no antihistamines are approved for use that affect the H_3 and H_4 receptors, but there is a potential for these receptors to be drug targets in treatments for sleeping disorders, attention-deficit/hyperactivity disorder (ADHD), and obesity, to name a few conditions.

H_1 antihistamines are typically the first drugs used to treat the symptoms of an allergic reaction or allergic rhinitis, but when used intranasally they are considered secondary agents, to be used after glucocorticoids. These antihistamines are also the drugs of choice for managing urticaria (itching) associated with an allergic response; they are effective in this indication even if given prior to an anticipated exposure. If allergic rhinitis (hay fever) presents with nasal congestion, antihistamines are not as efficacious as nasal decongestants, such as pseudoephedrine, or combination antihistamine–decongestants (frequently named with a "D" added after the drug name, such as loratidine-D). H_1 antihistamines are not effective for bronchial asthma and antihistamines are used only as adjuvant treatment for patients experiencing systemic anaphylaxis (epinephrine is the mainstay of treatment).

Many antihistamine formulations are also available for topical administration in the eye and nose. When ophthalmic preparations are used, contact lenses should be removed prior to application, and can be reinserted 10–15 minutes after administration, unless otherwise specified. Do not reinsert the lenses if the eyes are red, and separate administration of other ophthalmic topical agents by 5 minutes. With nasal preparations, the nasal spray must be primed prior to first use until a fine mist appears. Repriming is necessary when the product is unused for a number of days specified by the certain manufacturer.

1.1 First-Generation Antihistamine Agents

First-generation antihistamines are H_1 antagonists and are known for their strong sedating properties due to the easy penetration of the central nervous system (CNS). Since the sedating effect is so powerful with some agents, they are commonly used as sleep aids. However, children and some adults (though rare) may experience an excitation effect. Some medications in this class have antinausea and antiemetic effects and can be used to prevent motion sickness (though they are not as effective if used to treat an active episode). Some H_1 antagonists—predominantly diphenhydramine—can suppress extrapyramidal symptoms caused by antipsychotic use. The ethanolamine and ethylenediamine agent subgroups have antimuscarinic actions, which may help patients with non-allergic rhinorrhea, but also cause undesirable side effects of urinary retention and blurred vision.

First-generation antihistamines are largely anticholinergic and can cause dry mouth, dry eyes, urinary retention, constipation, and cognitive disturbances. Patients with a diagnosis of closed-angle glaucoma, urinary retention, peptic ulcer disease, or uncontrolled asthma should not use first-generation antihistamines. Anticholinergic side effects can be further exacerbated by other anticholinergic medications, such as tricyclic antidepressants (TCAs). Because monoamine oxidase inhibitors (MAOIs) can also exacerbate anticholinergic side effects, first-generation antihistamines should not be used during treatment or within 2 weeks of MAOI discontinuation.

Toxicities of the first-generation antihistamines include convulsions, postural hypotension (increasing the risk of falls in patients, especially the elderly), and cardiac arrhythmias. Central nervous system depression can be additive if first-generation antihistamines are combined with other medications with sedative properties or alcohol. Patients should be cautioned about driving and operating machinery while using these medications. There is also a potential for sedative properties to still be present the following morning if these agents are used for sleep. First-generation antihistamines are on the Beers list and are considered potentially harmful in elderly patients; other medication options should be explored if possible.

First-Generation Antihistamine Agents

Brompheniramine
Carbinoxamine
Chlorpheniramine
Clemastine
Cyproheptadine

Diphenhydramine
Doxylamine
Promethazine
Triprolidine
Dimenhydrinate *(see also the Antiemetic Agents section in the Gastrointestinal Agents chapter)*
Hydroxyzine *(see also the Anxiolytic, Sedative, and Hypnotic Agents section in the Central Nervous System Agents chapter)*
Meclizine *(see also the Antiemetic Agents section in the Gastrointestinal Agents chapter)*

Case Studies and Conclusions

Joanne was doing yard work over the weekend and is now covered in an itchy rash on both arms. She states she has not been able to sleep at night because she cannot stop scratching.

1. Which of the following would be the best option to manage Joanne's allergic reaction?
   a. Fexofenadine
   b. Epinephrine
   c. Diphenhydramine
   d. Ranitidine

Answer C is correct. Fexofenadine is a nonsedating second-generation antihistamine; this patient would benefit from a first-generation antihistamine to increase sedation at night. Epinephrine is used in cases of anaphylaxis, but this patient presents with a local rash. Ranitidine is an H_2 antihistamine that is used for gastrointestinal disorders, not allergies.

It has been a few days, and Joanne's rash has improved and has almost disappeared. She states that she is going on a cruise next week and is afraid she will get motion sickness. She wants a recommendation for an OTC product.

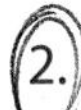

2. What is an OTC formulation of an antihistamine that can be used to prevent nausea?
   a. Doxylamine
   b. Promethazine
   c. Diphenhydramine
   d. Cetirizine

Answer C is correct. Doxylamine and cetirizine are not indicated for the treatment of nausea. Promethazine is a prescription-only medication. Diphenhydramine is OTC and has indications for nausea and vomiting as well as helping with the uticaria and insomnia.

Joanne returned from her cruise and came home just in time for allergy season. She states that she would like to take a first-generation antihistamine to manage her seasonal allergies.

3. Which of the following statements is FALSE?
   a. Counsel the patient about the morning "hangover" that may occur if she takes a first-generation antihistamine at bedtime.
   b. A common side effect with frequent use of a first-generation antihistamine is diarrhea.
   c. Many of the first-generation antihistamines should be used with caution in geriatric patients.
   d. First-generation antihistamines should not be used within 2 weeks of use of an MAOI.

Answer B is correct. First-generation antihistamines can cause daytime sleepiness, so patients should be warned about driving or operating machinery. The most common side effects with these drugs are anticholinergic, such as constipation, urinary retention, dry eyes, and dry mouth. First-generation antihistamines are on the Beers list, so second-generation antihistamines should be used instead if possible. The combination of MAOIs and first-generation antihistamines has the potential to cause hypertensive crisis due to the antihistamine's concurrent effects on neurotransmitters.

George is a 68-year-old patient being seen for his annual physical examination appointment. He mentions that he experiences seasonal allergies and in the past had success with diphenhydramine. His medical history includes depression, hypertension, dyslipidemia, and type 2 diabetes mellitus.

1. What is a concern with using a first-generation antihistamine in George?
   a. Many first-generation antihistamines are Beers list medications and may not be safe for all patients.
   b. First-generation antihistamines may cause excitation in geriatric patients instead of sedation.
   c. Use of antihistamines may exacerbate George's diabetes.
   d. All of the above are true.

Answer A is correct. First-generation antihistamines are on the Beers list, and alternative options for therapy should be explored if possible. In George's case, it would be appropriate to try a second-generation antihistamine first. Excitation—as opposed to sedation—is a possible side effect when first-generation antihistamines are used in pediatric patients. These antihistamines have anticholinergic properties and could exacerbate closed-angle glaucoma, urinary retention, and prostatic hypertrophy.

Despite your suggestion that a first-generation antihistamine may not be the best option, George says that he is used to these products and would rather take something with which he has had prior experience. George is currently being treated with fluoxetine (a selective serotonin reuptake inhibitor [SSRI]) for his depression.

2. Which of the following statements is true regarding possible drug interactions between the SSRI and first-generation antihistamines?
   a. George must wait 2 weeks between his last dose of fluoxetine and brompheniramine.
   b. Fluoxetine will exacerbate the anticholinergic side effects of the first-generation antihistamines.
   c. Fluoxetine may worsen the drowsiness/sedative effects of the first-generation antihistamines.
   d. Use of antidepressants is contraindicated with the first-generation antihistamines.

Answer C is correct. Use of MAOIs should be avoided when a patient is taking brompheniramine, with a 2-week washout period being recommended. TCAs have the potential to exacerbate anticholinergic side effects of the first-generation antihistamines; some SSRIs have the potential to cause anticholinergic effects, although this is not a common side effect of fluoxetine. Medications that have the potential to lead to CNS depression (including antidepressants) may also worsen the drowsiness and sedative effects of the first-generation antihistamines. Although use of antidepressants is not contraindicated with the first-generation antihistamines, MAOIs, TCAs, and other antidepressants with anticholinergic side effects should be used with caution.

George states that his biggest complaint about his allergies occurs when he is working in his garden. On top of the typical "hay fever"-like symptoms, he says that he almost always manages to come in contact with poison ivy or poison oak and breaks out in a rash.

3. Which product would be best to manage this patient's allergic rhinitis and the contact allergic reaction?
   a. Meclizine
   b. Chlorpheniramine
   c. Doxylamine
   d. Diphenhydramine

Answer D is correct. Meclizine is approved as an antiemetic drug. Chlorpheniramine will treat the allergic rhinitis but does not have contact allergic reactions as a labeled indication. Doxylamine is used for insomnia or allergic rhinitis. Diphenhydramine would manage both allergic rhinitis and the contact allergic reaction.

1.2 Second-Generation Antihistamine Agents

Both first and second generations of antihistamines have been found to have equal efficacy in the treatment of allergic responses. Unlike the first-generation antihistamines, however, the second-generation products do not cross the blood-brain barrier to the same extent and, therefore, do not have the same sedative properties; in addition, they have fewer antimuscarinic and anticholinergic effects. Nevertheless, the second-generation antihistamines may still cause drowsiness in some patients, especially if used concurrently with medications that cause CNS depression or alcohol. The second-generation products are most commonly used for chronic allergy symptoms due to their lack of sedation and amenability to daily use. This class is the preferred treatment in geriatric patients and children due to the favorable side-effect profile and minimal CNS penetration.

Second-Generation Antihistamines

Acrivastine
Cetirizine
Desloratadine
Fexofenadine
Levocetirizine
Loratadine
Azelastine *(see also the Antiallergic Agents section in the Eye, Ear, Nose, and Throat Preparations chapter)*

Case Studies and Conclusions

Ray is a construction worker and has complaints of seasonal allergies. He says that whenever the pollen level is high, he gets watery and itchy eyes, a runny nose, and persistent sneezing.

1. Which of the following would be the best first-choice option for managing Ray's allergies?
   a. Diphenhydramine by mouth
   b. Azelastine intranasally
   c. Loratadine by mouth
   d. Cimetidine by mouth

Answer C is correct. Ray is a construction worker, so he presumably operates machinery that requires full attention. Thus diphenhydramine would be too sedating for him. Azelastine intranasally is not a first-choice option; instead, intranasal antihistamines are used after the patient has tried an intranasal glucocorticoid. Cimetidine is an H_2 antihistamine and used to treat gastrointestinal upset.

Ray later adds that he typically is very congested, during especially bad pollen days.

2. What would the best advice be for the patient?
   a. An antihistamine is sufficient alone to manage nasal congestion.
   b. Use a combination antihistamine and decongestant.
   c. Use a decongestant alone.
   d. Use a combination oral and nasal antihistamine when symptoms are worse.

Answer B is correct. Antihistamines alone are not sufficient to manage nasal congestion with allergy symptoms; combination products with a decongestant, such as pseudoephedrine, are more effective. A decongestant alone would manage Ray's nasal symptoms, but the antihistamine would be required to help treat his other symptoms, such as watery eyes. While nasal antihistamines are effective for symptom management in patients with nasal congestion, they are not a first-line option and need to be used regularly to achieve their greatest efficacy.

Ray asks whether his medications might also be safe for his 72-year old father, who is having similar reactions.

3. Which of the following statements best summarizes the recommended use of antihistamines in older adults?
   a. First-generation antihistamines are a good option for geriatric patients with seasonal allergies because they can cause CNS excitation, which can help give them more energy.
   b. Second-generation antihistamines are the best option for geriatric patients with seasonal allergies because of their minimal CNS penetration.
   c. Geriatric patients should be offered only intranasal or ophthalmic preparations; oral medications are not recommended in older adults.
   d. No antihistamines are safe in geriatric patients under any circumstances.

Answer B is correct. Second-generation antihistamines have less CNS penetration and a safer side-effect profile for geriatric patients.

Sam presents to his doctor's appointment with complaints of a runny nose, watery eyes, and nasal congestion. He says that these symptoms occur every year around this time, but he usually just muddles his way through the allergy season without any medications. This year, however, his symptoms are worse than ever, and he would like to explore possible medication options.

1. Which of the following is NOT a benefit of Sam using a second-generation antihistamine as opposed to a first-generation antihistamine?
   a. The risk of sedation is less with the first-generation antihistamines, so using the second-generation products could help him sleep better at night.
   b. Many second-generation products come in combination products with a decongestant.
   c. Most second-generation medications are dosed once a day.
   d. All of the above are true.

Answer A is correct. Second-generation antihistamines are less sedating than the first-generation products. Second-generation antihistamines are available in many different combinations, including with pseudoephedrine, ibuprofen, or acetaminophen. Another appealing aspect of second-generation products is that most require only once-daily dosing, whereas most first-generation antihistamines are dosed multiple times a day.

Sam's medical history includes hypertension, and he has an extensive family history of cardiovascular disease. His blood pressure at the beginning of this visit was elevated, and he says he often forgets to take his blood pressure medication.

2. Which of the following products would be the least appropriate to recommend to Sam?
   a. Acrivastine
   b. Cetirizine
   c. Fexofenadine
   d. Loratadine

Answer A is correct. Acrivastine should be avoided in patients with severe hypertension or coronary artery disease. Cetirizine, fexofenadine, and loratidine do not have cardiovascular concerns and would be better recommendations for Sam to use.

Sam states that he frequently consumes alcoholic beverages and would like to avoid an allergy agent that is metabolized via the liver.

3. Which of the following medications requires dose adjustment or dose consideration with hepatic impairment?
   a. Cetirizine
   b. Desloratadine
   c. Levocetirizine
   d. Loratadine

Answer B is correct. Desloratadine requires dose adjustment for both hepatic and renal impairment (5 mg every other day). Cetirizine, levocetirizine, and loratadine require dose adjustment for renal impairment.

1.3 Other Antihistamine Agents

H_2 antihistamines (cimetidine, famotidine, nizatidine, and ranitidine) are used to inhibit the secretion of gastric acid in patients with gastrointestinal (GI) disorders. Intranasal products should be used after a patient has tried an intranasal glucocorticoid. Intranasal antihistamines are most effective when used regularly and do not cause rebound effects as nasal decongestants do.

Other Antihistamine Agents

Bepotastine *(see also the Antiallergic Agents section in the Eye, Ear, Nose, and Throat Preparations chapter)*
Cimetidine *(see also the Antiulcer Agents and Suppressants section in the Gastrointestinal Agents chapter)*
Emedastine *(see also the Antiallergic Agents section in the Eye, Ear, Nose, and Throat Preparations chapter)*

Famotidine *(see also the Antiulcer Agents and Suppressants section in the Gastrointestinal Agents chapter)*
Ketotifen *(see also the Antiallergic Agents section in the Eye, Ear, Nose, and Throat Preparations chapter)*
Nizatidine *(see also the Antiulcer Agents and Suppressants section in the Gastrointestinal Agents chapter)*
Olopatadine *(see also the Antiallergic Agents section in the Eye, Ear, Nose, and Throat Preparations chapter)*
Ranitidine *(see also the Antiulcer Agents and Suppressants section in the Gastrointestinal Agents chapter)*

Common Class Considerations

Anaphylaxis: A life-threatening allergic reaction. Signs and symptoms include an itchy rash, swelling of the tongue, bronchoconstriction, hypotension, and facial edema. Anaphylaxis presents suddenly, typically over a few minutes. Antihistamines alone are not a sufficient treatment, and patients should immediately receive epinephrine. Antihistamines and steroids are added as adjuvant treatments.

Excitation: In children, normal doses of first-generation antihistamines often result in an excitatory effect instead of a sedative effect. This phenomenon has also been infrequently reported in some adult cases at therapeutic doses, but is more common in overdose and toxic situations.

Sedation/somnolence: Increased sedation and somnolence are frequently reported with use of the first-generation antihistamines. When taken at bedtime, these drugs may also lead to a daytime "hangover" of drowsiness and somnolence. Second-generation antihistamines are referred to as "nonsedating" and have similar incidence of sedation as placebo in studies.

Toxicity: Toxicity of antihistamines has been reported in incidents of overdose or interactions with liver metabolism enzymes (CYP)-inhibiting medications (predominately macrolides and azole antifungal drugs), with patients experiencing higher than intended circulating antihistamine levels. Signs and symptoms of toxicity include hallucinations, incoordination, convulsions, cardiac arrhythmias, and fever.

Tips from the Field

1. Make sure your patients understand the difference between antihistamines and decongestants. Decongestants constrict nasal blood vessels, resulting in an improvement in nasal stuffiness but they do not affect histamine and won't impact any of the other symptoms associated with hay fever, such as sneezing, runny nose, and itching. Caution patients that if they use nasal spray decongestants for more than a few days, these agents can produce a rebound swelling of the nasal tissues, resulting in even greater congestion.

2. Suggest use of OTC products, such as Claritin D, which contain both an antihistamine and a decongestant if symptoms warrant use. Make sure they understand the side effects associated with this combination.

3. Help patients determine the right antihistamine for them, for example, daytime use avoid sedating agents like diphenhydramine (Benadryl). Newer generation antihistamines, such as loratadine (Claritin), fexofenadine (Allegra), and cetirizine (Zyrtec), are generally a better choice since they are less sedating.

4. Note that even the newer nonsedating generation antihistamines can cause drowsiness and other symptoms in some people, especially older adults, particularly if they take them at higher doses. Make sure they understand importance of starting the drug at the lowest dose and evaluate its effectiveness.

5. Most of these agents can be purchased OTC and there is no difference between the generic brand versus the name brand.

6. Explain to your elderly patients that antihistamines can cause other central nervous system effects, including coordination problems, fatigue, and temporary cognitive impairment. Research has shown an increased risk of long-term cognitive decline in older people who take the drugs regularly.
7. First-generation antihistamines are also more likely than the newer products to cause serious side effects, such as a rapid heart rate or urinary retention (which can be especially problematic in men who have BPH).
8. Several first-generation antihistamines can reduce motion sickness such as diphenhydramine, doxylamine, dimenhydrinate (as found in Dramamine), and meclizine (the active ingredient in Bonine) These are all OTC and are the most commonly used motion sickness medications. Make sure they understand that it can take at least 30 minutes for them to take effect.
9. People suffering closed or narrow-angle glaucoma, chronic obstructive pulmonary disease, kidney disease, prostate problems, hypertension, heart disease, and thyroid problems should not take *any* OTC antihistamines without first consulting with their provider.
10. The FDA Nonprescription Drug Advisory Committee and the Pediatric Advisory Committee has recommended that nonprescription cough and cold products should not be used in children less than 2 years of age and an official ruling regarding the use of these products in children older than 2 has not yet been announced. Refer to pediatric drug references for additional information (FDA, 2008).

Bibliography

American Geriatrics Society. Updated Beers criteria for potentially inappropriate medication use in older adults. *J Am Geriatr Soc.* 2015;63:2227-2246.

Haas HL, Sergeeva OA, Selbach O. Histamine in the nervous system. *Physiol Rev.* 2008;88:1183-1241.

Holgate ST, Canonica GW, Simons FE, et al. Consensus Group on New-Generation Antihistamines (CONGA): present status and recommendations. *Clin Exp Allergy.* 2003;33:1305-1324.

McEvoy GK, ed. *AHFS: Drug Information.* Bethesda, MD: American Society of Health-System Pharmacists; 2016.

Richardson GS, Roehrs TA, Rosenthal L, Koshorek G, Roth T. Tolerance to daytime sedative effects of H1 antihistamines. *J Clin Psychopharmacol.* 2002;22:511-515.

Skidgel RA, Kaplan AP, Erdös EG. Histamine, bradykinin, and their antagonists. In: Brunton LL, Chabner BA, Knollmann BC, eds. *Goodman & Gilman's The Pharmacological Basis of Therapeutics.* 12th ed. New York, NY: McGraw-Hill; 2011:911-936.

U.S. Food and Drug Administration (FDA). Public health advisory: FDA recommends that over-the-counter (OTC) cough and cold products not be used for infants and children under 2 years of age. 2008. http://www.fda.gov/NewsEvents/Newsroom/PressAnnouncements/2008/ucm051137.htm

Symbols

- ▲ Renal impairment: Dose adjustment is recommended.
- ◼ Hepatic impairment: Dose adjustment is recommended.
- ■ Black box warning exists for this drug.
- (QT) QTc prolongation effects have been reported.
- (BL) Beers list criteria (avoid in elderly).
- (PD) FDA-approved pediatric doses are available.
- (GD) FDA-approved geriatric doses are available.
-  See primary body system.

Antihistamine Agents

Universal prescribing alerts:

- Known serious hypersensitivity to the specific drug or any other component of the product/formulation selected warrants a contraindication for use.
- Adverse reactions associated with the use of some antihistamine agents include dizziness, drowsiness, vertigo, or fatigue; these drugs may also impair the ability to perform tasks requiring mental alertness. Caution should always be recommended when using any new drug for the first time, when there is a dose change, and with continued use of known offending agents.
- Doses expressed are for the usual adult dosage ranges only. "Geriatric doses" are assumed to be the same as the adult doses unless otherwise noted with a symbol. Where FDA-approved geriatric or pediatric dosing is available, a symbol will guide the reader to additional prescribing references. Refer to real-time prescribing references for these age-specific doses. Please also refer to the narrative chapter overview to learn more about the FDA Nonprescription Drug Advisory Committee and the Pediatric Advisory Committee recommendations for cough and cold products in pediatric patients.
- Use of antihistamines in pregnancy is based on clinical risk versus benefit; safety concerns are not represented in this grid. Refer to the package insert (PI) for more information. Clinicians should continue to provide education about the reproductive risks of any medication use and offer risk-reduction strategies (which may include contraceptive use) to women of childbearing age and understand that these reproductive risks may also extend to males.
- Brand names are provided for those agents still available on the market. Due to the ever-changing product availability, refer to Food and Drug Administration (FDA) resources to confirm the actual brands available This drug summary is for educational purposes only. Prescribing decisions should be based on real-time comprehensive drug databases that are updated on a regular basis.

First-Generation Antihistamine Agents

Universal prescribing alerts:

- Central nervous depression can be additive if first-generation antihistamines are combined with other medications with sedative properties or alcohol; patients should be cautioned about driving and operating machinery while using these medications.
- First-generation antihistamines are largely anticholinergic agents and can cause dry mouth, dry eyes, urinary retention, constipation, and cognitive disturbances; their use should be avoided in patients with underlying closed-angle glaucoma, urinary retention, peptic ulcer disease, and uncontrolled asthma. Anticholinergic side effects can be further exacerbated by other anticholinergic medications, such as tricyclic antidepressants and monoamine oxidase inhibitors (MAOIs).
- First-generation antihistamines should not be used within 2 weeks of MAOIs.
- There is a potential for sedative properties to still be present the following morning if these agents are used for sleep.
- First-generation antihistamines are on the Beers list and are considered potentially harmful in elderly patients; other medication options should be explored if possible.

Drug Name	FDA-Approved Indications	Dosage Range	Precautions and Clinical Pearls
Generic Name Brompheniramine maleate **Brand Name** J-Tan PD Respa-BR Bromax LoHist (BL) (PD)	Allergic rhinitis Common cold	Dose varies depending on product selected **Illustrative oral dose (maleate):** 6 to 12 mg every 12 hours	• Take with food, water, or milk to minimize gastric irritation • Dexbrompheniramine maleate is a chemically related ingredient • Use is generally "as needed" • Some brompheniramine containing products are OTC and others require a prescription • Different salt forms are available (maleate and tannate) requiring different dose schedules. • Available in multiple combination products; see individual product for indications, dosing, and name brand.
Generic Name Carbinoxamine maleate **Brand Name** Arbinoxa Karbinal ER (BL) (PD)	Allergies and related symptoms such as rhinitis, pruritus, rhinorrhea, and urticaria	**Usual oral dose:** IR: 4 to 8 mg 3 to 4 times daily ER: 6 to 16 mg every 12 hours (not to exceed 32 mg daily)	• Take on an empty stomach with water • Available by prescription only • Extended release and immediate release product dosing schedules are different, review directions prior to use
Generic Name Chlorpheniramine maleate **Brand Name** Aller-Chlor Chlor-Trimeton Allergy Chlor-Trimeton Chlorphen Ed ChlorPed Ed-Chlortan Pharbechlor (BL) (PD)	Allergic rhinitis, pruritus, rhinorrhea, and urticaria	Dose varies depending on product selected **Illustrative oral dose immediate release:** 4 mg every 4 to 6 hours (maximum daily dose [MDD]: 24 mg)	• Dexchlorpheniramine maleate is a chemically related ingredient • OTC and prescription (higher doses) are available • Extended release and immediate release product dosing schedules are different, review directions prior to use • Available in multiple combination products; see individual product for indications, dosing, and name brand.

Generic Name Clemastine fumarate **Brand Name** Dayhist Allergy 12 Hour Relief Tavist Allergy BL PD	Allergic rhinitis, pruritus, urticaria, symptoms of the common cold and angioedema	Dose varies depending on product selected **Illustrative OTC oral dose:** 1.34 mg twice daily (MDD: 8.04 mg including prescription dosing)	• Take with food or milk if patient experiences stomach upset • Prescription products available for use at higher doses • Available in multiple combination products; see individual product for indications, dosing, and name brand.
Generic Name Cyproheptadine hydrochloride BL PD	**Illustrative indications for use:** Allergic rhinitis, pruritus, urticaria, and angioedema	**Usual oral dose:** 4 to 20 mg daily in divided doses (MDD: 0.5 mg/kg per day or 32 mg whichever is less)	• Hepatic impairment dose adjustment recommended, however, no specific dose suggestion provided by manufacturer
Generic Name Diphenhydramine hydrochloride **Brand Name** Benadryl and various others BL PD QT ■	**Illustrative indications for use:** Allergic rhinitis, contact dermatitis, antitussive, drug-induced EPS, Parkinsonian syndromes, insomnia, motion sickness, adjunct treatment of anaphylaxis	Dose varies depending on combination product selected **Illustrative oral dose:** 25 to 50 mg every 4 to 8 hours (max 300 mg per 24 hours) **Usual parenteral dose:** **IM/IV:**10 to 50 mg per dose (max 100 mg per dose; max 400 mg per day)	• Topical application can cause an allergic-type contact dermatitis • Drug interactions may require dose adjustments • Available in multiple combination products; see individual product for indications, dosing, and name brand.
Generic Name Doxylamine succinate **Brand Name** Doxytex Nitetime Sleep-Aid Sleep Aid Unisom BL PD	Allergic rhinitis, insomnia	Dose varies depending on product selected **Illustrative oral dose:** 25 mg daily or at bedtime	• Optimal dose schedule for insomnia is take dose 30 minutes prior to planned 8-hour sleep (bedtime) • Available in multiple combination products; see individual product for indications, dosing, and name brand.

Drug Name	FDA-Approved Indications	Adult Dosage Range	Precautions and Clinical Pearls
Generic Name Promethazine hydrochloride **Brand Name** Phenadoz Phenergan Promethegan ■ QT BL PD	Allergic conditions, motion sickness, antiemetic, sedative	Dose varies depending on product selected **Illustrative oral dose for nausea/vomiting:** 12.5 mg before meals and HS **Illustrative rectal dose for nausea/vomiting:** 12.5 to 25 mg every 4 to 6 hours as needed **Illustrative IM dose for nausea/vomiting:** 12.5 to 25 mg every 4 to 6 hours as needed	• Mild to moderate akathisia and extrapyramidal symptoms possible after injection or long-term use • Use is associated with QT prolongation • Drug interactions may require dose adjustment • When treating nausea/vomiting; administer before meals or snack • Deep IM injection preferred route of parenteral administration • Available in multiple combination products; see individual product for indications, dosing, and name brand. Associated with: • Injection can cause severe tissue injury • Subcutaneous and intra-arterial administration • Use in patients in a coma • Use in patients with asthma
Generic Name Triprolidine hydrochloride **Brand Name** Histex PD Histex BL PD	Allergies, rhinitis, urticaria	Dose varies depending on product selected **Illustrative oral dose:** 2.5 mg every 4 to 6 hours (max 10 mg per 24 hours)	• May be administered without regard to meals, however may take with food or milk to minimize stomach upset • Available in multiple combination products; see individual product for indications, dosing, and name brand.
Dimenhydrinate	Refer to the Gastrointestinal Agents chapter.		
Hydroxyzine	Refer to the Central Nervous System Agents chapter.		
Meclizine	Refer to the Gastrointestinal Agents chapter.		

Second-Generation Antihistamine Agents

Universal prescribing alerts:

- Many of these second-generation agents cause CNS depression (albeit not to the same extent as the first-generation antihistamines). Patients should use caution when performing tasks that require mental alertness.

Drug Name	FDA-Approved Indications	Dosage Range	Precautions and Clinical Pearls
Generic Name Acrivastine **Brand Name** Semprex-D	Allergic rhinitis, nasal congestion	**Usual oral dose:** 8 mg every 4 to 6 hours (32 mg maximum per day)	• Avoid use in patients with CrCl less than 48 mL/min • Use in caution in patients with diabetes or thyroid dysfunction • Available in combination with pseudoephedrine only • 8 mg acrivastine tablets also contain 60 mg pseudoephedrine • Recommended for use as needed up to 14 days Contraindications: • Coronary artery disease • Uncontrolled hypertension • Drug interactions may preclude use (i.e., MAOIs)
Generic Name Cetirizine hydrochloride **Brand Name** All Day Allergy Zyrtec ■ (PD) (GD)	Allergies, rhinitis, urticaria	Dose varies depending on product selected **Illustrative oral dose:** 5 to 10 mg daily	• Cetirizine is not removed with hemodialysis • ISMP safety alert (may sound like or look like other medications, thus mistakes may be more common with this drug) • Available in multiple combination products; see individual product for indications, dosing, and name brand.
Generic Name Desloratadine **Brand Name** Clarinex ▲ ■ (PD)	Allergic rhinitis, chronic idiopathic urticaria, pruritus	Dose varies depending on product selected **Illustrative oral dose:** 5 mg daily	• Desloratadine is not removed by hemodialysis • Available in multiple combination products; see individual product for indications, dosing, and name brand.

Drug Name	FDA-Approved Indications	Adult Dosage Range	Precautions and Clinical Pearls
Generic Name Fexofenadine hydrochloride **Brand Name** Allegra ▲ (PD)	Allergic rhinitis Chronic idiopathic urticaria	Dose varies depending on product selected **Illustrative oral dose:** 60 mg twice daily or 180 mg once daily	• Available in multiple combination products; see individual product for indications, dosing, and name brand.
Generic Name Levocetirizine dihydrochloride **Brand Name** Xyzal ▲ (PD)	Allergic rhinitis Chronic idiopathic urticaria	**Usual oral dose:** 5 mg once daily	• Diarrhea and constipation common adverse effects Contraindications: • End-stage renal disease • Use of levocetirizine in patients undergoing dialysis
Generic Name Loratadine **Brand Name Alavert** Allergy Claritin Loradamed ▲ ■ (BL) (PD)	Allergic rhinitis, urticaria, pruritus	Dose varies depending on product selected **Illustrative oral dose:** 10 mg once daily or 5 mg twice daily	• Headache is the most common side effect • Orally dissolvable tablets are available (tablet disintegrates with or without water) • Loratadine is not removed by hemodialysis • Brand name Claritin oral products do not contain the same ingredient as Claritin eye products (ketotifen fumarate)—use care when prescribing • Available in multiple combination products; see individual product for indications, dosing, and name brand.
Azelastine	Refer to the Eye, Ear, Nose, and Throat Preparations chapter.		

Other Antihistamine Agents

Universal prescribing alerts:

- Intranasal antihistamines are most effective when used regularly and do not cause rebound effects as nasal decongestants do.

Drug Name	FDA-Approved Indications	Dosage Range	Precautions and Clinical Pearls
Bepotastine	Refer to the Eye, Ear, Nose, and Throat Preparations chapter.		
Cimetidine	Refer to the Gastrointestinal Agents chapter.		
Emedastine	Refer to the Eye, Ear, Nose, and Throat Preparations chapter.		
Famotidine	Refer to the Gastrointestinal Agents chapter.		
Ketotifen	Refer to the Eye, Ear, Nose, and Throat Preparations chapter.		
Nizatidine	Refer to the Gastrointestinal Agents chapter.		
Olopatadine	Refer to the Eye, Ear, Nose, and Throat Preparations chapter.		
Ranitidine	Refer to the Gastrointestinal Agents chapter.		

Chapter 2

Anti-infective Agents

Author: **Beatriz Manzor Mitrzyk, PharmD, BCPS, BCACP**

Editor: **Amy L. Wojciechowski, PharmD, BCPS-AQ ID, BCCCP**

Learning Objectives

- Identify current pharmacologic agents that are appropriate for each condition/diagnosis.
- Recommend optimal pharmacologic interventions based on patient-specific characteristics.
- Provide appropriate patient-specific counseling points and optimal overall medication management.

Key Terms: anthelmintic agents, antibacterial agents, aminoglycosides, cephalosporins, beta-lactams, carbapenems, cephamycins, monobactams, chloramphenicols, macrolides, erythromycins, ketolides, penicillins, aminopenicillins, penicillinase-resistant penicillins, extended-spectrum penicillins, quinolones, sulfonamides, tetracyclines, glycylcyclines, bacitracins, cyclic lipopeptides, glycopeptides, lincomycins, oxazolidinones, polymyxins, rifamycins, streptogramins, antifungal agents, allylamines, azoles, echinocandins, polyenes, pyrimidines, antimycobacterial agents, antituberculosis agents, antiviral agents, adamantanes, antiretroviral agents, HIV entry and fusion inhibitors, HIV protease inhibitors, HIV integrase inhibitors, HIV non-nucleoside reverse transcriptase inhibitors, HIV nucleoside and nucleotide reverse transcriptase inhibitors, interferons, monoclonal antibodies, neuraminidase inhibitors, nucleosides and nucleotides, HCV antiviral agents, HCV polymerase inhibitors, HCV protease inhibitors, HCV replication complex inhibitors, antiprotozoal agents

Overview of Anti-infective Agents

Antimicrobials are medications that prevent and treat infections; they are vital to the health and well-being of society. Often assisting the body's defenses, this wide variety of medications has been developed to manage infections caused by bacteria, viruses, and parasites. The clinical course of any infection is dependent on the interaction between the pathogen and a complex set of host defenses.

The first consideration in selecting antimicrobial therapy is whether an antimicrobial agent is truly needed. The differential diagnosis should indicate whether the cause requires treatment with an antimicrobial drug or whether the infection is self-limiting and will resolve without antimicrobial therapy. For self-limiting infections, supportive treatment and symptom management are recommended. If possible, antimicrobial use should be limited to highly suspicious, empiric, and definitive diagnoses of infection to avoid toxicity and the development of antimicrobial resistance.

Prior to beginning antimicrobial therapy, specimens for culture and sensitivity testing should be obtained. The exceptions to this care are septic patients, in whom prompt antimicrobial therapy should not be delayed if culture specimens cannot be obtained in a timely manner, because early administration of antibiotics in sepsis has shown to reduce mortality. Empiric antimicrobial therapy selection is based on the likely pathogens for the site or type of infection; the patient's medical, medication, and social history; prior antibiotic use; and local susceptibility patterns.

Monitoring includes assessing for resolution of signs and symptoms of infection (e.g., normalization of body temperature and white blood cell [WBC] count) and watching for adverse drug events. Ideally, the antibiotic with the narrowest effective spectrum of activity should be selected. The route of administration should be evaluated daily, and conversion to oral therapy should be made once the patient is clinically improving and able to tolerate it (i.e., functioning gastrointestinal [GI] tract; general exceptions are endocarditis and central nervous system [CNS] infections). Patients not responding to therapy within 2–3 days should be reevaluated to assess the diagnosis, determine whether therapeutic drug concentrations are being achieved, and identify if the patient is immunosuppressed. In addition, further investigation should be conducted to determine if there is an isolated infection (i.e., abscess, foreign body) or if resistance to the therapy has developed.

It is recommended that practitioners follow a systematic approach when selecting an antimicrobial regimen. This approach minimizes the development of resistance, the likelihood of superinfections, and the use of more expensive and potentially more toxic agents.

Systematic Approach for Selection of Antimicrobials

- Confirm the presence of infection.
- Perform a careful history and physical examination.
- Identify signs and symptoms.
- Identify predisposing factors.
- Identify the pathogen.
- Collect infected material.
- Perform Gram stain.
- Perform serologies.
- Perform culture and sensitivity tests.
- Select an empiric therapy considering every infected site.
- Assess host factors.
- Assess drug factors.
- Monitor therapeutic response.
- Perform clinical assessment.
- Perform laboratory tests.
- Assess for therapeutic failure.

Initial selection of antimicrobial therapy is typically empiric, meaning before the causative pathogen has been identified. Infections are usually acute cases, and delaying treatment can result in serious morbidity or possibly death. Patient-specific factors such as allergy history, age, pregnancy, renal function, liver function, type of infection, infection site, and the cost of medication must be considered when deciding which antimicrobial agent to use. The classic signs and symptoms of infection include fever, elevated WBCs, and pain; however, they may not always be present. Older adults, for example, may experience altered mental status with a urinary tract infection (UTI), so clinicians must always look past the expected and seemingly obvious symptoms.

After beginning antimicrobial therapy, the patient must be monitored for a therapeutic response. Tissue and fluid cultures should be obtained for infections such as pneumonia, meningitis, bacteremia, and pyelonephritis. Cultures can take days to weeks for results to become available, depending on the pathogen. Once a pathogen is confirmed, the patient can be switched to narrower-spectrum antimicrobial therapy based on the susceptibility results. If anaerobic bacteria are suspected but not identified, anaerobic therapy should be continued, as commonly used laboratory culture techniques are often unsuccessful in isolating and identifying anaerobic organisms. Patient monitoring should include similar parameters used for diagnosis. The WBC count and temperature should begin to normalize within 24 to 48 hours. Physical complaints from the patient should also begin to diminish (i.e., decreased pain, shortness of breath, cough, or sputum production) and appetite (if reduced) should improve. Resolution of radiologic changes may lag behind the patient's clinical improvement.

Serum (or other fluid) concentrations of antimicrobials may guide efficacy assessments and prevent toxicity. Antimicrobials that require serum concentration monitoring in patient-specific situations include the aminoglycosides, vancomycin, flucytosine, and some azole antifungals. More efficacious outcomes have been associated with therapeutic aminoglycoside concentrations; for example, for a gram-negative infection, therapeutic peak concentrations have been correlated with better clinical outcomes.

Patient education is critical to optimize efficacy, minimize adverse effects, and prevent the development of antibiotic resistance. If the infection worsens, the patient should report this status to the prescriber, who will then determine whether a different therapy is needed. Patients should be instructed to finish the entire medication regimen, even if they are feeling better, to prevent recurrence and/or the development of antibiotic resistance. They should also report any significant effects or possible "new" secondary infections such as yeast infection or severe diarrhea. They should report serious adverse effects and not stop taking the medication unless instructed to do so. Excess medication should be disposed of properly and not shared or saved for later. Clinicians should explain to their patients that antibiotic resistance is an increasing societal problem and educate them on the rationale for using antimicrobials exactly as prescribed. In addition, they should explain why prescribers reserve the use of these medications for patients who have a suspected or documented bacterial infection and do not prescribe them for self-limiting viral infections.

Prescribing practices involving antibiotics have changed significantly with the rise of antibiotic resistance and the emergence of "superbugs." Clinicians have begun to reserve use of antibiotics for cases where bacterial infection is most likely, and to avoid indiscriminate use in a patient with a suspected viral infection. Because antibiotic resistance is a growing public health issue, prescribers should reserve use of these medications for patients with true infections to avoid contributing to this problem. Antimicrobial stewardship programs have been implemented at hospitals and some outpatient settings, with the goals of optimizing treatment of infections and reducing inappropriate use of antibiotics.

2.1 Anthelmintic Agents

Infections with helminths or parasitic worms affect more than 2 billion people worldwide. Worms pathogenic for humans are classified as roundworms (intestinal and tissue nematodes) or as one of two types of flatworms, flukes (trematodes) and tapeworms (cestodes). Worldwide, several types of soil-transmitted helminths infect millions of people in developing countries and can negatively impact the health and well-being of school-aged children. Simultaneous infection with more than one type of helminth is common in tropical, poor, rural areas. In the United States, the most common helminthic infections are caused by intestinal nematodes: *Enterobius vermicularis* (pinworm), *Trichuris trichiura* (whipworm), *Ascaris lumbricoides* (roundworm), *Strongyloides stercoralis* (threadworm), and *Ancylostoma duodenale* and *Necator americanus* (hookworms). Anthelmintics are drugs that treat infections with parasitic worms.

Anthelmintics act either locally within the gut lumen to cause expulsion of worms from the GI tract or systemically against helminths residing outside the GI tract. Broad-spectrum anthelmintics, initially developed for veterinary use, are also used in humans. Unfortunately, treatment for many tissue-dwelling worms, such as filarial parasites, is not completely effective.

Anthelmintics are separated into classes on the basis of their chemical structure and mode of action. Anthelmintic resistance has been widely reported in livestock, and it may be only a matter of time before it emerges in human parasites.

Ascariasis

Ascariasis is caused by *Ascaris lumbricoides*, a giant roundworm that can grow to be 35 cm long. Endemic areas in the United States include the southeastern parts of the Appalachian range, the Gulf Coast states, and areas with poor sanitation. Symptoms of ascariasis include abdominal discomfort, abdominal obstruction, vomiting, and appendicitis; many patients, however, are asymptomatic. During migration of the larvae through the lungs, patients can present with pneumonitis, fever, cough, eosinophilia, and pulmonary infiltrates on chest x-ray.

Diagnosis is made by identifying the characteristic egg in the stool. Because of a very high egg burden, sample concentration techniques are generally not needed to make the diagnosis. Eosinophilia is marked during worm migration but may be absent during intestinal infection. Treatment of ascariasis is one dose of albendazole or pyrantel pamoate (refer to companion drug grid for detailed drug regimens).

Enterobiasis

Enterobiasis is caused by the small, threadlike pinworm, *Enterobius vermicularis*, which is approximately 1 cm long. It is a common helminthic infection and primarily affects children. Infection is manifested by a perianal cutaneous irritation caused by the migrating female worm or presence of eggs, which may result in dermatitis and secondary bacterial infections. Children may be restless and have difficulty sleeping. Appendicitis and intestinal perforation occur rarely.

Pinworm can be diagnosed by perianal swab using adhesive tape that is examined microscopically for eggs. Treatment includes two doses of pyrantel pamoate or albendazole with the second dose administered 2 weeks later. Following treatment, all bedding, underclothes, bathroom rungs, and toilet accessories should be sterilized by steaming or washing in the hot-water cycle of a regular washing machine to eradicate eggs. It is critical for all those in the household and those in close contact with the infected person be evaluated and also treated for infection.

Trichuriasis

Infections caused by *Trichuris trichiura* (whipworm) are typically asymptomatic, but heavy infections may cause gastrointestinal symptoms, malnourishment, and rectal prolapse. Such infections are most common among poor children from resource-poor regions. *Trichuris* worms live in the colon and cecum. Lemon-shaped eggs are easily detected on stool examination. Adult worms, which are typically 3–5 cm long, may be seen on proctoscopy.

The treatment of choice in the United States is albendazole (400 mg daily for 3 doses), which produces cure rates of 70% to 90%. Ivermectin (200 μg/kg daily for 3 doses) may also be used, but has a lower cure rate.

Anthelmintic Agents

Albendazole
Ivermectin
Praziquantel
Pyrantel

Case Studies and Conclusions

A 5-year-old boy presents for care, accompanied by his mother. The child is scratching between his legs and has been unable to sleep for the past 2 days. His perianal area is red and irritated and the prescriber has diagnosed the patient with pinworm (*Enterobius vermicularis*) infection. The mother describes she is experiencing similar symptoms.

1. What is the appropriate intervention for this mother once the pediatrician treats the child?
   a. One-time dose of pyrantel pamoate or albendazole
   b. One-time dose of mebendazole or albendazole
   c. One dose of pyrantel pamoate or albendazole, then a second dose 2 weeks later
   d. One dose of mebendazole or albendazole, then a second dose 2 weeks later

Answer C is correct. One dose of pyrantel pamoate or albendazole is given, then a second dose is administered 2 weeks later. Mebendazole is also an effective treatment but is no longer available in the United States.

The prescriber selects the optimal drug regimen.

2. What common side effect should you warn the mother of?
   a. Confusion
   b. Behavior changes
   c. Abdominal pain
   d. Seizures

Answer C is correct. Patients on pyrantel pamoate commonly develop abdominal pain and nausea (mild adverse effects).

3. What administration recommendation would you make for taking the drug selected?
   a. May take with food or juice
   b. Must take on empty stomach
   c. Must take only at night
   d. Must take every other day

Answer A is correct. May take with food or juice and none of the other factors are required for appropriate medication administration.

4. Should anyone else be treated for pinworm infection?
   a. No one else needs to be treated.
   b. Only household contacts should be treated.
   c. All individuals in close contact with an infected person should be treated.
   d. All individuals with any contact with an infected person should be treated.

Answer C is correct. All individuals in close contact with the infected person should be treated, including family members.

A 23-year-old female has just returned from her visit to Panama City, Florida, after volunteering with a medical mission group for a month. She has abdominal discomfort and she reports that she ate some undercooked pork and also went swimming in dark, dirty (brackish) water. She is concerned she may have contracted an infection involving pork tapeworm (Taenia solium [*Ascaris lumbricoides*]), which is a fear that is confirmed upon diagnosis by her healthcare provider.

1. What is the appropriate treatment for this patient's condition?
   a. Albendazole 400 mg, single dose
   b. Mebendazole 500 mg, daily for 3 days
   c. Pyrantel pamoate 2 g, single dose
   d. Albendazole 400 mg once, then repeat 2 weeks later

Answer A is correct. Albendazole 400 mg as a single dose is the appropriate treatment in the United States.

The prescriber selects the optimal drug regimen.

2. What common side effect would you want to prepare the family to observe for based on your previous answer?
   a. Confusion
   b. Behavior problems
   c. Abdominal pain
   d. Seizures

Answer C is correct. Patients on albendazole commonly develop abdominal pain and nausea (mild adverse effects). More common side effects include elevated liver enzymes and hepatotoxicity, which may also be associated with abdominal pain. Prescribers should monitor LFTS and discontinue therapy if liver enzymes are more than 2 times the upper limit of normal.

3. What administration recommendation would you make for taking the drug selected?
   a. Must take with high fat meal
   b. Must take on empty stomach
   c. Must take only at night
   d. Must take every other day

Answer A is correct. Optimal absorption of albendazole occurs in the presence of a high fat meal.

2.2 Antibacterial Agents

The development of new antibiotics has also evolved to "keep up" with bacterial mutations; thus the different categories of antibiotics described in this section have different mechanisms of action that are responsible for their bactericidal (and sometimes bacteriostatic) effects. As is the case with the cephalosporin antibiotics, the mechanism of action may be similar for drug classes, but progressive "generations" of the antibiotic may be developed to increase potency and/or reduce chances of bacterial resistance through mutation of the organism. Antibiotics are unique in their concentration and in the time of exposure required for bacterial killing. While each antibiotic category has a somewhat unique mechanism of action, generally all of these drugs target critical survival mechanisms of the bacteria (such as altering the cell wall or disrupting protein synthesis), resulting in death of the pathogenic organism. One example of recent resistance includes the ability of some bacteria to produce the enzyme penicillinase, which destroys the chemical structure of certain antibiotics (β-lactam ring). Penicillinase-resistant penicillins are an effective tool in our clinical toolbox; however we are aware of current and evolving resistance to these agents. Penicillinase-resistant penicillins include oxacillin, dicloxacillin, and nafcillin, and are the agents of choice for most staphylococcal disease. However, the recent emergence of methicillin-resistant (MRSA) organisms has reminded the clinical community of the need for heightened efforts to use antibiotics responsibly.

The absorption, distribution, metabolism, and elimination (ADME) of a medication are all critical elements for drug action with the body. One key aspect associated with the ADME process is the amount of drug found in the blood at any given time. Certain medications have a lower safety "tolerance" for large fluctuations of drug in the blood and are termed *narrow therapeutic* agents. Therapeutic drug monitoring is the process of using ADME predictions to estimate a safe range between efficacy and toxicity. It is critical that the ADME of antibacterial agents is accurately predicted to ensure the prescribed drug concentrations remain at therapeutic levels. Therapeutic levels of antibacterial agents are established during clinical trials and are based on specific microbiologic end points—including measurements such as the area under the curve (AUC):minimal inhibitory concentration (MIC) ratio, peak:MIC ratio, and time (T) that the concentration remains greater than MIC (T > MIC).

Aminoglycosides exhibit concentration-dependent bactericidal effects. High-dose, extended-interval aminoglycoside dosing maximizes the peak:MIC ratio through administration of a large dose once daily. Aminoglycosides have a postantibiotic effect (persistent suppression of organism growth after concentrations decrease to less than the MIC), which facilitates the efficacy of this regimen. Fluoroquinolones also exhibit concentration-dependent killing activity. For these antibiotics, the bactericidal effect is characterized by the AUC:MIC ratio. In contrast, beta-lactams (β-lactams) display time-dependent bactericidal effects. Bactericidal activity is most likely when the drug concentration is greater than the MIC (T > MIC) for at least 40% to 50% of the dosing interval. To achieve this effect, the antibiotic is typically administered as a continuous infusion, as a prolonged infusion, or as a series of small, frequent doses.

Many antimicrobials require dosage adjustment in patients with renal dysfunction (if the renal system is a substantial source of elimination) to minimize toxicity, and some may require dosage adjustment in patients with liver dysfunction. Food–drug or drug–drug interactions with certain antibacterial medications (such as occurs with the quinolones and calcium-containing foods or aluminum/magnesium-containing antacids) may decrease absorption of the antibacterial medication. This interaction is usually addressed by separating the administration times or avoiding the combination.

Patients who experience anaphylaxis (i.e., type 1 hypersensitivity reactions) to penicillin should not receive cephalosporins; however, patients with a delayed dermatologic reaction (rash) can generally still receive a cephalosporin without adverse effects. Although the likelihood of cross-reactivity is low, the severe consequences of an anaphylactic reaction outweigh the benefits of using another β-lactam antibiotic. Non-β-lactam options (depending on the targeted pathogen) include aztreonam, quinolones, sulfonamides, and vancomycin.

It is important to evaluate a patient's renal function prior to prescribing any medication; however, it is even more important when prescribing certain antibiotic agents that are renally eliminated. Calculating the creatinine clearance and estimating the glomerular filtration rate will help establish both the dose and frequency of the drug regimen. Additionally, as with any other drug therapy, hepatic function (and the potential for drug interactions) should be assessed and dosing adjusted accordingly if advised to do so by the manufacturer. Combination antibiotic therapy may be indicated where polymicrobial infection exists, such as often seen in intra-abdominal and gynecological infections, in order to prevent antimicrobial resistance and to produce synergistic bactericidal effects.

Aminoglycosides

Amikacin
Gentamicin
Neomycin
Streptomycin
Tobramycin
Paromomycin *(see also the Antiprotozoal Agents section)*

Cephalosporins

First-Generation Cephalosporins

Cefadroxil
Cefazolin
Cephalexin

Second-Generation Cephalosporins

Cefaclor
Cefprozil
Cefuroxime
Cefotetan *(see also the Cephamycins section)*
Cefoxitin *(see also the Cephamycins section)*

Third-Generation Cephalosporins

Cefdinir
Cefditoren
Cefixime
Cefotaxime
Cefpodoxime
Ceftazidime
Ceftazidime and avibactam
Ceftibuten
Ceftolozane and tazobactam
Ceftriaxone

Fourth-Generation Cephalosporins

Cefepime

Fifth-Generation Cephalosporins

Ceftaroline

Miscellaneous Beta Lactams

Carbapenems

Doripenem
Ertapenem
Imipenem and cilastatin sodium
Meropenem

Cephamycins

Cefotetan
Cefoxitin

Monobactams

Aztreonam

Chloramphenicols

Chloramphenicol

Macrolides

Erythromycins

Erythromycin
Erythromycin estolate
Erythromycin ethylsuccinate
Erythromycin lactobionate
Erythromycin stearate

Ketolides

Telithromycin

Other Macrolides

Azithromycin
Clarithromycin
Fidaxomicin

Penicillins

Natural Penicillins

Penicillin G (benzathine, potassium, procaine)
Penicillin V potassium

Aminopenicillins

Amoxicillin
Amoxicillin and clavulanate
Ampicillin
Ampicillin and sulbactam

Penicillinase-Resistant Penicillins

Dicloxacillin
Nafcillin
Oxacillin

Extended-Spectrum Penicillins

Piperacillin and tazobactam

Quinolones

Ciprofloxacin
Finafloxacin
Gemifloxacin
Levofloxacin
Moxifloxacin
Ofloxacin

Sulfonamides

Sulfadiazine
Sulfamthoxazole/Trimethoprim
Sulfasalazine

Tetracyclines

Demeclocycline
Doxycycline
Minocycline
Tetracycline

Glycylcyclines

Tigecycline

Miscellaneous Antibacterial Agents

Bacitracins

Bacitracin

Cyclic Lipopeptides

Daptomycin

Glycopeptides

Dalbavancin
Oritavancin
Telavancin
Vancomycin

Lincomycins

Clindamycin
Lincomycin

Oxazolidinones

Linezolid
Tedizolid

Polymyxins

Colistimethate/colistin
Polymyxin B

Rifamycins

Rifaximin
Rifabutin *(see also the Antimycobacterial Agents section)*
Rifampin *(see also the Antimycobacterial Agents section)*
Rifapentine *(see also the Antimycobacterial Agents section)*

Streptogramins

Quinupristin and dalfopristin

Miscellaneous Urinary Anti-infectives

Fosfomycin
Methenamine
Nitrofurantoin
Trimethoprim

Case Studies and Conclusions

A 56-year-old man diagnosed with a MRSA infection expresses concern that he has never "not finished" an antibiotic and has always followed the instructions.

1. Why is he now experiencing antibiotic resistance?
   a. He shares the societal problem of progressive mutation.
   b. His body must just be "born" to be resistant.
   c. He may grow out of resistance, so keep trying penicillin.
   d. He may never use penicillin again.

Answer A is correct. Antibacterial resistance is on the rise. The mechanism of penicillin resistance is as follows: β-Lactam antibiotics are capable of being inactivated by β-lactamases that are present in large quantities. The β-lactamases are grouped into four classes. Some Class A and D enzymes are inhibited by β-lactamase inhibitors such as clavulanate and tazobactam. Bacterial resistance to the β-lactam antibiotics may also develop by mechanisms other than destruction by β-lactamases.

A 68-year-old woman has contracted an *S. epidermidis* infection that is methicillin sensitive. An infectious diseases consultant recommends the use of a penicillinase-resistant penicillin. The patient wants to know which medications are included in this category so she can determine if they are "covered by her health plan."

1. Which of the following agents do you advise as being the list of potential penicillinase-resistant penicillins?
   a. Amoxicillin
   b. Dicloxacillin
   c. Moxifloxacin
   d. Azithromycin

Answer B is correct. The penicillinase-resistant penicillins (oxacillin, dicloxacillin, and nafcillin) are resistant to hydrolysis by staphylococcal penicillinase. These semisynthetic penicillins are effective against penicillinase-producing strains of *Staphylococcus*.

Your patient inquires further about which types of infections might be resistant to dicloxacillin.

2. Which infection type is resistant to penicillinase-resistant penicillins?
   a. *Candida* infections
   b. MSSA infections
   c. MRSA infections
   d. *C. difficile* infections

Answer C is correct. Vancomycin became the drug of choice for hospital-acquired resistant bacterial strains when penicillins—initially considered the agent of choice—were displaced with the increased incidence of MRSA that demonstrated resistance to penicillinase-resistant penicillins and cephalosporin. Hospital-acquired bacterial strains are also typically resistant to clindamycin, erythromycin, and tetracycline and are now also developing resistance to aminoglycoside antibiotics such as vancomycin.

2.3 Antifungal Agents

Fungal infections are becoming more common. Organ and bone marrow transplantation, cytotoxic chemotherapy, long-term indwelling IV catheters, and the increased use of potent broad-spectrum antibiotic agents have contributed to the increase in fungal infections. Immunocompromised patients are at increased risk for fungal infections.

Systemic fungal infections include histoplasmosis, coccidioidomycosis, cryptococcosis, blastomycosis, paracoccidioidomycosis, and sporotrichosis. Most systemic fungal infections are acquired via inhalation. Fungi are eukaryotes with unique cell walls containing glucans and chitin, and their eradication requires different strategies than those used for treatment of bacterial infections. Antifungals work by inhibiting synthesis of cell wall components, synthesis of nucleic acids, or microtubule/mitotic spindle function. As with most infections, host factors contribute greatly to the clinical outcome for patients with fungal infections. An antifungal agent may provide for cure of an infection despite in vitro resistance because the immune system may eradicate the infection, or the antifungal agent may achieve high concentrations at the infection site, allowing the drug to overcome high MICs.

Resistance can be categorized as clinical or microbiological. Clinical resistance refers to treatment failure because of factors other than microbial resistance; microbial resistance can refer to either primary or secondary resistance, as determined by in vitro susceptibility testing using standardized methodology. Primary (intrinsic) resistance is present prior to drug exposure. Secondary (acquired) resistance develops after exposure to an antifungal agent; it can be reversible in some cases. The clinical consequences of antifungal resistance can take the form of treatment failure and changes in the prevalence of the fungal species causing disease. Antifungal resistance has been reported in *Candida albicans* as well as *C. glabrata*, *C. tropicalis*, and *C. krusei* isolates.

Several antifungal classes are available. Amphotericin B, a polyene, binds to sterols in the fungal cell membrane, leading to alterations in cell permeability and cell death. It is available in four formulations; each has relative advantages and disadvantages. Newer liposomal formulations are associated with less toxicity than the older ones, however, renal toxicity remains one of the most prominent clinical concerns. Imidazoles and triazoles have a similar spectrum of activity and mechanism of action. The azoles are agents that require significant hepatic metabolism and often strongly compete with other drugs using the same pathway through the liver. For this reason, these agents are associated with drug–drug interactions that may limit their use. The echinocandins are used primarily for invasive candidiasis and aspergillosis. Griseofulvin is used for mycotic disease of the skin, hair, and nails due to *Microsporum*, *Trichophyton*, or *Epidermophyton* species. Topical antifungal treatment is useful for superficial infections that are confined to the stratum corneum, squamous mucosa, or cornea. In addition, creams for vaginal use are available to treat vaginal candidiasis.

Allylamines

Terbinafine

Azoles

Efinaconazole
Fluconazole
Isavuconazonium sulfate
Itraconazole
Ketoconazole
Luliconazole
Posaconazole
Voriconazole

Echinocandins

Anidulafungin
Caspofungin
Micafungin

Oxaboroles

Tavaborole

Polyenes

Amphotericin B
Nystatin

Pyrimidines

Flucytosine

Miscellaneous Antifungal Agents

Griseofulvin
Potassium iodide *(see also the Thyroid and Antithyroid Agents section in the Hormones and Synthetic Substitutes chapter)*

Case Studies and Conclusions

A 56-year-old woman is diagnosed with mucormycoses involving the maxillary sinuses. An infectious diseases consultant recommends that she be treated with amphotericin B.

1. Which formulations of amphotericin B are available for her treatment?
    a. C-AMB, L-AMB, ABLC, ABCD
    b. C-AAB, L-AAB, ABBC, AAAD
    c. C-BBA, LBBB, ABBA, ADDA
    d. CAAA, LAAB, ABBL, ADDD

Answer A is correct. Four formulations of amphotericin B are commercially available: conventional amphotericin B (C-AMB), liposomal amphotericin B (L-AMB), amphotericin B lipid complex (ABLC), and amphotericin B colloidal dispersion (ABCD).

The patient requests more information about the amphotericin options available to her.

2. What would you advise her about the major difference in these formulations?
    a. Degree of infusion reaction
    b. Blood concentration achieved
    c. Indications for use
    d. All of these are major differences.

Answer D is correct. C-AMB is insoluble in water, but is formulated for intravenous use by complexing it with a bile salt, deoxycholate. ABCD forms a colloidal solution when dispersed in water and is present in much lower blood concentrations than C-AMB. Infusion reactions of chills and fever are more commonly noted with ABCD than with C-AMB. L-AMB is supplied as a lyophilized powder and achieves blood concentrations equivalent to those for C-AMB. L-AMB is approved for empirical therapy of fever in the neutropenic host not responding to appropriate antibacterial agents, as well as for salvage therapy in patients with aspergillosis and candidiasis. ABLC provides blood concentrations of amphotericin B that are much lower than those achieved with the same dose of C-AMB. ABLC is approved for salvage therapy of deep mycoses. The lipid formulations appear to reduce the risk of nephrotoxicity during therapy. The costs of the lipid formulations of amphotericin B greatly exceed the cost of C-AMB.

The patient requests information on how these medications will "fight her infection."

3. How would you describe the mechanism of action of amphotericin?
    a. Binds to the membranes of fungi, increasing permeability
    b. Decreases permeability of the fungal membrane, causing fungal dehydration
    c. Forms a calcified cell membrane
    d. Triggers preprogrammed cell death

Answer A is correct. Polyene antifungal agents, such as amphotericin B, increase the permeability of the membrane of sensitive fungi, causing an outward leakage of small molecules and death of the organism.

The patient is concerned about side effects of amphotericin B.

4. Which serious, untoward effects should be watched for in this patient?
    a. Hepatic impairment
    b. Renal impairment
    c. Hair loss
    d. Constipation

Answer B is correct. Major untoward effects of amphotericin B are infusion-related reactions such as fever and chills. These are most severe with ABCD, slightly less severe with C-AMB, even less severe with ABLC, and least severe with L-AMB. Nephrotoxicity is a serious side effect reported with the use of amphotericin B that is generally transient and dose dependent, and the incidence is increased with concomitant use of other nephrotoxic drugs. Permanent functional renal impairment is uncommon in adults with normal renal function prior to treatment. Hypochromic, normocytic anemia commonly occurs during treatment with C-AMB.

A 19-year-old woman with coccidioidal meningitis is being treated with fluconazole. Her parents (who have received HIPAA clearance from the patient) and she request information about why fluconazole was chosen instead of amphotericin B.

1. Which of the following statements is the best response?
   a. Fluconazole is the least expensive antifungal drug available.
   b. Fluconazole is the drug of choice for this type of fungal infection.
   c. Fluconazole has less potential to cause stomach irritation.
   d. Fluconazole will not interfere with the patient's oral contraceptive.

Answer B is correct. Fluconazole is the drug of choice for the treatment of coccidioidal meningitis because of its good penetration into cerebrospinal fluid and its much lower morbidity compared to intrathecal amphotericin B.

The patient is a new pharmacy technician and is learning about medication side effects as she works in the pharmacy. She wants to know which major issues and limitations are involved with the use of fluconazole, an azole antifungal.

2. What do you tell her?
   a. There are none; fluconazole is 100% safe to use.
   b. Fluconazole has numerous drug interactions that must be considered.
   c. Fluconazole should not be used in patients older than age 50.
   d. Fluconazole is not covered by most insurance plans and is expensive.

Answer B is correct. Fluconazole competes with other drugs that are metabolized through the liver and for this reason drug–drug interactions limit its use.

2.4 Antimycobacterial Agents

Multiple-drug regimens are prescribed with prolonged duration when treating mycobacterial infections, such as tuberculosis (TB). Because these pathogenic organisms grow slowly, treatment requires a much longer course of therapy compared with most bacterial infections. Combination therapy is needed because of the high rate of intrinsic resistance mutations as well as mutations that develop during treatment.

The incidence of TB (i.e., *Mycobacterium tuberculosis* infection) has been declining in the United States; however, TB remains a leading cause of morbidity and mortality in developing countries. In addition to effective drug regimens, a well-organized infrastructure for diagnosis and treatment of TB, including both therapeutic and control efforts, is needed to ensure successful individual and public health outcomes. Infections with nontuberculous mycobacteria have become more common because of the increased number of immunocompromised hosts and persons with structural lung disease.

Even though a multiple-drug regimen is used, typically 3–6 months of treatment is required to eradicate drug-susceptible TB. Latent TB infection (LTBI) and active TB disease are diagnosed based on the patient's history, physical examination, radiographic imaging, tuberculin skin test (TST), interferon-γ release assays (IGRA), acid-fast staining, and/or mycobacterial cultures. Active TB disease is treated with regimens involving different phases. The initial treatment phase requires 2 months of daily treatment and includes isoniazid, rifampin, pyrazinamide, and ethambutol. Following the initial phase is the continuation phase, which can either be 4 or 7 months, generally using a combination of isoniazid with rifampin, for a total of 6 or 9 months of total treatment. Multiple drug combination treatment has decreased the risk of resistance and has also led to a reduction in total treatment duration. LTBI is treated with isoniazid (optimally given daily or twice weekly for 6–9 months), rifampin (daily for 4 months), or isoniazid plus rifapentine (weekly for 3 months). Directly observed therapy (DOT) is a strategy to ensure adherence to the drug regimen and is an especially critical element to regimens with any frequency less than daily dosing (i.e., once weekly or twice weekly administration). If the clinical status of the patient deteriorates or if there is no significant improvement in his or her condition, the clinician should investigate whether there may be drug resistance or other preventable treatment failures due to non-adherence or pharmacokinetic complications, such as impaired absorption of the drug or otherwise avoidable drug interactions. Because these agents are highly susceptible to drug–drug interactions, any exaggerated side effects or inadequate therapeutic responses when using isoniazid and rifamin should be considered in light of potential drug interactions with other medications the patient is taking concurrently.

Multidrug-resistant TB (MDR-TB) is resistant to both isoniazid and rifampin and the risk of this type of infection is greater in patients presenting from specific geographic areas and in any patient previously treated for TB. Treatment regimens for MDR-TB generally include a susceptible fluoroquinolone and an injectable second-line agent (such as capreomycin or amikacin). Regimens of at least five drugs are recommended for the treatment of MDR-TB. Extensively drug-resistant TB (XDR-TB) is MDR-TB with additional resistance to any fluoroquinolone and at least one of the second-line injectable agents. Treatment of XDR-TB is individualized on the basis of complete phenotypic and, if possible, genotypic antimicrobial susceptibility testing. Treatment of XDR-TB is individualized based on a complete phenotypic and, if possible, genotypic antimicrobial testing, and thus should be managed by clinicians experienced in the use of these agents and this type of infection.

Antituberculosis Agents

Aminosalicylic acid
Bedaquiline
Capreomycin
Cycloserine
Ethambutol
Ethionamide
Isoniazid
Pyrazinamide
Rifabutin
Rifampin
Rifapentine
Amikacin *(see also the Antibacterial Agents section)*
Ciprofloxacin *(see also the Antibacterial Agents section)*
Clarithromycin *(see also the Antibacterial Agents section)*
Levofloxacin *(see also the Antibacterial Agents section)*
Moxifloxacin *(see also the Antibacterial Agents section)*
Streptomycin *(see also the Antibacterial Agents section)*

Miscellaneous Antimycobacterial Agents

Dapsone

Case Studies and Conclusions

A 55-year-old male has returned from traveling to India for 3 months. He returns with a productive cough and chest x-ray indicative of TB.

1. Which medication(s) should be initiated in this patient?
   a. Isoniazid for 9 months
   b. Isoniazid and rifampin for 6 months
   c. Isoniazid, rifampin, and pyrazinamide for 6 months
   d. Isoniazid, rifampin, pyrazinamide, and ethambutol for up to 9 months

Answer D is correct. Regimens for treating TB disease are based on an initial phase lasting 2 months (daily isoniazid, rifampin, pyrazinamide, and ethambutol), followed by a choice of several options for the continuation phase—either 4 or 7 months (typically the combination of isoniazid and rifampin is used for drug-susceptible TB), for a total of 6 or 9 months for treatment. Combination anti-TB therapy is recommended for treatment of TB because resistance quickly develops when these medications are used alone. The probability that resistance will emerge when the regimen includes more than 2 drugs is small. Multidrug therapy has also led to a reduction in the length of therapy to 6–9 months.

TB disease is defined as the condition that results from TB bacteria multiplying in the body (becomes active) and is unable to be stopped by the immune system. Patients with TB disease can spread bacteria to other individuals with prolonged exposure. TB medication adherence is important to prevent treatment failure, TB spread, and resistance. MDR-TB is more difficult and more expensive to treat compared with susceptible strains.

2. Which drug interaction education should this patient be warned about with isoniazid?
    a. Isoniazid is a potent competitor (inhibitor) of drug metabolism and is responsible for many drug interactions.
    b. Isoniazid is not metabolized by the liver and therefore is not subject to drug interactions.
    c. Isoniazid is only a potential drug interaction problem when taken with rifampin.
    d. Isoniazid should never be taken with any other drug because it is dangerous to do so.

Answer A is correct. Isoniazid is a potent inhibitor of specific liver enzymes well known to be responsible for numerous drug interactions. Drugs metabolized by competing liver enzymes will potentially be affected by the patient's use of isoniazid.

A 37-year-old respiratory therapist with no past medical history has a positive (more than 10 mm) tuberculin skin test (TST) and normal chest x-ray. She is employed full time at the university hospital.

1. Which medication therapy, if any, should this patient receive?
    a. Isoniazid for 3 months
    b. Isoniazid for 9 months or rifampin for 4 months
    c. Isoniazid, rifampin, and pyrazinamide for 6 months
    d. No therapy is needed because TST is less than 15 mm.

Answer B is correct. Patients with latent TB infection should receive treatment to prevent the development of active TB disease. Latent TB infection is not associated with symptoms; however, controlling and eliminating TB (active or latent) is essential for controlling and eliminating the disease. Groups who should be given high priority for latent TB infection treatment (not a complete list) include HIV-infected persons, organ transplant recipients, and persons with a positive IGRA result or a TST reaction of 10 mm or more, including residents and employees of high-risk congregate settings (e.g., correctional facilities, nursing homes, homeless shelters, hospitals, and other healthcare facilities). An appropriate treatment intervention for patients with latent TB (positive TST, no symptoms, and normal chest x-ray) is drug therapy with isoniazid for 6–9 months, rifampin for 4 months, or combination isoniazid plus rifapentine for 3 months.

2. What is a potential adverse effect of isoniazid therapy in this otherwise healthy woman with adequate nutrition?
    a. Nephrotoxicity
    b. Cardiac toxicity
    c. Hepatotoxicity
    d. Peripheral neuropathy

Answer C is correct. Isoniazid is converted to acetyl isoniazid, which can be converted to acetyl hydrazine and hepatotoxic metabolites. Rapid acetylators will form diacetyl hydrazine, which is nontoxic; slow acetylators or CYP2E1 induction will lead to more hepatotoxic metabolites. Rifampin, a potent inducer of CYP2E1, potentiates isoniazid hepatotoxicity. Isoniazid also can cause a peripheral neuropathy in patients who are deficient in vitamin B_6 (pyridoxine).

3. Which adverse effect(s) from rifampin use should this patient be warned about?
    a. Orange-tan discoloration of skin, urine, and contact lenses
    b. Peripheral neuritis
    c. Cardiac toxicity
    d. Nephrotoxicity

Answer A is correct. Orange-tan discoloration of the skin, urine, feces, saliva, tears, and contact lenses is possible with rifampin.

2.5 Antiviral Agents

Viruses use host cells to make additional viral particles; therefore, optimal antiviral agents must be able to differenciate between the cell functions of the host and the viral functions of the invader in order to create specificity of drug action to avoid toxicity too significant for clinical use.

Viruses are simple microorganisms made up of double- or single-stranded DNA or RNA enclosed in a protein coat (capsid). Effective antiviral agents inhibit virus-specific replicative events or inhibit virus-directed nucleic acid or protein synthesis. Nonspecific antiviral agents (e.g., interferons) have multiple mechanisms of action that include modulation of the host's immune responses. DNA viruses include poxviruses (smallpox), herpesviruses (chickenpox, shingles, herpes), adenoviruses (conjunctivitis, sore throat), hepadnaviruses (hepatitis B [HBV]), and papillomaviruses (warts). Antiviral agents work best when administered early (when infection is first recognized). As is the case with antibiotics, antiviral agents are also susceptible to mutation and resistance. For example, with some miscellaneous antivirals, such as foscarnet, resistant clinical isolate of herpes viruses have emerged during therapeutic use and may be associated with poor clinical response.

Interferons

Interferons (IFNs) are biological response modifiers with antiviral and immunomodulatory activity. IFN-α (leukocyte interferon) and IFN-β (fibroblast interferon) are released by human cells infected with certain viruses, whereas IFN-γ (immune interferon) is produced by natural killer cells (T-cell lymphocytes) in response to antigen exposure. These cytokines then act on uninfected host tissue cells to induce a state of relative resistance to viral infections. IFNs bind to cell-surface receptors that initiate the induction of certain enzymes, inhibition of cell proliferation, enhancement of immune activities (including increased phagocytosis by macrophages), and augmentation of cytotoxicity by T cells. IFNs are not absorbed orally because of their large amino acid sequence, which is digested by proteolytic enzymes in the digestive tract.

IFN-α is rapidly absorbed after both intramuscular and subcutaneous injection, and frequent injections are needed to maintain adequate serum concentrations. The available products are now chemically modified with polyethylene glycol (PEG) to extend their half-life and allow for once-weekly dosing. In addition, adverse effects are reduced because of the lowered peak concentration. IFN-α is used to treat chronic hepatitis C infections.

IFN-β products have antiviral properties but are used for multiple sclerosis, not infections. IFN-γ1b injection is used for prevention of infections in patients with chronic granulomatous disease in combination with antibacterials and antifungals. In rare cases, IFN-γ is used as salvage therapy for mycobacterial infections.

Topical imiquimod creams do not have inherent antiviral activity alone, but instead induce IFN-α, IFN-β, and IFN-γ plus tumor necrosis factor alpha (TNF-α). Local application of these medications to external genital and perianal warts stimulates an immunomodulatory response that produces cytokines, which have antiviral action and reduce viral load and wart size.

Monoclonal Antibodies

Antibodies (immunoglobulins) are produced by B cells of the immune system. Antibodies neutralize and eliminate the infectious agents and toxins produced by pathogens. They are found in blood, plasma, and extracellular fluids. Antibodies' Y-shaped structures contain two identical variable-region antigen binding sites, with the lower (constant) region being responsible for the initiation of effector functions that lead to the removal and destruction of the pathogen or cells harboring the pathogen. The antigen binding sites on an antibody can bind to and neutralize bacterial toxins and viruses, thereby preventing them from binding to their target cells or receptors and thereby causing toxic effects or spread of the infection.

Antibodies being developed for treatment of diseases in humans are highly purified and are mostly fully human monoclonal antibodies. The term *monoclonal antibody* (mAb) refers to the cell cultures used—that is, a single cell line that produces one specific antibody. Antibodies are specific to a single virus, bacterium, or bacterial subtype. Mutations can render the antibody ineffective; however, the mutation would not affect other similar agents and would not cause resistance to spread. Only one monoclonal antibody, palivizumab, is approved for treatment of infection—that is, for the prevention and treatment of respiratory syncytial virus (RSV) infection in high-risk children.

Antiretroviral Agents

Patients become infected with the human immunodeficiency virus (HIV) through sexual, parenteral, or perinatal routes. Once infected, HIV targets T-helper lymphocytes, macrophages, and monocytes among others. Untreated or advanced infections increase the risk of the patient experiencing opportunistic infections (OIs), which is one of the main causes of morbidity and mortality.

The current goal of antiretroviral therapy (ART) is to achieve maximum and durable suppression of HIV replication or a level of HIV RNA in plasma (viral load) less than the lower limit of quantification. Another, equally important outcome is an increase in CD4 lymphocytes, as their number closely correlates with the risk for developing OIs. Prophylaxis with antiretroviral agents in at-risk persons lowers HIV acquisition risk.

Current treatment guidelines for the initial treatment of HIV infection support the use of no less than three active antiretroviral agents from no fewer than two different therapeutic classes of drugs. The maximum benefit of the HIV regimen can be diminished, or the potentially increased serum concentration of others can lead to exaggerated toxic effects, by the impact of drug–drug interactions. However, there are cases where the use of purposeful interactions can boost the clinical effects of other drugs within the HIV regimen.

The typical HIV regimen consists of two nucleoside/nucleotide analogues plus either a "boosted" protease inhibitor (PI)—utilizing a purposeful drug interaction that results in an increased blood concentration of the PI—a non-nucleoside reverse transcriptase inhibitor, or an integrase strand transfer inhibitor. Suboptimal viral suppression has been identified as a major factor limiting the intended action of antiretroviral drugs to inhibit viral replication. Current treatment recommendations for drug resistant HIV includes prescribing two (preferably three) agents to which the patient's virus is susceptible. To assess susceptibility, use either virtual genotypic or phenotypic resistance testing.

The longer life span conferred by antiretroviral treatment has given rise to other medical issues. Complications associated with older age have become common, some of which are adverse effects from antiretroviral drugs. The management of medical complications, including hepatitis C virus (HCV) coinfection, continues to evolve but is recognized to be a significant cause of morbidity and mortality in these patients.

Adamantanes

Amantadine
Rimantadine

Antiretroviral Agents

HIV Entry and Fusion Inhibitors

Enfuvirtide
Maraviroc

HIV Protease Inhibitors

Atazanavir
Darunavir
Fosamprenavir
Indinavir
Lopinavir and ritonavir
Nelfinavir
Ritonavir
Saquinavir
Tipranavir

HIV Integrase Inhibitors

Dolutegravir
Elvitegravir and cobicistat
Raltegravir

HIV Non-nucleoside Reverse Transcriptase Inhibitors

Delavirdine
Efavirenz
Etravirine
Nevirapine
Rilpivirine

HIV Nucleoside and Nucleotide Reverse Transcriptase Inhibitors

Abacavir
Didanosine
Emtricitabine
Lamivudine
Stavudine
Tenofovir
Zidovudine

Interferons

Interferon alfa
Peginterferon alfa

Neuraminidase Inhibitors

Oseltamivir
Peramivir
Zanamivir

Nucleosides and Nucleotides

Acyclovir
Adefovir
Cidofovir
Entecavir
Famciclovir
Ganciclovir
Ribavirin
Telbivudine
Valacyclovir
Valganciclovir

HCV Antiviral Agents

NS5B Polymerase inhibitors

Dasabuvir
Sofosbuvir

NS3/4A Protease Inhibitors

Grazoprevir
Paritaprevir
Simeprevir

NS5A Replication Complex Inhibitors

Daclatasvir
Elbasvir
Ledipasvir
Ombitasvir

Miscellaneous Antiviral Agents

Foscarnet

Case Studies and Conclusions

A 73-year-old man with no other health issues developed a rash on his back yesterday. He now complains of considerable pain in the area. You suspect varicella zoster virus (VZV) infection (shingles).

1. What is the best treatment option for this patient?
   a. Acyclovir within 7 days of rash presentation
   b. Valacyclovir within 24 hours of rash presentation
   c. Penciclovir within 5 days of rash presentation
   d. Famciclovir within 3 days of rash presentation

Answer B is correct. The two drugs most commonly used for VZV infections are acyclovir and penciclovir, or their prodrugs, valacyclovir and famciclovir, respectively. Both drugs are most effective if started within 24 hours of the rash's appearance.

A 23-year-old man with AIDS has begun to develop blurred vision in his left eye. The diagnosis of cytomegalovirus (CMV) retinitis is made. The patient is started on intravenous foscarnet.

1. Regardless of the initial choice of IV foscarnet, which treatment option is not recommended for the treatment of CMV retinitis?
   a. Ganciclovir
   b. Famciclovir
   c. Fomivirsen
   d. Cidofovir

Answer B is correct. The treatment options for CMV retinitis include foscarnet, ganciclovir, fomivirsen, and cidofovir. Fomivirsen is given by intravitreal injection for patients intolerant of or unresponsive to other therapies.

2. Which of the following statements is true regarding development of resistance to foscarnet?
   a. Resistant clinical isolates of adenoviruses have emerged during therapeutic use of foscarnet and may be associated with poor clinical response.
   b. CMV strains that are resistant to foscarnet have point mutations in the viral DNA polymerase and are associated with 3- to 7-fold reductions in foscarnet activity in vitro.
   c. Herpesviruses that are resistant to foscarnet have point mutations in the viral DNA polymerase and are associated with 3- to 7-fold reductions in foscarnet activity in vitro.
   d. Resistant clinical isolates of noroviruses have emerged during therapeutic use of foscarnet and may be associated with poor clinical response.

Answer C is correct. Poor clinical response has been associated with the therapeutic use of foscarnet and the emergence of resistant clinical specimens. Herpesviruses resistant to foscarnet have point mutations in the viral DNA polymerase and are associated with 3- to 7-fold reductions in foscarnet activity in vitro.

3. This patient should be monitored for which major adverse effects while on foscarnet?
   a. Nephrotoxicity and symptomatic hypocalcemia
   b. Nephrotoxicity and hyponatremia
   c. Hepatoxicity and hyponatremia
   d. Hepatoxicity and symptomatic hypocalcemia

Answer A is correct. Serious kidney-related adverse effects have been associated with foscarnet, including nephrogenic diabetes insipidus, interstitial nephritis, symptomatic hypocalcemia, and acute tubular necrosis. Some of these side effects would be considered dose-limiting toxicities and saline loading may reduce the risk of such nephrotoxicity. Patients using foscarnet may also experience arrhythmias, seizures, and other CNS disturbances while using foscarnet if there are significant changes in serum calcium and phosphate due to the highly ionized nature of foscarnet at physiological pH.

2.6 Antiprotozoal Agents

Antiprotozoal drugs are a class of medications used to treat infections caused by protozoa (single-cell organisms) that can act as parasites. Amebiasis, giardiasis, trichomoniasis, toxoplasmosis, cryptosporidiosis, trypanosomiasis, and leishmaniasis are common protozoal infections seen worldwide. Protozoa multiply rapidly, and effective vaccines against them are not available. Therapy of protozoal infections often requires multiple drugs, but antiprotozoal drugs have severe toxicities that require careful monitoring.

Giardiasis is the most commonly reported protozoal infection in the United States. Trichomoniasis is a sexually transmitted disease that is common in the United States. Treatment of patients with giardiasis or trichomoniasis using either metronidazole or tinidazole is usually successful.

Malaria infection is caused by transmission of tissue parasites (sporozoites) into the bloodstream by infected mosquitos, which can have life stages allowing these organisms to remain in the liver and require antiparasitic drugs to treat this infection.

Giardiasis

The acute presentation of giardiasis is characterized by diarrhea, cramping abdominal pain, bloating, flatulence, malaise, anorexia, nausea, and belching. Chronic presentation includes diarrhea (foul-smelling, copious, light-colored, fatty stools) and weight loss. Periods of diarrhea may alternate with constipation. Steatorrhea, lactose intolerance, and vitamin B_{12} and fat-soluble vitamin deficiencies may also be present. For patients with prolonged diarrhea and malabsorption with a history of recent travel to an endemic area, rapid identification based on ova and parasites examination or an antigen detection test should be performed so as to institute appropriate therapy.

Giardiasis can be prevented with good personal hygiene and avoiding potentially contaminated food and drink. All symptomatic adults and children (older than 8 years) with giardiasis can be treated with metronidazole 250 mg 3 times daily for 5–10 days or tinidazole 2 g once or nitazoxanide 500 mg twice daily for 3 days. Metronidazole cures 80% to 90% of cases and is the agent most commonly used to treat giardiasis. This treatment regimen also prevents the infected person from shedding infection to others which is described as the development of a carrier state. Diarrhea should cease within 2–3 days, although it may take as long as 2 weeks to end. Patients who do not respond to the initial therapy with metronidazole should be switched to a drug from a different class, such as nitazoxanide (500 mg twice daily for 3 days).

Malaria

Malaria is a devastating disease in terms of its burden of human suffering and economics. As many as 500 million new infections and 2 million deaths are reported annually worldwide. Deaths occur in patients because of lack of access to or failure to take chemoprophylaxis, inappropriate chemoprophylaxis, delay in seeking medical care, or misdiagnosis.

Symptoms of malaria vary based on the course of the disease. At their initial presentation, patients may complain of nonspecific fever, chills, rigors, diaphoresis, malaise, vomiting, and lightheadedness. During the erythrocytic phase (when the plasmodia attack erythrocytes), patients may complain of headache, anorexia, malaise, fatigue, and myalgia as well as abdominal pain, diarrhea, chest pain, and arthralgia. Complications such as hypoglycemia, pulmonary edema, and renal failure are associated with increased mortality. Blood smears should be obtained every 12–24 hours for 3 consecutive days. The presence of parasites in the blood 3–5 days after initiation of therapy suggests drug resistance. Recent advances in detecting malaria parasite have included DNA or RNA probes that utilize polymerase chain reaction (PCR) and rapid dipstick tests. The dipstick is reported to have a sensitivity of 88% and a specificity of 97%; however, microscopy is still considered the optimal test.

Chloroquine phosphate 300 mg (base) taken once a week starting 1 or 2 weeks before departing to affected area and continuing for 4 weeks after leaving the area has been the traditionally accepted chemoprophylaxis. When departing an area where *P. vivax* or *P. ovale* is endemic, primaquine phosphate 30 mg (base) daily for 14 days, beginning during the last 2 weeks of chloroquine prophylaxis, should be added to the regimen. When advising potential travelers on prophylaxis for malaria, be aware of the incidence of chloroquine-resistant *P. falciparum* (CRPF) and the countries where in which this variant is prevalent. In these areas, commonly recommended drugs for malaria prophylaxis include mefloquine, atovaquone/proguanil, or doxycycline.

Adults should take 250 mg mefloquine once a week and should start therapy 1 week before departure. They should continue taking mefloquine for the full period of exposure, and should continue taking mefloquine for 4 additional weeks after last exposure. Neuropsychiatric symptoms have been reported, therefore patients should be monitored for these reactions which might include psychosis, anxiety, insomnia, sleep disturbances, and dizziness.

Doxycycline is an alternative option for chemoprophylaxis that avoids the central nervous system side effects. However, it requires daily dosing, can increase sun sensitivity, and should be avoided in children and pregnant women.

Atovaquone/proguanil is generally well tolerated and preferred by many travelers. This regimen is more expensive than most malaria prophylaxis medications, which may be a barrier to its use.

Detailed recommendations for prevention of malaria may be obtained by checking the Centers for Disease Control and Prevention's (CDC) website: www.cdc.gov/travel.

Amebicides

Iodoquinol
Paromomycin
Metronidazole (*see also the Miscellaneous Antiprotozoal Agents section*)

Antimalarial Agents

Artemether and lumefantrine
Atovaquone and proguanil
Chloroquine
Hydroxychloroquine
Mefloquine
Primaquine
Pyrimethamine
Quinine
Quinidine (*see also the Cardiac Agents section in the Cardiovascular Agents chapter*)

Miscellaneous Antiprotozoal Agents

Atovaquone
Metronidazole
Nitazoxanide
Pentamidine
Tinidazole
Dapsone (*see also the Antimycobacterial Agents section*)

Case Studies and Conclusions

A 35-year-old woman presents with a history of diarrhea and abdominal pain for the past 3 days. She recently returned from a whitewater rafting trip. During the trip, she fell out of the boat; although she had a life preserver on, she swallowed considerable amounts of river water. She is diagnosed with giardiasis, and treatment should begin after obtaining appropriate specimens.

1. How is the diagnosis of giardiasis made?
   a. Identification of cysts or trophozoites in feces
   b. Based on history and clinical presentation
   c. Microscopic analysis of blood sample
   d. Identification of cysts in duodenal contents

Answer A is correct. Giardiasis is the most common protozoal infection in the United States and is also prevalent around the world. The clinical consequences of this infection are highly variable with some patients experiencing acute diarrhea, chronic diarrhea, or an asymptomatic carrier state.

2. What is the most appropriate therapy to limit the acute diarrhea, prevent the development of chronic diarrhea, and prevent the development of a "carrier state" in patients with giardiasis?
    a. Nitazoxanide
    b. Pentamidine
    c. Metronidazole
    d. Co-trimoxazole

Answer C is correct. Chemotherapy with a 5-day course of metronidazole or a single dose of tinidazole is usually successful in eradicating giardiasis. Paromomycin has been used to treat pregnant women to avoid any possible mutagenic effects of the other drugs.

A 38-year-old male with no significant past medical history has returned from traveling to Nicaragua. He forgot to take chemoprophylaxis for malaria and now presents with fever, chills, rigors, and diaphoresis.

1. Which therapy should be initiated in this patient?
    a. Chloroquine 600 mg
    b. Quinine 648 mg
    c. Mefloquine 250 mg
    d. Quinidine 300 mg

Answer A is correct. In an uncomplicated attack of malaria (for all plasmodia except CRPF), the recommended regimen is chloroquine 600 mg (base) initially, followed by 300 mg (base) 6 hours later, and then 300 mg (base) daily for 2 days.

Tips from the Field

Worms

1. Diagnosis of tape worms and pinworms is generally made by detection of eggs in stool. Stool should be analyzed for the characteristic eggs, such as for the Ascaris lumbricoides-"round worm." Because of a very high egg burden, sample concentration techniques are generally not needed to make the diagnosis.

2. Patients may assist in diagnosis of pinworms with cellophane tape used to collect the eggs from the perianal area and collected in the morning before bathing or using the toilet. The tape is removed and brought in for examination under a microscope. The sensitivity of the tape test is about 50% for a one-time collection and 90% for three collections.

Other Pearls

1. Remember:
    - Systematic Approach for Selection of Antimicrobials (details provided in this chapter).
    - Refer to guidelines prior to ordering/administering subacute bacterial endocarditis (SBE) prophylaxis to patients as the criteria for use have become more restrictive in order to reduce the overuse and unnecessary use of antibiotics.

2. For most agents that require nebulized inhalation administration (such as tobramycin):
    - The solution for nebulization should not be administered parenterally (i.e., IM, SQ, or IV) as it is intended for inhaled administration only.
    - Do not dilute or mix with other medicines in the nebulizer (unless there are specific manufacturer's directions that offer these administration alternatives).
    - Administer *nebulized solution for inhalation* while the patient is sitting or standing upright and breathing normally through the mouthpiece of the nebulizer.
    - Encourage gradual inhalation over approximately 15 minutes, using a hand-held nebulizer as recommended by the specific product manufacturer. Full treatment dose has been administered when the mouthpiece makes a spitting noise for at least 1 minute and the nebulizer cup is empty.

3. For most agents that require administration of the powder for inhalation:
   - Capsules are for oral inhalation only; do not swallow the capsules.
   - Devices to use for powder inhalation are specific to product used.
   - Clean, store, and/or replace device according to manufacturer recommendations.
   - Encourage patients to keep a back-up device in reserve should the device they are currently using fails. Remind patients that capsules should not be removed from the package until ready to use.
   - Become familiar with stewardship programs and appropriate prescribing (refer to http://www.cdc.gov/getsmart/community/improving-prescribing/outpatient-stewardship.html).
4. For most agents that require reconstitution prior to use:
   - Many of these anti-infective agent injections are supplied as powder that must be reconstituted prior to administration.
   - It is important to read instructions on the specific diluent to use, and how long the product is good for once reconstituted.
   - Keep in mind that refrigerated storage of reconstituted injections often allows a longer beyond use date.
   - Always label and indicate date of reconstitution.

Bibliography

Acosta EP, Flexner C. Antiviral agents (nonretroviral). In: Brunton LL, Chabner BA, Knollmann BC, eds. *Goodman and Gilman's The Pharmacological Basis of Therapeutics*. 12th ed. New York, NY: McGraw-Hill; 2011:1593-1622.

American Geriatrics Society. 2015 updated Beers criteria for potentially inappropriate medication use in older adults. *J Am Geriatr Soc.* 2015;63:2227-2246.

American Thoracic Society, Centers for Disease Control and Prevention, Infectious Diseases Society of America. Treatment of tuberculosis. *MMWR.* 2003;52(No. RR-11):1-88. http://www.cdc.gov/mmwr/pdf/rr/rr5211.pdf. Accessed June 14, 2016.

Anandan JV. Parasitic diseases. In: DiPiro JT, Talbert RL, Yee GC, Matzke GR, Wells BG, Posey LM, eds. *Pharmacotherapy: A Pathophysiologic Approach*. 9th ed. New York, NY: McGraw-Hill; 2014:1835-1848.

Anderson PL, Kakuda TN, Fletcher CV. Human immunodeficiency virus infection. In: DiPiro JT, Talbert RL, Yee GC, Matzke GR, Wells BG, Posey LM, eds. *Pharmacotherapy: A Pathophysiologic Approach*. 9th ed. New York, NY: McGraw-Hill; 2014:2031-2054.

Arguin PM, Tan KR. Infectious diseases related to travel. Malaria. In: Centers for Disease Control and Prevention, ed. *2014 Yellow Book - Traveler's Health*. Atlanta, GA: U.S. Department of Health and Human Services, Public Health Service. 2014. http://wwwnc.cdc.gov/travel/yellowbook/2014/chapter-3-infectious-diseases-related-to-travel/malaria

Baden LR, Dolin R. Antiviral chemotherapy, excluding antiretroviral drugs. In: Kasper DL, Fauci AS, Hauser SL, Longo DL, Jameson JL, Loscalzo J, eds. *Harrison's Principles of Internal Medicine*. 19th ed. New York, NY: McGraw-Hill; 2016.

Bennett JE. Antifungal agents. In: Brunton LL, Chabner BA, Knollmann BC, eds. *Goodman and Gilman's The Pharmacological Basis of Therapeutics*. 12th ed. New York, NY: McGraw-Hill; 2011:1571-1592.

Bergman SJ, Ferguson MC, Santanello C. Interferons as therapeutic agents for infectious diseases. *Infect Dis Clin North Am.* 2011;25(4):819-834. doi: 10.1016/j.idc.2011.07.008.

Carver PL. Invasive fungal infections. In: DiPiro JT, Talbert RL, Yee GC, Matzke GR, Wells BG, Posey LM, eds. *Pharmacotherapy: A Pathophysiologic Approach*. 9th ed. New York, NY: McGraw-Hill; 2014:1931-1962.

Centers for Disease Control and Prevention. Deciding when to treat latent TB infection. http://www.cdc.gov/tb/topic/treatment/decideltbi.htm. Accessed June 14, 2016.

Centers for Disease Control and Prevention. Fact sheet: treatment options for latent tuberculosis infection. August 31, 2016. https://www.cdc.gov/tb/publications/factsheets/treatment/ltbitreatmentoptions.htm. Accessed January 20, 2017.

Centers for Disease Control and Prevention. Treatment for TB disease. http://www.cdc.gov/tb/topic/treatment/tbdisease.htm. Accessed January 20, 2017.

Centers for Disease Control and Prevention. Treatment regimens for latent TB infection (LTBI). April 5, 2016. http://www.cdc.gov/tb/topic/treatment/ltbi.htm. Accessed January 20, 2017.

Dellinger RP, Levy MM, Rhodes A, et al. Surviving sepsis campaign: international guidelines for management of severe sepsis and septic shock: 2012. *Crit Care Med.* 2013;41(2):580-637.

Flexner C. Antiviral agents and treatment of HIV infection. In: Brunton LL, Chabner BA, Knollmann BC, eds. *Goodman and Gilman's The Pharmacological Basis of Therapeutics.* 12th ed. New York, NY: McGraw-Hill; 2011:1623-1664.

Food and Drug Administration. FDA drug safety communication: FDA to review study examining use of oral fluconazole (Diflucan) in pregnancy. http://www.fda.gov/Drugs/DrugSafety/ucm497482.htm. Accessed September 18, 2016.

Gumbo T. Chemotherapy of tuberculosis, *Mycobacterium avium* complex disease, and leprosy. In: Brunton LL, Chabner BA, Knollmann BC, eds. *Goodman and Gilman's The Pharmacological Basis of Therapeutics.* 12th ed. New York, NY: McGraw-Hill; 2011:1549-1570.

Hey A. History and practice: antibodies in infectious diseases. *Microbiol Spectr.* 2015;3(2):AID-0026-2014. doi: 10.1128/microbiolspec.AID-0026-2014

Lee GC, Burgess DS. Antimicrobial regimen selection. In: DiPiro JT, Talbert RL, Yee GC, Matzke GR, Wells BG, Posey LM, eds. *Pharmacotherapy: A Pathophysiologic Approach.* 9th ed. New York, NY: McGraw-Hill; 2014:1661-1674.

McCarthy J, Loukas A, Hoetz PJ. Chemotherapy of helminth infections. In: Brunton LL, Chabner BA, Knollmann BC, eds. *Goodman and Gilman's The Pharmacological Basis of Therapeutics.* 12th ed. New York, NY: McGraw-Hill; 2011:1443-1462.

McEvoy GK, ed. *AHFS: Drug Information.* Bethesda, MD: American Society of Health-System Pharmacists; 2016.

O'Donnell MR, Reddy D, Saukkonen JJ. Antimycobacterial agents. In: Kasper DL, Fauci AS, Hauser SL, Longo DL, Jameson JL, Loscalzo J, eds. *Harrison's Principles of Internal Medicine.* 19th ed. New York, NY: McGraw-Hill; 2016.

PDR. Tobramycin: drug summary. http://www.pdr.net/drug-summary/Tobi-tobramycin-446. Accessed January 20, 2017.

Phillips MA, Stanley SL Jr. Chemotherapy of protozoal infections: amebiasis, giardiasis, trichomoniasis, trypanosomiasis, leishmaniasis, and other protozoal infections. In: Brunton LL, Chabner BA, Knollmann BC, eds. *Goodman and Gilman's The Pharmacological Basis of Therapeutics.* 12th ed. New York, NY: McGraw-Hill; 2011:1419-1442.

Weller PF, Nutman TB. Intestinal nematode infections. In: Kasper DL, Fauci AS, Hauser SL, Longo DL, Jameson JL, Loscalzo J, eds. *Harrison's Principles of Internal Medicine.* 19th ed. New York, NY: McGraw-Hill; 2016.

Symbols

▲	Renal impairment: Dose adjustment is recommended.	(BL)	Beers list criteria (avoid in elderly).
▢	Hepatic impairment: Dose adjustment is recommended.	(PD)	FDA-approved pediatric doses are available.
■	Black box warning exists for this drug.	(GD)	FDA-approved geriatric doses are available.
(QT)	QTc prolongation effects have been reported.		See primary body system.

Anti-infective Agents

Universal prescribing alerts:

- Known serious hypersensitivity to the specific drug or any other component of the product/formulation selected warrants a contraindication for use.
- Adverse reactions associated with the use of some **anti-infective agents** include dizziness, drowsiness, vertigo, or fatigue; these agents may also impair the ability to perform tasks requiring mental alertness. Caution should always be recommended when using any new drug for the first time, when there is a dose change, and for continued use of known offending agents.
- Doses expressed are for usual adult dosage ranges only. "Geriatric doses" are assumed to be the same as adult doses unless otherwise noted with a symbol. Where FDA approved geriatric or pediatric dosing is available, a symbol will guide the reader to additional prescribing references. Refer to real-time prescribing references for these age specific doses.
- Use of anti-infective agents in pregnancy is based on clinical risk versus benefit; safety concerns are not represented in this grid. Refer to the package insert (PI) for more information. Clinicians should continue to provide education about the reproductive risks of any medication and offer risk reduction strategies (which may include contraceptive use) to women of childbearing age and understand that these reproductive risks may also extend to males. Anti-infective agents, as well as a number of other medications, may decrease the effectiveness of oral contraceptives. Where necessary, an alternative means of birth control should be explored.
- Brand names are provided for those agents that are still available on the market. Due to the ever-changing product availability, refer to Food and Drug Administration (FDA) resources to confirm the actual brands available. This drug summary is for educational purposes only. Prescribing decisions should be based on real-time, comprehensive drug databases that are updated on a regular basis.

Anthelmintic Agents

Drug Name	FDA-Approved Indications	Adult Dosage Range	Precautions and Clinical Pearls
Generic Name * Albendazole **Brand Name** Albenza (PD)	Parenchymal neurocysticercosis *Taenia solium* (pork tapeworm) Cystic hydatid disease of the liver, lung, or peritoneum *Echinococcus granulosus* (dog tapeworm)	**Usual oral dose:** Patients weighing less than 60 kg: 15 mg/kg per day in 2 divided doses (max 800 mg per day) Patients weighing 60 kg or more: 800 mg per day in 2 divided doses	• Can cause severe bone marrow suppression, especially in hepatic impairment; discontinue if clinically significant decreases in complete blood count (CBC) occur • May elevate liver function tests (LFTs); discontinue if LFTs rise to more than 2 times the upper limit of normal • Take with high-fat meal for optimal bioavailability • When treating neurocysticercosis, use anticonvulsants and corticosteroids during first week • Monitor: fecal specimens for ova and parasites 3 weeks after treatment, LFTs, CBC with differential, and perform ophthalmic exam if treating neurocysticercosis to determine eye involvement

Drug Name	FDA-Approved Indications	Adult Dosage Range	Precautions and Clinical Pearls
Generic Name Ivermectin **Brand Name** Stromectol Soolantra Sklice	Strongyloidiasis of intestinal tract (*Strongyloides stercoralis* [nematode]) Onchocerciasis (*Onchocerca volvulus* [immature nematode]) Head lice (*Pediculus capitis*) Rosacea	**Usual oral dose for onchocerciasis:** 150 mcg/kg single dose **Usual oral dose for strongyloidiasis:** 200 mcg/kg single dose (alternatively, once daily for 2 days per CDC) **Topical lotion for head lice:** Apply enough to cover dry scalp and hair for single use **Topical cream for rosacea:** Apply to affected area daily	• Systemic exposure can cause cutaneous and systemic reactions, especially in hyper-reactive onchodermatitis • Assess for loiasis if has traveled to West and Central Africa, and pretreat before systemic exposure (serious/fatal encephalopathy has been reported in patients with *Loa loa* infection) • Take oral on empty stomach with water for optimal bioavailability (bioavailability increased 2.5-fold when administered with a high-fat meal) • No activity against adult *Onchocerca volvulus* • Monitor (systemic): skin and eye microfilarial counts, ophthalmologic exams, stool exam post treatment • Leave lotion on for 10 minutes, then rinse out; recommend washing clothing, bedding, and hair accessories
Generic Name Praziquantel **Brand Name** Biltricide	Treatment of all species of *Schistosoma* (blood flukes) *Clonorchis sinensis* (liver fluke) *Opisthorchis viverrini* (liver fluke)	**Usual oral dose for schistosomiasis:** 20 mg/kg per dose 3 times per day separated by 4 to 6 hours for 1 day **Usual oral dose for clonorchiasis/ opisthorchiasis:** 25 mg/kg per dose 3 times per day separated by 4 to 6 hours for 1 day	• Use with caution in patients with cardiac abnormalities • Systemic exposure can increase in patients with moderate to severe hepatic impairment • Not recommended for use if patient has a history of seizures or infection involves the CNS • Swallow tablets quickly with water to avoid potent bitter taste • Caution patients about driving and operating machinery (adverse effects may last for 2 days) • Drug interactions may require dose adjustments • Patients with cerebral cysticercosis should be hospitalized during treatment • May not be effective in migrating schistosomiasis and can potentiate severe reactions caused by a sudden inflammatory immune response • Monitor: LFTs, seizures, patients with cardiac abnormalities, and a feces exam for ova prior to use

Generic Name Pyrantel **Brand Name** Pamix Pin-X Reese's Pinworm Medicine	Pinworms (*Enterobius vermicularis*)	**Usual oral dose:** 11 mg/kg single dose (max 1 g per dose)	• Use with caution in patients with hepatic impairment owing to risk of increased exposure • Alternative agent; not first-line therapy • Treat family members who were in close contact with the patient • Monitor: feces for eggs, worms, and occult blood • Usual oral dose is based on pyrantel base

Antibacterial Agents

Aminoglycosides

Universal prescribing alerts:

- Can cause *C. difficile*–associated diarrhea and pseudomembranous colitis with extended use.

Drug Name	FDA-Approved Indications	Adult Dosage Range	Precautions and Clinical Pearls
Generic Name Amikacin **Brand Name** Amikin (See also Antituberculosis Agents) ▲ ■ (PD)	Treatment of serious gram-negative bacilli bacteria that cause bone infections, respiratory tract infections, endocarditis, and septicemia that is resistant to gentamicin and tobramycin *(for example: Pseudomonas, Proteus, Serratia)*	**Usual parenteral dose:** IM/IV: 5 to 7.5 mg/kg per dose every 8 hours	• Low therapeutic index: individualize dosing • Use with caution if patient has low calcium • Monitor: urinalysis, blood urea nitrogen (BUN), serum creatinine (SCr), peaks and troughs (usually after third dose), vital signs, temperature, weight, input and output (I&O); audiograms at baseline, during, and after treatment if used for an extended period of time Associated with: • Nephrotoxicity; use caution when using with other nephrotoxic agents • Neuromuscular blockade and paralysis; do not give after using anesthesia or a muscle relaxant • Neurotoxicity; ototoxicity can occur with high doses at extended use and is irreversible
Generic Name Gentamicin **Brand Name** Garamycin ▲ ■ (PD)	Treatment of susceptible bacteria that cause bone infections, respiratory tract infections, skin and soft-tissue infections, abdominal and urinary tract infections, septicemia, and endocarditis *(for example: Pseudomonas, Proteus, Serratia, Staphylococcus)*	**Usual parenteral dose:** IM/IV: Conventional: 1 to 2.5 mg/kg per dose every 8 to 12 hours Extended dosing interval: 4 to 7 mg/kg per dose once daily Intrathecal: 4 to 8 mg per day	• May cause neuromuscular blockade and paralysis; do not give after using anesthesia or a muscle relaxant • Low therapeutic index: individualize dosing • Decreased absorption in atrophic muscles • Suitable solutions for administration are clear to slight yellow • Use with caution if patient has low calcium • Monitor: urinalysis, urine output, BUN, SCr, troughs and peaks (usually after third dose); audiograms at baseline, during, and after treatment if using for 2 weeks or more • Inconclusive data show certain penicillins, when administered with gentamicin, may result in loss of efficacy

Drug Name	FDA-Approved Indications	Adult Dosage Range	Precautions and Clinical Pearls
			Associated with: • Nephrotoxicity; use caution when using with other nephrotoxic agents • Neurotoxicity; ototoxicity can occur with high doses at extended use and is irreversible
Generic Name Neomycin **Brand Name** Neo-Fradin ■	Portal-systemic encephalopathy as adjunct Perioperative prophylaxis as adjunct with erythromycin EC	**Usual oral dose for perioperative prophylaxis:** 1 g at 1:00 pm, 2:00 pm, and 11:00 pm on the day before 8:00 am surgery as an adjunct **Usual oral dose for hepatic encephalopathy:** 4 to 12 g daily in divided dose every 4 to 6 hours for 5 to 6 days **Chronic hepatic insufficiency:** 4 g daily	• Doses greater than 12 g per day may cause malabsorption of certain nutrients, fats, and glucose • Do not administer parenterally or as surgical irrigation due to toxicity from increased systemic absorption • Monitor: SCr and BUN at baseline and throughout therapy; audiograms if symptoms develop • Contraindicated in intestinal obstruction, inflammatory or ulcerative bowel disease Associated with: • Nephrotoxicity; use caution when using with other nephrotoxic agents • Neuromuscular blockade and paralysis; do not give after using anesthesia or a muscle relaxant • Neurotoxicity; ototoxicity can occur with high doses at extended use and is irreversible
Generic Name Streptomycin ■ (PD)	Treatment of tuberculosis in combination with other antibiotic agents Treatment of numerous infections involving the following susceptible bacteria: plague *(Yersinia pestis)*, tularemia *(Francisella tularensis), Brucella, K. granulomatis, Haemophilus ducreyi, H. influenza, K. pneumoniae, E. coli, Proteus, E. aerogenes, E. faecalis, S. viridans, E. faecalis*	**Usual parenteral dose:** IM: 15 to 30 mg/kg per day in divided doses or 1 to 2 g daily	• Adjusted doses for renal impairment are suggested, although the manufacturer does not provide specific dosing recommendations; refer to PI • Specific dosing recommendations for patients undergoing intermittent dialysis; refer to PI • Often used as second-line therapy due to the high risk of toxicities • Administer in mid lateral thigh muscle or upper gluteal muscle • Exposure to light can darken the solution without loss of efficacy • Monitor: audiograms at baseline and periodically during treatment; BUN, SCr, troughs and peaks after third dose Associated with: • Nephrotoxicity; use caution when using with other nephrotoxic agents • Neuromuscular blockade and paralysis; do not give after using anesthesia or a muscle relaxant • Neurotoxicity; ototoxicity can occur with high doses at extended use and is irreversible • Parenteral infusions: need appropriate audiometric and laboratory testing facility in place

Generic Name Tobramycin **Brand Name** Tobi Tobi Podhaler Kitabis Pak Bethkis ▲ ■ (PD) (GD)	Treatment of infections by gram-negative bacilli *P. aeruginosa* Cystic fibrosis with *P. aeruginosa* Treatment of susceptible bacteria that cause brucellosis, cholangitis, complicated diverticulitis, meningitis, pelvic inflammatory disease, plague *(Yersinia pestis)*, pneumonia, tularemia, urinary tract infections, ocular infections Prophylaxis against endocarditis	**Usual parenteral dose:** IM/IV: Conventional dosing: 1 to 2.5 mg/kg per dose every 8 to 12 hours Extended interval dosing: 4 to 7 mg/kg per dose daily **Usual nebulized dose for cystic fibrosis:** 300 mg of solution for inhalation nebulized every 12 hours in 28-day cycles **Usual oral inhalation dose for cystic fibrosis:** Powder for inhalation: 112 mg (four 28 mg capsules) every 12 hours in 28-day cycles **Usual ophthalmic dose:** Ointment: ½ inch, 2 to 6 times per day Solution: 1 to 2 drops every 2 to 4 hours	• May cause neuromuscular blockade and paralysis; do not give after using anesthesia or a muscle relaxant • Low therapeutic index: individualize dosing • Specific dosing recommendations for patients undergoing intermittent dialysis; refer to PI • Use caution if patient has low calcium • If patient uses a multiple dose inhaler for cystic fibrosis, use tobramycin last: 15 to 90 minutes after bronchodilator • Exposure of drug to light can darken the solution without loss of efficacy: normal solution for inhalation is clear to pale yellow • Monitor: urinalysis, urine output, BUN, SCr, peaks and troughs after third dose; audiograms at baseline and during treatment if used for extended period of time • Inconclusive data show certain penicillins, when administered with tobramycin, may result in loss of efficacy • Injectable aminoglycoside dosing is highly variable and dependent on several factors Associated with: • Nephrotoxicity; use caution when using with other nephrotoxic agents • Neuromuscular blockade and paralysis; do not give after using anesthesia or a muscle relaxant • Neurotoxicity; ototoxicity can occur with high doses at extended use and is irreversible
Paromomycin	Refer to the Antiprotozoal Agents section.		

Cephalosporins

Universal prescribing alerts:

- Known serious allergic reaction: use with caution if the patient is allergic to penicillin agents due to cross-reaction.
- Cephalosporins have been associated with seizures, especially in patients with renal impairment given unadjusted doses. Dosage reductions are recommended in these patients for certain cephalosporin agents.
- Can cause false-positive urinary glucose if the patient is using cupric sulfate (Benedict's solution, Clinitest, Fehling's solution).

First-Generation Cephalosporins

Drug Name	FDA-Approved Indications	Adult Dosage Range	Precautions and Clinical Pearls
Generic Name Cefadroxil **Brand Name** Duricef ▲ (PD)	Pharyngitis or tonsillitis *Streptococcus pyogenes* Skin and skin structure infections caused by staphylococci or streptococci Urinary tract infection *(for example: E. coli, Proteus mirabilis, Klebsiella)*	**Usual oral dose:** 1 to 2 g daily as single dose or 2 divided doses	• Use with caution in patients with colitis due to increased absorption • Monitor: renal function
Generic Name Cefazolin **Brand Name** Ancef ▲ (PD)	Treatment of susceptible bacteria that cause biliary tract infections, bone and joint infections, endocarditis, genital infections, respiratory tract infections, septicemia, skin and skin structure infections, and urinary tract infections *(for example: E. coli,* streptococci, *P. mirabilis, Klebsiella, S. aureus, H. influenza)* Perioperative prophylaxis	**Usual parenteral dose for treatment of endocarditis:** IM/IV: 1 to 1.5 g ever 6 hours (max of 12 g per day) **Perioperative prophylaxis:** 1 g, 30 to 60 minutes prior to surgery; additional doses are often required postoperatively depending on type of surgery (refer to PI for specific details)	• May increase international normalized ration (INR) • High levels in patients with poor renal function can increase risk for seizures • Reconstitution of powder formulation is required prior to administration • Stability of reconstituted solution vary based on storage location (longer beyond use date when refrigerated; refer to PI • Suitable solutions for administration range in color from light yellow to yellow • Monitor: renal function, LFTs, CBC

Drug Name	FDA-Approved Indications	Adult Dosage Range	Precautions and Clinical Pearls
Generic Name Cephalexin **Brand Name** Keflex ▲ (PD)	Treatment of susceptible gram-positive bacteria that cause respiratory tract infections, otitis media, skin and skin structure infections, bone infections, and genitourinary tract infections Prophylaxis for acute infective endocarditis	**Usual oral dose:** 250 to 1000 mg every 6 hours (max 4 g per day)	• May increase INR • Store suspension in the refrigerator • Monitor: renal, hepatic, and hematologic function with extended use
Second-Generation Cephalosporins			
Universal prescribing alerts: • Can cause *C. difficile*–associated diarrhea and pseudomembranous colitis with extended use. • Some cephalosporins have been associated with seizures, especially in patients with renal impairment given unadjusted doses. Dosage reductions are recommended in these patients for certain cephalosporin agents. • Can cause false-positive urinary glucose if the patient is using cupric sulfate (Benedict's solution, Clinitest, Fehling's solution).			
Drug Name	**FDA-Approved Indications**	**Adult Dosage Range**	**Precautions and Clinical Pearls**
Generic Name Cefaclor **Brand Name** Ceclor (PD)	Treatment of susceptible bacteria that cause exacerbations of chronic bronchitis (ER only), lower respiratory tract infections (capsules and suspension only), otitis media (capsules and suspension only), pharyngitis and tonsillitis, secondary infection of acute bronchitis (ER only), skin and skin structure infections, urinary tract infections (for example: *H. influenza, M. catarrhalis, S. pneumoniae, S. pyogenes, E. coli, P. mirabilis, Klebsiella*, coagulase-negative staphylococci)	**Usual oral dose:** Immediate release (IR): 250 to 500 mg every 8 hours Extended release (ER): 500 mg every 12 hours	• Use with caution in patients with colitis due to increased absorption • Use with caution in patients with poor renal function • Beta-lactamase–negative, ampicillin-resistant (BLNAR) strains of *H. influenza* should be considered resistant to cefaclor • Administer ER tablets with food or within 1 hour of food • Extended release (ER) 500 mg can be ordered 2 times per day as an alternative to immediate release (IR) 250 mg 3 times per day • Monitor: renal function

Drug Name	FDA-Approved Indications	Adult Dosage Range	Precautions and Clinical Pearls
Generic Name Cefprozil **Brand Name** Cefzil ▲ (PD)	Treatment of susceptible bacteria that cause pharyngitis/tonsillitis, otitis media, acute bronchitis secondary infection or exacerbation, skin and skin structure infections *(for example: S. pyogenes, S. pneumoniae, H. influenza, M. catarrhalis, S. aureus)*	**Usual oral dose for uncomplicated skin infections:** 250 to 500 mg every 12 to 24 hours for 10 days	• Use with caution in patients with colitis due to increased absorption • Store reconstituted suspension in a refrigerator • Monitor: renal function
Generic Name Cefuroxime **Brand Name** Ceftin Zinacef ▲ (PD)	Treatment of susceptible bacteria that cause bone and joint infections, lower respiratory infections, septicemia, skin and skin structure infections, urinary tract infections, and early Lyme disease *(for example: S. pneumoniae, H. influenza, Klebsiella, S. aureus, S. pyogenes, E. coli, Enterobacter)* Perioperative prophylaxis	**Usual oral dose for uncomplicated skin infections:** 250 to 500 mg every 12 hours for 10 days **Usual parenteral dose for uncomplicated skin infections:** IM/IV: 750 mg every 8 hours **Perioperative prophylaxis:** IV: 1.5 g 30 to 60 minutes prior to procedure; additional doses are often required postoperatively depending on type of surgery (refer to PI for specific details)	• May increase INR • Use with caution in patients with colitis due to increased absorption • High levels in patients with poor renal function can increase risk for seizures • Swallow tablets whole due to potent bitter taste • Administer suspension with food and store reconstituted suspension in a refrigerator • Tablets and suspension are not bioequivalent and not equal on a milligram-to-milligram basis • Transition patients to oral administration as soon as medically appropriate. • Monitor: renal, hepatic, and hematologic function with extended use; prothrombin time if extended use, poor renal or hepatic function, or malnourished
Cefotetan	Refer to the Cephamycins section.		
Cefoxitin	Refer to the Cephamycins section.		

Third-Generation Cephalosporins

Universal prescribing alerts:

- Can cause *C. difficile*–associated diarrhea and pseudomembranous colitis with extended use.
- Can cause false-positive urinary glucose if patient is using cupric sulfate (Benedict's solution, Clinitest, Fehling's solution).
- Some cephalosporins have been associated with seizures, especially in patients with renal impairment given unadjusted doses. Dosage reductions are recommended in these patients for certain cephalosporin agents.

Drug Name	FDA-Approved Indications	Adult Dosage Range	Precautions and Clinical Pearls
Generic Name Cefdinir **Brand Name** Omnicef ▲ (PD)	Treatment of susceptible bacteria that cause acute otitis media, acute exacerbations of chronic bronchitis, sinusitis, community-acquired pneumonia, pharyngitis/tonsillitis, and skin and skin structure infections *(for example: H. influenza, S. pneumoniae, M. catarrhalis, H. parainfluenzae, S. pyogenes, S. aureus)*	**Usual oral dose for acute sinusitis:** 300 mg twice daily for 5 to 10 days or 600 mg once daily for 10 days	• Use with caution in patients with colitis due to increased absorption • Administer 2 hours before or after antacids or iron supplements • Monitor: renal function • Specific recommendations provided for patients undergoing dialysis
Generic Name Cefditoren **Brand Name** Spectracef ▲	Treatment of susceptible bacteria that cause exacerbation of chronic bronchitis or community-acquired pneumonia, pharyngitis, tonsillitis, and skin and skin structure infections *(for example: H. influenzae, H. parainfluenzae, S. pneumoniae, M. catarrhalis, S. pyogenes, S. aureus)*	**Usual oral dose for community acquired pneumonia:** 400 mg twice daily for 14 days	• Contraindicated if patient is carnitine deficient due to worsening of condition • May increase INR • Use with caution in patients with hepatic impairment; cefditoren has not been studied in patients with severe hepatic disease. No dose adjustment is required with mild hepatic impairment (Child-Pugh Class A or B) per PI • High levels in patients with poor renal function can increase risk for seizures • Administer with food to increase absorption • Monitor: renal function

Drug Name	FDA-Approved Indications	Adult Dosage Range	Precautions and Clinical Pearls
Generic Name Cefixime **Brand Name** Suprax ▲ (PD)	Treatment of susceptible bacteria that cause uncomplicated urinary tract infections (UTI), otitis media, pharyngitis/tonsillitis, acute exacerbations of chronic bronchitis, and uncomplicated cervical/urethral gonorrhea *(for example: E. coli, P. mirabilis, H. influenzae, M. catarrhalis, S. pyogenes, S. pneumoniae, N. gonorrhoeae)*	**Usual oral dose for uncomplicated UTI:** 400 mg daily in divided doses every 12 to 24 hours	• Chewable tablets and suspensions achieve higher peak blood concentrations compared with an equivalent dose of the capsule; otitis media should be treated with the chewable tablet or suspension • No longer considered first-line therapy for uncomplicated gonorrhea in the United States because of resistance; ceftriaxone is preferred • Monitor: renal and hepatic function with prolonged therapy • Specific recommendations for patients undergoing dialysis; refer to PI
Generic Name Cefotaxime **Brand Name** Claforan ▲ (PD)	Treatment of susceptible bacteria that cause bacteremia/septicemia, bone and joint infections; CNS infections, genitourinary infections, gynecologic infections, intra-abdominal infections, lower respiratory tract infections, and skin and skin structure infections *(for example: E. coli, Klebsiella, S. marcescens, S. aureus, Streptococcus, Pseudomonas, P. mirabilis, N. meningitides, H. influenzae, S. pneumoniae, Enterococcus, S. epidermidis, Citrobacter, P. vulgaris, P. stuartii, M. morganii, P. rettgeri, S. marcescens, N. gonorrhoeae, Enterobacter, Bacteroides,* Clostridium, anaerobic cocci, *Fusobacterium, S. pyogenes, H. parainfluenzae)* Surgical prophylaxis for contaminated or potentially contaminated procedure	**Usual parenteral dose for severe infection:** IM/IV: 1 to 2 g every 8 hours	• Infuse bolus slowly; arrhythmias have been reported when infusing the bolus in less than 1 minute • May cause granulocytopenia with extended use greater than 10 days • Use with caution in patients with colitis due to increased absorption • If administering 2 g, divide into 2 doses and give into different IM injection sites • To limit inflammation. change infusion sites when applicable • Monitor: CBC with differential and renal function

Generic Name Cefpodoxime **Brand Name** Vantin ▲ (PD)	Treatment of susceptible bacteria that cause chronic bronchitis exacerbations, gonorrhea, otitis media, pharyngitis/tonsillitis, community-acquired pneumonia, sinusitis, skin and skin structure infections, and uncomplicated urinary tract infections *(for example: S. pneumoniae, H. influenzae, M. catarrhalis, N. gonorrhoeae, S. pyogenes, S. aureus, E. coli, K. pneumoniae, P. mirabilis, S. saprophyticus)*	**Usual oral dose for community acquired pneumonia:** 200 mg every 12 hours for 14 days	• Administer tablets with food to increase bioavailability • Monitor: renal function • Specific recommendations for patients undergoing dialysis; refer to PI
Generic Name Ceftazidime **Brand Name** Fortaz Tazicef ▲ (PD)	Treatment of susceptible bacteria that cause septicemia, bone and joint infections, CNS infections, gynecologic infections, intra-abdominal infections, lower respiratory infections, skin and skin structure infections, and urinary tract infections (complicated and uncomplicated) *(for example: P. aeruginosa, Klebsiella, H. influenzae, E. coli, Serratia, S. pneumoniae, S. aureus, Enterobacter, N. meningitides, Bacteroides, P. mirabilis, Serratia, Citrobacter, S. pyogenes, Proteus)* Empiric treatment in immunocompromised patients	**Usual parenteral dose for uncomplicated lower respiratory tract infections:** IM/IV: 500 mg to 1000 mg every 8 hours	• May increase INR • Neurotoxicity can develop in patients with poor renal function due to increased levels: decrease dose • Use with caution in patients with history of seizures; high levels can increase risk for seizure • With some organisms (such as *Enterobacter* and *Serratia*), resistance can develop during treatment; consider combination therapy or intermittent susceptibility testing for bacteria with inducible resistance • Monitor: renal function • Specific recommendations for patients undergoing dialysis; refer to PI

Drug Name	FDA-Approved Indications	Adult Dosage Range	Precautions and Clinical Pearls
Generic Name Ceftazidime and avibactam **Brand Name** Avycaz ▲	Treatment of susceptible bacteria that cause complicated intra-abdominal infections (when used with metronidazole) and complicated urinary tract infections *(for example: C. freundii, C. koseri, E. aerogenes, E. cloacae, E. coli, K. pneumoniae, Proteus* species, *P. aeruginosa, K. oxytoca, P. mirabilis, P. stuartii)*	**Usual parenteral dose for complicated urinary tract infections:** IV: 2.5 g every 8 hours for 7 to 14 days	• May cause neurotoxicity, such as seizures and encephalopathy: may worsen in renal impairment • Infuse over 2 hours • Suitable solutions for administration range in color from clear to light yellow • Monitor: renal function • Specific recommendations for patients undergoing dialysis; refer to PI
Generic Name Ceftibuten **Brand Name** Cedax ▲ (PD)	Treatment of susceptible bacteria that cause exacerbations of chronic bronchitis, otitis media, and pharyngitis/tonsillitis	**Usual oral dose for otitis media:** 400 mg daily for 10 days	• Use with caution in patients with colitis due to increased absorption • Administer suspension 2 hours before or 1 hour after meals (empty stomach) • Refrigerate suspension • Monitor: renal, hepatic, and hematologic function with extended use • Specific recommendations for patients undergoing dialysis; refer to PI
Generic Name Ceftolozane and tazobactam **Brand Name** Zerbaxa ▲	Treatment of susceptible bacteria that cause complicated intra-abdominal infections (when used with metronidazole) and complicated UTI including pyelonephritis *(for example: B. fragilis, S. anginosus, S constellatus, S. salivarius, E. cloacae, E. coli, K. pneumoniae, P. aeruginosa, K. oxytoca, P. mirabilis)*	**Usual parenteral dose for complicated UTI:** IV: 1.5 g every 8 hours for 7 days	• Administer suspension 2 hours before or 1 hour after meals • Suitable solutions for administration range in color from clear to slight yellow • Monitor: renal function • Specific recommendations for patients undergoing dialysis; refer to PI

Generic Name Ceftriaxone **Brand Name** Rocephin (PD)	Treatment of susceptible bacteria that cause lower respiratory tract infections, otitis media, skin and skin structure infections, bone and joint infections, intra-abdominal infections, urinary tract infections, pelvic inflammatory disease, uncomplicated gonorrhea, septicemia, and meningitis Perioperative prophylaxis	**Usual parenteral dose for skin and skin structure infections:** IM/IV: 1 to 2 g every 12 to 24 hours	• Contraindicated in IV solutions with lidocaine • May increase INR • Rarely causes hemolytic anemia • Use with caution if patient has biliary stasis or sludge; can cause pancreatitis • Use with caution in patients with colitis due to increased absorption • Do not administer concurrently with calcium due to precipitation; flush lines before and after infusion • In patients with renal and hepatic impairment, do not use doses greater than 2 g daily • Monitor: prothrombin time and INR

Fourth-Generation Cephalosporins

Universal prescribing alerts:

- Cephalosporins have been associated with seizures, especially in patients with renal impairment given unadjusted doses. Dosage reductions are recommended in these patients for certain cephalosporin agents.

Drug Name	FDA-Approved Indications	Adult Dosage Range	Precautions and Clinical Pearls
Generic Name Cefepime **Brand Name** Maxipime ▲ (PD)	Treatment of susceptible bacteria that cause intra-abdominal infections, pneumonia, skin and skin structure infections, and complicated and uncomplicated urinary tract infections *(for example: E. coli, viridans group streptococci, P. aeruginosa, K. pneumoniae, Enterobacter, B. fragilis, S. pneumoniae, S. aureus, S pyogenes, P. mirabilis)* Empiric treatment of febrile neutropenia	**Usual parenteral dose for moderate to severe pneumonia:** IV: 1 to 2 g every 12 hours for 10 days	• May increase INR • Neurotoxicity can develop in patients with poor renal function due to increased levels: decrease dose • Use with caution in patients with colitis due to increased absorption • Use with caution in patients with history of seizures; high levels can increase risk for seizure • Decrease dose in elderly patients, who often have impaired renal function; increased risk of encephalopathy, myoclonus, and seizures • The intramuscular (IM) administration is only indicated by the FDA for UTI due to *E. coli* when the IM route is considered a more appropriate route of administration • Monitor: renal function • Specific recommendations for patients undergoing dialysis; refer to PI

Fifth-Generation Cephalosporins

Universal prescribing alerts:

- Can cause *C. difficile*–associated diarrhea and pseudomembranous colitis with extended use.
- Cephalosporins have been associated with seizures, especially in patients with renal impairment given unadjusted doses. Dosage reductions are recommended in these patients for certain cephalosporin agents.

Drug Name	FDA-Approved Indications	Adult Dosage Range	Precautions and Clinical Pearls
Generic Name Ceftaroline **Brand Name** Teflaro ▲	Community-acquired pneumonia *(for example those caused by: S. pneumoniae, S. aureus, H. influenzae, K. pneumoniae, K. oxytoca, E. coli)* Complicated skin and skin structure infections *(for example those caused by: S. aureus* (MSSA and MRSA), *S. pyogenes, S. agalactiae, E. coli, K. pneumoniae, K. oxytoca)*	**Usual parenteral dose for skin and skin structure infections:** IV: 600 mg every 12 hours for 5 to 14 days	• Rarely can cause hemolytic anemia • Administer by slow infusion over 5 to 60 minutes • Suitable solutions for administration range in color from clear to dark yellow • Monitor: renal function and for allergic reaction • Specific recommendations for patients undergoing dialysis; refer to PI

Miscellaneous Beta-Lactams

Carbapenems

Universal prescribing alerts

- Can cause *C. difficile*–associated diarrhea and pseudomembranous colitis with extended use
- Contraindicated if patient has a known serious allergic reaction to carbapenems; use caution if patient is allergic to beta-lactams

Drug Name	FDA-Approved Indications	Adult Dosage Range	Precautions and Clinical Pearls
Generic Name Doripenem **Brand Name** Doribax ▲	Treatment of susceptible bacteria that cause complicated intra-abdominal infections, and complicated urinary tract infections Aerobic gram-positive, aerobic gram-negative *(P. aeruginosa)*, and anaerobic organisms	**Usual parenteral dose for complicated intra-abdominal infections:** IV: 500 mg every 8 hours for 5 to 14 days	• Can cause confusion and seizures in high doses; use with caution in patients with poor renal function and CNS disorders • Monitor: renal function; hematologic function with extended use • Switch to oral therapy when clinical improvement is appropriate for conversion.

Generic Name Ertapenem **Brand Name** Invanz ▲ (GD)	Treatment of susceptible bacteria that cause pelvic infections, community-acquired pneumonia, complicated intra-abdominal infections, complicated skin and skin structure infections, and complicated UTI Colorectal surgery prophylaxis *(for example: S. agalactiae, E, coli, Bacteroides, P. asaccharolytica, Peptostreptococcus, P. bivia, S. pneumoniae, H. influenzae, M. catarrhalis, C. clostridioforme, E. lentim, S. aureus, S pyogenes, K. pneumoniae, P. mirabilis)* Sensitive to beta-lactamase–producing bacteria	**Usual parenteral dose for complicated UTI:** IV: 1 g daily for 10 to 14 days IM administration may be used as an alternative to IV, however only administer IM injection for 7 days **Usual dose for surgical prophylaxis:** IV: 1 g 1 hour before surgery	• Can cause confusion and seizures in high doses; use with caution in patients with poor renal function and CNS disorders • IM is diluted with lidocaine • Can increase risk of breakthrough seizures if used with valproic acid and derivatives: avoid combination use if possible • Monitor: renal, hepatic, and hematologic function with extended use; conduct neurologic assessment before use
Generic Name Imipenem and cilastatin sodium **Brand Name** Primaxin ▲ (PD)	Treatment of susceptible bacteria that cause lower respiratory tract infections, urinary tract infections, intra-abdominal infections, gynecologic infections, bone and joint infections, skin and skin structure infections, endocarditis, polymicrobic infections, and septicemia *(for example: S. aureus, Streptococcus, E. coli, Klebsiella, Enterobacter, P. aeruginosa,* anaerobes*)* Sensitive to beta-lactamase–producing bacteria	**Usual parenteral dose for UTI:** IV: 250 to 500 mg every 6 hours. Duration of treatment is based on severity of the infection	• Can cause confusion and seizures in high doses; use with caution in patients with poor renal function and CNS disorders • Do not administer IV push • If nausea/vomiting develops during administration, lower the infusion rate • May cause glucose monitoring by Clinitest to be inaccurate • Monitor: renal, hepatic, and hematologic function throughout therapy • Specific recommendations for patients undergoing dialysis; refer to PI • Adults with lower body weight require dose adjustments (less than 70 kg)

Drug Name	FDA-Approved Indications	Adult Dosage Range	Precautions and Clinical Pearls
Generic Name Meropenem **Brand Name** Merrem ▲ (PD)	Treatment of infections caused by susceptible bacteria such as: meningitis, complicated skin and skin structure infections, and intra-abdominal infections *(for example: S. pneumoniae, H. influenzae, N. meningitides, S. aureus, S. pyogenes, S. agalactiae, E. faecalis, viridans group streptococci, P. aeruginosa, E. coli, P. mirabilis, B. fragilis, Peptostreptococcus, K. pneumoniae, B. thetaiotaomicron)*	**Usual parenteral dose for complicated skin and skin structure infections:** IV: 500 to 1000mg daily every 8 hours. Duration of treatment is based on severity of infection	• Can cause confusion and seizures in high doses; use with caution in patients with poor renal function and CNS disorders • Outpatients should not operate machinery or drive until it is determined that the patient can tolerate the therapy • Monitor: renal and liver function and CBC during extended use • Specific recommendations for patients undergoing dialysis; refer to PI • Age-specific dose/indications; refer to PI

Cephamycins

Universal prescribing alerts:

- Known serious allergic reaction: contraindicated if patient has had an allergic reaction to a cephalosporin agent; use caution if patient has had an allergic reaction to a penicillin agent due to cross-reaction.
- Can cause *C. difficile*–associated diarrhea and pseudomembranous colitis with extended use.
- Can cause false-positive urinary glucose if patient is using cupric sulfate (Benedict's solution, Clinitest, Fehling's solution).

Drug Name	FDA-Approved Indications	Adult Dosage Range	Precautions and Clinical Pearls
Generic Name Cefotetan **Brand Name** Cefotan ▲	Treats susceptible bacteria that cause respiratory tract infections, skin and skin structure infections, bone and joint infections, UTI and gynecologic infections, septicemia, intra-abdominal infections, and mixed infections Active against gram-negative bacilli: *E. coli, Klebsiella, Proteus;* anaerobes Less active against staphylococci and streptococci Perioperative prophylaxis	**Usual parenteral dose for complicated UTI:** IM/IV: 1 to 2g every 12 hours	• Alcohol use may cause a disulfiram-like reaction • Monitor: renal, hepatic, and hematologic function with extended use; prothrombin time if poor renal/hepatic function, nutritionally deficient, or extended use of treatment; for hemolytic anemia • Specific recommendations for patients undergoing dialysis; refer to PI • Perioperative doses are given 30 to 60 minutes prior to surgery Contraindications: • Previous cephalosporin-associated hemolytic anemia (threefold increased risk compared to other cephalosporins)

Drug Name	FDA-Approved Indications	Adult Dosage Range	Precautions and Clinical Pearls
Generic Name Cefoxitin **Brand Name** Mefoxin ▲ PD	Treatment of susceptible bacteria that cause bone and joint infections, gynecologic infections, intra-abdominal infections, lower respiratory infections, lower respiratory tract infections, septicemia, skin and skin structure infections, and urinary tract infections *(for example: S. aureus, E. coli, N. gonorrhoeae, B. fragilis, Clostridium, P. niger, Peptostreptococcus, S. agalactiae, Klebsiella, S. pneumoniae, H. influenzae, S. epidermidis, S. pyogenes, P. mirabilis, Morganella morganii, P. vulgaris, Providencia)* Perioperative prophylaxis for uncontaminated GI surgery, hysterectomy, and cesarean section	**Usual parenteral dose for lower respiratory infection:** IV/IM: 1 to 2 g every 6 to 8 hours (max 12 g per day)	• Use with caution in patients with colitis due to increased absorption • Powder for solution requires reconstitution prior to use • Cephalosporin agents, including cefoxitin, have been associated with seizures, especially in patients with renal impairment given unadjusted doses • High levels in patients with poor renal function can increase risk for seizures • IV is preferred route since IM is painful • Solution for injection can darken depending on storage conditions with no loss in efficacy • Monitor: renal function and prothrombin time • Specific recommendations for patients undergoing dialysis; refer to PI
Monobactams			
Drug Name	**FDA-Approved Indications**	**Adult Dosage Range**	**Precautions and Clinical Pearls**
Generic Name Aztreonam **Brand Name** Azactam Cayston ▲ PD	Treatment of susceptible gram-negative bacilli bacteria that cause urinary tract infections, lower respiratory tract infections, septicemia, skin and skin structure infections, intra-abdominal infections, and gynecologic infections Inhalation via nebulizer improves respiratory symptoms in cystic fibrosis (CF). *P. aeruginosa*	**Usual parenteral dose for lower respiratory infections:** IM/IV: 1 to 2 g every 8 to 12 hours (max 8 g per day) **Usual nebulized dose for CF:** 75 mg 3 times per day for 28 days	• Rarely can cause toxic epidermal necrolysis (TEN): use with caution in bone marrow transplant patients who have risks for TEN • Suitable solutions for administration range in color from clear to light yellow to pink • Administer a bronchodilator before using the nebulizer to prevent bronchospasm • Special pharmacies distribute Cayston; contact Cayston Access Program • Monitor: liver function periodically • Specific recommendations for patients undergoing dialysis; refer to PI

Chloramphenicols

Universal prescribing alerts:

- Can cause *C. difficile*–associated diarrhea and pseudomembranous colitis with extended use.
- Can cause false-positive urinary glucose if patient is using cupric sulfate (Benedict's solution, Clinitest, Fehling's solution).

Drug Name	FDA-Approved Indications	Adult Dosage Range	Precautions and Clinical Pearls
Generic Name Chloramphenicol **Brand Name** Chloromycetin ■	Treatment of severe infections when other antibiotics are unable to eradicate the bacteria *(for example: Bacteroides, H. influenzae, N. meningitides, Salmonella, Rickettsia)* Active against most vancomycin-resistant enterococci	**Usual parenteral dose for CNS infections:** IV: 50 to 100 mg/kg per day in divided doses every 6 hours	• Drug interactions may require dose adjustment • May cause gray syndrome, which causes circulatory collapse: do not let blood levels reach or exceed 50 mcg/mL; use with caution in patients with poor renal or hepatic function • Use with caution in patients with glucose 6-phosphate dehydrogenase (G6PD) deficiency: greater risk for hemolytic anemia • Can deplete vitamin B in patients: may need to supplement • Use caution in preparing and disposing of infusion • Aplastic anemia may develop weeks or months after use: caution patients on symptoms • Monitor: CBC with differential at baseline and every 2 days during treatment; renal and liver function periodically; chloramphenicol blood levels (greater risk of high levels with poor renal or hepatic function) Contraindicated: • In patients with viral infections or mild or moderate bacterial infections • When used for bacterial prophylaxis and other minor infections due to potential for toxicity Associated with: • Serious and fatal blood dyscrasia events when used on a short-term or long-term basis

Macrolides

Erythromycins

Universal prescribing alerts:

- Can cause *C. difficile*–associated diarrhea and pseudomembranous colitis with extended use.
- Drug interactions may require dose adjustments.

Drug Name	FDA-Approved Indications	Adult Dosage Range	Precautions and Clinical Pearls
Generic Name Erythromycin **Brand Name** Ery-Tab (delayed release)	Treatment of infections caused by susceptible bacteria *(for example: S. pyogenes, S. pneumoniae, S. aureus, M. pneumoniae, L. pneumophila,* diphtheria, pertussis, *Chlamydia, erythrasma, N. gonorrhoeae, E. histolytica,*	**Usual oral dose:** 250 to 500 mg every 6 to 12 hours (max 4 g per day) Delayed release tablet/ capsule	• Rarely can cause QTc prolongation and ventricular arrhythmias: use with caution in patients who already have prolongation, hypokalemia, or hypomagnesemia • Can cause hepatic impairment: use with caution in patients with existing poor hepatic function

PCE Dispertab (delayed release, contains polymer-coated particles) ERYC (delayed release) Ilotycin (ophthalmic) Romycin (ophthalmic) Erygel Akne-Mycin Ery	syphilis, *Campylobacter)* Nongonococcal urethritis Colorectal preoperative prophylaxis in combination with neomycin Conjunctivitis (ophthalmic only) Acne (topical only)	**Ophthalmic:** ½ inch, 2 to 6 times per day on the underlid of the eye **Gel (for acne):** Apply 1 to 2 times daily; response should be seen in 6 to 8 weeks **Ointment, solution, pads (for acne):** Apply 2 times daily	• High doses may cause ototoxicity • Do not administer with milk or acidic beverages • Administer with food if nausea/vomiting develops • May worsen weakness caused by myasthenia gravis • Elderly patients are at increased risk of adverse events • Alcohol may decrease absorption: avoid use • Gel is flammable: do not put near heat source • Monitor: for adverse events
Generic Name Erythromycin estolate **Brand Name** Ilosone QT PD	See Erythromycin	**Usual oral dose:** 250 mg every 6 hours 500 mg every 12 hours	• See Erythromycin • More acid-stable compared to base • Available as capsules, tablets and suspension
Generic Name Erythromycin ethylsuccinate **Brand Name** E.E.S. granules EryPed E.E.S. Liquid E.E.S. Filmtab QT PD	See Erythromycin	**Usual oral dose for moderately severe lower respiratory tract infections:** 400 to 800 mg every 6 to 12 hours (max 4 g erythromycin base per day)	• See Erythromycin • Refrigerate after reconstituting • More acid-stable compared to base • 400mg EES is roughly equal to 250mg base/stearate • Available as a tablet and suspension

Drug Name	FDA-Approved Indications	Adult Dosage Range	Precautions and Clinical Pearls
Generic Name Erythromycin lactobionate QT PD	See Erythromycin	**Usual parenteral dose for lower respiratory tract infections:** IV: 15 to 20 mg/kg per day in divided doses every 6 hours (max 4 g erythromycin base per day)	• See Erythromycin • Administer IV slowly to minimize irritation to the vein
Generic Name Erythromycin stearate **Brand Name** Erythrocin Filmtab QT PD	See Erythromycin	**Usual oral dose for lower respiratory tract infections:** 250 to 500 mg every 6 to 12 hours (max 4 g erythromycin base per day)	• See Erythromycin • More acid-stable than base • Better bioavailability on empty stomach; however, most people take it with food to avoid nausea

Ketolides

Universal prescribing alerts

- Can cause *C. difficile*–associated diarrhea and pseudomembranous colitis with extended use

Drug Name	FDA-Approved Indications	Adult Dosage Range	Precautions and Clinical Pearls
Generic Name Telithromycin **Brand Name** Ketek ▲ ■ QT	Treatment of infections caused by susceptible bacteria that cause community-acquired pneumonia *(for example: S. pneumoniae, H. influenzae, M. catarrhalis, Chlamydophila pneumoniae, M. pneumoniae)*	**Usual oral dose for community acquired pneumonia:** 800 mg once daily for 7 to 10 days	• Rarely can cause QTc prolongation and ventricular arrhythmias: use with caution in patients with existing prolongation, hypokalemia, or hypomagnesemia • Can cause hepatic impairment: use with caution in patients with existing poor hepatic function and discontinue therapy if signs and symptoms of liver damage occur • Can cause syncope, loss of consciousness, and visual disturbances: caution patients about operating machinery and driving until tolerance of the therapy is established • Monitor: hepatic function including liver enzymes and signs and symptoms of liver failure, visual changes • Drug interactions may require dose adjustments Contraindications: • Myasthenia gravis • History of hepatitis with macrolide use • Associated with life-threatening respiratory failure in myasthenia gravis; avoid use in patients with this condition

Other Macrolides

Universal prescribing alerts:

- Drug interactions may require dose adjustments.

Drug Name	FDA-Approved Indications	Adult Dosage Range	Precautions and Clinical Pearls
Generic Name Azithromycin **Brand Name** Zithromax Tri-Pak Zithromax Z-Pak Zmax AzaSite QT PD	Treatment of susceptible bacteria that cause infections such as: otitis media, pharyngitis/tonsillitis, community-acquired pneumonia (CAP), pelvic inflammatory disease, genital ulcer disease in males, exacerbations of chronic obstructive pulmonary disease, sinusitis, uncomplicated skin and skin structure infections, urethritis, and cervicitis *(for example: H. influenzae, M. catarrhalis, S. pneumoniae, Chlamydia pneumoniae, S. pyogenes, M. pneumoniae, C. trachomatis, N. gonorrhoeae, M. hominis, H. ducreyl, S. aureus, S. agalactiae)* Prophylaxis against and treatment of Mycobacterium avium complex in HIV patients Conjunctivitis	**Usual oral dose for CAP:** 500 mg day 1, then 250 mg daily on days 2 through 5 Alternatively may give ER: 2 g once as a single dose Alternatively may give usual parenteral dose for CAP: IV: 500 mg daily for at least 2 days then convert to oral dose to complete 7 to 10 day course ***M. avium* complex disease prophylaxis in HIV patients:** 1200 mg once weekly 600 mg twice weekly 500 to 600 mg daily with ethambutol **Ophthalmic:** 1 drop into affected eye 2 times per day for 2 days, then once daily for 5 days	• Rarely can cause QTc prolongation and ventricular arrhythmias: use with caution in patients with existing prolongation, hypokalemia, or hypomagnesemia • Use with caution in patients with hepatic impairment: can cause cholestatic hepatitis and hepatic dysfunction • Can delay or mask symptoms of gonorrhea or syphilis; assess for these diseases before initiating treatment • Use with caution if GFR less than 10 mL per minute; increased gastrointestinal side effects are possible in such cases • Immediate-release forms are not interchangeable with the extended-release suspension • Administer extended-release suspension on an empty stomach • May cause worsening of existing myasthenia gravis symptoms or create new symptoms • Increased macrolide resistance is occurring in syphilis; macrolides are not recommended for early syphilis • Monitor: hepatic function, CBC with differential; if used for gonorrhea, test for cure 7 days after treatment Contraindications: • Prior azithromycin use was associated with cholestatic jaundice or hepatic dysfunction

Drug Name	FDA-Approved Indications	Adult Dosage Range	Precautions and Clinical Pearls
Generic Name Clarithromycin **Brand Name** Biaxin ▲ QT PD	Treatment of susceptible bacteria that cause infections such as: pharyngitis/tonsillitis, sinusitis, chronic bronchitis, community-acquired pneumonia (CAP), uncomplicated skin and skin structure infections, and duodenal ulcer disease Prophylaxis against and treatment of *Mycobacterium avium* complex in HIV patients *(for example: H. influenzae, S. pneumoniae, M. catarrhalis, M. pneumoniae, Chlamydophila pneumoniae, S. pyogenes, H. parainfluenzae, S. aureus, H. pylori)*	**Usual oral dose for CAP:** 250 every 12 hours for 7 to 14 days Alternatively may give: 1000 mg ER once daily for 7 days	• Rarely can cause QTc prolongation and ventricular arrhythmias: use with caution in patients with existing prolongation, hypokalemia, or hypomagnesemia • Can cause hepatic impairment: use with caution in patients with existing poor hepatic function and discontinue therapy if signs and symptoms of liver damage occur • Can cause TEN, Stevens–Johnson syndrome (SJS), and drug reaction with eosinophilia and systemic symptoms (DRESS): discontinue if patient develops rash or other symptoms • Administer ER formulation with food • ER tablets may appear in stools: consider alternative dosage form • May cause worsening of existing myasthenia gravis symptoms or create new symptoms • Use with caution in patients with coronary artery disease: associated with an increase in cardiovascular mortality • Do not use with ranitidine if patient has a history of porphyria or if CrCl less than 25 mL per minute • Monitor: CBC with differential, BUN, SCr Contraindications: • History of QTc prolongation or ventricular arrhythmias • Prior clarithromycin use was associated with cholestatic jaundice or hepatic dysfunction
Generic Name Fidaxomicin **Brand Name** Dificid	Treatment of *C. difficile*-associated diarrhea (CDAD)	**Usual oral dose for CDAD:** 200 mg 2 times per day for 10 days	• Minimal absorption: not effective against systemic infections
Penicillins			
Natural Penicillins			
Universal prescribing alerts: • Can cause *C. difficile*–associated diarrhea and pseudomembranous colitis with extended use. • May cause false-positive or negative urinary glucose if patient is using Clinitest.			

Drug Name	FDA-Approved Indications	Adult Dosage Range	Precautions and Clinical Pearls
Generic Name Penicillin G **Brand Name** Benzathine Bicillin L-A ■ (PD)	Treatment of susceptible bacteria that cause respiratory tract infections caused by streptococci Treatment of syphilis, yaws, bejel, and pinta Secondary prophylaxis against glomerulonephritis, rheumatic fever, chorea, and rheumatic heart disease	**Usual parenteral dose for upper respiratory tract infections:** IM: 600,000 to 1.2 million units once daily for at least 10 days (duration is based on severity of infection)	• Use with caution in patients with poor renal function • May increase risk of seizures in patients with history of seizure disorder • To reduce the pain of injection, warm the medication to room temperature • Inject in the upper outer quadrant of the gluteal muscle; avoid injecting near an artery or nerve to prevent neurologic damage • Not recommended to treat congenital syphilis and neurosyphilis due to treatment failures • Assess the patient's renal function and identify any history of seizures • Associated with cardiopulmonary arrest and death with IV use (never administer IV) • May be give every 1 to 4 weeks for secondary prevention or latent syphilis • Benzathine recommended for syphyllis
Generic Name Penicillin G **Brand Name** Potassium Pfizerpen-G ▲ (PD)	Treatment of susceptible bacteria that cause infections such as sepsis, pneumonia, pericarditis, endocarditis, meningitis, anthrax, botulism, gas gangrene, and tetanus	**Usual parenteral dose for pneumonia:** IV: 5 to 24 million units per day in divided doses every 4 to 6 hours	• High levels may increase risk of seizures: use with caution in patients with history of seizures • Neurovascular damage may occur if administered via an artery or near peripheral nerves or blood vessels • May increase potassium in serum • 1 million units is approximately equal to 625 mg • Monitor: electrolytes periodically; hepatic, renal, cardiac, and hematologic function if extended use or high doses
Generic Name Penicillin G **Brand Name** Procaine Wycillin (PD)	Treatment of susceptible bacteria that cause infections such as: anthrax, diphtheria, endocarditis, erysipeloid, fusospirochetosis, respiratory tract infections, rat-bite fever, skin and soft-tissue infections, syphilis, yaws, bejel, and pinta Prophylaxis against anthrax Treatment of susceptible streptococci and staphylococci	**Usual parenteral dose for upper respiratory tract infections:** IM: 600,000 to 1.2 million units once daily for at least 10 days (duration is based on severity of infection)	• May cause fibrosis and atrophy with repeated injections in the anterolateral thigh • Transient neuropsychiatric reactions such as confusion and hallucinations have occurred after receiving a large dose; they typically last for 15 to 30 minutes • Use with caution in patients with poor renal function or history of seizures • Neurovascular damage may occur if administered via the intra-arterial, intravascular, or IV route • If the patient has an allergy to procaine, test with 0.1 mL of procaine to determine if there is an allergic reaction; do not use if an allergic reaction occurs • Monitor: injection-site reactions; mental status after injection; renal and hematologic function with extended use

Drug Name	FDA-Approved Indications	Adult Dosage Range	Precautions and Clinical Pearls
Generic Name Penicillin V potassium **Brand Name** Potassium Pen-Vee K Veetids (PD)	Treatment of susceptible bacteria that cause respiratory tract infections, otitis media, sinusitis, and skin and soft-tissue infections Prophylaxis in rheumatic fever Strong activity in streptococcal species	**Usual oral dose for upper tract infections:** 250 to 500 mg every 6 hours	• Use with caution in patients with poor renal function or history of seizures • Administer on an empty stomach to increase absorption • Store reconstituted suspension in the refrigerator • Monitor: renal and hematologic function periodically with extended use • Treatment duration depends on severity of infection

Aminopenicillins

Universal prescribing alerts:

- Can cause *C. difficile*–associated diarrhea and pseudomembranous colitis with extended use.
- Can cause false-positive urinary glucose if patient is using cupric sulfate (Benedict's solution, Clinitest, Fehling's solution).

Drug Name	FDA-Approved Indications	Adult Dosage Range	Precautions and Clinical Pearls
Generic Name Amoxicillin **Brand Name** Moxatag ▲ (PD)	Treatment of susceptible bacteria that cause genitourinary tract infections, *H. pylori* infections, lower respiratory infections, pharyngitis/tonsillitis, otitis media, rhinosinusitis, and skin and skin structure infections *(for example: E. coli, P. mirabilis, E. faecalis, Streptococcus, S. pneumoniae, Staphylococcus, H. influenzae)* ER: *S. pyogenes*	**Usual oral dose for upper respiratory tract infections:** 250 to 500 mg every 8 hours Alternatively may give: 500 to 875 mg twice daily ER: 775 mg once daily	• Administer extended-release tablets within 1 hour after a meal • Monitor: renal, hepatic, and hematologic function with extended use
Generic Name Amoxicillin and clavulanate **Brand Name** Augmentin Amoclan ▲ (PD)	Treatment of susceptible bacteria that cause community-acquired pneumonia (XR only), otitis media, lower respiratory tract, sinusitis, skin and skin structure infections, and urinary tract infections *(for example: H. influenzae,*	**Usual oral dose for acute otitis media:** 500 mg every 8 to 12 hours Alternatively may give: 875 mg every 12 hours For sinusitis and other infections may alternatively give: XR: 2000 mg every 12 hours	• More likely to cause diarrhea than amoxicillin due to the amounts of clavulanic acid used • Can cause hepatic dysfunction (though rare) • Dosed based on the amoxicillin component • Administer XR tablets with food; may administer other formulations with food to decrease stomach upset • Refrigerate suspension after reconstitution

	M. catarrhalis, H. parainfluenzae, K. pneumoniae, S. aureus, S. pneumoniae, E. coli, Klebsiella, Enterobacter) Sensitive to beta-lactamase–producing bacteria		• Different formulations may contain different amounts of clavulanic acid and are not interchangeable • Monitor: renal, hepatic, and hematologic function with extended use • Specific recommendations for patients undergoing dialysis; refer to PI Contraindications: • Prior use caused hepatic dysfunction • XR tablets are contraindicated if CrCl less than 30 mL per minute
Generic Name Ampicillin **Brand Name** Principen ▲ (PD)	Treatment of susceptible bacteria that cause the following infections: Oral: genitourinary tract infections, gastrointestinal tract infections, respiratory tract infections Parenteral (IM, IV): meningitis, gastrointestinal infections, respiratory tract infections, septicemia, endocarditis, urinary tract infections *(for example: E. coli, P. mirabilis,* enterococci, *Shigella, Salmonella, N. gonorrhoeae, H. influenzae,* staphylococci, streptococci, *L. monocytogenes, N. meningitides, S. pneumoniae, S. aureus)*	**Usual oral dose for respiratory tract infections:** 250 to 500 mg every 6 hours **Usual parenteral dose for respiratory tract infections:** IM/IV: 250 to 500 mg every 6 hours	• May cause a rash that is not associated with hypersensitivity reaction; appears 3 to 14 days after first dose • Rapid infusion may cause seizures: infuse slowly • Administer on an empty stomach to increase absorption • Monitor: renal, hepatic, and hematologic function with extended use • Specific recommendations for patients undergoing dialysis Contraindications: • Infection with penicillinase-producing bacteria
Generic Name Ampicillin and sulbactam **Brand Name** Unasyn ▲ (PD)	Treatment of susceptible bacteria that cause skin and skin structure infections, intra-abdominal infections, and gynecologic infections *(for example: S. aureus, H. influenzae, E. coli, Klebsiella, Acinetobacter, Enterobacter,* anaerobes) Sensitive to beta-lactamase–producing bacteria	**Usual parenteral dose for skin and skin structure infections:** IM/IV: 1.5 to 3 g every 6 hours (max 12 g per day)	• May cause hepatic dysfunction: use with caution in patients with hepatic impairment • May cause a rash that is not associated with hypersensitivity reaction; appears 3 to 14 days after first dose • Dose represents the combination of ampicillin and sulbactam • Monitor: renal, hepatic, and hematologic function with extended therapy; if hepatic impairment exists, monitor LFTs periodically Contraindications: • Prior use caused hepatic dysfunction

Penicillinase-Resistant Penicillins

Universal prescribing alerts:

- Can cause *C. difficile*–associated diarrhea and pseudomembranous colitis with extended use.
- Can cause false-positive urinary glucose if patient is using cupric sulfate (Benedict's solution, Clinitest, Fehling's solution).

Drug Name	FDA-Approved Indications	Adult Dosage Range	Precautions and Clinical Pearls
Generic Name Dicloxacillin **Brand Name** Dynapen PD	Treatment of susceptible bacteria that cause pneumonia, skin and soft-tissue infections, and osteomyelitis Sensitive to penicillinase-producing staphylococci	**Usual oral dose:** 125 to 500 mg every 6 hours for 7 to 14 days	• Administer on an empty stomach
Generic Name Nafcillin **Brand Name** Nallpen PD	Treatment of susceptible bacteria that cause osteomyelitis, bacteremia, septicemia, endocarditis, and CNS infections *Staphylococcus*	**Usual parenteral dose for osteomyelitis:** IV: 1 to 2 g every 4 hours Treatment duration based on severity of infection	• Can cause neurotoxic effects: use caution when giving large doses or if patient has renal/hepatic impairment • Administer IM injections deep in the gluteal muscle • IV formulation is a vesicant: avoid extravasation; if extravasation occurs, stop the infusion immediately and give hyaluronidase • Monitor: CBC with differential at baseline and throughout treatment, urinalysis, BUN, SCr, aspartate transaminase (AST), alanine aminotransferase (ALT) • May administer for a longer period of time for more serious infections (6 weeks)
Generic Name Oxacillin **Brand Name** Bactocill PD	Treatment of infections caused by penicillinase-producing staphylococci Not for use if organism is susceptible to penicillin G	**Usual parenteral dose for mild to moderate severity skin infections:** IM/IV: 250 to 500 mg every 4 to 6 hours	• Can cause acute (but reversible) hepatitis 2 to 3 weeks after first dose • Use with caution in patients with poor renal function, although no specific dosage reductions are recommended • May contain a significant amount of sodium: use with caution in elderly patients and patients on salt-restricted diets • Can cause false-positive results for urinary and serum proteins • Monitor: CBC, urinalysis, BUN, renal and liver function

Extended-Spectrum Penicillins

Universal prescribing alerts:

- Can cause *C. difficile*–associated diarrhea and pseudomembranous colitis with extended use.
- Can cause false-positive urinary glucose if patient is using copper reduction (Clinitest).

Drug Name	FDA-Approved Indications	Adult Dosage Range	Precautions and Clinical Pearls
Generic Name Piperacillin and tazobactam **Brand Name** Zosyn ▲ (PD)	Treatment of susceptible bacteria that cause community-acquired pneumonia, intra-abdominal infections, nosocomial pneumonia, pelvic infections, and skin and skin structure infections *(for example: H. influenzae, P. aeruginosa, E. coli, B. fragilis, B. ovatus, B. thetaiotaomicron, B. vulgatus, S. aureus, Acinetobacter baumanii, K. pneumoniae)* Treatment of moderate to severe susceptible infections Sensitive to beta-lactamase–producing bacteria	**Usual parenteral dose for skin and skin structure infections:** IV: 3.375 g every 6 hours Higher dose recommendations for more severe infections (max 18 g per day)	• May cause severe skin reactions such as TEN, SJS, or DRESS; discontinue if rash progresses • Monitor electrolytes, especially if patient has low potassium • Abnormal prothrombin time, platelet aggregation, and clotting times have occurred: use with caution in patients with renal impairment; discontinue if bleeding occurs • Use with caution in patients with cystic fibrosis: increases the risk of fever and rash • Use with caution in patients with renal impairment • May increase risk of seizures: use with caution in patients with preexisting seizure disorders or renal impairment • Specific recommendations for patients undergoing dialysis • Ratio of piperacillin to tazobactam is 8:1 • 1 g contains 2.79 mEq of sodium • Can cause false-positive results with the Platelia *Aspergillus* enzyme immunoassay • Monitor: SCr, BUN, CBC with differential, prothrombin time (PT), partial thromboplastin time (PTT), serum electrolytes, LFTs, urinalysis, signs of bleeding

Quinolones

Universal prescribing alerts:

- Can cause *C. difficile*–associated diarrhea and pseudomembranous colitis with extended use.
- Can cause false-positive results with commercially available immunoassay kits for opioids.
- May cause photosensitivity.
- May cause QTc prolongation: use with caution in patients at high risk for arrhythmias.
- May cause CNS effects such as tremor, restlessness, confusion, hallucinations, seizures, and pseudotumor cerebri: discontinue if severe adverse effects occur.
- Because of the risk for serious and potentially permanent side effects associated with fluoroquinolone antibiotics, it is recommended that these agents be used only when alternative treatment options cannot be used.
- Pediatric dose symbols are not included for these agents. Specific cautions are noted in the PI for anyone under the age of 18. Refer to additional references when treating this population.

Associated with:

- Tendon inflammation or rupture: increased risk with concurrent corticosteroids, organ transplant, and age greater than 60 years.
- Worsening weakness in myasthenia gravis: avoid use in patients with this condition.

Drug Name	FDA-Approved Indications	Adult Dosage Range	Precautions and Clinical Pearls
Generic Name Ciprofloxacin **Brand Name** Cipro Ciloxan Cextraxal ▲ ■ QT	Treatment of susceptible bacteria that cause plague, UTI, uncomplicated cystitis in females, chronic prostatitis, lower respiratory tract infections, sinusitis, skin and skin structure infections, bone and joint infections, complicated intra-abdominal infections, infectious diarrhea, typhoid fever, uncomplicated cervical and urethra gonorrhea, and nosocomial pneumonia To prevent anthrax or prevent progression of disease Empiric treatment of febrile neutropenic patients Ophthalmic: bacterial conjunctivitis and corneal ulcer Otic: otitis externa	**Usual oral dose for complicated UTI:** 250 to 500 mg every 12 hours Alternatively may give: Usual ER dose: 1000 mg once daily Alternatively may give: Usual IV dose: 200 to 400 mg every 12 hours Duration 7 to 14 days depending on severity of UTI infection **Usual ophthalmic dose:** Solution: 1 to 2 drops every 15 minutes to 4 hours **Usual topical dose:** Ointment: apply ½ inch under eye 2 to 3 times per day **Usual otic dose:** Instill contents of "single dose" container twice per day for 7 days	• Rarely causes crystalluria: keep patient well hydrated • May cause serious hypoglycemia: greater risk in diabetes and elderly • Can cause hepatotoxicity: discontinue if signs of hepatitis occur • Rarely can cause peripheral neuropathy: discontinue if symptoms occur • Use with caution in patients with rheumatoid arthritis or seizure disorder • Hemolytic anemia is more likely to occur with G6PD deficiency • Immediate-release and extended-release tablets are not interchangeable • Administer IV via slow infusion over 60 minutes and in a large vein to reduce venous irritation • Administer at least 2 hours before or 6 hours after using antacids, calcium, iron, zinc, and dairy products • Do not administer suspension through feeding tubes to avoid adherence to the tube • Drug interactions may require doses adjustments or avoidance of certain drug combinations • May mask symptoms of syphilis: test patients for syphilis when treating them for gonorrhea • Warm the otic solution to room temperature before use • Monitor: CBC, renal and hepatic function with extended use
Generic Name Finafloxacin **Brand Name** Xtoro	Treatment of susceptible bacteria that cause acute otitis externa *P. aeruginosa*, *S. aureus* (including MRSA)	**Usual otic dose:** 4 drops twice daily for 7 days; may increase dose to 8 drops for first dose with use of otowick	• Before instilling drops into affected ears, warm the bottle by holding it in the hand for 1 to 2 minutes • Shake well before administration

Generic Name Gemifloxacin **Brand Name** Factive ▲ ■ QT	Treatment of susceptible bacteria that cause exacerbation of chronic bronchitis and community-acquired pneumonia Treatment of multidrug-resistant strains of *S. pneumoniae*	**Usual oral dose:** 320 mg once daily	• May cause serious hypoglycemia: greater risk in patients with diabetes and elderly patients • Rarely can cause peripheral neuropathy: discontinue if symptoms occur • Use with caution in patients with rheumatoid arthritis or seizure disorder • Hemolytic anemia is more likely to occur in patients with G6PD deficiency • Administer 3 hours before or 2 hours after using iron, zinc, or magnesium supplements • May cause photosensitivity • Monitor: WBC, renal function • Specific recommendations for patients undergoing dialysis
Generic Name Levofloxacin **Brand Name** Levaquin Quixin (See also Antituberculosis Agents) ▲ ■ QT	Treatment of susceptible bacteria that cause community-acquired pneumonia, nosocomial pneumonia, chronic bronchitis exacerbation, rhinosinusitis, prostatitis, urinary tract infections (complicated and uncomplicated), pyelonephritis, and skin and skin structure infections (complicated and uncomplicated) Reduce progression of anthrax Treatment and prophylaxis of plague Treatment of multidrug-resistant strains of *S. pneumoniae* Ophthalmic: bacterial conjunctivitis	**Usual dose for sinusitis:** Oral/IV: 500 mg every 24 hours for 10 to 14 days Alternatively may give: 750 mg daily for 5 days **Usual ophthalmic dose:** 1 to 2 drops 4 to 8 times per day	• May cause serious hypoglycemia: greater risk in patients with diabetes and elderly patients • Can cause hepatotoxicity: discontinue if signs of hepatitis occur • Rarely can cause peripheral neuropathy: discontinue if symptoms occur • Use with caution in patients with rheumatoid arthritis or seizure disorder • Hemolytic anemia is more likely to occur in patients with G6PD deficiency • Infuse slowly to prevent hypotension • Keep patients well hydrated to prevent crystalluria or cylindruria • Administer oral medication 1 hour before or 2 hours after meals • Administer 2 hours before or after antacids, magnesium, aluminum, iron, and zinc supplements • Monitor: renal, hepatic, and hematopoietic function periodically during therapy; WBC • Specific recommendations for patients undergoing dialysis.

Drug Name	FDA-Approved Indications	Adult Dosage Range	Precautions and Clinical Pearls
Generic Name Moxifloxacin **Brand Name** Avelox Vigamox Moxeza ■ QT	Treatment of susceptible bacteria that cause community-acquired pneumonia, chronic bronchitis exacerbation, sinusitis, complicated and uncomplicated skin and skin structure infections, and complicated intra-abdominal infections Treatment of multidrug-resistant *S. pneumoniae* Prophylaxis and treatment of plague Ophthalmic: conjunctivitis	**Usual dose for sinusitis:** Oral/IV: 400 mg every 24 hours for 10 days **Usual ophthalmic dose:** 1 drop 2 to 3 times per day for 7 days	• May cause serious hypoglycemia: greater risk in patients with diabetes and elderly patients • Can cause hepatotoxicity: discontinue if signs of hepatitis occur • Rarely can cause peripheral neuropathy: discontinue if symptoms occur • Use with caution in patients with rheumatoid arthritis or seizure disorder • Hemolytic anemia is more likely to occur in patients with G6PD deficiency • Administer 4 hours before or 8 hours after antacids, magnesium, aluminum, iron, and zinc supplements • Infusion contains 34.2 mEq of sodium • Monitor: WBC, ECG in patients with cirrhosis of the liver
Generic Name Ofloxacin **Brand Name** Oflox Ocuflox Floxin ▲ ■ ■ QT	Treatment of susceptible bacteria that cause chronic bronchitis exacerbation, community-acquired pneumonia, uncomplicated skin and skin structure infections, gonorrhea, urethritis and cervicitis, mixed infections of the urethra and cervix, pelvic inflammatory disease, uncomplicated cystitis, complicated urinary tract infections, and prostatitis Ophthalmic: conjunctivitis and corneal ulcer Otic: otitis media, chronic otitis media, and otitis externa	**Usual oral dose:** 200 to 400 mg every 12 to 24 hours **Usual ophthalmic dose:** 1 to 2 drops every 2 to 6 hours **Usual otic dose:** 10 drops 1 to 2 times per day	• May cause serious hypoglycemia: greater risk in patients with diabetes and elderly patients • Rarely can cause peripheral neuropathy: discontinue if symptoms occur • Use with caution in patients with hepatic impairment • Use with caution in patients with rheumatoid arthritis or seizure disorder • Drug interactions may require dose adjustment or avoidance of certain drug combinations • Hemolytic anemia is more likely to occur in patients with G6PD deficiency • Do not administer 2 hours before or after food, antacids, zinc, magnesium, and aluminum supplements • Can delay or mask symptoms of syphilis: assess for this infection before initiating treatment for gonorrhea • Warm the otic solution to room temperature before administering it • Monitor: CBC, renal and hepatic function with extended use

Sulfonamides

Universal prescribing alerts

- Can cause *C. difficile*–associated diarrhea and pseudomembranous colitis with extended use

Drug Name	FDA-Approved Indications	Adult Dosage Range	Precautions and Clinical Pearls
Generic Name Sulfadiazine ▲ (PD)	Treatment of susceptible bacteria that cause chancroid, trachoma, inclusion conjunctivitis, nocardiosis, UTI, toxoplasmosis encephalitis, malaria, meningococcal meningitis, otitis medias, and meningitis Prophylaxis against rheumatic fever	**Usual oral dose for UTI:** 2 to 4 g per day divided into 3 to 6 doses	• May cause blood dyscrasias, including fatal agranulocytosis • Drug interactions may require dose adjustment or avoidance of certain drug combinations • Can cause SJS or TEN: discontinue if rash develops • May cause hepatic necrosis: monitor and discontinue if adverse event becomes severe • Use with caution in patients with asthma, hepatic impairment, or renal impairment • Hemolytic anemia is more likely to occur in patients with G6PD deficiency • Administer with 8 ounces of water • Avoid concomitant intake of vitamins or acidic foods due to increased risk of crystalluria • May give leucovorin to prevent adverse effects from folate deficiency • Monitor: CBC, urinalysis, CD4+ count if treating for toxoplasmosis in HIV patients, sulfonamide blood levels if severe infection
Generic Name Sulfamthoxazole/ Trimethoprim **Brand Name** Bactrim Septra Sulfatrim ▲ (PD)	Oral formulations treat susceptible bacteria that cause urinary tract infections, otitis media, chronic bronchitis exacerbations, prophylaxis and treatment of *Pneumocystis* pneumonia (PCP), traveler's diarrhea, and enteritis *(for example: E. coli, Klebsiella, Enterobacter, M. morganii, P. mirabilis, P. vulgaris, H. influenzae, S. pneumoniae, S. flexneri, S. sonnei)* IV treats susceptible bacteria that cause PCP, enteritis, and complicated or severe urinary tract infections	**Usual oral dose:** 1 to 2 double-strength (DS) every 12 to 24 hours **Usual parenteral dose:** IV: 8 to 20 mg/kg per day divided into doses every 6 to 12 hours	• May cause blood dyscrasias, including fatal agranulocytosis and thrombocytopenia • Can cause SJS or TEN: discontinue if rash develops • May cause hepatic necrosis, hyperkalemia, hypoglycemia, hyponatremia: monitor and discontinue if adverse event becomes severe • Use with caution in patients with asthma, thyroid dysfunction, folate deficiency, porphyria, and slow acetylators • Do not use with leucovorin when treating PCP in HIV patients: increases risk of failure and death • Hemolytic anemia is more likely to occur in patients with G6PD deficiency • Dosing is based on the trimethoprim component • Double-strength: sulfamethoxazole 800 mg and trimethoprim 160 mg • Administer oral formulations with 8 ounces of water • Some dosage forms contain propylene glycol; large amounts are toxic • Monitor: CBC, potassium blood level, SCr, BUN • May cause sun sensitivity Contraindications: • Megaloblastic anemia caused by folate deficiency • Severe hepatic or renal impairment

Drug Name	FDA-Approved Indications	Adult Dosage Range	Precautions and Clinical Pearls
Generic Name Sulfasalazine **Brand Name** Azulfidine Sulfazine (PD)	Treatment of susceptible bacteria that cause juvenile rheumatoid arthritis (EC), rheumatoid arthritis (EC), and ulcerative colitis (IR and EC)	**Usual oral dose for ulcerative colitis:** Uncoated tablets: 1 g every 6 to 8 hours Enteric coated tablets: 3 to 4 g per day divided doses and given every 8 hours.	• May cause blood dyscrasias, including fatal agranulocytosis • Rarely can cause death from irreversible neuromuscular and CNS changes or from fibrosing alveolitis • Can cause SJS or TEN: discontinue if rash develops • May decrease folate absorption • May cause hepatic necrosis: monitor and discontinue if adverse event becomes severe • Reports of serious infections have occurred, including sepsis and pneumonia: monitor CBC with differential and watch for signs and symptoms of infection during and after treatment • Use with caution in patients with asthma, hepatic impairment, or renal impairment, and slow acetylators • Hemolytic anemia is more likely to occur in patients with G6PD deficiency • Administer in evenly divided doses after meals • Keep patients well hydrated to prevent crystalluria • To prevent common gastrointestinal adverse effects, use EC or titrate dose to goal • If EC tablets are found in stool, discontinue and use IR formulation • Monitor: CBC with differential and LFTs at baseline and throughout therapy, urinalysis, renal function tests, stool frequency Contraindications: • Intestinal or urinary obstruction • Porphyria

Tetracyclines

Universal prescribing alerts:

- Can cause *C. difficile*–associated diarrhea and pseudomembranous colitis with extended use.
- Can cause permanently discolored teeth; refer to pediatric medication management guidelines.
- May cause photosensitivity; protect skin from direct sunlight.
- Some agents require administration 2 hours before or 4 hours after antacids, aluminum, and magnesium supplements to maintain absorption; refer to PI.

Drug Name	FDA-Approved Indications	Adult Dosage Range	Precautions and Clinical Pearls
Generic Name Demeclocycline **Brand Name** Declomycin (PD)	Treatment of susceptible bacteria that cause acne, urinary tract infections, and respiratory infections Covers gram-negative and gram-positive organisms	**Usual oral dose:** 150 mg 4 times per day 300 mg twice daily	• Can cause nephrogenic diabetes insipidus: dose dependent • May increase BUN: use with caution in patients with renal impairment • Rarely causes pseudotumor cerebri: resolves when discontinued • Use with caution in patients with hepatic and renal impairment: specific recommendations are not stated, but dose decrease or less frequent dosing interval is advised • Administer 1 hour before or 2 hours after food or milk intake • Administer with fluids to prevent esophageal irritation • Monitor: CBC, renal and hepatic function

Generic Name Doxycycline **Brand Name** Adoxa Vibramycin Acticlate Avidoxy Doryx Monodox Morgidox TargaDOX Oracea Targadox (PD)	Treatment of susceptible bacteria that cause syphilis, gonorrhea, community-acquired pneumonia, anthrax, plague, tularemia, Q fever, intestinal amebiasis, severe acne, and the following organisms: *Rickettsia, Chlamydia, Chlamydophila, Mycoplasma, Listeria, A. israelii, Clostridium, B. recurrentis, U. urealyticum, H. decreyi, V. cholera, C. fetus, Brucella, B. bacilliformis, K. granulomatis* Prophylaxis against malaria Oracea: inflammatory lesions due to rosacea Excels at treating uncommon gram-negative and gram-positive bacteria	**Usual oral dose for lower respiratory tract infections:** 100 to 200 mg per day in 1 to 2 divided doses IV dose is the same	• Rarely can cause hepatotoxicity: discontinue if signs and symptoms occur • May cause hypersensitivity syndromes such as DRESS, angioneurotic edema, and systemic lupus erythematosus exacerbation • May increase BUN: use with caution in patients with renal impairment • Rarely causes pseudotumor cerebri: do not use with isotretinoin; will resolve when discontinued • Can cause hyperpigmentation in various body tissues, including nails and skin • IV and oral formulations are bioequivalent except for Oracea • Oral formulation is preferred; needs to be infused slowly, but prolonged administration can cause thrombophlebitis • Administer oral formulations with 8 ounces of water while sitting up for 30 minutes to decrease esophageal irritation • Administer Oracea on an empty stomach • Can take with food to lessen stomach upset • Drug interactions may require dose adjustment or avoidance of certain drug combinations. • IV formulations with ascorbic acid may cause a false-negative urine glucose when using glucose oxidase tests (Clinistix, Diastix, Tes-Tape) • Monitor: CBC; hepatic and renal function with extended use; test of cure 7 days after treatment for gonorrhea
Generic Name Minocycline **Brand Name** Minocin Solodyn ▲ (PD)	Treatment of susceptible bacteria that cause intestinal amebiasis, acne, actinomycosis, anthrax, cholera, listeriosis, meningitis, ophthalmic infections, relapsing fever, respiratory tract infections, Rocky Mountain spotted fever, typhus fever, Q fever, rickettsialpox, tick fevers, sexually transmitted infections, skin and skin structure infections, urinary tract infections, Vincent infection, yaws, psittacosis, plague, tularemia, brucellosis, and bartonellosis *(for example:*	**Usual dose for lower respiratory tract infections:** IV/oral : 200 mg, then 100 mg every 12 hours	• Can cause autoimmune syndromes such as lupus-like, hepatitis, and vasculitis autoimmune syndromes: discontinue and monitor LFT, antinuclear antibodies (ANA), and CBC • Rarely can cause hepatotoxicity when using for acne: discontinue if signs and symptoms occur • May cause severe skin reactions such as SJS and DRESS: discontinue if rash or other signs and symptoms appear • May increase BUN: use with caution in patients with renal impairment • Rarely causes pseudotumor cerebri: do not use with isotretinoin; will resolve when discontinued • Can cause hyperpigmentation in various body tissues, including nails and skin • Oral formulation is preferred; needs to be infused slowly, but prolonged administration can cause thrombophlebitis • Administer oral formulations with 8 ounces of water while sitting up for 30 minutes to decrease esophageal irritation

Drug Name	FDA-Approved Indications	Adult Dosage Range	Precautions and Clinical Pearls
	Campylobacter fetus, Clostridium, Acinetobacter, E. coli, E. aerogenes, Shigella, N. meningitides, C. trachomatis, H. influenzae, Klebsiella, M. pneumoniae, S. pneumoniae, U. urealyticum, K. granulomatis, Treponema pallidum, S. aureus, Klebsiella) Treatment of asymptomatic carriers of *N. meningitides*		• Can take with food to lessen stomach upset • Caution patients about operating machinery and driving until effects of the medication are known: may cause dizziness • IV formulation contains magnesium: use with caution in patients with renal impairment • Monitor: liver and renal function tests and BUN with extended use; magnesium in patients with renal impairment; if symptoms of an autoimmune disorder occur, ANA and CBC; visual exams, if visual disturbances occur; if treating for syphilis, follow up with a serologic test 3 months after treatment
Generic Name Tetracycline **Brand Name** Sumycin ▲ (PD)	Treats susceptible bacteria that cause acne, chronic bronchitis exacerbations, gonorrhea syphilis, tularemia Gram-positive organisms, gram-negative organisms, *Mycoplasma, Chlamydia, Rickettsia* Treats *H. pylori* when used with additional medications to reduce duodenal ulcer recurrence	**Usual oral dose for upper respiratory tract infections:** 250 to 500 mg 2 to 4 times per day	• Rarely can cause hepatotoxicity: use with caution in patients with renal and hepatic impairment • May increase BUN: use with caution in patients with renal impairment • Drug interactions may require dose adjustment or avoidance of certain drug combinations • Expired medications can cause nephropathy • Rarely causes pseudotumor cerebri: do not use with isotretinoin; will resolve when discontinued • Administer on an empty stomach to increase absorption • Monitor: renal, hepatic, and hematologic function; temperature; WBC

Glycylcyclines

Universal prescribing alerts

- Can cause *C. difficile*–associated diarrhea and pseudomembranous colitis with extended use.

Drug Name	FDA-Approved Indications	Adult Dosage Range	Precautions and Clinical Pearls
Generic Name Tigecycline **Brand Name** Tygacil ■ ■	Treatment of susceptible bacteria that cause community-acquired pneumonia, complicated skin and skin structure infections, and complicated intra-abdominal infections *(for example: S. pneumoniae,*	**Usual parenteral dose for skin and skin structure infections:** 100 mg one-time dose, then 50 mg every 12 hours for 7 to 14 days	• Can cause antianabolic effects (increase in BUN, azotemia, acidosis, hyperphosphatemia) • Hepatotoxic • Can cause pancreatitis • Can cause pseudotumor cerebri • Suitable solutions for administration are yellow-orange in color • Can cause significant nausea/vomiting; may need to premedicate patients with antiemetics

	H. influenzae, L. pneumophila, Citrobacter, Enterobacter, E. coli, Klebsiella, E. faecalis, S. aureus (MSSA/ MRSA), *S. anginosus, Bacteroides, Clostridium, Peptostreptococcus S. agalactiae, S. pyogenes, E. cloacae)*		• Can cause photosensitivity • Monitor: CBC, allergic reactions • Associated with an increase in all-cause mortality (0.6%) compared to other antibiotics • Switch to appropriate oral therapy as soon as medically appropriate.

Miscellaneous Antibacterial Agents

Bacitracins

Drug Name	FDA-Approved Indications	Adult Dosage Range	Precautions and Clinical Pearls
Generic Name Bacitracin **Brand Name** Baciim Ocu-Tracin AK-Tracin Baciguent (PD)	Treatment of susceptible bacteria that cause superficial ocular infections Topical ointment prevents infection in minor cuts, scrapes, and burns: not recommended to use for longer than 1 week	**Usual ophthalmic dose:** Apply 1 to 3 times daily on the lower eyelid **Topical:** Apply 1 to 3 times daily on affected area	• Extended use may lead to overgrowth of nonsusceptible bacteria, such as fungi: treat if new infection develops • Systemic formulation use is indicated only in specific age populations; refer to PI • Ointment: 1 unit = 0.026 mg

Cyclic Lipopeptides

Universal prescribing alerts:

- Can cause *C. difficile*–associated diarrhea and pseudomembranous colitis with extended use.

Drug Name	FDA-Approved Indications	Adult Dosage Range	Precautions and Clinical Pearls
Generic Name Daptomycin **Brand Name** Cubicin ▲	Treatment of susceptible bacteria that cause complicated skin and skin structure infections and bloodstream infections *(for example: S. aureus including MRSA, S. pyogenes, S. agalactiae, S. dysgalactiae subspecies equismilis, E. faecalis)*	**Usual parenteral dose for skin and skin structure infections:** IV: 4 mg/kg once daily for 7 to 14 days Duration of treatment depends on severity of infection. Longer treatment may be warranted in certain cases	• May cause eosinophilic pneumonia, usually 2 to 4 weeks after initiating therapy • May cause myopathy: discontinue if creatine phosphokinase (CPK) 10 times upper normal limit (UNL) or higher or CPK more than 5 times ULN with signs and symptoms • May cause peripheral neuropathy • Do not use with ReadyMED elastomeric infusion pumps due to leaching of an impurity into the solution • May falsely increase both PT and INR • Monitor: CPK weekly or more often if using a statin, compromised renal function, or unexpected rise in CPK levels • Specific recommendations for patients undergoing dialysis

Glycopeptides			
Drug Name	FDA-Approved Indications	Adult Dosage Range	Precautions and Clinical Pearls
Generic Name Dalbavancin **Brand Name** Dalvance ▲	Treatment of susceptible bacteria that cause acute skin and skin structure infections *(for example: S. aureus* including MRSA, *S. pyogenes, S. agalactiae, S. dysgalactiae, S. anginosus* group, *E. faecalis)*	**Usual parenteral dose:** IV: 1500 mg single dose 1000 mg on day 1, then 500 mg 1 week later	• May cause reversible increase in transaminase levels • May cause an infusion reaction resembling red man syndrome (hypotension, flushing, and/or maculopapular rash): slowing the infusion may alleviate symptoms • Suitable solutions for administration range in color from colorless to yellow • Monitor: BUN, renal and liver function, infusion-related reaction symptoms
Generic Name Oritavancin **Brand Name** Orbactiv	Treatment of susceptible bacteria that cause acute skin and skin structure infections *(for example: S. aureus* including MRSA, *S. pyogenes, S. agalactiae, S. dysgalactiae, S. anginosus* group, *E. faecalis)*	**Usual parenteral dose:** IV: 1200 mg single dose	• May cause infusion reactions, which are resolved by slowing or discontinuing the infusion • May cause osteomyelitis • Infuse over 3 hours • Suitable solutions for administration range in color from colorless to pale yellow • Monitor: serum urea nitrogen, renal and liver function Contraindication: • If heparin is used 120 hours after oritavancin dose due to false elevation of activated partial thromboplastin time (aPTT)
Generic Name Telavancin **Brand Name** Vibativ ■ QT	Treatment of susceptible bacteria that cause complicated skin and skin structure infections, hospital-acquired pneumonia (HAP), and ventilator-associated pneumonia (VAP) *S. aureus* (including MRSA), *E. faecalis, S. pyogenes, S. agalactiae, S. anginosus*	**Usual parenteral dose for HAP:** IV: 10 mg/kg every 24 hours for 1 to 3 weeks	• May cause red man syndrome indicated by hypotension, flushing, and/or maculopapular rash: slow or discontinue infusion • May cause QTc prolongation: use with caution in patients with preexisting prolongation or heart conditions • Handle as a hazardous agent • May interfere with coagulation tests: perform levels as close to the next dose as possible (at least 18 hours after previous dose) • Monitor: renal function at baseline, during therapy, and 48 to 72 hours after last dose • Infuse over 60 minutes Associated with nephrotoxicity: • Use with caution in patients with risk factors and monitor renal function throughout therapy and 48 to 72 hours after last dose • Increased all-cause mortality compared to vancomycin when CrCl 50 mL per minute or less when treating for HAP/VAP

Generic Name Vancomycin **Brand Name** Vancocin ▲ (PD)	IV treats infection caused by staphylococci or streptococci, including meningitis, pneumonia, and prophylaxis against endocarditis Oral dosing: *C. difficile*–associated diarrhea and enterocolitis from *S. aureus* (including MRSA)	**Usual parenteral dose for lower respiratory infections:** IV: 15 to 20 mg/kg per dose every 8 to 12 hours Alternatively may give: 500 mg every 6 hours Dose should be based on actual body weight **Usual oral dose:** 500 mg daily in divided doses every 6 hours	• May cause nephrotoxicity: use with caution if patient has risk factors • May cause neurotoxicity • May cause neutropenia: higher risk if use is greater than 1 week and total dose exceeds 25 g • May cause ototoxicity • May cause red man syndrome indicated by hypotension, flushing, and/or maculopapular rash: slow infusion, dilute further, and treat with antihistamines and steroids • Oral vancomycin use in inflammatory bowel disease may cause systemic absorption (IV product may be used orally) • Vancomycin is an irritant: avoid extravasation; if extravasation does occur, stop the infusion as soon as possible and aspirate the solution • Monitor: IV: renal function tests, urinalysis, WBC, troughs if therapy extends for more than 3 days with high-intensity dosing

Lincomycins

Drug Name	FDA-Approved Indications	Adult Dosage Range	Precautions and Clinical Pearls
Generic Name Clindamycin **Brand Name** Cleocin Clindacin Clindagel ClindaMax Clindesse Evoclin ■ (PD)	Treatment of susceptible bacteria that cause bone and joint infections, gynecologic infections, intra-abdominal infections, lower respiratory tract infections, septicemia, and skin and skin structure infections *S. aureus* (including community-acquired MRSA), anaerobes, *S. pneumoniae*, streptococci (not *E. faecalis*), *S. pyogenes* Treatment of serious infections caused by streptococci, pneumococci, and staphylococci Topical agents: acne Vaginal agents: bacterial vaginosis	**Usual oral dose for skin and skin structure infections:** 150 to 450 mg every 6 hours **Usual parenteral dose:** IM/IV: 600 to 2700 mg in 2 to 4 divided doses daily (IV max 4800 mg per day) **Topical:** apply 1 to 2 times daily **Vaginal cream:** insert 1 applicatorful once daily for 1 to 7 days (product specific durations)	• Use with caution in patients with severe allergy to tartrazine; reaction is more likely to occur if patients have allergy to aspirin • May cause severe skin reactions such as TEN: discontinue if severe rash occurs • Use with caution in patients with hepatic impairment: less accumulation occurs if dose is given every 8 hours • Use with caution in patients with atopy • Do not administer undiluted solution as a bolus • Do not administer more than 600 mg in a single IM dose • Administer oral dosage forms with plenty of water to decrease the risk of esophageal ulceration • Do not refrigerate oral solution: will thicken • Not for meningitis: does not penetrate cerebrospinal fluid (CSF) adequately • If bacteria are erythromycin resistant, perform D-zone test to ensure the pathogen is not clindamycin-resistance inducible • Monitor: LFTs in patients with severe hepatic impairment; CBC, renal tests, and LFTs with extended use; signs and symptoms of colitis • Associated with severe colitis that can be fatal: use only if necessary, and use with caution in patients with preexisting gastrointestinal disease • Vaginal creams are generally recommended for installation just prior to bedtime (Clindesse brand is only 1 single dose at any time of the day)

Drug Name	FDA-Approved Indications	Adult Dosage Range	Precautions and Clinical Pearls
Generic Name Lincomycin **Brand Name** Lincocin ▲ ■ (PD)	Treatment of severe bacterial infections caused by susceptible strains of streptococci, pneumococci, and staphylococci For patients who have severe allergy to penicillins	**Usual parenteral dose:** IM: 600 mg every 12 to 24 hours IV: 600 to 1000 mg every 8 to 12 hours (max 8 g IV per day)	• Extended use can cause overgrowth of bacteria or fungi • Use with caution in patients with asthma, gastrointestinal diseases (especially colitis), or poor hepatic or renal function • Do not give IV bolus of undiluted solution • Infuse over 1 hour per gram to avoid cardiopulmonary arrest and hypotension • Not for meningitis: does not penetrate CSF adequately • Monitor: baseline SCr and LFTs; renal tests, LFTs, and CBC with differential with extended use; bowel changes throughout therapy
Oxazolidinones			
Universal prescribing alerts: • Can cause *C. difficile*–associated diarrhea and pseudomembranous colitis with extended use.			
Drug Name	**FDA-Approved Indications**	**Adult Dosage Range**	**Precautions and Clinical Pearls**
Generic Name Linezolid **Brand Name** Zyvox (PD)	Enterococcal vancomycin-resistant infections Pneumonia: Community-acquired (CAP): *S. pneumoniae*, *S. aureus* Hospital-acquired: *S. aureus* (MSSA/MRSA), *S. pneumoniae* Skin and skin structure infections Complicated: *S. aureus* (MSSA/MRSA), *S. pyogenes*, *S. agalactiae* Uncomplicated: *S. aureus*, *S. pyogenes*	**Usual dose for CAP:** Oral/IV: 600 mg every 12 hours for 10 to 14 days Longer treatment durations may be warranted based on severity and extent of infection.	• Can cause lactic acidosis • Myelosuppression may be dependent on length of use • Peripheral and optic neuropathy with extended use • Rarely can cause serotonin syndrome • Monitor for hypoglycemia in patients with diabetes • Use with caution in patients with history of seizures • Do not mix or infuse with other medications; flush line before and after use • Yellow color of the solution can intensify over time • Avoid consumption of large amounts of tyramine-containing foods • Protect tablets, suspensions, and infusions from light • Do not shake the suspension • Monitor: CBC weekly; visual function; hematopoietic/neuropathic adverse events in patients with poor renal function • Specific recommendations for patients undergoing dialysis
Generic Name Tedizolid **Brand Name** Sivextro	Treatment of susceptible bacteria that cause acute skin and skin structure infections (for example: *S. aureus* including MRSA, *S. pyogenes*, *S. agalactiae*, *S. anginosus* group, *E. faecalis*)	**Usual dose:** Oral/IV: 200 mg once daily for 6 days	• Do not use if neutrophil count is less than 1000 cells/mm^3 • Suitable solutions for administration range in color from colorless to pale yellow • Inhibits monoamine oxidase, which can cause drug interactions • Monitor: CBC with differential

Polymyxins

Universal prescribing alerts:

- Can cause *C. difficile*–associated diarrhea and pseudomembranous colitis with extended use.

Drug Name	FDA-Approved Indications	Adult Dosage Range	Precautions and Clinical Pearls
Generic Name Colistimethate/ colistin **Brand Name** Coly-Mycin ▲	Sensitive to certain gram-negative bacilli that are typically resistant to other antibiotics *P. aeruginosa* Used in meningitis if bacteria are resistant and/or patient is allergic to first-line agents	**Usual dose expressed as colistin base:** IM/IV: 2.5 to 5 mg/kg per day in 2 to 4 divided doses (max 5 mg/kg per day)	• Can cause transient CNS adverse effects such as dizziness, numbness, slurred speech, and tingling: reducing dose may alleviate symptoms • Dose-dependent renal toxicity may develop: interrupt therapy if signs and symptoms of renal impairment occur • Reports of respiratory arrest have occurred: use with caution in patients with poor renal function • Colistimethate is the prodrug of colistin (equivalence data are available in the package insert) • In obese patients, use ideal body weight to calculate the dose • Caution patients about operating machinery and driving until tolerance of the medication is established • Monitor: renal function test at baseline; for nephrotoxicity, neurotoxicity, and pulmonary toxicity throughout therapy
Generic Name Polymyxin B ▲ ■ (PD)	Treatment of susceptible strains of *P. aeruginosa*	**Usual otic dose:** 1 to 2 drops 3 to 4 times daily **Usual ophthalmic dose:** 1 to 3 drops every 1 to 6 hours daily **Usual parenteral dose:** IM: 25,000 to 30,000 units/ kg per day divided every 4 to 6 hours IV: 15,000 to 25,000 units/ kg per day divided every 12 hours **Intrathecal:** 50,000 units daily or every other day **Topical irrigation:** 0.1 to 0.25% solution as part of wet dressings or as a wound irrigation	• IM formulation is not recommended due to the severe pain it causes • IV formulation is reserved for patients in whom other antibiotics fail • Monitor: renal function tests, neurotoxicity signs/symptoms Associated with: • Nephrotoxicity: avoid use with other nephrotoxic agents • Neurotoxicity that can cause respiratory paralysis: use with caution in patients with renal impairment and high polymyxin serum levels • Need for giving only IM/intrathecal formulations in the hospital

Rifamycins

Universal prescribing alerts:

- Can cause *C. difficile*–associated diarrhea and pseudomembranous colitis with extended use.

Drug Name	FDA-Approved Indications	Adult Dosage Range	Precautions and Clinical Pearls
Generic Name Rifaximin **Brand Name** Xifaxan	Hepatic encephalopathy Irritable bowel syndrome with diarrhea Traveler's diarrhea caused by *E. coli*	**Usual oral dose for irritable bowel syndrome:** 550 mg 3 times daily for 14 days	• Use with caution in patients with severe hepatic impairment: efficacy may be diminished in preventing encephalopathy • Do not use for diarrhea if blood appears in the stool or the patient has a fever • Some dosage forms contain propylene glycol: large amounts are toxic • Not for systemic infections: not adequately absorbed • Monitor: body temperature and for presence of blood in the patient's stool
Rifabutin	Refer to the Antimycobacterial Agents section.		
Rifampin	Refer to the Antimycobacterial Agents section.		
Rifapentine	Refer to the Antimycobacterial Agents section.		
Streptogramins			
Universal prescribing alerts: • Can cause *C. difficile*–associated diarrhea and pseudomembranous colitis with extended use.			
Drug Name	FDA-Approved Indications	Adult Dosage Range	Precautions and Clinical Pearls
Generic Name Quinupristin and dalfopristin **Brand Name** Synercid	Treatment of susceptible bacteria that cause complicated skin and skin structure infections *(for example: S. aureus, S. pyogenes)*	**Usual parenteral dose for skin and skin structure infections:** IV: 7.5 mg/kg every 12 hours for at least 7 days.	• Can cause arthralgia or myalgia: decrease dosing frequency in such cases • May cause hyperbilirubinemia • May cause phlebitis if used peripherally: hydrocortisone and diphenhydramine do not relieve symptoms • Drug interactions may require dose adjustment or avoidance of certain drug combinations • Infuse over 60 minutes to decrease toxicity: if venous irritation occurs, dilute further • Monitor: culture and sensitivity, periodically check infusion site
Miscellaneous Urinary Anti-infective Agents			
Universal prescribing alerts: • Can cause *C. difficile*–associated diarrhea and pseudomembranous colitis with extended use.			
Drug Name	FDA-Approved Indications	Adult Dosage Range	Precautions and Clinical Pearls
Generic Name Fosfomycin **Brand Name** Monurol	Treatment of susceptible bacteria that cause uncomplicated urinary tract infections in women *(for example: E. coli, E. faecalis)*	**Usual oral dose:** 3 g single dose in 3 to 4 ounces of water	• Always mix powder with water before administering • High concentrations persist for up to 48 hours in the urine • Monitor: urine culture with sensitivity

Generic Name Methenamine **Brand Name** Hiprex Urex Mandelamine (PD)	Treatment of susceptible bacteria that cause recurrent urinary tract infections Prophylaxis against urinary tract infections Decreases urinary tract discomfort secondary to hypermotility	**Usual oral dose:** Hippurate: 1 g twice daily Mandelate: 1 g 4 times per day after meals and at bedtime	• Use with caution in patients with gout • Use with caution in elderly patients • Foods or dinks that may alkalinize the urine can decrease the activity of methenamine • Monitor: urinalysis, hepatic function periodically Contraindications: • Severe renal or hepatic impairment • Severe dehydration
Generic Name Nitrofurantoin **Brand Name** Furadantin Macrobid Macrodantin (BL) (PD)	Treatment of susceptible bacteria that cause urinary tract infections *(for example: E. coli,* enterococci, *S. aureus, Klebsiella, Enterobacter)* Macrobid: indicated only for acute uncomplicated urinary tract infections *(for example: E. coli, S. saprophyticus)*	**Usual oral dose for UTI:** 50 to 100 mg every 6 hours Alternatively may give: **Macrobid products:** 100 mg twice daily Treatment usually for 7 days or 3 days after obtaining sterile urine **Prophylaxis (all products except Macrobid):** 50 to 100 mg at bedtime	• Macrobid formulation and oral suspension are not interchangeable with other nitrofurantoin products • May cause optic neuritis • May cause peripheral neuropathy: use with caution if patient has risk factors • Pulmonary toxicity has occurred: discontinue immediately if signs and symptoms occur • Administer with meals to increase absorption • Suspension may be mixed with water, milk, or fruit juice • Protect suspension from light to prevent darkening of nitrofurantoin • Patients with G6PD deficiency are at higher risk of hemolytic anemia • Monitor: signs of pulmonary toxicity, signs of numbness or tingling of the extremities, CBC, hepatic function periodically, renal function with extended use Contraindications: • In patients with CrCl less than 60 mL per minute • Previous hepatic dysfunction associated with nitrofurantoin

Drug Name	FDA-Approved Indications	Adult Dosage Range	Precautions and Clinical Pearls
Generic Name Trimethoprim **Brand Name** Primsol ▲ QT PD	Treatment of susceptible bacteria that cause UTI (*for example: E. coli, P. mirabilis, K. pneumoniae, Enterobacter*, coagulase-negative *Staphylococcus, S. saprophyticus*) Treatment of otitis media *S. pneumoniae, H. influenzae*	**Usual oral dose for UTI:** 100 mg every 12 hours Alternatively may give: 200 mg every 24 hours Treatment is generally recommended for 10 to 14 day duration	• May cause hyperkalemia: use with caution if administering high doses or in patients with renal impairment • Use with caution in patients with hepatic or renal impairment • Administer with milk or food • Drug interactions may require dose adjustment or avoidance of certain drug combinations • May need to supplement with folic acid • Monitor: CBC and potassium with extended use Contraindications: • Megaloblastic anemia due to folate deficiency

Antifungal Agents

Allylamines

Drug Name	FDA-Approved Indications	Adult Dosage Range	Precautions and Clinical Pearls
Generic Name Terbinafine **Brand Name** Lamisil Terbinex PD	Onychomycosis (tablets) caused by dermatophytes Tinea capitis (granules) Topical formulations: tinea pedis, tinea cruris, and tinea corporis	**Usual oral dose:** 250 mg once daily for at least 6 weeks **Topical:** Cream: apply 2 times daily for 1 to 2 weeks Gel or solution: apply once daily for at least 1 week	• Not recommended for use in chronic or active hepatic disease or if CrCl 50 mL per minute or less • May cause depression • May cause taste and smell disturbances: discontinue if symptoms occur • Drug interactions may require dose adjustments or avoidance of certain drug combinations • Can cause transient hematologic effects: monitor CBC in immunosuppressed patients if therapy lasts longer than 6 weeks • Rare cases of hepatic failure have occurred: assess the patient for this condition if signs and symptoms occur; discontinue if LFTs are significantly elevated • Serious skin reactions have been reported, such as SJS and DRESS: discontinue if rash progresses • Rarely can cause ocular changes in the lens and retina • Can exacerbate or precipitate lupus: discontinue if signs and symptoms develop • Administer granules with food: sprinkle on soft food that is not acidic, such as pudding or mashed potatoes, and swallow without chewing • When administering topical solution, hold 4 to 6 inches away from skin • Monitor: LFTs at baseline and again if duration of therapy exceeds 6 weeks; changes in taste or smell

Azoles			
Drug Name	**FDA-Approved Indications**	**Adult Dosage Range**	**Precautions and Clinical Pearls**
Generic Name Efinaconazole **Brand Name** Jublia	Treatment of onychomycosis caused by *T. rubrum* or *T. mentagrophytes*	**Usual topical dose:** Apply to affected toenails once daily for 48 weeks	• May cause local irritation • Toenails should be dry and clean before administration • Avoid nail products, such as nail polish, while using medication
Generic Name Fluconazole **Brand Name** Diflucan ▲ QT PD	Treatment of candidiasis infections: esophageal, oropharyngeal, peritoneal, urinary tract, vaginal, candidemia, pneumonia, and disseminated candidiasis Treatment of cryptococcal meningitis Prophylaxis against candidiasis in allogenic bone marrow transplant recipients	**Usual dose for oropharyngeal candidiasis:** Oral/IV: 200 mg once, then 100 daily for 2 weeks after the resolution of symptoms	• Can cause arrhythmias and QTc prolongation: use with caution in patients with preexisting arrhythmias and with concurrent use of agents that have a similar effect • Drug interactions may require dose adjustments • May cause hepatotoxicity that can be fatal: discontinue if signs and symptoms occur • Rarely causes exfoliative skin disorders: discontinue if rash develops • Do not use IV solution if cloudy or precipitated • Hazardous agent: use caution in preparing and disposing of medication • Caution patients about operating machinery and driving until tolerance of the medication is established due to the potential for dizziness or seizures • Monitor: liver and renal function tests periodically, potassium
Generic Name Isavuconazonium sulfate **Brand Name** Cresemba QT	Invasive aspergillosis Invasive mucormycosis	**Usual dose for treatment:** Oral/IV: 372 mg every 8 hours for 6 doses then once daily	• Drug interactions may require dose adjustments • May cause hepatotoxicity that can be fatal: discontinue if signs and symptoms occur • Infusion-related reactions may occur such as hypotension, chills, and paresthesia: discontinue if they occur • IV solution may contain clear to white particulates of isavuconazole: use 0.2- to 1.2-micron in-line filter • Monitor: LFTs at baseline and during therapy, infusion-related reactions during infusion Contraindications: • Familial short QT syndrome
Generic Name Itraconazole **Brand Name** Sporanox Onmel ■ QT	Treatment of aspergillosis, blastomycosis, and histoplasmosis in immunocompromised and non-immunocompromised patients (capsule)	**Usual oral dose for allergic bronchopulmonary aspergillosis:** 600 mg in divided doses for 3 days, then 400 mg daily in divided doses	• Can cause transient or permanent hearing loss: usually resolves upon discontinuation • May cause hepatotoxicity that can be fatal: discontinue if signs and symptoms occur • May cause neuropathy • Drug interactions may require dose adjustments or avoidance of certain drug combinations

Drug Name	FDA-Approved Indications	Adult Dosage Range	Precautions and Clinical Pearls
	Onychomycosis caused by dermatophytes (capsule), *Trichophyton rubrum* (tablet), or *Trichophyton mentagrophytes* (tablet) Oral solution: oropharyngeal/esophageal candidiasis		• Use with caution in patients with cystic fibrosis: displays erratic pharmacokinetics; use alternative therapy if infection does not improve • Do not give more than 200 mg at one time • Do not administer with antacids: capsules and tablets need gastric acidity for proper absorption • Capsules and oral solutions are not bioequivalent • Administer capsules and tablets with food; administer oral suspension on an empty stomach • Swish and swallow oral solution if treating for oropharyngeal and esophageal candidiasis • Caution patients about operating machinery and driving until tolerance of the medication is established due to the potential for CNS depression • Monitor: LFTs if preexisting impairment and duration is greater than 1 month; itraconazole blood levels, especially for oral therapy; renal function tests; signs and symptoms of heart failure Associated with: • Heart failure: discontinue if signs and symptoms develop • Ventricular dysfunction if treating patients for onychomycosis
Generic Name Ketoconazole **Brand Name** Nizoral Extina Ketodan Nizoral A-D Xolegel ■ QT PD	Treatment of systemic fungal infections including blastomycosis, histoplasmosis, paracoccidoidomycosis, coccidoidomycosis, and chromomycosis when other therapies have failed Cream: tinea corporis, tinea cruris, tinea versicolor, cutaneous candidiasis, and seborrheic dermatitis Foam/gel: seborrheic dermatitis Shampoo: dandruff, seborrheic dermatitis, and tinea versicolor	**Usual oral dose:** 200 to 400 mg once daily **Usual topical dose:** Cream: apply 1 to 2 times daily (dose varies on affected area targeted for treatment) OTC 1% shampoo: apply and rinse once or twice weekly Foam: apply twice daily Gel: apply once daily	• Drug interactions may require dose adjustments • May cause adrenocortical dysfunction that resolves upon discontinuation • Can cause increased long bone fragility • Administer 2 hours before antacid use to maintain gastric acidity for absorption • In patients with achlorhydria, administer with acidic liquids • Poorly penetrates the brain and should not be used for fungal meningitis • Gel and foam preparations are flammable • Shampoo may remove curls, discolor hair, and change hair texture • Monitor: LFTs at baseline and throughout therapy, calcium and phosphorus with extended use, adrenal function as needed Contraindications: • Acute or chronic liver disease Associated with: • QTc prolongation: do not use with other medications that can cause QTc prolongation • Hepatotoxicity that can be fatal: discontinue if signs and symptoms occur • Use only if other therapies have failed and the benefit outweighs the risk

Generic Name Luliconazole **Brand Name** Luzu	Treatment of susceptible fungi that cause tinea pedis, tinea cruris, and tinea corporis *T. rubrum, E. floccosum*	**Usual topical dose:** Apply to affected area and 1 inch of surrounding area once daily for 1 to 2 weeks	• Topical use only
Generic Name Posaconazole **Brand Name** Noxafil QT	Prophylaxis against invasive *Aspergillus* and *Candida* infections in severely immunocompromised patients Suspension: oropharyngeal candidiasis	**Usual dose for oral candidiasis:** Oral suspension: 100 to 400 mg 1 to 3 times daily **Usual dose for candiasis prophylaxis:** IV/Oral (DR tablets): 300 mg 2 times per day on the first day, then once daily Duration of therapy is based on clinical progress and recovery	• Can cause QTc prolongation and arrhythmias: use with caution in patients at high risk for arrhythmias • Drug interactions may require dose adjustments • Can cause hepatotoxicity that can be fatal: discontinue if signs and symptoms occur; effects are usually reversible upon discontinuation • DR tablets and oral suspensions are not interchangeable on a mg per mg basis • If glomerular filtration rate (GFR) less than 50 mL per minute, do not use IV due to accumulation of cyclodextrin • Limit peripheral IV infusion to one 30-minute infusion due to increased chance of infusion-site reactions • Administer suspension and DR tablets with food • Suitable IV solution color is clear to yellow • Monitor for breakthrough fungal infections in patients weighing more than 120 kg due to lower blood levels • Monitor: LFTs at baseline ad throughout therapy, renal function tests, electrolytes, CBC, breakthrough fungal infections
Generic Name Voriconazole **Brand Name** Vfend ■ QT	Treatment of invasive aspergillosis; esophageal candidiasis; candidemia (if non-neutropenic); disseminated *Candida* infections of the skin and abdomen, kidney, bladder wall, and wounds Used in serious infections caused by *Scedosporium apiospermum* and *Fusarium* if other treatments failed	**Usual parenteral dose:** IV: 3 to 6 mg/kg every 12 hours **Usual oral dose:** Adjusted body weight (ABW) 40 kg or greater: 200 mg every 12 hours	• Can cause QTc prolongation and arrhythmias: caution in patients at high risk for arrhythmias, correct electrolytes prior to use • Drug interactions may require dose adjustments • Can cause severe dermatologic reactions including melanoma and SJS: avoid exposure to direct sunlight, perform skin examinations for lesions periodically, and discontinue if signs and symptoms appear • Oral dosing based on adjusted body weight • Can cause hepatotoxicity that can be fatal: discontinue if signs and symptoms occur; effects are usually reversible upon discontinuation • Can cause ocular adverse effects such as change in visual acuity, blurred vision, and photophobia: reversible if duration of therapy is 28 days or less; long-term effects have not been studied • May cause renal toxicity in severely ill patients: use with caution if administering concurrently with other nephrotoxic agents

Drug Name	FDA-Approved Indications	Adult Dosage Range	Precautions and Clinical Pearls
			• Can cause fluorosis or periostitis with extended use: discontinue if bone pain develops and is supported by radiologic findings • Can cause pancreatitis (rare) • Infusion reactions presenting as anaphylactoid may occur: discontinue if reaction occurs • If CrCl is less than 50 mL per minute, recommend using oral formulations due to accumulation of cyclodextrin in the IV formulation • Do not infuse IV in same line with other medications; do not infuse at the same time (even when using separate lines) as concentrated electrolytes and blood products • Administer oral formulations 1 hour before or after meals to increase absorption • Caution patients about operating machinery and driving until tolerance of the medication is established due to the potential for visual changes • A small increase in dose can cause toxicity leading to neurologic and dermatologic effects • Monitor: hepatic and renal function and electrolytes at baseline and throughout therapy; eye exams if duration is greater than 28 days; voriconazole blood levels on day 5, then weekly if treating severe infections, and otherwise as needed; full-body skin examination yearly; phototoxic adverse events
Echinocandins			
Drug Name	FDA-Approved Indications	Adult Dosage Range	Precautions and Clinical Pearls
Generic Name Anidulafungin **Brand Name** Eraxis	Treatment of *Candida* infections including intra-abdominal, peritoneal, esophageal, and candidemia	**Usual parenteral dose for invasive candidiasis:** IV: 200 mg dose for day 1, then 100 mg once daily	• May cause hepatic impairment: discontinue if impairment progresses • Infusion reactions such as bronchospasm, hypotension, and rash may occur if the rate of infusion is too high • Monitor: LFTs
Generic Name Caspofungin **Brand Name** Cancidas ■ (PD)	Treatment of invasive *Aspergillus* infections when other agents fail Treatment of candidemia and *Candida* infections, including intra-abdominal abscesses, peritonitis, and pleural space infections	**Usual parenteral dose for invasive candidiasis:** IV: 70 mg dose for day 1, then 50 mg once daily	• May cause hepatic impairment: discontinue if impairment progresses • Dose interactions may require dose adjustment or avoidance of certain drug combinations • Histamine-related reactions may occur, such as rash, flushing, and facial edema • Monitor: hepatic function, hypersensitivity reactions

	Treatment of esophageal candidiasis Empiric treatment in patients with febrile neutropenia		
Generic Name Micafungin **Brand Name** Mycamine (PD)	Treatment of candidemia, disseminated candidiasis, *Candida* peritonitis and abscesses, and esophageal candidiasis Prophylaxis against *Candida* infections during hematopoietic stem cell transplant	**Usual parenteral dose for invasive candidiasis:** IV: 100 mg once daily Treatment duration depends on severity of infection and patient's clinical progress	• Hemolytic anemia and hemoglobinuria have been reported • May cause hepatic and renal impairment: discontinue if impairment progresses • Monitor: hepatic function
Oxaboroles			
Drug Name	**FDA-Approved Indications**	**Adult Dosage Range**	**Precautions and Clinical Pearls**
Generic Name Tavaborole **Brand Name** Kerydin	Treatment of onychomycosis due to *T. rubrum* or *T. mentagrophytes*	**Usual topical dose:** Apply to affected toenails once daily for 48 weeks	• May cause local irritation • Before applying, make sure toenails are dry and clean • Discard 3 months after opening bottle
Polyenes			
Drug Name	**FDA-Approved Indications**	**Adult Dosage Range**	**Precautions and Clinical Pearls**
Generic Name Amphotericin B **Brand Name** Amphocin *Conventional* Amphotec *Cholesteryl sulfate complex*	Conventional: Treats life-threatening fungal infections including aspergillosis, cryptococcosis, North American blastomycosis, systemic candidiasis, coccidioidomycosis, histoplasmosis, zygomycosis, *Conidiobolus, Basidiobolus,* and sporotrichosis	**Usual parenteral dose:** **Conventional:** IV: 0.3 to 1.5 mg/kg per day (max 1.5 mg/kg per day) **Amphotec:** IV: 3 to 4 mg/kg per day (max 6 mg/kg per day)	• Use extra care when selecting amphotericin products. Liposomal product doses are generally HIGHER than conventional doses. Use extra care to check if conventional product ordered exceeds 1.5 mg/kg (this may have been intended for liposomal administration). • Amphotericin B conventional is Amphocin • Amphotericin B cholesterol sulfate complex (ABCD) is Amphotec • Amphotericin B lipid complex (ABLC) is Abelcet • Amphotericin B liposomal injection (LAmB) is AmBisome • Administer the first dose with careful observation for respiratory distress • Can cause severe infusion reactions (fever, chills, shaking, hypotension, nausea, vomiting, headache, tachypnea) 1 to 3 hours after initiating the infusion: pretreat with medication or decrease the rate; with subsequent doses, the reactions become more tolerable

Drug Name	FDA-Approved Indications	Adult Dosage Range	Precautions and Clinical Pearls
Abelcet *Lipid complex* AmBisome *Liposomal* ■ (PD)	Can be used in leishmaniasis, but is not first choice Abelcet: invasive aspergillosis after failure to respond to amphotericin B deoxycholate Amphotec: invasive aspergillosis after failure to respond to amphotericin B deoxycholate and in patients with poor renal function AmBisome: invasive aspergillosis after failure to respond to amphotericin B deoxycholate and in patients with poor renal function Treatment of *Aspergillus*, *Candida*, and *Cryptococcus* infections that are refractory to amphotericin B deoxycholate; cryptococcal meningitis in HIV patients; visceral leishmaniasis Empiric therapy in febrile, neutropenic patients	**Abelcet:** IV: 5 mg/kg once daily **AmBisome:** IV: 3 to 6 mg/kg per day	• Can cause nephrotoxicity: interrupt therapy, decrease the dose, or decrease the frequency of dosing to help improve renal function; use with caution in high-risk patients • If renal impairment is due to use of the conventional infusion, decrease the dose by 50% • Separate dosing from leukocyte transfusions to prevent pulmonary reactions in neutropenic patients (conventional, lipid complex) • Rarely causes leukoencephalopathy (conventional) • Conventional formulation is thought to have the highest rate of infusion-related reactions and nephrotoxicity • If infusion-related reactions such as chills, fever, hypotension, and nausea occur, pretreat the patient 30 to 60 minutes before infusion with a nonsteroidal anti-inflammatory drug (NSAID) with or without diphenhydramine or acetaminophen (APAP) with or without diphenhydramine or hydrocortisone 50 to 100 mg with or without NSAID and diphenhydramine • If the patient experiences rigors during the fusion, meperidine may be administered • To reduce nephrotoxicity, give a bolus of normal saline before the infusion or before and after the infusion; doses greater than 1 mg/kg per day (conventional) have a higher risk of nephrotoxicity • If therapy is interrupted for more than 7 days, restart at the lowest dose and titrate up gradually • Monitor: LFTs, electrolytes, renal function, BUN, SCr, CBC, PTT, temperature, I/O, signs and symptoms of hypokalemia Associated with: • Check product name and dose if conventional dose exceeds 1.5 mg/kg • Use in progressive, life-threatening infections only
Generic Name Nystatin **Brand Name** Bio-Statin Nyamyc Nystop Pediaderm AF Complete (PD)	Treatment of susceptible fungus that cause cutaneous, mucocutaneous, and oral cavity infections *Candida*	**Usual oral dose:** 400,000 to 600,000 units 3 to 4 times per day **Usual topical dose:** Cream/ointment: apply twice daily Powder: apply 2 to 3 times per day	• Swish the suspension in the mouth as long as possible before swallowing (a few minutes) • Refrigerate suspension • Apply powder in the shoes when treating tinea pedis

Pyrimidines

Drug Name	FDA-Approved Indications	Adult Dosage Range	Precautions and Clinical Pearls
Generic Name Flucytosine **Brand Name** Ancobon ■ ▲	An adjunctive to treat systemic fungal infections (septicemia, endocarditis, urinary tract infections, meningitis, pulmonary infections) *Candida, Cryptococcus*	**Usual oral dose:** 50 to 150 mg/kg per day in divided doses every 6 hours	• Use with caution in patients with preexisting bone marrow depression or hematologic disease: can cause irreversible bone toxicity • Can cause hepatotoxicity: use with caution in patients with preexisting hepatic dysfunction • To diminish nausea and vomiting, administer a couple of capsules at once over 15 minutes • Interferes with SCr measurements when using the Ektachem analyzer • Monitor: perform baseline tests on electrolytes, CBC with differential, BUN, renal function, and blood culture; during treatment, monitor CBC with differential and LFTs frequently, flucytosine blood levels, renal function Associated with: • Renal dysfunction • Need to monitor renal, hepatic, and hematologic function

Miscellaneous Antifungal Agents

Drug Name	FDA-Approved Indications	Adult Dosage Range	Precautions and Clinical Pearls
Generic Name Griseofulvin **Brand Name** Grifulvin V (microsize) Gris-PEG (ultramicrosize) (PD)	Treatment of susceptible fungi that cause tinea infections of the skin, hair, and nails *Microsporum, Epidermophyton, Trichophyton*	**Usual oral dose for tinea corporis:** Microsize: 500 mg once daily (or in divided doses) for 2 to 4 weeks Ultramicrosize: 300 to 375 mg once daily (or to or in divided doses) for 2 to 4 weeks	• May cause granulocytopenia: discontinue if reaction occurs • May cause hepatic dysfunction • Rarely causes SJS or TEN: discontinue if reaction occurs • Administer with a fatty meal to increase absorption • Causes increased photosensitivity: wear sunscreen and avoid direct sunlight • Avoid ethanol use: will cause a disulfiram-like reaction • Monitor: renal, hepatic, and hematopoietic function periodically Contraindications: • Liver failure • Porphyria
Potassium iodide	Refer to the Hormones and Synthetic Substitutes chapter.		

Antimycobacterial Agents

Antituberculosis Agents

Universal prescribing alerts:

- Can cause *C. difficile*–associated diarrhea and pseudomembranous colitis with extended use.

Drug Name	FDA-Approved Indications	Adult Dosage Range	Precautions and Clinical Pearls
Generic Name Aminosalicylic acid **Brand Name** Paser PD	Treatment of tuberculosis in combination with other agents	**Usual oral dose:** 8 to 12 g per day in 2 to 3 divided doses	• Use with caution in patients with gastric ulcer or hepatic impairment • Do not use granules if color is brown or purple or if packet is swollen • When dispensed, store in refrigerator or freezer • Monitor: hepatic function at baseline, thyroid function at baseline and every 3 months with extended use Contraindications: • Severe renal impairment
Generic Name Bedaquiline **Brand Name** Sirturo ■ QT	Treatment of susceptible strains of multidrug-resistant pulmonary tuberculosis when other agents cannot be used Use with 3 or more agents active against the patient's tuberculosis strand	**Usual oral dose:** 400 mg once daily for 2 weeks then 200 mg 3 times per week for weeks 3 to 24 Directly observe therapy	• May cause hepatic dysfunction and increase in hepatic enzymes • Use with caution in patients with poor renal function • Administer with food to increase absorption • For weeks 3 to 24 of regimen, doses should be administered at least 48 hours apart from each other • Store in original container or discard within 3 months • Monitor: ECG at baseline and weeks 2, 12, and 24 or weekly if patient has risk factors; baseline potassium, calcium, and magnesium; hepatic function tests at baseline and monthly; weekly for arthralgia, chest pain, headache, hemoptysis, nausea, and rash • Drug interactions may require dose adjustments Associated with: • Arrhythmias and QTc prolongation; discontinue if interval is greater than 500 ms • Increased risk of death: use as last-line therapy
Generic Name Capreomycin **Brand Name** Capastat Sulfate ▲ ■ GD	Treatment of pulmonary tuberculosis with concurrent use of other agents when primary agents are ineffective	**Usual parenteral dose:** IM/IV: 1 g once daily for 5 to 7 days a week, reduced to 2 to 3 times a week after the first 2 to 4 months Total duration of treatment often requires culture conversion	• Can cause electrolyte imbalances: monitor calcium, potassium, and magnesium • May cause nephrotoxicity: if BUN greater than 30 mg/dL or renal function is falling, adjust dosing or discontinue • Can cause permanent hearing impairment: monitor using audiometric assessment • Dosing per weight is based on ideal body weight • Specific doses for those 60 years and older • Monitor: audiometric assessment and vestibular function at baseline and throughout therapy, renal function at baseline and weekly during treatment, electrolytes at baseline and throughout therapy, hepatic function tests Associated with: • Hearing impairment and/or renal impairment • Increased risk with concurrent use of other ototoxic or nephrotoxic agents • Increased risk with concurrent use with other IV antituberculous agents due to high risk of toxic effects

Generic Name Cycloserine **Brand Name** Seromycin	Treatment of pulmonary or extrapulmonary tuberculosis with concurrent use of other agents when primary agents are inadequate Treatment-susceptible bacteria causing urinary tract infections when organism is resistant *Enterobacter, E. coli*	**Usual oral dose:** 250 mg every 12 hours for 14 days, then 500 to 1000 mg per day in 2 divided doses	• Dose-related CNS effects, such as seizures, psychosis, depression, and confusion have occurred: pyridoxine can help prevent/treat CNS adverse effects • Can cause allergic dermatitis: decrease dose or discontinue if rash develops • May need to supplement with folic acid and vitamin B_{12} • Monitor: hepatic, renal, and hematologic function; cycloserine blood levels; neuropsychiatric status at least every month Contraindications: • Severe renal function • Epilepsy • Depression • Severe anxiety • Psychosis • Excessive use of alcohol
Generic Name Ethambutol **Brand Name** Myambutol ▲ (PD)	Treatment of pulmonary tuberculosis with concurrent use of other agents	**Usual oral dose:** 15 to 25 mg/kg once daily	• May cause hepatotoxicity: monitor LFTs • Dosing strategy is based on whether patient is treatment naïve or if they have already received therapy • Can cause optic neuritis: discontinue immediately if changes in vision occur; usually reversible over a period of time • Use with caution in patients with ocular disease: determine if visual changes are due to ocular disease or ethambutol use • Can administer with food to decrease stomach irritation • Monitor: visual examination at baseline and monthly if receiving more than 15 mg/kg per day (test in both eyes separately and together); hepatic, renal, and hematopoietic function at baseline and throughout therapy Contraindications: • Optic neuritis • Unconscious patients • Patients who cannot communicate visual changes due to ethambutol
Generic Name Ethionamide **Brand Name** Trecator (PD)	Treatment of tuberculosis along with other mycobacterial diseases with concurrent use of other agents when primary agents fail	**Usual oral dose:** 15 to 30 mg/kg per day (max 1 g per day in divided doses)	• Can cause hypoglycemia: use with caution in patients with diabetes • Can cause porphyria and hypothyroidism • Use with cycloserine has resulted in seizures • Can increase isoniazid blood levels if used concurrently and cross-resistance may develop if *inhA* mutation is present • Administering with food, at bedtime, or with an antiemetic may alleviate gastrointestinal adverse events

Drug Name	FDA-Approved Indications	Adult Dosage Range	Precautions and Clinical Pearls
			• Concurrent use of pyridoxine can prevent or treat the neurotoxic effects • Do not drink alcohol: can cause psychotic adverse events • Monitor: LFTs at baseline and throughout therapy, blood glucose, thyroid-stimulating hormone (TSH) every 6 months, ophthalmic exams at baseline and throughout therapy Contraindications: • Severe hepatic impairment due to risk of hepatotoxicity
Generic Name Isoniazid **Brand Name** Nydrazid ■ (PD)	Treatment of tuberculosis and latent tuberculosis with concurrent use of other agents	**Usual dose:** Oral/IM: 5 mg/kg per dose once daily or 5 times per week (maximum 300 mg per day) Dosing recommendations by the CDC may change with changes in resistance patterns Oral is preferred route of administration	• If ALT or AST is more than 3 times the UNL, then temporarily hold isoniazid • Use with caution in patients with severe renal impairment • Drug interactions may require dose adjustments • May need to supplement folic acid, niacin, and magnesium • If IV vials crystalize, warm the vial to room temperature to dissolve the precipitates • Pyridoxine use can help prevent peripheral neuropathies in high-risk groups such as patients with HIV, malnourished patients, and patients with diabetes • Isoniazid is a weak monoamine oxidase (MAO) inhibitor and may cause adverse effects with tyramine-containing food • Avoid histamine-containing foods (tuna, tropical fish) due to potential adverse effects of headache, sweating, palpitations, flushing, diarrhea, wheezing, itching, dyspnea, and hypotension: treat with corticosteroids and antihistamines • May cause a false-positive urinary glucose result with Clinitest • Monitor: LFTs at baseline and throughout therapy, sputum cultures monthly until 2 consecutive cultures are negative, signs and symptoms of hepatitis, regular ophthalmic exams • Specific recommendations for patients undergoing dialysis Contraindications: • Acute liver disease • History of drug-induced hepatitis • History of hepatic injury due to isoniazid • Previous severe reaction to isoniazid Associated with: • Hepatitis, which can be fatal: monitor for signs and symptoms and liver function regularly
Generic Name Pyrazinamide ▲ (PD)	Treatment of tuberculosis with concurrent use of other agents	**Usual oral dose:** 15 to 30 mg/kg per dose once daily (max 3g per day) or 50 to 70 mg/kg per dose 2 times per week	• Hepatotoxicity is dose dependent and rarely can cause liver atrophy • Use with caution in patients with history of alcoholism, concurrent use of hepatotoxic medications, porphyria, and renal impairment • May inhibit secretion of uric acid, leading to gout attacks

			• Can cause a pink-brown color when used with Acetest and Ketostix • Monitor: LFTs, uric acid blood levels, sputum culture, chest x-ray 2 to 3 months after first dose and upon completion of therapy • Specific recommendations for patients undergoing dialysis Contraindications: • Severe hepatic impairment • Active gout flare
Generic Name Rifabutin **Brand Name** Mycobutin ▲	Prevents *Mycobacterium avium* complex (MAC) in patients with HIV	**Usual oral dose:** 300 mg once daily 150 mg twice daily	• Can cause hematologic toxicity: discontinue if signs of thrombocytopenia occur • May cause uveitis: increased risk with concurrent macrolide or azole use; refer the patient to an ophthalmologist if signs and symptoms of uveitis occur • Drug interactions may require dose adjustment or avoidance of certain drug combinations • Use with caution in patients with hepatic impairment: discontinue if significant elevation in LFTs occurs • Do not administer if patient has active TB: may cause resistance to rifampin • Can be administered with meals to reduce nausea • A brown/orange discoloration of bodily fluids and the skin may occur: remove contact lenses to prevent staining • Monitor: LFTs, CBC with differential, platelet count
Generic Name Rifampin **Brand Name** Rifadin	Treatment of active tuberculosis in combination with other agents Eradicates meningococci from asymptomatic carriers	**Usual dose:** Oral/IV: 10 mg/kg per dose given once daily or 2, 3 or 5 times per week (max 600 mg per day)	• May cause flu-like symptoms: more likely if patient takes more than 600 mg 1 to 2 times per week • Can cause hematologic adverse events including thrombocytopenia: more likely if patient takes more than 600 mg 1 to 2 times per week • Drug interactions may require dose adjustment or avoidance of certain drug combinations • May cause hyperbilirubinemia: discontinue if signs and symptoms develop • Use with caution in patients with hepatic impairment and alcoholism: dose adjustments may be necessary • Use with caution in patients with porphyria: exacerbations can occur • Administer oral formulations on an empty stomach with 8 ounces of water to increase absorption • Separate administration time of oral formulations from antacids • A brown/orange discoloration of bodily fluids may occur: remove contact lenses to prevent staining • Can cause false-positive detection of opioids in the urine • Interferes with standard microbiological assays for measuring folate and vitamin B12 blood levels • Monitor: LFTs at baseline and every 2 to 4 weeks during therapy; CBC; CNS effects; sputum culture; chest x-ray 2 to 3 months after first dose

Drug Name	FDA-Approved Indications	Adult Dosage Range	Precautions and Clinical Pearls
Generic Name Rifapentine **Brand Name** Priftin (PD)	Treatment of active tuberculosis in combination with other agents Not recommended in HIV patients during the continuation phase due to increased failure rate Treatment of latent tuberculosis in combination with other agents	**Usual oral dose for treatment of TB:** 600 mg 2 times per week for 2 months with interval of no less than 3 days (72 hours) between doses Must be administered with at least one other antituberculosis agent	• Use with caution in patients with hepatic impairment: use only when necessary and monitor LFTs • Use with caution in patients with porphyria: exacerbations can occur; use in this population is not recommended • Administer with food to increase absorption • Ensure compliance before starting therapy or resistance may develop • A brown/orange discoloration of bodily fluids, skin, and teeth may occur: remove contact lenses to prevent staining • Drug interactions may require dose adjustment or avoidance of certain drug combinations • Interferes with standard microbiological assays for measuring folate and vitamin B12 blood levels • Monitor: LFTs at baseline and every 2 to 4 weeks if preexisting hepatic impairment exists; LFTs at baseline and as needed if treating latent disease in HIV patients, patients with hepatic impairment, and patients with constant alcohol consumption
Amikacin	Refer to the Antibacterial Agents section.		
Ciprofloxacin	Refer to the Antibacterial Agents section.		
Clarithromycin	Refer to the Antibacterial Agents section.		
Levofloxacin	Refer to the Antibacterial Agents section.		
Moxifloxacin	Refer to the Antibacterial Agents section.		
Streptomycin	Refer to the Antibacterial Agents section.		

Miscellaneous Antimycobacterial Agents

Drug Name	FDA-Approved Indications	Adult Dosage Range	Precautions and Clinical Pearls
Generic Name Dapsone **Brand Name** Avlosulfon Aczone (PD)	Leprosy Dermatitis herpetiformis Acne vulgaris	**Usual oral dose for dermatitis herpetiformis:** 50 once daily; maintenance doses may range 25 to 300 mg daily **Usual topical dose:** Apply once daily	• May cause severe blood dyscrasias: monitor • Rarely serious skin reactions can occur, such as TEN • May cause peripheral neuropathy • Use with caution in patients with G6PD deficiency: higher risk for anemia • Use lowest effective dose possible • Drug interactions may require dose adjustment or avoidance of certain drug combinations • Use with caution in patients with hemoglobin M or methemoglobin reductase deficiency: higher risk of methemoglobinemia • Can cause *C. difficile*–associated diarrhea and pseudomembranous colitis with extended use • Separate the time it is given from intake of antacids, alkaline foods, or alkaline medications • If using with benzoyl peroxide, may cause reversible yellow/orange color to the skin • Monitor: G6PD levels baseline; CBC weekly for first month, monthly for 6 months, then semiannually; reticulocyte counts; LFTs

Antiviral Agents

Adamantanes

Drug Name	FDA-Approved Indications	Adult Dosage Range	Precautions and Clinical Pearls
Generic Name Amantadine **Brand Name** Symmetrel QT PD GD	Prophylaxis and treatment of influenza A Drug-induced extrapyramidal symptoms Parkinson's disease	**Usual oral dose for treatment of influenza A virus infection:** 200 mg daily 100 mg 2 times per day	• May cause compulsive behavior such as gambling, hypersexuality, and binge eating if used for Parkinson's disease: reduce dose or discontinue • Increased risk of developing melanoma in patients with Parkinson's disease: monitor for new/changed skin lesions • May cause neuroleptic malignant syndrome if dose is decreased or discontinued • May worsen psychiatric illness: monitor for suicidal ideation • Use with caution in patients with the following conditions: cardiovascular disease, eczema, glaucoma, poor hepatic or renal function, seizure history • Influenza A is highly resistant to therapy, and resistance can develop during therapy • Administer within 48 hours of flu symptoms' appearance • Caution patients about operating machinery and driving until tolerance of the medication is established • May cause withdrawal syndrome: taper slowly, especially in patients with Parkinson's disease • Tolerance can develop over time • Elderly patients are at an increased risk of experiencing CNS adverse effects such as dizziness and weakness • May lead to false-positive results for amphetamines • Monitor: renal function, mental status, blood pressure, and symptoms of Parkinson's disease or influenza • Special recommendations for patients undergoing dialysis • Additional reference to drug use in Central Nervous System Agents chapter
Generic Name Rimantadine **Brand Name** Flumadine PD GD	Prophylaxis and treatment of influenza A	**Usual oral dose:** 100 mg 2 times per day	• Use with caution in patients with hepatic and/or renal impairment • Avoid use in patients with psychosis • Use with caution in patients with history of seizures: increased risk of seizures • Influenza A is highly resistant to therapy, and resistance can develop during therapy • Administer within 48 hours of flu symptoms' appearance • Elderly patients are at an increased risk of experiencing CNS adverse effects such as dizziness and weakness • Monitor for CNS and gastrointestinal symptoms in elderly patients, patients with impaired renal function, and patients with impaired hepatic function

Antiretroviral Agents

HIV Entry and Fusion Inhibitors

Drug Name	FDA-Approved Indications	Adult Dosage Range	Precautions and Clinical Pearls
Generic Name Enfuvirtide **Brand Name** Fuzeon (PD)	Treatment of HIV-1 infection when used with other antiretroviral agents in treatment-experienced patients	**Usual parenteral dose:** SQ: 90 mg 2 times a day	• May cause immune reconstitution syndrome, in which an inflammatory reaction develops due to a residual opportunistic infection or activation of an autoimmune disorder • Commonly causes injection-site reactions • Patients are more likely to develop pneumonia: use with caution in patients with a high viral load • Increased risk of bleeding in patients with preexisting coagulation disorders • Rotate injection sites • Powder for injection may take up to 45 minutes to completely dissolve • Do not inject near a nerve to avoid nerve pain • Monitor: viral load, CD4 count
Generic Name Maraviroc **Brand Name** Selzentry ▲ ■	Treatment of CCR5-tropic HIV-1 infection when used with other antiretroviral agents	**Usual oral dose:** 300 mg twice daily	• May cause immune reconstitution syndrome, in which an inflammatory reaction develops due to a residual opportunistic infection or activation of an autoimmune disorder • Can cause postural hypotension: use with caution in patients with poor renal function and cardiovascular disease • Hypersensitivity reactions such as SJS and DRESS have occurred: discontinue use • Caution patients about operating machinery and driving until tolerance of the medication is established due to the potential for dizziness • Monitor: viral load, CD4 count, LFTs, and bilirubin before treatment and during therapy; tropism testing before initiation • Contraindicated in patients with CrCl less than 30 mL per minute with other factors that add risk, such as drug interactions that may require dose adjustments • Dose recommendations are specific for CYP inhibitors and inducers; refer to PI Associated with: • Drug-induced hepatotoxicity with allergic-type features: use with caution in patients with hepatic impairment; discontinue if signs and symptoms occur

HIV Protease Inhibitors

Universal prescribing alerts:

- Can cause fat redistribution, elevated bilirubin, prolonged PR interval, diabetes, hepatic impairment, nephrolithiasis, hemolytic anemia, elevated triglycerides, and elevated cholesterol.
- Contraindicated in patients who experience specific drug-induced hypersensitivity reactions (including SJS and DRESS) and drug interactions that may require dose adjustments.

Drug Name	FDA-Approved Indications	Adult Dosage Range	Precautions and Clinical Pearls
Generic Name Atazanavir **Brand Name** Reyataz ■ QT PD	Treatment of HIV infection when used with other antiretroviral agents	**Usual oral dose:** 300 mg once daily with ritonavir 100 mg or cobicistat 150 mg Additional adjustments when used with H_2 antagonist or proton pump inhibitor (i.e., increase to 400 mg once daily)	• May cause immune reconstitution syndrome, in which an inflammatory reaction develops due to a residual opportunistic infection or activation of an autoimmune disorder • Not recommended for use in antiretroviral-experienced patients with end-stage renal disease (ESRD) • Administer with food, and separate administration from that of antacids and buffered medications • Limit dose of H_2 blocker (see PI) AND when using H_2 blockers, administer at the same time as atazanavir or at least 10 hours after the atazanavir dose. • Patients with hemophilia A or B are at an increased risk of bleeding • Specific recommendations for patients undergoing dialysis • Confirm that baseline/pretreatment HIV RNA greater than 100,000 copies/mL • Monitor: viral load, CD4 count, blood glucose, LFTs, bilirubin, atazanavir levels if used with interacting medications, ECG in patients with preexisting prolonged PR interval or concurrent use of atrioventricular (AV) nodal-blocking medications
Generic Name Darunavir **Brand Name** Prezista PD	Treatment of HIV infection when used with other antiretroviral agents	**Usual oral dose:** 800 mg once daily with ritonavir 100 mg or cobicistat 150 mg **Suspected resistance:** 600 mg twice daily Treatment experienced patients may require higher doses	• Can cause fat redistribution, diabetes, hepatic impairment, pancreatitis, and elevated cholesterol • Drug interactions may require dose adjustments • May cause hypersensitivity reactions such as SJS or DRESS: discontinue if rash appears • May cause immune reconstitution syndrome, in which an inflammatory reaction develops due to a residual opportunistic infection or activation of an autoimmune disorder • Not recommended in patients with severe hepatic impairment: discontinue if hepatic function worsens during therapy • Administer with food • Patients with hemophilia A or B are at an increased risk of bleeding • Do not use darunavir/ritonavir if CD4 count is less than 200 cells/mm3 and/or HIV RNA greater than 100,000 copies/mL • Monitor: viral load, CD4 count, baseline genotyping in treatment-experienced patients, blood glucose, LFTs at baseline and throughout therapy, cholesterol, triglycerides

Drug Name	FDA-Approved Indications	Adult Dosage Range	Precautions and Clinical Pearls
Generic Name Fosamprenavir **Brand Name** Lexiva ■ (PD)	Treatment of HIV infection when used with other antiretroviral agents	**Usual oral dose:** 1400 mg with ritonavir 100 to 200 mg once daily Alternatively may give: 700 mg with ritonavir 100 mg twice daily	• May cause immune reconstitution syndrome, in which an inflammatory reaction develops due to a residual opportunistic infection or activation of an autoimmune disorder • Drug interactions may require dose adjustments • Administer suspension without food in adults; if vomiting occurs within 30 minutes, readminister • Administer tablet with food if taken with ritonavir • Twice-daily dosing is recommended in protease inhibitor–experienced adults • Patients with hemophilia A or B are at an increased risk of bleeding • Monitor: viral load, CD4 count, blood glucose, LFTs in patients with hepatitis B or C, cholesterol, triglycerides • Regimens without ritonavir are available, but not recommended by guidelines
Generic Name Indinavir **Brand Name** Crixivan ■	Treatment of HIV infection when used with other antiretroviral agents	**Usual oral dose:** 800 mg with ritonavir 100 to 200 mg 2 times per daily Alternative dose schedules using other antiretrovirals are available; refer to PI	• May cause tubulointerstitial nephritis: monitor for leukocytopenia (rare) • May cause immune reconstitution syndrome, in which an inflammatory reaction develops due to a residual opportunistic infection or activation of an autoimmune disorder • Use with caution in patients with preexisting hepatic disease: can exacerbate symptoms • Drug interactions may require dose adjustments • Administer with water on an empty stomach when unboosted • Keep patients well hydrated: drink 48 ounces of water daily to help prevent nephrolithiasis • Dispense in original container • Patients with hemophilia A or B are at an increased risk of bleeding • Monitor: viral load, CD4 count, blood glucose, LFTs, cholesterol, triglycerides, CBC, urinalysis (especially monitor for leukocyturia) • Regimens without ritonavir are available, but not recommended by guidelines
Generic Name Lopinavir and ritonavir **Brand Name** Kaletra (QT) (PD)	Treatment of HIV infection when used with other antiretroviral agents	**Usual oral dose:** lopinavir 400 mg with ritonavir 100 mg twice daily Alternatively may give: Lopinavir 800 mg with ritonavir 200 mg once daily	• May cause QTc prolongation and other conduction abnormalities, and patients may have a higher risk of myocardial infarction (MI): use with caution in patients with preexisting cardiac disease • May cause immune reconstitution syndrome, in which an inflammatory reaction develops due to a residual opportunistic infection or activation of an autoimmune disorder • Administer solution with food • Drug interactions may require dose adjustments • Patients with hemophilia A or B are at an increased risk of bleeding • Use with caution in patients with poor renal function to ensure accumulation and toxicity do not occur

			• Monitor: viral load, CD4 count, baseline genotyping or phenotypic testing before starting therapy, blood glucose, LFTs, electrolytes, cholesterol, triglycerides • Specific recommendations for patients undergoing dialysis
Generic Name Nelfinavir **Brand Name** Viracept QT PD	Treatment of HIV infection when used with other antiretroviral agents	**Usual oral dose:** 750 mg 3 times per day 1250 mg 2 times per day	• May cause immune reconstitution syndrome, in which an inflammatory reaction develops due to a residual opportunistic infection or activation of an autoimmune disorder • Not recommended in patients with moderate to severe hepatic impairment: discontinue if hepatic function worsens during therapy • Administer with food; mixing a crushed tablet with acidic foods or juices will cause a bitter taste • Patients with hemophilia A or B are at an increased risk of bleeding • Monitor: viral load, CD4 count, blood glucose, LFTs, cholesterol, triglycerides, CBC with differential
Generic Name Ritonavir **Brand Name** Norvir ■ QT PD	Treatment of HIV infection when used with other antiretroviral agents	**Usual oral dose:** 600 mg 2 times per day (titrate up from 300 mg 2 times per day and increase by 100 mg 2 times per day every 2 to 3 days)	• Use dose escalation strategy to reduce nausea • Can cause fat redistribution, QT interval prolongation, diabetes, hepatic impairment, pancreatitis, and elevated cholesterol • Drug interactions may require dose adjustments • Use with caution in patients with preexisting cardiovascular disease • May cause immune reconstitution syndrome, in which an inflammatory reaction develops due to a residual opportunistic infection or activation of an autoimmune disorder • Not recommended in patients with severe hepatic impairment: discontinue if hepatic function worsens during therapy • Tablets are not bioequivalent to capsules • Administer with food and advise patients to stay well hydrated • Mix solution with chocolate to mask bad taste • Contains 43% ethanol and 26.57% propylene glycol: monitor for toxicity • Patients with hemophilia A or B are at an increased risk of bleeding • Monitor: viral load, CD4 count, blood glucose, LFTs, cholesterol, triglycerides, CBC, CPK, uric acid, amylase and lipase serum levels • Lower doses of ritonavir are used to enhance or "boost" the serum concentrations of other antiretroviral agents (purposeful drug interaction)

Drug Name	FDA-Approved Indications	Adult Dosage Range	Precautions and Clinical Pearls
Generic Name Saquinavir **Brand Name** Invirase QT	Treatment of HIV infection when used with other antiretroviral agents	**Usual oral dose:** 1000 mg with ritonavir 100 mg 2 times per day	• Can cause QTc prolongation, fat redistribution, photosensitivity, diabetes, hepatic impairment, electrolyte imbalances, and elevated cholesterol • May cause immune reconstitution syndrome, in which an inflammatory reaction develops due to a residual opportunistic infection or activation of an autoimmune disorder • Administer within 2 hours after a meal; do not take with grapefruit juice • Patients with hemophilia A or B are at an increased risk of bleeding • Monitor: viral load, CD4 count, blood glucose, cholesterol and triglycerides at baseline and throughout treatment; ECG at baseline and 3-4 days after starting therapy; potassium and magnesium blood levels • Contraindicated for use in patients with severe hepatic impairment
Generic Name Tipranavir **Brand Name** Aptivus ■ PD	Treatment of HIV infection when used with other antiretroviral agents in treatment-experienced or multiple protease inhibitor–resistant patients	**Usual oral dose:** 500 mg with ritonavir 200 mg 2 times per day for 7 days, then may increase to standard dose of 1000 mg with ritonavir 100 mg 2 times per day	• Can cause fat redistribution, skin reactions such as rash and photosensitivity, impaired platelet aggregation, diabetes, hepatic impairment, and elevated cholesterol • May cause immune reconstitution syndrome, in which an inflammatory reaction develops due to a residual opportunistic infection or activation of an autoimmune disorder • Not recommended in patients with severe hepatic impairment: discontinue if hepatic function worsens during therapy • Administer with food when administering with ritonavir tablets • Solution contains vitamin E; capsules contain dehydrated ethanol • Patients with hemophilia A or B are at an increased risk of bleeding • Monitor: viral load, CD4 count, blood glucose, LFTs (including bilirubin) at baseline and frequently throughout therapy, cholesterol and triglycerides at baseline and throughout treatment; monitor patients coinfected with hepatitis B or C carefully Associated with: • Hepatotoxicity when used with certain other drugs, which can be fatal • Use with caution in patients with preexisting hepatic impairment • Rare cases of intracranial hemorrhage when used with certain other drugs

HIV Integrase Inhibitors

Drug Name	FDA-Approved Indications	Adult Dosage Range	Precautions and Clinical Pearls
Generic Name Dolutegravir **Brand Name** Tivicay	Treatment of HIV infection when used with other antiretroviral agents	**Usual oral dose:** 50 mg once a day, may increase to 50 mg 2 times daily when coadministered with specific antiretrovirals; refer to PI	• Risk of lactic acidosis when used in combination with higher doses of metformin • Avoid co-administration with multivitamins or supplements containing calcium, magnesium, or iron

Drug Name	FDA-Approved Indications	Adult Dosage Range	Precautions and Clinical Pearls
Generic Name Elvitegravir and cobicistat **Brand Name** Vitekta	Treatment of HIV infection when used with other antiretroviral agents in adults who are antiretroviral experienced	**Usual oral dose:** 85 mg (with ritonavir 100 mg and atazanavir 300 mg) once a day	• Higher dose options are available in combination with other agents • May cause elevations in serum creatinine • Avoid in renal dysfunction
Generic Name Raltegravir **Brand Name** Isentress (PD)	Treatment of HIV infection when used with other antiretroviral agents	**Usual oral dose:** 400 mg twice daily	• Can cause myopathy: use with caution in patients who are at risk for elevated CK • Severe skin and hypersensitivity reactions have occurred, including SJS and TEN: discontinue if rash occurs • May cause immune reconstitution syndrome, in which an inflammatory reaction develops due to a residual opportunistic infection or activation of an autoimmune disorder • Store chewable tablets and oral suspensions in their original containers • Chewable tablets, oral suspensions, and film-coated tablets are not bioequivalent • Do not use darunavir/ritonavir and raltegravir if the patient's pre-antiretroviral therapy (ART) CD4 count less than 200 cells/mm^3 and/or HIV RNA greater than 100,000 copies/mL • Monitor: viral load, CD4 count, complete lipid profile • Drug interactions may require dose adjustment or avoidance of certain drug combinations
HIV Non-nucleoside Reverse Transcriptase Inhibitors			
Drug Name	FDA-Approved Indications	Adult Dosage Range	Precautions and Clinical Pearls
Generic Name Delavirdine **Brand Name** Rescriptor	Treatment of HIV-1 infection when used with other antiretroviral agents	**Usual oral dose:** 400 mg 3 times per day	• May cause fat redistribution or a rash that requires interruption of therapy • Use with caution in patients with hepatic and renal impairment • May cause immune reconstitution syndrome, in which an inflammatory reaction develops due to a residual opportunistic infection or activation of an autoimmune disorder • Do not administer with antacids to ensure gastric acidity for absorption • Drug interactions may require dose adjustments or avoidance of certain drug combinations • Monitor: viral load, CD4 count, LFTs if used with saquinavir

Drug Name	FDA-Approved Indications	Adult Dosage Range	Precautions and Clinical Pearls
Generic Name Efavirenz **Brand Name** Sustiva (PD)	Treatment of HIV infection when used with other antiretroviral agents	**Usual oral dose:** 600 mg once per day	• Not recommended in patients with moderate to severe hepatic impairment; avoid use in patients with HIV-associated dementia • May cause immune reconstitution syndrome, in which an inflammatory reaction develops due to a residual opportunistic infection or activation of an autoimmune disorder • Administer on an empty stomach; recommended to take at bedtime due to increased tolerability of CNS effects • Drug interactions may require dose adjustments or avoidance of certain drug combinations • Oral solution is available only through an expanded access program • Do not use efavirenz with abacavir and lamivudine if the patient's pre-ART HIV RNA greater than 100,000 copies/mL • Can cause false-positive tests for cannabinoids if using the CEDIA DAU Multilevel THC assay • Can cause false-positive tests for benzodiazepines • Monitor: LFTs, cholesterol and triglycerides, psychiatric adverse effects
Generic Name Etravirine **Brand Name** Intelence (PD)	Treatment of HIV infection when used with other antiretroviral agents in treatment-experienced patients with NNRTI resistance	**Usual oral dose:** 200 mg 2 times per day	• May cause fat redistribution or a rash (SJS, TEN, DRESS): discontinue if rash becomes severe • May cause immune reconstitution syndrome, in which an inflammatory reaction develops due to a residual opportunistic infection or activation of an autoimmune disorder • Administer after meals • Can disperse in water; do not use grapefruit juice, carbonated drinks, or warm water when taking etravirine • Drug interactions may require dose adjustments or avoidance of certain drug combinations • Monitor: cholesterol and triglycerides, blood glucose, LFTs if signs and symptoms of hypersensitivity occur
Generic Name Nevirapine **Brand Name** Viramune Viramune XR ■ (PD)	Treatment of HIV infection when used with other antiretroviral agents	**Usual oral dose:** IR: 200 mg once daily for 14 days, then increase to twice daily XR: 400 mg once daily for maintenance (must have received 200 mg IR formulation before XR; refer to PI for details)	• May cause fat redistribution or rhabdomyolysis • Not recommended in combination with nevirapine due to increased adverse effects • May cause immune reconstitution syndrome, in which an inflammatory reaction develops due to a residual opportunistic infection or activation of an autoimmune disorder • Drug interactions may require dose adjustments or avoidance of certain drug combinations • Do not administer in antiretroviral-naïve patients if CD4+ cell counts greater than 250 cells/mm3 in females or CD4+ cell counts greater than 400 cells/mm3 in males • If rash appears during first 14 days of use, do not increase dose until it disappears; use alternative therapy if rash duration exceeds 28 days

			• Monitor: viral load; CD4 count; CBC; baseline LFTs, then every 2 weeks for the first 4 weeks and monthly for the first 18 weeks, then every 3 to 4 months; signs of rash Contraindications: • Moderate to severe hepatic impairment • Use in postexposure prophylaxis Associated with: • Severe hepatotoxicity: risk is greatest in the first 6 weeks; monitor intensely for the first 18 weeks • Life-threatening skin reactions such as SJS and TEN: risk is greatest in the first 6 weeks; monitor intensely for the first 18 weeks
Generic Name Rilpivirine **Brand Name** Edurant (QT)	Treatment of HIV infection when used with other antiretroviral agents in treatment-naïve patients if HIV RNA 100,000 copies per mL or less and/or pre-ART CD4 or count of 200 cells/mm^3 or greater	**Usual oral dose:** 25 mg once daily	• May cause depressive disorders, fat redistribution, hepatotoxicity, or hypersensitivity reaction such as DRESS: discontinue if severe or rash develops • Drug interactions may require dose adjustments • Use with caution in patients with severe renal impairment • Doses greater than 25 mg per day can cause QTc prolongation • May cause immune reconstitution syndrome, in which an inflammatory reaction develops due to a residual opportunistic infection or activation of an autoimmune disorder • Administer with a meal—not just a protein shake • Keep in original container • Monitor: viral load, CD4, cholesterol and triglycerides, LFTs

HIV Nucleoside and Nucleotide Reverse Transcriptase Inhibitors

Universal prescribing alerts:

Associated with:

- Lactic acidosis and severe hepatomegaly with steatosis: use with caution in patients at risk for liver disease.
- Pancreatitis: discontinue upon diagnosis.

Drug Name	FDA-Approved Indications	Adult Dosage Range	Precautions and Clinical Pearls
Generic Name Abacavir **Brand Name** Ziagen ■ ■ (PD)	Treatment of HIV infection when used with other antiretroviral agents	**Usual oral dose:** 300 mg twice daily 600 mg once daily	• Use with caution in patients with coronary heart disease • May cause fat redistribution • May cause immune reconstitution syndrome, in which an inflammatory reaction develops due to a residual opportunistic infection or activation of an autoimmune disorder • Ethanol can increase the risk of toxicity; avoid use • Monitor: CBC with differential, CK, CD4 count, HIV RNA levels, LFTs, triglycerides, amylase, HLA-B*5701 genotype testing before starting therapy, signs and symptoms of hypersensitivity reactions

Drug Name	FDA-Approved Indications	Adult Dosage Range	Precautions and Clinical Pearls
			Associated with: • Serious hypersensitivity reactions; testing for HLA-B*5701 allele is recommended before treatment as these patients are at an increased risk • Severe hepatotoxicity and/or lactic acidosis
Generic Name Didanosine **Brand Name** Videx Videx EC ▲ ■ (PD)	Treatment of HIV infection when used with other antiretroviral agents	**Usual oral dose:** For patients weighing 60 kg or more: Oral solution: 200 mg twice daily (preferred) or 400 mg once daily Capsule: 400 mg once daily	• May cause noncirrhotic portal hypertension: discontinue if signs and symptoms occur • May cause retinal changes and optic neuritis, peripheral neuropathy, and fat redistribution • Use with caution in patients with hepatic and renal impairment • Specific recommendations for patients undergoing dialysis • Drug interactions may require dose adjustments or avoidance of certain drug combinations • Dosing for patients weighing less than 60 kg is available; refer to PI • May cause immune reconstitution syndrome, in which an inflammatory reaction develops due to a residual opportunistic infection or activation of an autoimmune disorder • Administer on an empty stomach • Oral suspension needs to be mixed with antacid solution before dispensing • Monitor: viral load, CD4 count, potassium, uric acid, SCr, hemoglobin, CBC with neutrophil and platelet count, LFTs, bilirubin, albumin, INR, amylase, retinal exam every 6 months, ultrasonography if portal hypertension is suspected Associated with: • Hepatotoxicity and/or lactic acidosis • Pancreatitis
Generic Name Emtricitabine **Brand Name** Emtriva ▲ ■ (PD)	Treatment of HIV infection when used with other antiretroviral agents Recommended as initial therapy with other agents	**Usual oral dose:** Capsule: 200 mg once daily Solution: 240 mg once daily	• May cause fat redistribution • Use with caution in patients with renal impairment • Avoid use with lamivudine due to potential for cross-resistance • Capsules and solution are not interchangeable on a mg per mg basis • May cause immune reconstitution syndrome, in which an inflammatory reaction develops due to a residual opportunistic infection or activation of an autoimmune disorder • Monitor: viral load, CD4 count, LFTs, hepatitis B screening before initiating therapy • Specific recommendations for patients undergoing dialysis Associated with: • Coinfection with hepatitis B: severe exacerbations of HBV have occurred when discontinuing HIV therapy • Hepatotoxicity and/or lactic acidosis

Generic Name Lamivudine **Brand Name** Epivir Epivir HBV ▲ ■ (PD)	Treatment of HIV-1 infection when used with other antiretroviral agents Recommended for initial therapy (including in patients coinfected with HBV) when used with other agents Treatment of chronic hepatitis B (has not been studied in coinfected patients with HIV and is not recommended as first-line therapy)	**Usual oral dose:** 150 mg twice per day or 300 mg once per day	• May cause fat redistribution and pancreatitis • Use with caution in patients with renal impairment, not recommended in patients with impaired renal function. • Use caution when lamivudine is used in patients on interferon alfa (i.e., HIV/HBV-coinfected patients) due to increased risk of hepatotoxicity. Not recommended for use in patients with impaired hepatic function • Avoid use with emtricitabine due to potential for cross-resistance • May cause immune reconstitution syndrome, in which an inflammatory reaction develops due to a residual opportunistic infection or activation of an autoimmune disorder • Monitor: viral load; CD4 count; amylase; bilirubin; LFTs every 3 months; hematologic parameters; HBV DNA if treating for HBV; HBeAg and anti-HBe 1 year after starting HBV therapy, then every 3 to 6 months; signs/symptoms of relapse after stopping HBV treatment for several months Associated with: • Need to monitor patients after discontinuing therapy for hepatitis B: exacerbations may develop that require retreatment • HIV-1 resistance development if treating for chronic hepatitis B: if patients are unaware they have HIV-1, resistance can develop • Need to use Epivir HBV tablets or solution only for hepatitis B and not HIV infection • Hepatotoxicity and/or lactic acidosis
Generic Name Stavudine **Brand Name** Zerit ▲ ■ (PD)	Treatment of HIV infection when used with other antiretroviral agents	**Usual oral dose:** For patients weighing 60 kg or more: 40 mg every 12 hours	• May cause fat redistribution and peripheral neuropathy • May cause motor weakness: discontinue if it develops • Use with caution in patients with renal and hepatic impairment or preexisting bone marrow suppression • Avoid use with didanosine, hydroxyurea, and zidovudine due to increased risk of adverse events; use with caution when patients are also receiving interferon alfa • May cause immune reconstitution syndrome, in which an inflammatory reaction develops due to a residual opportunistic infection or activation of an autoimmune disorder • Doses for those weighing less than 60 kg are available; refer to PI Associated with: • Pancreatitis when used with certain other drugs upon diagnosis • Hepatotoxicity and/or lactic acidosis

Drug Name	FDA-Approved Indications	Adult Dosage Range	Precautions and Clinical Pearls

Generic Name
Tenofovir
 	
Brand Name
Viread
▲ ■ (PD)
	Treatment of HIV infection when used with other antiretroviral agents
	
	Recommended in initial regimen when used with other agents
	
	Treatment of chronic hepatitis B infection
		Usual oral dose:
		300 mg once daily
			• May cause fat redistribution, decrease in bone mineral density, osteomalacia, pancreatitis, or renal toxicity: avoid use in high-risk patients
			• Use with caution in patients with hepatic and renal impairment
			• If treating the patient for HBV, screen for HIV to ensure resistance will not develop to HIV
			• May cause immune reconstitution syndrome, in which an inflammatory reaction develops due to a residual opportunistic infection or activation of an autoimmune disorder
			• Mix powder with 2 to 4 ounces of soft food to avoid bitter taste
			• May need to supplement with calcium and vitamin D due to decrease in bone mineral density
			• Monitor:
			  • HIV: viral load, CD4 count, CBC with differential, reticulocyte count, CK, HIV RNA levels, phosphorus, SCr at baseline and throughout therapy, urine glucose and protein if at risk for renal impairment, LFTs, bone density if at risk, screen for HBV before use
			  • HBV: phosphorus, SCr, urine glucose and protein, bone density, HBV DNA every 3 to 6 months, HBeAg and anti-HBe, LFTs every 3 months and several months after therapy
			Associated with:
			• Severe exacerbations of HBV upon discontinuation
			• Monitor for relapse for several months
			• Hepatotoxicity and/or lactic acidosis

Generic Name Zidovudine **Brand Name** Retrovir ▲ ■ (PD)	Treatment of HIV infection when used with other antiretroviral agents	**Usual parenteral dose:** 1 mg/kg per dose every 4 hours around the clock **Usual oral dose:** 300 mg twice per day Oral therapy is preferred	• May cause fat redistribution • Use with caution in patients with hepatic and renal impairment • Specific recommendations for patients undergoing dialysis • May cause immune reconstitution syndrome, in which an inflammatory reaction develops due to a residual opportunistic infection or activation of an autoimmune disorder • If assay is negative for HIV in an infant who received preventive therapy, retest in 2 to 4 weeks to confirm diagnosis • The injection vial's stopper contains latex • Monitor: viral load, CD4 count, CBC with differential every 3 to 6 months, LFTs every 6 to 12 months, lipid profile, blood glucose levels Associated with: • Hematologic toxicity, including neutropenia and anemia; may need to interrupt therapy • Myopathy over prolonged use • Hepatotoxicity and/or lactic acidosis

Interferons

Drug Name	FDA-Approved Indications	Adult Dosage Range	Precautions and Clinical Pearls

Generic Name
Interferon alfa
 	
Brand Name
Intron
Alferon N
▲ ■ (PD)
	Alfa-2b: AIDS-related Kaposi sarcoma, chronic hepatitis B, chronic hepatitis C with other agents, condylomata acuminata, follicular lymphoma with other agents, and hairy cell leukemia; adjunct therapy for malignant melanoma
	
	Alferon N: condylomata acuminata
		Usual parenteral dose for AID's related Kaposi's sarcoma:
		IM/SQ: 30 million units/m^2 3 times per week until disease progression is confirmed or achievement of maximum response after 16 weeks of treatment
			• Causes bone marrow suppression, which can lead to anemia, neutropenia, and thrombocytopenia
			• In combination with ribavirin can cause dental and periodontal disorders, including dry mouth
			• Can cause hypertriglyceridemia, changes in vision and other eye disorders, pulmonary infections and other disorders, arrhythmias, thyroid disorders, strokes, and diabetes
			• Use with caution in patients with coagulation and pulmonary disorders
			• Recommended to administer acetaminophen before injection to reduce adverse effects
			• If dose is 10 million units/m^2 or greater, recommend using an antiemetic concurrently
			• Administration in the evening results in increased tolerability
			• Inject IM into the anterior thigh, deltoid, and superlateral buttock
			• IM injection is preferred; use SubQ administration if concerned about bleeding or thrombocytopenia
			• Continue to use the same brand for in the patient due to differences in dosages
			• Monitor:
			  • Baseline and as needed: chest x-ray, SCr, albumin, PTT
			  • Baseline and during therapy: CBC with differential; platelets (PLT); hemoglobin; LFTs; electrolytes; TSH; ophthalmic exams; ECG if preexisting cardiac conditions or advanced cancer; bilirubin; lactate dehydrogenase (LDH) at 2, 8, and 12 weeks, then every 6 months
			  • During therapy: weight, neuropsychiatric changes
			Contraindications:
			• Autoimmune hepatitis
			• Severe liver disease
			Associated with:
			• Causing or exacerbating neuropsychiatric disorders, including depression, psychosis, mania, suicidal ideation, and homicidal ideation: discontinue if symptoms worsen; usually is reversible upon discontinuation
			• Causing or exacerbating autoimmune diseases infectious disorders, and ischemic disorders: discontinue if symptoms worsen
			• Fever and flu-like symptoms associated with interferon administration requires extra caution in patients with cardiac disease
			• Hepatotoxicity, which can be fatal: discontinue if severe injury develops

Drug Name	FDA-Approved Indications	Adult Dosage Range	Precautions and Clinical Pearls
Generic Name Peginterferon alfa **Brand Name** Pegasys (2a) Peg-Intron (2b) Sylatron (2b) ▲ ■ ■ (PD)	Alfa-2a: chronic hepatitis B and chronic hepatitis C Hepatitis C should also be treated concurrently with antiviral medications Alfa-2b: chronic hepatitis C; adjunct therapy for melanoma	**Usual parenteral dose:** **Alfa-2a (Pegasys):** SQ: 180 mg once weekly **Alfa-2b PegIntron:** Max doses: SQ 1 mcg/kg per week for monotherapy or 1.5 mcg/kg per week for combination therapy **Alfa-2b Sylatron:** Max doses: SQ 6 mcg/kg per week	• Causes bone marrow suppression, which can lead to anemia, neutropenia, and thrombocytopenia • Can cause hepatotoxicity, which can be fatal: discontinue if severe injury develops • In patients with hepatitis B, flares may occur for ALT levels: reduce the dose and discontinue if ALT does not drop • Can cause serious skin reactions such as SJS and exfoliative dermatitis, flu-like symptoms, gastrointestinal ulcerative colitis and other serious disorders, hypertriglyceridemia, changes in vision and other eye disorders, pancreatitis, pulmonary infections and other disorders, arrhythmias, thyroid disorders, dental/periodontal disorders in combination therapy, and diabetes • Do not drink alcohol • Do not shake vial, syringe, or autoinjector • Warm by rolling between the palms of the hands for a vial and syringe; let the autoinjector warm by setting it outside the refrigerator • Caution patients about operating machinery and driving due to the potential for CNS depression • Continue to use the same brand for the patient due to differences in dosages • Monitor: CBC, hemoglobin, PLT, LFTs, and uric acid at weeks 1, 2, 4, 6, and 8, and every 4 to 6 weeks after; TSH every 12 weeks; ECG if preexisting cardiac disease; neuropsychiatric symptoms Contraindications: • Autoimmune hepatitis • Severe liver disease Associated with: • Causing or exacerbating neuropsychiatric disorders, including depression, psychosis, mania, suicidal ideation, and homicidal ideation: discontinue if symptoms worsen; usually is reversible upon discontinuation • Causing or exacerbating autoimmune diseases infectious disorders, and ischemic disorders: discontinue if symptoms worsen • Drug interactions that require dose adjustments or avoidance of certain drug combinations • Myocardial infarction and stroke

Neuraminidase Inhibitors			
Drug Name	**FDA-Approved Indications**	**Adult Dosage Range**	**Precautions and Clinical Pearls**
Generic Name Oseltamivir **Brand Name** Tamiflu ▲ (PD)	Prophylaxis against and treatment of influenza A and B Recommended to be used in patients at a higher risk for complications from influenza	**Usual oral dose:** 75 mg 1 to 2 times daily for 5 to 10 days Start within 48 hours of symptoms or contact with an infected individual	• Rarely causes neuropsychiatric adverse events, including confusion and hallucinations • Use with caution in patients with cardiovascular disease, severe hepatic impairment, renal impairment, and respiratory disease • Safety and efficacy have not been proved in immunocompromised patients • Monitor: signs and symptoms of neuropsychiatric changes
Generic Name Peramivir **Brand Name** Rapivab ▲	Treatment of acute influenza when patient has been symptomatic for 2 or fewer days	**Usual parenteral dose:** IV: 600 mg single dose	• May cause severe skin reactions, such as SJS • Infuse over 15 to 30 minutes • Administer within 48 hours of onset of flu symptoms • May cause neuropsychiatric events, such as delirium and hallucination: usually symptoms appear soon after use and in pediatric patients • Hypersensitivity reactions have been reported when peramivir is used with other neuraminidase inhibitors: caution is advised • Monitor: BUN and SCr, rash after administration
Generic Name Zanamivir **Brand Name** Relenza Diskhaler	Prophylaxis against and treatment of influenza A and B Recommended to be used in patients at a higher risk for complications from influenza	**Usual oral inhaled dose:** 2 inhalations 1 to 2 times daily for 5 days Treatment: begin within 2 days of symptoms Prophylaxis: begin within 36 hours to 5 days after contact with an infected person	• May cause neuropsychiatric adverse events, including confusion, seizures, and hallucinations • May cause bronchospasm: not recommended for use in patients with respiratory disease; discontinue if lung function decreases • Efficacy has not been established for use as prophylaxis in nursing homes • If patient needs a bronchodilator, use it before administering zanamivir • Monitor: signs and symptoms of neuropsychiatric changes and bronchospasm

Nucleosides and Nucleotides			
Drug Name	**FDA-Approved Indications**	**Adult Dosage Range**	**Precautions and Clinical Pearls**
Generic Name Acyclovir	Oral therapy: herpes zoster (shingles), genital herpes simplex virus, varicella (chickenpox)	**Usual oral dose for herpes zoster in immunocompetent patients:** 800 mg every 4 hours (5 times per day) for 7 to 10 days	• Can cause renal impairment: use with caution in patients at high risk • May cause thrombocytopenic purpura/hemolytic uremic syndrome in immunocompromised patients • Treatment for chickenpox should start within 24 hours of rash appearance if patient is at an increased risk of complications • Treatment for shingles should start within 72 hours of rash appearance

Drug Name	FDA-Approved Indications	Adult Dosage Range	Precautions and Clinical Pearls
Brand Name Zovirax Sitavig ▲ (PD)	Parenteral (IV) therapy: herpes simplex virus in immunocompromised patients, severe genital herpes simplex virus, herpes simplex encephalitis, herpes zoster (shingles) in immunocompromised patients Buccal tablet/cream: recurrent herpes labialis (cold sores) Ointment: genital herpes simplex virus and mild mucocutaneous herpes simplex virus infections in immunocompromised patients	**Usual parenteral dose for immunocompromised patients:** IV: 10 mg/kg per dose every 8 hours for 7 days **Topical:** Ointment: apply ½-inch ribbon per 4-inch square surface every 3 hours for 7 days Cream/ointment: apply 5 times per day for 4 days to lesions	• Use IV acyclovir with caution in patients with neurologic abnormalities, severe hepatic dysfunction, serious electrolyte imbalances, or significant hypoxia • If patient is obese, dose based on ideal body weight (IBW) • Keep well hydrated to help protect the kidneys • Infuse IV formulation over 1 hour to avoid kidney damage • Available also as a buccal tablet • If buccal tablet falls out within 6 hours of placement, replace the tablet or apply a new tablet: for maximum effect, apply 1 hour after prodromal symptoms are noted • Apply ointment while wearing a glove to prevent transmission of virus to other parts of the body • Monitor: urinalysis, BUN, SCr, LFTs, CBC
Generic Name Adefovir **Brand Name** Hepsera ▲ ■	Treatment of chronic hepatitis B if there is evidence of active viral replication	**Usual oral dose:** 10 mg once daily	• Do not use with tenofovir, as it decreases the efficacy of tenofovir • Not a first-line treatment • Monitor: HIV status before starting therapy, SCr at baseline and throughout therapy, LFTs for several months after stopping therapy, HBV DNA every 3 to 6 months while using adefovir, HBeAg and anti-HBe Associated with: • Severe lactic acidosis and hepatomegaly with steatosis when using nucleoside analogues: use with caution in patients with risk factors for liver dysfunction; interrupt therapy if signs and symptoms occur • Severe exacerbation of hepatitis B upon discontinuation: usually occurs within the first 12 weeks and may dissipate or resolve with initiating treatment • Risk of developing HIV resistance in patients who do not realize they are HIV infected: determine status before treatment • Nephrotoxicity: use with caution in patients at high risk for toxicity or with preexisting renal impairment

Generic Name Cidofovir **Brand Name** Vistide ▲ ■	Treatment of cytomegalovirus (CMV) retinitis in patients infected with AIDS	**Usual parenteral dose:** IV: 5 mg/kg per dose every other week while receiving maintenance therapy	• Reports of metabolic acidosis have been reported: monitor for signs and symptoms including low bicarbonate and renal wasting syndrome • Ensure proper hydration throughout • Can cause ocular dysfunction: monitor intraocular pressure; treat the patient with a topical steroid if uveitis or iritis occurs • Monitor: SCr and urine protein at baseline and within 48 hours prior to administering a dose, WBC with differential before each dose, intraocular pressure and visual acuity, signs and symptoms of uveitis/iritis and metabolic acidosis Contraindications: • Use of nephrotoxic agents with the last 7 days • Direct intraocular injection • SCr greater than 1.5 mg/dL, CrCl 55 mL per minute or less, or 2+ proteinuria Associated with: • Categorized as a possible carcinogen and teratogen based on animal data; can cause hypospermia • Renal failure and death when administering 1 to 2 doses: monitor renal function within 48 hours before administering a dose; must administer with probenecid and saline • Neutropenia
Generic Name Entecavir **Brand Name** Baraclude ▲ ■ (PD)	Treatment of chronic hepatitis B with evidence of active viral replication in patients with elevated transaminase or histologically active disease	**Usual oral dose:** 0.5 to 1 mg once daily	• Use with caution in patients with hepatic impairment • Administer on an empty stomach: food delays absorption • Available as tablet and solution • Cross-resistance may develop in patients who have failed lamivudine therapy: resistance can develop quickly • Monitor: HIV status before starting therapy; hepatic and renal function tests; if coinfected with HIV, monitor HIV viral load and CD4 count; HBV DNA every 3 months; HBeAg Associated with: • Severe lactic acidosis and hepatomegaly with steatosis when using nucleoside analogues: use with caution in patients with risk factors for liver dysfunction; interrupt therapy if signs and symptoms occur • Severe exacerbation of hepatitis B upon discontinuation: may dissipate or resolve with initiating treatment • Risk of developing HIV resistance in patients who do not realize they are HIV infected: determine status before treatment

Drug Name	FDA-Approved Indications	Adult Dosage Range	Precautions and Clinical Pearls
Generic Name Famciclovir **Brand Name** Famvir ▲	Treatment of herpes zoster (shingles), herpes labialis (cold sores), and recurrent orolabial/genital herpes simplex in HIV-infected patients Treatment and suppression of recurrent genital herpes	**Usual oral dose for treatment of herpes zoster:** 500 mg every 8 hours for 7 days Cold sores: 1500 mg once as single dose	• Use with caution in patients with renal impairment: dose appropriately • Treatment for shingles should start within 72 hours of rash's appearance • Monitor: CBC with extended use
Generic Name Ganciclovir **Brand Name** Cytovene Zirgan ▲ ■	Treatment of susceptible viruses that cause CMV retinitis in immunocompromised patients Prophylaxis against CMV infection in transplant patients	**Usual parenteral dose for CMV retinitis:** IV: 5 mg/kg per dose every 12 hours for a minimum of 14 days	• When handling, use hazardous precautions due to its extreme basic nature • Administer via slow IV infusion over 1 hour • Monitor: CBC with differential, platelet count, SCr Associated with: • Blood dyscrasias: may need to adjust or interrupt therapy until white blood cell levels increase • Carcinogenic and potential teratogenic effects
Generic Name Ribavirin **Brand Name** Copegus Moderiba Rebetol Ribasphere Virazole ▲ ■ (PD)	Chronic hepatitis C infection:	**Usual oral dose (tablets) for chronic hepatitis C with concurrent use of other recommended medications:** 1000 to 1200 mg per day in 2 divided doses daily Treatment duration and formulation selected is individualized based on patient's clinical status and dose is based on weight (patients weighing less than 75 kg are recommended to get lower dose)	• Use with caution in patients with hepatic and renal impairment • Risk of autoimmune/infectious disorders, bone marrow suppression, dental and periodontal disorders, dermatologic reactions such as SJS, diabetes, serious ophthalmic disorders, pancreatitis, psychiatric disorders, and pulmonary adverse events • Administer with food to increase absorption • Inhalation monitoring: respiratory function, hemoglobin, reticulocyte count, CBC with differential, ins and outs (I&O) • Oral monitoring: hematologic and biochemical tests before administration and during therapy, dental exam, ECG if preexisting cardiac disease exists, ophthalmic exam, TSH at week 12, pregnancy screening and tests monthly, HCV RNA before administration and at 12, 24, and 24 weeks after completion • Formulations have different indications for use; refer to PI prior to prescribing Contraindications: • Hemoglobinopathy and concurrent use of didanosine • CrCl less than 50 mL per minute • Hepatic decompensation in cirrhosis (when used with other specific agents) • Autoimmune hepatitis

			Associated with: • Hemolytic anemia: can worsen cardiac diseases; use with caution in patients at risk for anemia • Should not be used as monotherapy in patients with chronic hepatitis C • Sudden respiratory deterioration when initiating via inhalation in infants • Interference with effective ventilation; use of inhalation formulation in patients with assisted ventilation may increase risk
Generic Name Telbivudine **Brand Name** Tyzeka ▲ ■	Treatment of chronic hepatitis B with evidence of active viral replication in patients with elevated transaminase or histologically active disease	**Usual oral dose:** 600 mg once daily	• May cause myopathy and peripheral neuropathy: discontinue if either condition is diagnosed • Safety and efficacy have not been studied in African American and Hispanic subpopulations; in patients coinfected with HIV, hepatitis C, or hepatitis D; or in liver transplant patients • Cross-resistance may develop in patients who failed to respond to lamivudine • Not considered first-line therapy due to the high rate of resistance • Monitor: LFTs during therapy and post therapy, renal function tests before initiating and during use, CK, HBV DNA every 3 to 6 months, HBeAg and anti-Hbe • Specific recommendations for patients undergoing dialysis. Associated with: • Severe lactic acidosis and hepatomegaly with steatosis when using nucleoside analogues: use with caution in patients with risk factors for liver dysfunction; interrupt therapy if signs and symptoms occur • Severe exacerbation of hepatitis B upon discontinuation: may dissipate or resolve with initiating treatment
Generic Name Valacyclovir **Brand Name** Valtrex ▲ (PD)	Treatment of susceptible viruses that cause shingles, genital herpes, suppression of genital herpes in immunocompetent and HIV-infected patients, cold sores, and chickenpox	**Usual oral dose:** 1 to 2 g 2 times per day for 1 to 7 days Dose and duration are individualized based on type of episode and severity of infection	• May cause CNS effects such as hallucinations, delirium, seizures, and encephalopathy • Thrombotic thrombocytopenic purpura/hemolytic uremic syndrome has occurred in immunocompromised patients: use caution with doses of 8 g per day • Has not been studied in severely immunocompromised patients: use with caution when CD4 is less than 100 cells/mm3 • Start treatment as soon as symptoms arise: treatment for shingles and genital herpes should begin within 72 hours (24 hours if recurrent genital herpes) • Monitor: urinalysis, BUN, SCr, LFTs, CBC

Drug Name	FDA-Approved Indications	Adult Dosage Range	Precautions and Clinical Pearls
Generic Name Valganciclovir **Brand Name** Valcyte ▲ ■ (PD)	Treatment of cytomegalovirus (CMV) retinitis in patients with AIDS Prevention of CMV disease in high-risk patients who are getting a kidney, heart, or pancreas transplant	**Usual oral dose:** 900 mg once or twice per day depending on indication for use and severity of infection	• Can cause renal failure: keep patient well hydrated and use with caution with other nephrotoxic agents • Manufacturer recommends tablets over solution in adults • Administer with meals to increase absorption • Use gloves to avoid contact with crushed tablets, powder from solution, and oral solution due to their carcinogenic and mutagenic potential • Monitor: ophthalmic exam every 4 to 6 weeks when treating CMV retinitis, CBC, platelet count, SCr at baseline and throughout therapy Associated with: • Blood dyscrasias: may need to adjust or interrupt therapy until white blood cell levels increase • Carcinogenic and potential teratogenic effects
HCV Antiviral Agents			
NS5B Polymerase Inhibitors			
Drug Name	**FDA-Approved Indications**	**Adult Dosage Range**	**Precautions and Clinical Pearls**
Generic Name Dasabuvir **Brand Name** Viekira Pak (in combination with ombitasvir, paritaprevir, and ritonavir)	Treatment of chronic hepatitis C with or without coinfection of HCV/HIV-1 when used with other medication For genotypes 1b and 1a without cirrhosis or with compensated cirrhosis	**Usual oral dose:** 250 mg 2 times per day	• May cause hepatic decompensation, and ALT elevation • Drug interactions may require dose adjustments • Viekira Pak and Viekira SR are not interchangeable on a mg per mg basis • Take with food for optimal absorption • Dispense in original container • Monitor: hepatic function tests, serum HCV RNA, hepatic decomposition if patient has cirrhosis
Generic Name Sofosbuvir **Brand Name** Sovaldi	Treatment of chronic hepatitis C with or without infection of HCV/HIV-1 with other medications Genotypes 1, 2, 3, and 4	**Usual oral dose:** 400 mg daily with ribavirin and with or without peginterferon alfa for 12 to 24 weeks or until liver transplant for patients with hepatocellular carcinoma	• Can cause bradycardia when used with amiodarone • Dispense in original container • Monitor: bilirubin, LFTs, SCr, inpatient EKG monitoring for 48 hours when on amiodarone and self-monitoring for 2 weeks of heart rate, serum HCV RNA • Can be used for treatment naïve patients and those with prior relapse able to receive interferon products

NS3/4A Protease Inhibitors

Drug Name	FDA-Approved Indications	Adult Dosage Range	Precautions and Clinical Pearls
Generic Name Grazoprevir **Brand Name** Zepatier (in combination with elbasvir)	Treatment of chronic hepatitis C infection with or without cirrhosis and with or without infection of HCV/HIV-1 Genotypes 1a, 1b, and 4	**Usual oral dose:** 100 mg once per day for 12 to 16 weeks	• Keep in original container until use • Drug interactions may require dose adjustments • May cause elevated ALT: discontinue if ALT remains higher than 10 times the upper limit of normal • Monitor: hepatic function tests at baseline, week 8, and week 12; testing for NS5A resistance for genotype 1a; serum HCV RNA at baseline, weeks 4, 8, and 12, and during follow-up
Generic Name Paritaprevir **Brand Name** Technivie (in combination with ombitasvir and ritonavir) Viekira Pak (in combination with ombitasvir, ritonavir, and dasabuvir) ■	Treatment of chronic hepatitis C with or without coinfection of HCV/HIV-1 when used with other medication Genotypes 1b and 1a without cirrhosis or with compensated cirrhosis (Viekira) Genotype 4 without cirrhosis (Technivie)	**Usual oral dose:** Technivie: 2 tablets every morning for 12 weeks Viekira Pak: 2 tablets every morning for 12 to 24 weeks	• May cause hepatic decompensation, and ALT elevation • Drug interactions may require dose adjustments • Take with food for optimal absorption • Dispense in original container • Monitor: hepatic function tests, serum HCV RNA, hepatic decomposition if patient has cirrhosis • Discontinue Technivie if ALT is continuously greater than 10 times ULN
Generic Name Simeprevir **Brand Name** Olysio	Treatment of chronic hepatitis C for 12 to 24 weeks in combination with other medications Genotypes 1 and 4	**Usual oral dose:** 150 mg once daily	• May cause hepatic decomposition; photosensitivity when used with peginterferon alfa and ribavirin, which has led to hospitalization; and rash, which usually appears within 4 weeks of therapy initiation • Drug interactions may require dose adjustments • Administer with food • Dispense in original container • Monitor: bilirubin and liver enzymes; serum HCV RNA at baseline and weeks 4, 12, and 24; screen for NS3 Q80K polymorphism for genotype 1a; inpatient EKG monitoring for 48 hours when on amiodarone and self-monitoring for 2 weeks of heart rate

NS5A Replication Complex Inhibitors

Drug Name	FDA-Approved Indications	Adult Dosage Range	Precautions and Clinical Pearls
Generic Name Daclatasvir **Brand Name** Daklinza	Treatment of chronic hepatitis C with or without compensated cirrhosis Genotypes 1 and 3	**Usual oral dose:** 60 mg once daily with sofosbuvir for 12 to 24 weeks and with or without ribavirin	• May cause bradycardia when used with amiodarone; use with caution in patients with cardiovascular diseases and hepatic disease • Drug interactions may require dose adjustments • Monitor: screen for NS5A polymorphisms for genotype 1a in patients with cirrhosis; LFTs; SCr; inpatient EKG monitoring for 48 hours when on amiodarone and self-monitoring for 2 weeks of heart rate
Generic Name Elbasvir **Brand Name** Zepatier (in combination with grazoprevir)	Treatment of chronic hepatitis C infection with or without cirrhosis and with or without infection of HCV/HIV-1 Genotypes 1a, 1b, and 4	**Usual oral dose:** 50 mg once daily for 12 to 16 weeks	• Keep in original container until use • Drug interactions may require dose adjustments • May cause elevated ALT: discontinue if ALT remains higher than 10 times the upper limit of normal (moderate to severe hepatic impairment) • Monitor: hepatic function tests at baseline and weeks 8 and 12; testing for NS5A resistance for genotype 1a; serum HCV RNA at baseline, weeks 4, 8, and 12, and during follow-up
Generic Name Ledipasvir **Brand Name** Harvoni (in combination with sofosbuvir)	Treatment of chronic hepatitis C with or without infection of HCV/HIV with or without ribavirin Genotypes 1, 4, 5, and 6	**Usual oral dose:** 90 mg once daily for 12 to 24 weeks	• Can cause bradycardia when used with amiodarone • Dispense in original container • Monitor: bilirubin, LFTs, SCr, inpatient EKG monitoring for 48 hours when on amiodarone and self-monitoring for 2 weeks of heart rate, serum HCV RNA
Generic Name Ombitasvir **Brand Name** Technivie (in combination with paritaprevir and ritonavir)	Treatment of chronic hepatitis C with or without coinfection of HCV/HIV when used with other medication Genotypes 1b and 1a without cirrhosis or with compensated cirrhosis (Viekira)	**Usual oral dose:** Technivie: 2 tablets every morning for 12 weeks Viekira Pak: 2 tablets every morning for 12 to 24 weeks	• Contraindicated in patients with moderate to severe hepatic impairment and ribavirin use • May cause QTc prolongation that is concentration dependent (Viekira only), hepatic decompensation, and ALT elevation • Drug interactions may require dose adjustments • Take with food for optimal absorption • Dispense in original container • Monitor: hepatic function tests, serum HCV RNA, hepatic decomposition if patient has cirrhosis

Viekira Pak (in combination with paritaprevir, ritonavir, and dasabuvir)	Genotype 4 without cirrhosis (Technivie)		• Discontinue Technivie if ALT is continuously greater than 10 times ULN • Viekira Pak and Viekira XR are not interchangeable on a mg per mg basis

Miscellaneous Antiviral Agents

Drug Name	FDA-Approved Indications	Adult Dosage Range	Precautions and Clinical Pearls
Generic Name Foscarnet **Brand Name** Foscavir	Treatment of acyclovir-resistant mucocutaneous herpes simplex virus infections in immunocompromised patients Treatment of CMV retinitis in patients with AIDS	**Usual parenteral dose for herpes simplex indication:** IV: 40 mg/kg per dose every 8 to 12 hours for 2 to 3 weeks or until lesions are healed	• May cause anemia, and granulocytopenia • May cause electrolyte imbalances: correct before initiating treatment • Some products contain sodium: use with caution in patients with heart failure • Foscarnet is a vascular irritant; administer into a vein with adequate blood flow • Monitor: 24-hour CrCl at baseline and throughout therapy; during induction, monitor CBC and electrolytes twice weekly, then weekly during maintenance therapy; hydration status Associated with: • Renal impairment: most patients will experience some degree of renal impairment; reduce dose if needed and monitor carefully • Seizures associated with electrolyte imbalance

Antiprotozoal Agents

Amebicides

Drug Name	FDA-Approved Indications	Adult Dosage Range	Precautions and Clinical Pearls
Generic Name Iodoquinol **Brand Name** Yodoxin	Treatment of intestinal amebiasis Trophozoite and cyst forms of *Entamoeba histolytica*	**Usual oral dose:** 650 mg 3 times per day for 20 days (max 1.95 g per day)	• May cause optic atrophy/neuritis: avoid extended use at high doses and use with caution in elderly patients • May cause peripheral neuropathy: avoid extended use at high doses • Use with caution in patients with thyroid abnormalities • Administer after meals • Monitor: ophthalmologic exam with extended use Contraindications: • Hepatic impairment

Drug Name	FDA-Approved Indications	Adult Dosage Range	Precautions and Clinical Pearls
Generic Name Paromomycin **Brand Name** Humatin	Intestinal amebiasis Hepatic coma adjunct or encephalopathy	**Usual oral dose for hepatic coma:** 4 g daily in divided doses for 5 to 10 days **Intestinal amebiasis:** 25 to 35 mg/kg per day in 3 divided doses for 7 to 10 days	• Patients with ulcerative bowel lesions may experience renal toxicity due to increased absorption • Administer with food • Alternative agent; not first-line therapy • Not effective for extra-intestinal amebiasis • Contraindicated in: intestinal obstruction
Metronidazole	Refer to the Miscellaneous Antiprotozoal Agents section.		
Antimalarial Agents			
Drug Name	FDA-Approved Indications	Adult Dosage Range	Precautions and Clinical Pearls
Generic Name Artemether and lumefantrine **Brand Name** Coartem QT PD	Treatment of uncomplicated malaria due to *Plasmodium falciparum* Sensitive to regions with chloroquine resistance	**Usual oral dose:** 4 tablets per dose (20 mg artemether/120 mg lumefantrine per tablet); treat with a 3-day oral regimen with a total of 6 doses including the initial dose, then a second dose 8 hours later, then 1 dose PO twice daily (morning and evening) for the next 2 days for a total course of 24 tablets	• May cause QTc prolongation • Drug interactions may require dose adjustment: avoid use of grapefruit juice because it increases the concentration of the medication • Use with caution in patients with hepatic and renal impairment • Administer with a full meal to increase absorption: if vomiting occurs within 2 hours of swallowing tablets, readminister • If malaria returns, treat with a different medication • Monitor: adequate food intake with medication, ECG if patients is concurrently taking other medications that can cause QTc prolongation
Generic Name Atovaquone and proguanil **Brand Name** Malarone ▲ PD	Treatment of uncomplicated malaria due to *Plasmodium falciparum* Sensitive to regions with chloroquine resistance Malaria prophylaxis due to *Plasmodium falciparum*	**Usual oral dose:** Prevention: 250 mg/100 mg once daily starting 1 to 2 days before entering malaria region, throughout stay, and 7 days after leaving Treatment: 1000 mg/400 mg once daily for 3 days	• Can cause hepatic impairment and rarely hepatic failure: use with caution in patients with preexisting renal function impairment • Diarrhea/vomiting can decrease the absorption of the medication: use an antiemetic or alternative therapy • Administer with food or milk: if patient vomits within 1 hour after taking dose, readminister • In patients who weigh more than 100 kg, treatment failure has been reported: follow up after completion of therapy to ensure cure • Monitor: hepatic and renal function, cure in patients weighing more than 100 kg Contraindications: • Use as prophylaxis if CrCl less than 30 mL per minute

Generic Name Chloroquine **Brand Name** Aralen QT PD	Suppressive treatment and acute treatment of malaria *P. vivax*, *P. malariae*, *P. ovale*, *P. falciparum* Several regions have highly resistant strands of *P. falciparum* Treatment of extraintestinal amebiasis	**Usual oral dose (phosphate):** Chemoprophylaxis: 500 mg weekly 1 to 2 weeks before exposure, during travel, and 4 weeks after Treatment: 1 g on day 1, then 500 mg 6 hours, 24 hours, and 48 hours after first dose Amebiasis: 1 g daily for 2 days, then 500 mg daily for 2 to 3 weeks	• Can cause ECG changes along with QTc prolongation: use with caution in patients with preexisting QTc prolongation • Can cause extrapyramidal effects that resolve after finishing therapy or treating the symptoms • May can cause hematologic effects, including agranulocytosis: discontinue if severe • May can cause myopathy or neuromyopathy: discontinue if weakness occurs • Can cause severe ophthalmic damage, including macular degeneration: monitor closely and discontinue if signs and symptoms occur • Patients with G6PD deficiency are at higher risk of hemolytic anemia • Use with caution in patients with hepatic impairment, porphyria, psoriasis, and seizures due to exacerbations • Chloroquine phosphate to base equivalence data are available in the package insert • Monitor: ophthalmic exams at baseline and with extended use, CBC with extended use • Drug interactions may require dose adjustments Contraindications: • History of retinal or visual changes due to 4-aminoquinoline compounds or due to other etiology
Generic Name Hydroxychloroquine **Brand Name** Plaquenil ■ PD	Suppressive treatment and acute treatment of malaria Treatment of systemic lupus erythematosus Treatment of rheumatoid arthritis (RA) Not effective against chloroquine-resistant *P. falciparum*	**Usual oral dose:** Chemoprophylaxis: 400 mg once weekly starting 2 weeks before and continuing for 8 weeks after exposure Treatment: 800 mg, then 400 mg at 6, 24, and 48 hours after first dose	• May cause cardiomyopathy with extended use • May cause hematologic effects, including agranulocytosis: discontinue if severe • May cause myopathy or neuromyopathy: discontinue if weakness occurs • May cause severe ophthalmic damage, including loss of visual acuity: monitor closely and discontinue if signs and symptoms occur • Patients with G6PD deficiency are at higher risk of hemolytic anemia • Use with caution in patients with hepatic impairment, porphyria, and psoriasis, due to exacerbations • Hydroxychloroquine sulfate to base (and chloroquine phosphate) equivalence data are available in the package insert • Chloroquine is preferred to hydroxychloroquine • Refer to CDC guidelines for alternative schedules and dosing based on infection surveillance • Administer with food or milk • Monitor: CBC at baseline and throughout therapy, LFTs, ophthalmic exam at baseline and every 3 months with extended use, muscle strength with extended use

Drug Name	FDA-Approved Indications	Adult Dosage Range	Precautions and Clinical Pearls
			Contraindications: • History of retinal or visual changes due to 4-aminoquinoline compounds Associated with: • Should be prescribed only by clinicians familiar with the medication (requires experienced clinician)
Generic Name Mefloquine **Brand Name** Lariam ■ PD QT	Treatment of mild to moderate malaria infections due to *P. falciparum* and *P. vivax* Sensitive to chloroquine-resistant *P. falciparum* Prophylaxis against malaria	**Usual oral dose:** Chemoprophylaxis: 250 mg once weekly beginning 1 or 2 weeks prior to exposure, continuing weekly during exposure and 4 weeks after exposure Treatment: 1250 mg once	• Reports of agranulocytosis and anemia have occurred • Can cause ECG changes and QTc prolongation: use with caution in patients with preexisting QTc prolongation • Drug interactions may require dose adjustments • Use with caution in patients with cardiovascular disease, impaired hepatic function, and seizures • Administer with food and at least 8 ounces of water: if vomiting occurs 30 minutes after dose, readminister; if vomiting occurs 30 to 60 minutes after dose, administer half the dose • If treating for *P. vivax*, also give an 8-aminoquinoline derivative to prevent relapse • Resistance has developed in Southeast Asia: do not use mefloquine in this region • Monitor: LFTs, ophthalmic exams, and for neuropsychiatric adverse events with extended use • Refer to CDC guidelines for alternative schedules and dosing based on infection surveillance Contraindications: • Use as prophylaxis in patients with a history of seizure or major psychiatric disorder Associated with: • Neuropsychiatric adverse events that can outlast therapy (including but not limited to seizures and psychosis): discontinue if they occur during use
Generic Name Primaquine Primaquine phosphate QT	Used to prevent relapse of *P. vivax* malaria	**Usual oral dose:** 15 mg once daily with chloroquine for 14 days	• Can cause ECG changes and QTc prolongation: use with caution in patients with preexisting QTc prolongation • Can cause hematologic effects, including anemia, methemoglobinemia, and leukopenia: discontinue if signs and symptoms occur • Patients with G6PD deficiency are at higher risk of hemolytic anemia • Use with caution in patients with hepatic impairment, porphyria, psoriasis, and seizures due to exacerbations • Primaquine base to phosphate equivalence data are available in the package insert • Administer with meals to lessen gastrointestinal upset: if patient vomits within 30 minutes of taking dose, readminister

			• May have cross-resistance with other aminoquinolines • Use with caution in patients with NADH methemoglobin reductase deficiency: methemoglobinemia is more likely to occur • Monitor: screen for G6PD deficiency before initiating therapy, CBC, check urine for darkening color (hematologic symptom), glucose, electrolytes, ECG in patients at high risk for QTc prolongation • If hemolysis is suspected during treatment, monitor CBC, haptoglobin, peripheral smear, and urinalysis dipstick for occult blood Contraindications: • Acutely ill patients who may develop granulocytopenia (systemic lupus erythematosus, rheumatoid arthritis) • Concurrent use of medications that can cause hemolytic anemia or bone marrow suppression • Concurrent or recent use of quinacrine
Generic Name Pyrimethamine **Brand Name** Daraprim (PD)	Chemoprophylaxis of malaria Resistance to pyrimethamine has developed worldwide Treatment of malaria and toxoplasmosis in combination with a sulfonamide	**Usual oral dose for toxoplasmosis:** 50 to 75 mg once per day, in combination with sulfonamide for 1 to 3 weeks	• Can cause hematologic effects, including megaloblastic anemia, thrombocytopenia, and leukopenia: monitor CBC and PLT twice weekly when treating for toxoplasmosis; discontinue if signs and symptoms occur • Patients with G6PD deficiency are at higher risk of hemolytic anemia • Use with caution in patients with folate deficiency, hepatic impairment, renal impairment, and seizures • Administer with meals to decrease gastrointestinal upset • Pyrimethamine can cause folic acid deficiency: supplement with leucovorin • Monitor: CBC; CBC and platelet count twice weekly when treating for toxoplasmosis; liver and renal function tests • Drug interactions may require dose adjustments Contraindications: • Megaloblastic anemia due to folate deficiency
Generic Name Quinine **Brand Name** Qualaquin ▲ ■ (QT)	Treatment of uncomplicated chloroquine-resistant *P. falciparum* malaria with the use of other agents	**Usual oral dose:** 648 mg every 8 hours for 7 days; administer with tetracycline, doxycycline, or clindamycin	• Drug interactions may require dose adjustments • Can cause severe hypersensitivity reactions such as SJS: discontinue if signs and symptoms occur • Can cause hypoglycemia • Immune-related thrombocytopenia, including hemolytic uremic syndrome/thrombotic thrombocytopenic purpura, has been reported: usually resolves within 1 week of discontinuation • Can cause QTc prolongation: use with caution in patients with preexisting arrhythmias • Do not use in patients with severe hepatic or renal impairment

Drug Name	FDA-Approved Indications	Adult Dosage Range	Precautions and Clinical Pearls
			• Do not take with antacids containing aluminum or magnesium due to decreased absorption • Swallow tablet whole to avoid bitter taste • Can cause false-positive results for opioids in the urine • Can cause false-positive results for steroids in the urine when using Zimmerman assay • Monitor: CBC, platelet count, LFTs, blood glucose, ECG, ophthalmic exam • Refer to CDC guidelines for alternative schedules and dosing based on infection surveillance Contraindications: • Prolonged QTc interval • Myasthenia gravis • Optic neuritis • G6PD deficiency Associated with: • Serious and life-threatening hematologic reactions • Benefit does not outweigh risk for the treatment of nocturnal leg cramps
Quinidine	Refer to the Cardiovascular Agents chapter.		

Miscellaneous Antiprotozoal Agents			
Drug Name	FDA-Approved Indications	Adult Dosage Range	Precautions and Clinical Pearls
Generic Name Atovaquone **Brand Name** Mepron	Treatment of mild to moderate *Pneumocystis jirovecii* pneumonia (PCP) in patients who cannot take trimethoprim–sulfamethoxazole (TMP-SMZ) Prophylaxis against PCP in patients who cannot use TMP-SMZ	**Usual oral dose:** 1500 mg once daily or 750 mg twice daily	• Use with caution in patients with gastrointestinal disorders: may impair absorption • Use with caution in patients with hepatic impairment • Must be administered with food, preferably high fat • Absorption may be inadequate if patient has diarrhea/vomiting: give with an antiemetic • Monitor: hepatic function tests at baseline and as needed, CD4 count for maintenance treatment in toxoplasmosis, patient's tolerability to ingest atovaquone

Generic Name Metronidazole **Brand Name** Flagyl Metro MetroCream Metrogel MetroLotion Noritate Nuvessa Rosadan Vandazole ■ ■ (PD)	Treatment of susceptible organisms that cause intestinal amebiasis, amebic liver abscess, anaerobic bacterial infections, bacterial septicemia, bone and joint infections, CNS infections, endocarditis, gynecologic infections, intra-abdominal infections, lower respiratory infections, skin and skin structure infections, bacterial vaginosis, and trichomoniasis *(for example: Bacteroides, Clostridium, Peptococcus, Peptostreptococcus, Fusobacterium, Eubacterium, Trichomonas vaginalis)* Perioperative colorectal surgery prophylaxis Topical: bacterial vaginosis and rosacea	**Usual oral dose for trichomoniasis:** 500 mg twice daily, or may alternatively use 250 mg 3 times daily for 7 days (max oral/IV: 4 g per day) **Usual vaginal dose for bacterial vaginosis (product dependent):** One applicatorful 1 to 2 times per day for 5 days day for 1 to 5 days **Usual topical dose:** Apply 1 to 2 times per day	• May cause CNS effects including aseptic meningitis, encephalopathy, seizures, peripheral neuropathy, and optic neuropathy: avoid chronic therapy with high doses • May cause leukopenia: use with caution in patients with history of blood dyscrasias • Use with caution in patients with ESRD: accumulation may occur • Can cause *C. difficile*–associated diarrhea and pseudomembranous colitis with extended use • IV solution should not come in contact with aluminum equipment • Administer ER formulation on an empty stomach • Avoid use of ER tablets in patients with severe hepatic impairment if possible • Injection contains 28 mEq sodium/g: use with caution in patients with sodium-retaining states (e.g., heart failure, edema) • May disrupt AST, ALT, TAG, glucose, and LDH results • Monitor: CBC with differential at baseline and with extended use • IV formulations are available for specific FDA approved indications including surgical prophylaxis Contraindications: • Use of disulfiram in the previous 2 weeks • Ethanol use during therapy and 3 days after the last dose Associated with: • Carcinogenicity in animal data: use only if needed
Generic Name Nitazoxanide **Brand Name** Alinia (PD)	Treatment of diarrhea caused by *Cryptosporidium parvum* or *Giardia lamblia*	**Usual oral dose:** 500 mg every 12 hours for 3 days	• Use with caution in patients with hepatic and renal impairment • Safety and efficacy have not been established in HIV-infected and immunocompromised patients • Administer with food
Generic Name Pentamidine **Brand Name** Nebupent Pentam (QT)	Treatment of pneumonia caused by *Pneumocystis jirovecii* (IM, IV)	**Usual parenteral dose:** IM/IV: 4 mg/kg once daily for 14 to 21 days	• May cause hypotension: monitor after infusion • May cause QTc prolongation: use with caution in patients with preexisting cardiovascular disease • May cause anemia, leukopenia, thrombocytopenia, pancreatitis, and SJS • Use with caution in patients with diabetes: can cause abnormal glucose levels • Use with caution in patients with hepatic and renal impairment, hypocalcemia, and asthma (when using the nebulizer)

Drug Name	FDA-Approved Indications	Adult Dosage Range	Precautions and Clinical Pearls
	Prophylaxis against PCP in high-risk, HIV-infected patients with a history of PCP or with a CD4+ count less than or equal to 200/mm^3 (inhalation)	**Usual inhalation dose:** 300 mg nebulized once every 4 weeks	• Do not dilute with normal saline • Refer to PI for specific nebulizing equipment (Respirgard II nebulizer) • Pentamidine is vesicant-like: avoid extravasation • Drug interactions may require dose adjustments • Monitor: liver and renal function tests, blood glucose, potassium and calcium, CBC and platelets, ECG, blood pressure
Generic Name Tinidazole **Brand Name** Tindamax ■ (PD)	Treatment of trichomoniasis caused by *T. vaginalis*, giardiasis caused by *G. duodenalis*, intestinal amebiasis and amebic liver abscess caused by *E. histolytica*, bacterial vaginosis caused by Bacteroides, Gardnerella vaginalis, and Prevotella in nonpregnant women	**Usual oral dose:** 2 g per day for 1 to 5 days; duration is dependent on type and severity of infection	• May cause seizures or peripheral neuropathy • Use with caution in patients with hepatic impairment or history of blood dyscrasia • Can cause *C. difficile*–associated diarrhea and pseudomembranous colitis with extended use • Administer with food • Avoid ethanol during treatment and 3 days after to prevent a disulfiram-like reaction • May interfere with AST, ALT, triglycerides, glucose, and LDH testing Associated with: • Carcinogenic properties; avoid unnecessary use
Dapsone	Refer to the Antimycobacterial Agents section.		

Chapter 3

Antineoplastic Agents

Author: **Jeffrey Lombardo, PharmD, BCOP**

Co-author: **Shannon Gowen, PharmD**

Editor: **Gene D. Morse, PharmD, FCCP, BCPS**

Learning Objectives

- Identify current pharmacologic agents that are appropriate for each condition/diagnosis.
- Recommend optimal pharmacologic interventions based on patient-specific characteristics.
- Provide appropriate patient-specific counseling points and optimal overall medication management.

Key Terms: antineoplastic agents, antibiotic agents, antimetabolite, folate antagonist, purine antagonist, pyrimidine antagonist, DNA agents, alkylating agents, nitrosourea, DNA cross-linking agents, enzymes, histone deacetylase inhibitors, hormone, hormone modifier, immunosuppressant, monoclonal antibody, tyrosine kinase inhibitor, topoisomerase inhibitor, anthracycline, camptothecin, podophyllotoxin, platinum complex, retinoid, taxane, vinca alkaloid

Overview of Antineoplastic Agents

Cancer Chemotherapy

Antineoplastic agents are any of several drugs that control or kill neoplastic cells and are used in chemotherapy to kill cancer cells. To understand the pharmacology of antineoplastic agents, it is important to first understand a basic background of how normal cells behave and what can—and often does—go wrong. In normal cells, the rates of cell division and cell death are tightly regulated. However, cancerous cells are able to evade these regulatory mechanisms and proliferate uncontrollably. The transformation of normal cells into cancerous cells can result from genetic mutations, exposure to chemicals in an occupation or from lifestyle habits such as cigarette smoking, or through exposure to environmental factors such as ultraviolet light. Many cancers present in an advanced stage; at this point, the purpose of treatment is palliation of symptoms emanating from the tumor. For this reason, screening is very important for early detection and treatment.

Chemotherapy is the use of drugs to slow the growth of, or kill, cancerous cells. Traditional chemotherapy agents target rapidly dividing cells, which include many types of normal cells. The cells in the body that are primarily affected by traditional chemotherapy include those that line the mouth and gastrointestinal tract, those found in bone marrow, and those in the hair follicles. Their targeting results in the common side effects of traditional chemotherapy—namely, nausea, diarrhea, bone marrow suppression, and hair loss. A decrease in the number of white blood cells caused by chemotherapy can increase the patient's risk for infections, fewer red blood cells can contribute to feelings of fatigue, and a lowered platelet count can increase the risk of bleeding.

While traditional chemotherapy is still the treatment of choice for many types of cancer, development of targeted therapies has led to new options for patients in recent years. These agents are specific for a certain tumor marker or molecule involved in the abnormal signaling process that leads to cancer cell growth and proliferation. When these antineoplastic agents are used, the side effects seen with traditional chemotherapy agents occur less frequently, but are replaced by other drug-specific side effects, such as acneiform rash as seen with the use of epidermal growth factor receptor (EGFR) inhibitors. Nevertheless, targeted therapies generally have a more tolerable side-effect profile in comparison to the traditional agents.

Many physical, chemical, and biologic agents are known to cause cancer by damaging DNA. Ionizing radiation and ultraviolet light are environmental factors that lead to the formation of free radicals that damage the body's DNA. Ultraviolet light exposure from the sun and tanning booths increases the risk of skin cancers. In addition, certain occupations can increase a person's risk of cancer through prolonged exposure to high levels of carcinogenic chemicals such as asbestos, formaldehyde, benzene, and arsenic. Lifestyle choices such as tobacco smoking and heavy alcohol consumption can also increase one's cancer risk. Some viruses are associated with cancer, such as Epstein-Barr virus with Burkitt lymphoma and human papillomavirus (HPV) with cervical cancer. Conventional anticancer agents, such as cyclophosphamide, etoposide, and doxorubicin, can increase the risk of secondary malignancies. Other risk factors for the development of cancer include age, diet, obesity, genetics, and chronic inflammation.

There are three major classes of genes that, when altered, can contribute to uncontrolled cell growth: tumor suppressor genes, proto-oncogenes, and DNA repair genes.

- Tumor suppressor genes normally inhibit inappropriate cell growth and division. If a tumor suppressor gene is mutated or inactivated, this state can lead to uncontrolled cell proliferation. Mutation of *p53* is one of the most common forms of tumor suppressor gene modifications seen and is associated with many malignancies.
- Proto-oncogenes normally play a role in regulating cellular functions. Their genetic alteration can lead to activation of an oncogene, which results in overexpression or abnormality of the gene product. The human epidermal growth factor receptor (HER) family comprises a variety of oncogenes associated with cancers of the breast, prostate, ovary, and colon.
- DNA repair genes are responsible for correcting errors that occur during DNA replication or from environmental factors. An alteration in these genes can lead to the accumulation of mutations over time, which increases the risk of cancer developing.

Cancer Treatment Modalities

Surgery, radiation, chemotherapy, hormonal therapy, targeted therapy, and biologic therapy are the cancer treatment modalities that are currently available. In many cases, patients will receive a combination of these modalities, either concurrently or sequentially, to optimize their outcomes.

Chemotherapy is a systemic treatment, administered through a variety of routes including oral, IM, SQ, IV, and intrathecally (the latter in some very specific cases). The use of systemic treatment to eliminate micrometastatic disease after surgery or radiation is called adjuvant therapy. When it is administered, the goal is to prevent recurrence of the cancer and improve survival. Systemic therapy can also be given prior to surgery or radiation; in this case, it is called neoadjuvant therapy. The purpose of neoadjuvant therapy is to reduce the tumor burden and to increase the effectiveness of the local treatment.

Biologic therapy is unique in that it uses the body's own immune system to facilitate the killing of cancerous cells. Promising and ongoing research is investigating PD-1 inhibitors, a class of immunotherapy drugs that are currently approved to treat melanoma, non-small cell lung cancer (NSCLC), and renal cell cancer. Side effects of the PD-1 inhibitors include immune-mediated reactions, such as hepatitis, colitis, pneumonitis, rash, hyperthyroidism or hypothyroidism, and infusion-related reactions. These agents will likely be approved for additional indications in the future as more research is conducted into their effects.

Cell-Cycle Kinetics and Anticancer Effects

The cell cycle entails a series of phases that a cell must undergo to reproduce. Both normal and cancerous cells must proceed through the cell cycle if they are to grow and divide. The four major phases of the cell cycle are designated as G_1, S, G_2, and M. During G_1, cells are growing and preparing for the S phase, in which DNA synthesis occurs. Cells in the G_2 phase are preparing for the M phase, in which mitosis (cell division) occurs. There is also a resting phase in the cell cycle in which the cells are not actively dividing; it is called G_0. The longest phases of the cell cycle are the S phase, which can last 18–20 hours, and the G_1 phase, which can last 18–30 hours. Various mechanisms present throughout the cell cycle ensure that any damaged DNA is repaired before the cell moves on to the next phase; if the damage cannot be fixed, the cell is forced to undergo apoptosis (preprogrammed cell death).

Two types of cytotoxic chemotherapy agents are available: those that are cell-cycle phase specific and those that are cell-cycle phase nonspecific. Examples of phase-specific agents include methotrexate and capecitabine, which exert most of their activity on cells that are in the S phase of the cell cycle. To ensure that as many cells as possible in the phase for which the agent is selective are exposed to a chemotherapeutic drug, it is important to administer these agents as a continuous infusion or via frequent infusions. Administering the agents in this manner optimizes the cytotoxic effects of the phase-specific or "schedule-dependent" agents.

Cell-cycle phase-specific drugs are more effective for treating tumors that are rapidly dividing. Conversely, cell-cycle nonspecific agents work in multiple phases of the cell cycle and can target cells that are either actively dividing or in the resting, dormant phase. The efficacy of these agents is more dependent on the total dose given, rather than the timing of the infusion. Alkylating agents and anthracyclines are examples of such cell-cycle nonspecific agents. The cell-cycle nonspecific agents are useful for treating slower-growing tumors, such as breast cancer.

Mechanisms of Drug Resistance

Tumors are able to acquire resistance to chemotherapy, as is evident in patients whose tumors initially showed a response to chemotherapy, but then stopped responding over time. In an effort to mitigate and overcome chemoresistance, combinations of drugs from different classes and with different mechanisms of action are often used.

Researchers have proposed many mechanisms by which drug resistance might occur. In some cases, a small portion of the cancer cells might have inherent resistance to the chemotherapy; over time, as these cells survive the chemotherapy assault and reproduce, they become able to spread their resistance mechanism to a new population of cells.

Resistance may also develop from altered membrane transporters. In normal cells, the membrane transporter P-glycoprotein (P-gp) serves a protective function and expels harmful substances out of the cell. In cancer cells, overexpression of this transporter can lead to resistance by extruding the chemotherapy agents out of the cell and preventing the agents from reaching a cytotoxic concentration inside the cell.

Another mechanism of resistance may be increased production or alteration of the target, so that the chemotherapy is no longer effective. Resistance could also be gained from a mutation in or inactivation of *p53*, which normally mediates apoptosis of cells that contain damaged DNA. Without functioning *p53*, cancer cells with DNA that has been damaged from chemotherapy can continue to proliferate.

Additionally, tumors can acquire resistance by increasing the production of DNA repair enzymes, which fix the damage caused by chemotherapy. Sometimes tumors may start to overexpress drug-metabolizing enzymes, which leads to increased drug degradation, or reduce the production of drug-metabolizing enzymes, when prodrugs need to be converted to their active metabolite to have a tumor-killing effect. It has also been found that tumors amplify their production of drug-conjugating molecules such as glutathione; the conjunction of glutathione to the chemotherapy leads to an inactive form of the drug.

Safe Handling of Antineoplastic Chemotherapeutic Agents

Occupational exposure to chemotherapy agents can put healthcare personnel at increased risk of adverse health events. Because these agents are teratogenic, mutagenic, and carcinogenic, it is imperative that precautionary measures be established and enforced to protect personnel from unintentional exposure. Those at risk include any staff involved in the preparation or administration of chemotherapy, disposing of patient waste, or cleaning of chemotherapy spills. Exposure may occur in many ways, such as through inhalation of an aerosolized drug, needle sticks, direct skin contact with the agent, or ingestion. Fortunately, by following proper standards and procedures, accidental exposure can be avoided. In addition to these safety precautions, it is recommended that providers participate in a medical surveillance program that includes physical examinations and laboratory tests to monitor for any abnormalities or changes.

3.1 Antibiotic Agents

The antitumor antibiotics bleomycin, dactinomycin, and mitomycin are derived from the *Streptomyces* bacteria. These agents work by causing DNA single- and double-strand breaks, intercalating between DNA, and causing DNA cross-linking.

Bleomycin is unique in that it causes minimal myelosuppression, but it does carry the risk of pulmonary toxicity; this risk increases with cumulative lifetime doses greater than 400 units. Pulmonary toxicity may present as pneumonitis, which then progresses to pulmonary fibrosis. Pulmonary function should be monitored prior to and throughout treatment.

Both dactinomycin and mitomycin are vesicants; these agents should be administered only by the intravenous route to prevent extravasation. If extravasation does occur, the infusion should be stopped immediately and proper management should be initiated. Dactinomycin and mitomycin can also cause dose-limiting myelosuppression; patients should be monitored for signs of an infection and bleeding. The onset of myelosuppression from mitomycin is delayed and cumulative, so blood counts should be monitored up to 8 weeks following treatment. Antiemetics are recommended with dactinomycin due to its high emetic potential.

Antibiotic Agents

Bleomycin
Dactinomycin
Mitomycin

Case Studies and Conclusions

RT is a 73-year-old female with non-Hodgkin lymphoma. She has been receiving treatment for the past 4 months and has recently started complaining of shortness of breath, dry cough, and chest pain.

1. RT has developed pneumonitis. Which of the following agents most likely caused this side effect?
   a. Bleomycin
   b. Dactinomycin
   c. Mitomycin
   d. All of the above

Answer A is correct: Pulmonary toxicity from bleomycin is very serious and can occur in as many as 10% of treated patients. It most frequently presents as pneumonitis, which can then progress to pulmonary fibrosis.

2. Pulmonary toxicity from bleomycin is more common in patients who are older than age 70 and in those who have received a cumulative lifetime dose greater than:
   a. 100 units.
   b. 200 units.
   c. 300 units.
   d. 400 units.

Answer D is correct. The incidence of pulmonary toxicity has been found to be greater in the elderly population and in those who have received a total lifetime dose greater than 400 units.

BR is currently receiving chemotherapy when she starts to complain of pain and swelling near the infusion site. The chemotherapy agent she is receiving is a vesicant and she is experiencing extravasation.

1. Which of the following are potent vesicants?
   a. Bleomycin
   b. Bleomycin and dactinomycin
   c. Dactinomycin and mitomycin
   d. Bleomycin and mitomycin

Answer C is correct. Both dactinomycin and mitomycin are potent vesicants; proper needle or catheter placement need to be ensured prior to and throughout their infusion. If extravasation does occur, the infusion should be stopped immediately. Treat by placing a dry, cold compress at the site of extravasation for 20 minutes, four times a day for the first 1-2 days.

BR recovers from the extravasation and continues receiving treatment, but recently her platelet count has been trending downward.

2. Which of the following agents is NOT likely the cause of the decreased platelet count?
   a. Bleomycin
   b. Dactinomycin
   c. Mitomycin
   d. All of the above

Answer A is correct. Bleomycin causes minimal myelosuppression. Dactinomycin and mitomycin can cause dose-limiting myelosuppression.

3.2 Antimetabolite Agents

The folate antimetabolites work by inhibiting the enzyme dihydrofolate reductase (DHFR), thereby preventing DNA synthesis. Side effects associated with all agents in this class include bone marrow suppression, mucositis, dermatologic toxicity, and renal toxicity. Pemetrexed and pralatrexate require the use of folic acid and vitamin B_{12} prior to and throughout treatment to lessen bone marrow suppression and gastrointestinal (GI) toxicities. Each of these agents is eliminated largely through the kidneys and need dose adjustments in patients with renal impairment to prevent increased toxicity.

The purine antagonists disrupt the synthesis of purines (adenosine and guanine) and DNA. These agents are indicated in treating various types of leukemia. Patients with leukemia may have a high tumor burden, and their treatment can result in tumor lysis syndrome (TLS). TLS is a group of metabolic abnormalities that can occur as a complication during the treatment of cancer. Patients should be monitored for signs of TLS and given adequate IV hydration as well as allopurinol if hyperuricemia is anticipated. A major dose-limiting toxicity of this class is bone marrow suppression.

The pyrimidine antagonists are structurally similar to cytosine and uracil—nucleobases within DNA and RNA—and these agents inhibit the synthesis of nucleotide, inserting themselves into DNA structures, preventing DNA from being copied. A common dose-limiting toxicity is bone marrow suppression. Capecitabine, fluorouracil, and cytarabine can cause hand-foot syndrome, diarrhea, and oral mucositis, which may require treatment disruption and dose reduction. These agents are organized based on mechanism of action and the specific indications for use as well as recommendations for dosing; administration and monitoring are included in the companion drug grid at the end of this chapter.

Folate Antagonists

Methotrexate
Pemetrexed
Pralatrexate

Purine Antagonists

Cladribine
Clofarabine
Fludarabine

Mercaptopurine
Nelarabine
Pentostatin
Thioguanine

Pyrimidine Antagonists

Azacitidine
Capecitabine
Cytarabine
Decitabine
Floxuridine
Fluorouracil
Gemcitabine
Hydroxyurea

Case Studies and Conclusions

TL is a 59-year-old male with metastatic nonsquamous NSCLC. He is going to be treated with the combination of cisplatin and pemetrexed.

1. Which of the following should the patient receive intramuscularly 1 week prior to the administration of pemetrexed (Alimta) to reduce gastrointestinal and hematologic toxicity?
   a. Vitamin D
   b. Vitamin A
   c. Potassium
   d. Vitamin B_{12}

Answer D is correct. Administer vitamin B_{12} 1 mg intramuscularly 1 week prior to the first dose of ALIMTA and every 3 cycles thereafter. Subsequent vitamin B_{12} injections may be given on the same day as treatment with ALIMTA.

2. In addition to vitamin B_{12}, which other supplement should TL start taking?
   a. Magnesium
   b. Sodium
   c. Folic acid
   d. Iron

Answer C is correct. Patients receiving treatment with pemetrexed should take folic acid 400-1000 mcg orally once daily, beginning 7 days before the first dose of pemetrexed. Folic acid should be continued during the full course of therapy and for 21 days after the last dose of pemetrexed.

TL begins to develop painful sores in his mouth that limit his ability to eat and drink.

3. For which agent should the doctor consider reducing the dose?
   a. Cisplatin
   b. Pemetrexed
   c. Both agents
   d. Neither agent

Answer B is correct. It is recommended that the dose of pemetrexed be reduced to 50% of the previous dose if the patient develops grade 3 or 4 mucositis. Cisplatin may be continued at its full dose because it is not the cause of mucositis.

MF has metastatic breast cancer. She has been receiving treatment for the past 2 months, and has recently noticed that the soles of her feet have become swollen, tender, and painful.

1. Which of the following medications is most likely causing this side effect?
   a. Docetaxel
   b. Doxorubicin
   c. Capecitabine
   d. Gemcitabine

Answer C is correct. Hand-foot syndrome is a potentially dose-limiting toxicity of capecitabine. Udderly Smooth cream can be applied to the hands and feet to manage this side effect. It is also recommended that patients avoid prolonged exposure to heat and friction on their hands and feet, which may cause capillary leakage of the drug.

Capecitabine is a member of the class of compounds called pyrimidine antagonists.

2. Which of the following side effects should patients who are receiving a pyrimidine antagonist be monitored for?
   a. Infection
   b. Unusual bruising or bleeding
   c. Fatigue
   d. All of the above

Answer D is correct. Pyrimidine antagonists can cause myelosuppression, and patients receiving these agents should be monitored appropriately.

Purine antagonists are similar to the pyrimidine antagonists in that they also cause dose-limiting myelosuppression. Purine antagonists are often used in the treatment of leukemia.

3. What is another adverse effect of treatment with purine antagonists that may require prophylaxis with allopurinol?
   a. Hypercalcemia
   b. Hypernatremia
   c. Hyperuricemia
   d. Hyperglycemia

Answer C is correct. The risk of tumor lysis syndrome increases in patients with a large tumor burden prior to treatment. Signs of tumor lysis syndrome include fast heartbeat, trouble passing urine, muscle weakness or cramps, upset stomach, throwing up, loose stools, or feeling sluggish.

3.3 DNA Agents

Alkylating agents work by covalently bonding an alkyl group to DNA, most commonly with the 7-nitrogen on guanine. This results in cross-linking between DNA strands, which ultimately inhibits DNA replication because the DNA strands are unable to separate. Alkylating agents are cell-cycle nonspecific. They are myelosuppressive, carcinogenic, mutagenic, and teratogenic.

Carmustine, lomustine, and streptozocin belong to the subclass of alkylating agents called nitrosoureas. Carmustine and lomustine are unique in that they are able to cross the blood-brain barrier and, therefore, can be used in the treatment of brain tumors. Dose-related and delayed pulmonary toxicity has occurred with their use; pulmonary function tests should be obtained at baseline and frequently throughout the patient's course of treatment.

Cyclophosphamide and ifosfamide can cause hemorrhagic cystitis due to their toxic metabolite, acrolein. Mesna is in a class of drugs known as chemoprotectants and is used to reduce the side effects of chemotherapy drugs. Mesna should be administered with high doses of cyclophosphamide and with any dose of ifosfamide to prevent bladder toxicity. Dacarbazine has a high emetic potential, so aggressive prophylaxis with antiemetics is recommended when this agent is administered. Because *Pneumocystis jirovecii* pneumonia (PCP) may occur with temozolomide treatment, all patients receiving this agent should be monitored for the development of dyspnea, fever, chills, and nonproductive cough. Prophylaxis with sulfamethoxazole and trimethoprim (Bactrim) is required in patients receiving the 42-day temozolomide treatment regimen with radiation. Providers need to know types of antineoplastic agents, how to select a specific one to meet the patient's needs, the potential side effects, and the strategies used to counteract adverse effects. These agents are organized based on mechanism of action and the specific indications for use as well as recommendations for dosing; administration and monitoring are included in the companion drug grid at the end of this chapter.

DNA Alkylating Agents: Nitrosoureas

Carmustine
Lomustine
Streptozocin

DNA Cross-linking/Alkylating Agents

Altretamine
Bendamustine
Busulfan
Chlorambucil
Cyclophosphamide
Dacarbazine
Estramustine
Ifosfamide
Mechlorethamine (nitrogen mustard)
Melphalan
Procarbazine
Temozolomide
Thiotepa

Case Studies and Conclusions

JK is a 36-year-old female who has been diagnosed with a brain tumor. Treatment options including surgery, radiation, and chemotherapy are discussed.

1. Which of the following is a chemotherapy agent that belongs to the nitrosoureas class and is used in the treatment of brain tumors?
   a. Lomustine
   b. Streptozocin
   c. Cyclophosphamide
   d. Temozolomide

Answer A is correct. Lomustine and carmustine are nitrosoureas used in the treatment of brain tumors. Streptozocin is a nitrosourea but is not used to treat brain tumors. Temozolomide is used to treat brain tumors but is not a nitrosourea.

One of JK's treatment options is carmustine. She wants to know which side effects she may experience with this treatment.

2. Which of the following tests should be conducted at baseline and frequently throughout treatment?
   a. Liver
   b. Pulmonary
   c. Renal
   d. Ophthalmic

Answer B is correct. Carmustine's label carries a black box warning for pulmonary toxicity, which is dose related and can occur years after treatment; the risk of delayed pulmonary toxicity is higher in children. Liver and renal function tests should be conducted periodically throughout treatment.

JK wants to know which other chemotherapy treatment options are available for her brain tumor. Her medical oncologist mentions a chemotherapy agent that can be given concurrently with radiation.

3. Which of the following regimens includes a chemotherapy agent used in the treatment of brain tumors and the prophylactic antibiotic it must be given with?

   a. Temozolomide–ciprofloxacin
   b. Temozolomide–Bactrim
   c. Lomustine–Bactrim
   d. Carmustine–ciprofloxacin

Answer B is correct. The 42-day temozolomide regimen requires prophylaxis for PCP; Bactrim is the antibiotic used for prevention of PCP.

MN is a 42-year-old male with testicular cancer. He will be receiving treatment with ifosfamide.

1. Ifosfamide should be given with which of the following to prevent hemorrhagic cystitis?

   a. Dexamethasone
   b. Mesna
   c. Benadryl
   d. Acrolein

Answer B is correct. Mesna inactivates the urotoxic metabolite of ifosfamide. Dexamethasone, prednisone, and Benadryl are not used in the prevention of hemorrhagic cystitis. Acrolein is the name of the urotoxic metabolite.

2. Which of the following agents, when given in high doses, also requires prophylaxis with mesna?

   a. Dacarbazine
   b. Cyclophosphamide
   c. Temozolomide
   d. Carmustine

Answer B is correct. Cyclophosphamide also produces the toxic metabolite acrolein, and in high doses it requires prophylaxis with mesna. The other agents listed do not cause hemorrhagic cystitis.

3. Which of the following DNA agents requires pretreatment with antiemetics due to its high emetic potential?

   a. Chlorambucil
   b. Dacarbazine
   c. Cetuximab
   d. Dasatinib

Answer B is correct. Dacarbazine is the only one of these agents with a high emetic risk.

3.4 Enzymes

Asparaginase is an enzyme that converts asparagine to L-aspartic acid and ammonia. Asparagine is a non-essential amino acid for normal cells because they are capable of synthesizing it. Leukemic cells, however, lack the enzyme that is required for production of this amino acid; thus, they rely on exogenous asparagine. Asparaginase depletes this source and deprives leukemic lymphoblasts of asparagine, which is needed for protein synthesis and cell survival, thereby leading to apoptosis. Asparaginase works in the G_1 phase of the cell cycle.

Asparaginase is indicated for acute lymphoblastic leukemia (ALL). Three formulations are available, but should not be used interchangeably: Elspar (L-asparaginase), Erwinzia (asparaginase), and Oncaspar (pegaspargase). Elspar is derived from *Escherichia coli*, Erwinaze is derived from *Erwinia chrysanthemi*, and Oncaspar is a modified form of L-asparaginase conjugated with polyethylene glycol. Asparaginase is indicated for patients who develop allergic reactions to the *E. coli*-derived formulation. Pegasparagase allows for doses to be given every 2 weeks and has a lower incidence of allergic reactions. Major class side effects include hypersensitivity reactions, pancreatitis, and coagulation deficiencies.

Enzymes

Asparaginase (*Erwinia chrysanthemi*)
Pegaspargase

Case Studies and Conclusions

RO is an 18-year-old male with ALL. After 3 weeks of treatment with asparaginase, he developed pancreatitis.

1. Is this patient a candidate for treatment with pegaspargase?
    a. Yes
    b. No

Answer B is correct. Pegaspargase is contraindicated in patients with past or present pancreatitis.

2. Can this patient be retreated with asparaginase?
    a. Yes
    b. No

Answer B is correct. Retreatment with asparaginase after a patient has had pancreatitis is associated with a high risk of recurrence.

3. Which of the following drugs is associated with the lower occurrence of hypersensitivity?
    a. Erwinzia
    b. Elspar
    c. Oncaspar
    d. Pegasparagase

Answer D is correct. PEG-asparaginase has a relatively lower immunogenicity due to the covalent conjugation to monomethoxy polyethylene glycol.

3.5 Histone Deacetylase Inhibitors

Histones are positively charged proteins that associate with negatively charged DNA to condense the DNA into units called nucleosomes, which make up chromatin. Both the acetylation and de-acetylation of histones play major roles in regulating gene expression. Histone deacetylase (HDAC) inhibitors lead to hyper-acetylation of histones and transcription factors, which halts cell growth and causes apoptosis.

Vorinostat and romidepsin are indicated for the treatment of cutaneous T-cell lymphoma, and romidepsin is also indicated for peripheral T-cell lymphoma. Vorinostat is supplied as an oral capsule, whereas romidepsin is supplied as a powder for reconstitution to be administered intravenously. Both of these agents are myelosuppressive and can cause QT prolongation. Patients should have a baseline and periodic ECG, and their electrolyte levels (especially potassium, magnesium, and calcium) should be monitored throughout treatment and corrected if abnormal. Vorinostat may increase the risk of pulmonary embolism or deep vein thrombosis; patients should be monitored for shortness of breath, chest pain, and tenderness or swelling in their legs. The most common side effects reported for these agents include fatigue, nausea, diarrhea, anorexia and altered taste.

Histone Deacetylase Inhibitors

Belinostat
Panobinostat
Romidepsin
Vorinostat

Case Studies and Conclusions

KD is a 66-year-old female with T-cell lymphoma who has been receiving treatment with vorinostat. Her potassium level is 3.1 mmol/L and her magnesium level is 1.3 mEq/L.

1. Given her current treatment regimen and electrolyte values, which of the following side effects is KD at risk of developing at this time?
   a. Myelosuppression
   b. QT prolongation
   c. Pulmonary embolism
   d. Diarrhea

Answer B is correct. Vorinostat may prolong the QT interval. Hypomagnesemia and hypokalemia may also increase the chance of this side effect, so patients receiving this medication should have their magnesium and potassium levels monitored prior to and throughout treatment, and corrected if abnormal.

2. Which of the following is/are side effect(s) of vorinostat about which KD should be counseled?
   a. Pain and swelling in leg
   b. Chest pain and shortness of breath
   c. Diarrhea
   d. All of the above

Answer D is correct. Vorinostat can cause pulmonary embolism, deep vein thrombosis, and diarrhea.

KD reports difficulty swallowing the capsules and asks if they can be opened and dissolved in something before she takes her dose.

3. What do you tell her?
   a. Yes, vorinostat capsules can be opened and dissolved in water.
   b. Yes, vorinostat capsules can be opened and sprinkled on applesauce.
   c. No, the capsules must never be crushed or opened.
   d. The manufacturer does not provide recommendations about this issue.

Answer C is correct. Direct contact of the powder in the capsules with the skin or mucous membranes should be avoided. If this happens, wash the area thoroughly.

3.6 Hormone/Hormone Modifiers

Drugs that influence hormonal balance and activity may also have antineoplastic effects. Conventional nonsteroidal antiandrogens, including bicalutamide, flutamide, and nilutamide, competitively bind to androgen receptors, causing altered growth and often preprogrammed cell death. Other agents target estrogen—for example, tamoxifen, which is a nonsteroidal estrogen agonist/antagonist. Tamoxifen is used as primary treatment for breast cancer in pre-menopausal women and post-menopausal women. Conversely, aromatase inhibitors are only for post-menopausal women. Aromatase inhibitors include anastrozole, letrozole, and exemestane, all of which cannot be used in pre-menopausal women. Aromatase inhibitors work by blocking the enzyme aromatase, which turns the hormone androgen into small amounts of estrogen in the body. This means that less estrogen is available to stimulate the growth of hormone-receptor-positive breast cancer cells.

In addition to the direct hormonal effects of these agents, other side effects may include secondary negative influences on lipids, bone integrity, and other tissues subject to hormonal effects. Additionally, LHRH agonists, such as triptorelin, can initially cause an increase in testosterone and, therefore, a tumor flare. This tumor flare can be blocked if an antiandrogen is used for the first few weeks of treatment with an LHRH agonist. Tumor flare is a side effect that may occur during the initial phase of hormonal treatment and symptoms include a sudden and painful increase in the tumor size, rash, low grade fever, hypercalcemia, bone pain, and an increase in the tumor marker levels.

Providers need to know types of these hormone modifying agents, how to select a specific one to meet the needs of the patient, the potential side effects, and the strategies used to counteract adverse effects. These agents are organized based on mechanism of action and the specific indications for use as well as recommendations for dosing; administration and monitoring are included in the companion drug grid at the end of this chapter.

Hormone/Hormone Modifiers

Abiraterone
Aldesleukin
Anastrozole
Bicalutamide
Degarelix
Enzalutamide
Exemestane
Flutamide
Fulvestrant
Goserelin
Histrelin
Letrozole
Leuprolide
Megestrol
Mitotane
Nilutamide
Tamoxifen
Toremifene
Triptorelin

Case Studies and Conclusions

LT is a 74-year-old male with metastatic prostate cancer. He is being treated with Trelstar and Casodex.

1. Which of the following correctly pairs the agent with its appropriate class?
   a. Bicalutamide (Casodex)—LHRH agonist
   b. Triptorelin (Trelstar)—antiandrogen
   c. Triptorelin (Trelstar)—LHRH agonist
   d. Bicalutamide (Casodex)—LHRH antagonist

Answer C is correct. Trelstar is an LHRH agonist and Casodex is an antiandrogen.

2. LHRH agonists, such as Trelstar, can initially cause an increase in testosterone and therefore a tumor flare. Which of the following medications can be used to block this initial flare?
   a. Goserelin (Zoladex)
   b. Bicalutamide (Casodex)
   c. Leuprolide (Eligard)
   d. Degarelix (Firmagon)

Answer B is correct. Casodex belongs to the antiandrogens class; these medications are often used during the first few weeks of treatment with an LHRH agonist to block tumor flares. Goserelin and leuprolide are both LHRH agonists that can cause tumor flares. Degarelix is an LHRH antagonist.

3. Which of the following is NOT a side effect commonly associated with the hormone therapy used to treat prostate cancer?
   a. Impotence
   b. Hot flashes
   c. Osteoporosis
   d. Pulmonary embolism

Answer D is correct. Pulmonary embolism is not a common side effect of hormone therapy, whereas the other conditions listed are frequently associated with these treatments.

DD is a 43-year-old female with stage II, estrogen receptor–positive breast cancer. Her last menses was 1 week ago.

1. Which of the following hormone therapies would be an appropriate treatment option for this patient's breast cancer?
    a. Anastrozole
    b. Letrozole
    c. Tamoxifen
    d. Exemestane

Answer C is correct. Tamoxifen is the only agent listed here that is approved for the treatment of breast cancer in premenopausal patients.

2. Which of the following is a black box warning associated with tamoxifen?
    a. Thromboembolic events
    b. Osteoporosis
    c. Myelosuppression
    d. Renal failure

Answer A is correct. Thrombotic events are rare but they have occurred; thus, caution is advised in patients with a history of thromboembolic events.

DD has been taking tamoxifen for 3 years and is now postmenopausal. She is switching from tamoxifen to letrozole.

3. Which of the following must be measured at baseline and routinely throughout her treatment?
    a. Bone density
    b. Vitamin D level
    c. Pulmonary function
    d. TSH

Answer A is correct. Aromatase inhibitors can cause bone loss and osteoporosis. Bone density scans should be performed at baseline and throughout treatment.

3.7 Immunosuppressant Agents

The categorization of antineoplastics based on their mechanism of action is challenging. Some immunosuppressant agents, such as temsirolimus and everolimus, inhibit T-lymphocyte activity but also inhibit tyrosine kinase, thereby exerting a multifactorial therapeutic action. Other agents within this class include recombinant humanized monoclonal antibodies, such as bevacizumab, which is an immunoglobulin G (IgG) antibody that contains both human framework regions and murine (mouse) complementary-determining regions; it binds to human vascular growth factor receptors, preventing growth of new blood vessels, reducing microvascular growth of tumors, and inhibiting metastatic disease progression. Immunosupressant antineoplastic agents may offer an alternative to treatment failures of more traditional interventions; for example, everolimus is approved for adults who have advanced renal cell carcinoma after failing sunitinib or sorafenib. Everolimus (and temsirolimus) are also mTOR inhibitors that have been shown to reduce cell proliferation, angiogenesis, and glucose uptake. The mammalian target of rapamycin (mTOR) signaling pathway integrates both intracellular and extracellular signals and serves as a central regulator of cancer and non-cancer cell growth and survival. Providers need to know how to select a specific immunosuppressant antineoplastic agent to meet the needs of the patient and to understand the potential side effects and the strategies used to counteract adverse effects. The specific indications for use as well as recommendations for dosing, administration and monitoring are included in the companion drug grid at the end of this chapter.

Immunosuppressant Agents

Everolimus
Temsirolimus

Monoclonal Antibodies

Ado-trastuzumab
Alemtuzumab
Bevacizumab
Brentuximab
Cetuximab
Erbitux
Ibritumomab
Ipilimumab
Nivolumab
Obinutuzumab
Ofatumumab
Panitumumab
Pembrolizumab
Pertuzumab
Ramucirumab
Rituximab
Siltuximab
Trastuzumab

Case Studies and Conclusions

AF is a 71-year-old female with renal cell carcinoma. She has been taking Sutent (Sunitinib) for the past 7 months, but a recent CT scan was highly suspicious for progression.

1. Which of the following is a treatment option for patients with advanced renal cell carcinoma after failing therapy with Sutent?
    a. Crizotinib
    b. Everolimus
    c. Erlotinib
    d. Imatinib

Answer B is correct. Everolimus is approved for adults who have advanced renal cell carcinoma after failing sunitinib or sorafenib. Crizotinib is approved for ALK-positive NSCLC. Erlotinib is approved for EGFR-positive NSCLC. Imatinib is approved for chronic lymphocytic leukemia (CLL).

2. For which of the following side effects should a patient taking Afinitor (everolimus) be monitored?
    a. Pulmonary toxicity
    b. Seizures
    c. Renal failure
    d. Both A and C
    e. Both A and B

Answer D is correct. Interstitial lung disease (ILD) and renal failure are two very serious side effects of Afinitor. Afinitor is not known to cause seizures.

3. What is the specific classification of everolimus?
   a. Tyrosine kinase inhibitor
   b. Monoclonal antibody
   c. PDL-1 inhibitor
   d. mTOR kinase inhibitor

Answer D is correct. Everolimus and temsirolimus are mTOR inhibitors and have been shown to reduce cell proliferation, angiogenesis, and glucose uptake.

LP is a 55-year-old female with ER/PR-negative, HER-2/neu-positive invasive ductal carcinoma. Today is her second cycle of chemotherapy. Her chemotherapy regimen includes a combination of docetaxel, carboplatin, trastuzumab and pertuzumab given every 3 weeks for 6 cycles.

1. Trastuzumab and pertuzumab belong to which class of medications?
   a. Monoclonal antibodies
   b. Aromatase inhibitors
   c. Topoisomerase inhibitors
   d. Anthracyclines

Answer A is correct. Monoclonal antibodies, such as trastuzumab and pertuzumab, work by targeting various antigens and receptors that are present on the surface of malignant cells or on the surface of the body's own immune cells.

Fifteen minutes after the pertuzumab infusion begins, LP experiences difficulty breathing, flushing, and angioedema.

2. Which action should the nurse take?
   a. Slow the infusion rate.
   b. Continue the infusion at the same rate because this is a minor reaction.
   c. Administer acetaminophen to the patient.
   d. Immediately discontinue the infusion.

Answer D is correct. Anaphylaxis is a life-threatening reaction and the infusion should be stopped immediately. Signs of an anaphylactic reaction include hives, angioedema, shortness of breath, hypotension, dizziness, and syncope.

LP's next line of treatment is a combination of paclitaxel and bevacizumab. Bevacizumab is a monoclonal antibody indicated in the treatment of many types of cancer, including metastatic colorectal cancer, cervical cancer, glioblastoma, NSCLC, ovarian cancer, and metastatic renal cell cancer. It works by inhibiting angiogenesis.

3. Which of the following is (are) a side effect of bevacizumab therapy?
   a. Hypotension
   b. Impaired wound healing
   c. Hypertension
   d. Both A and B
   e. Both B and C

Answer E is correct. Side effects from bevacizumab include bleeding, hypertension, heart failure, thrombosis, GI perforation, and delayed wound healing.

3.8 Tyrosine Kinase Inhibitors

Tyrosine kinase inhibitors are further differentiated by their "generation." First-generation agents include erlotinib and gefitinib, which are reversible tyrosine kinase inhibitors. While these agents can produce improved outcomes in some patients with small cell lung cancer, for example, they are prone to secondary resistance, with mutations being the most common cause of this resistance. This tendency resulted in the development of newer generations of tyrosine kinase inhibitors. For example, afatinib is a second-generation inhibitor of receptor tyrosine kinase. The second-generation agents form covalent bonds with kinase domains of the epidermal growth factor receptors, causing downregulation of signaling and inhibition of cell proliferation and are associated with skin toxicities when used for treatment. Epidermal growth factor receptor (EGFR) inhibitors, such as afatinib (Gilotrif) and erlotinib (Tarceva), are used in the treatment of metastatic NSCLC, in contrast to axitinib (Inlyta), which is also tyrosine kinase and a vascular endothelial growth factor (VEGF) inhibitor approved for the treatment of advanced renal cell cancer. Topical and oral antibiotics and steroids are all treatment options for EGFR-induced skin toxicity.

Tyrosine Kinase Inhibitors

Afatinib
Axitinib
Bosutinib
Cabozantinib
Ceritinib
Crizotinib
Dasatinib
Erlotinib
Gefitinib
Ibrutinib
Imatinib
Lapatinib
Lenvatinib
Nilotinib
Pazopanib
Ponatinib
Regorafenib
Ruxolitinib
Sorafenib
Sunitinib
Vandetanib
Vemurafenib
Vismodegib

Case Studies and Conclusions

AK has stage IV non-small cell lung cancer. EGFR mutation testing shows that he has an exon 19 deletion.

1. Which EGFR inhibitor(s) can be used to treat AK's lung cancer?
    a. Afatinib
    b. Axitinib
    c. Erlotinib
    d. Both A and C
    e. Both B and C

Answer D is correct. Afatinib (Gilotrif) and erlotinib (Tarceva) are EGFR inhibitors used in the treatment of metastatic NSCLC. Axitinib (Inlyta) is a tyrosine kinase and VEGF inhibitor approved for the treatment of advanced renal cell cancer.

AK begins treatment with an EGFR inhibitor and a few weeks later develops a rash on his back and upper chest.

2. Which of the following treatments may be used to manage this rash?

   a. 2% clindamycin gel
   b. 1% hydrocortisone
   c. Doxycycline 100 mg by mouth twice daily
   d. Both A and B
   e. All of the above

Answer E is correct. Topical and oral antibiotics and steroids are all treatment options for EGFR-induced skin toxicity.

AK calls a few days later complaining of diarrhea.

3. Which of the following is NOT an appropriate recommendation for managing this side effect?

   a. Drink at least 8 cups of water per day.
   b. Limit intake of foods high in fiber.
   c. Eat small, frequent meals and snacks.
   d. Limit intake of bananas, white rice, applesauce, and toast.

Answer D is correct. The BRAT (bananas, rice, applesauce, and toast) is recommended to help manage diarrhea because it can help solidify stools.

MF is an 81-year-old female with chronic myeloid leukemia (CML). After 5 months of treatment with the tyrosine kinase inhibitor imatinib, her CML has progressed.

1. Additional treatment options for CML include:

   a. Pazopanib (Votrient).
   b. Dasatinib (Sprycel).
   c. Bosutinib (Bosulif).
   d. Both A and B.
   e. Both B and C.

Answer E is correct. Votrient is indicated for the treatment of renal cell carcinoma and soft-tissue sarcoma. Additional treatment options include Sprycel, Bosulif, and Iclusig.

2. Identify the correct pairing of tyrosine kinase inhibitor and indication.

   a. Sunitinib (Sutent)—chronic lymphocytic leukemia
   b. Lapatinib (Tykerb)—breast cancer
   c. Regorafenib (Stivarga)—renal cell carcinoma
   d. Imbruvica (Ibrutinib)—colorectal cancer

Answer B is correct. Sutent is indicated for gastrointestinal stromal tumors (GIST), pancreatic neuroendocrine tumors (PNET), and renal cell cancer. Stivarga is indicated for metastatic colorectal cancer and GIST. Ibrutinib is indicated for chronic lymphocytic leukemia (CLL), mantle cell lymphoma, and Waldenström macroglobulinemia.

3. Which of the following tyrosine kinase inhibitors is NOT a treatment option for thyroid cancer?

   a. Tasigna (nilotinib)
   b. Lenvima (lenvatinib)
   c. Caprelsa (vandetanib)
   d. Cometriq (cabozantinib)

Answer A is correct. Tasigna is indicated only for the treatment of CML.

3.9 Topoisomerase Inhibitors

Topoisomerase inhibitors are agents that modify the action of topoisomerase enzymes that control changes in DNA structure by altering the phosphodiester structure of the strands during the normal life cycle of the cell. Topoisomerase enzymes are common targets for antineoplastic therapy, due to the theorized mechanism of action that alters the integrity of the genome and subsequently leads to cellular death.

Topoisomerase inhibitors can also function as antibacterial agents; daunorubicin, for example, can be considered an antineoplastic antibiotic. Topoisomerase inhibitors are often classified according to which type of enzyme they inhibit. Topoisomerase I inhibitors include irinotecan, topotecan, and camptothecin, all of which target type IB topoisomerases. Some of these topoisomerase I inhibitors, namely irinotecan, can cause acute or delayed diarrhea. Acute diarrhea, which develops within 24 hours of receiving irinotecan, should be treated with loperamide. Delayed diarrhea from irinotecan can be managed with loperamide and octreotide. Topoisomerase II inhibitors include etoposide, teniposide, doxorubicin, daunorubicin, and mitoxantrone.

Use of topoisomerase inhibitors for antineoplastic therapy may lead to secondary malignancies because of the DNA-damaging properties of these compounds. The risk of myocardial toxicity from the anthracycline topoisomerase inhibitors increases as the cumulative lifetime dose approaches a certain level; for doxorubicin, the risk significantly increases as the lifetime dose approaches 550 mg/m^2.

Anthracyclines

Daunorubicin
Doxorubicin
Epirubicin
Idarubicin
Valrubicin

Camptothecins

Irinotecan
Topotecan

Podophyllotoxins

Etoposide
Mitoxantrone
Teniposide

Case Studies and Conclusions

NM is a 68-year-old patient with metastatic colorectal cancer who has just received her first infusion of irinotecan this morning. Later in the day, she calls the office complaining of severe diarrhea.

1. Which agent should be administered to the patient for management of this side effect?
   a. Loperamide
   b. Atropine
   c. Zofran
   d. Compazine

Answer A is correct. Irinotecan can cause acute or delayed diarrhea. Acute diarrhea, which develops within 24 hours of receiving irinotecan, should be treated with loperamide. Delayed diarrhea from irinotecan can be managed with loperamide.

2. All of the following agents are considered topoisomerase II inhibitors EXCEPT:
   a. Etoposide.
   b. Daunorubicin.
   c. Topotecan.
   d. Mitoxantrone.

Answer C is correct. Topotecan is a topoisomerase I inhibitor. Etoposide, daunorubicin, and mitoxantrone are topoisomerase II inhibitors.

3. Which of the following is not classified as an anthracycline?
   a. Doxorubicin
   b. Daunorubicin
   c. Idarubicin
   d. Mitoxantrone

Answer D is correct. Mitoxantrone is not an anthracycline.

MF is a 68-year-old female who presents with a large palpable mass in her left breast. Her comorbidities include hypertension and congestive heart failure. The results from a core needle biopsy show grade 3 triple-negative breast cancer.

1. Which of the following classes of medications has a black box warning on the product label for cardiotoxicity and should be used with caution in patients with preexisting heart disease?
   a. Taxanes
   b. Anthracyclines
   c. Platinum agents
   d. Topoisomerase inhibitors

Answer B is correct. Doxorubicin, daunorubicin, and idarubicin are members of the anthracycline class. The label of each of these agents carries a black box warning for cardiotoxicity, with the risk of this side effect increasing with increasing cumulative lifetime doses.

MF has recently been diagnosed with bone metastases. As additional treatment options are discussed, MF asks which side effects she may experience.

2. What is the most common dose-limiting toxicity of the traditional chemotherapy agents, including topoisomerase inhibitors?
   a. Hepatotoxicity
   b. Rash
   c. Myelosuppression
   d. Cardiotoxicity

Answer C is correct. Patients should be monitored for signs of infection, fatigue, or unusual bruising or bleeding, which can indicate reduced white blood cell counts.

3. Which of the following medications should have the cumulative lifetime dose monitored due to dose-related adverse effects?
   a. Topotecan
   b. Etoposide
   c. Irinotecan
   d. Doxorubicin

Answer D is correct. The risk of myocardial toxicity from the anthracyclines increases as the cumulative lifetime dose approaches a certain level; for doxorubicin, the risk significantly increases as the lifetime dose approaches 550 mg/m^2.

3.10 Other Antineoplastic Agents

This section of platinum complex, spindle poisons (taxanes and vinca alkyloids), and miscellaneous antineoplastic agents completes the current story of the available pharmacotherapeutic interventions of antineoplastic agents. The types of chemotherapy drugs and combinations that may be needed are selected based on a variety of factors. Once initially considered investigational, prescribers have documented past response rates that are used today to tailor the type of drug, dose, and schedule that make up a "protocol" for specific types of cancer. Currently, most types of cancer have some standard protocols that help guide the prescribers in selecting the right chemotherapy for an individual with cancer. There is no one correct choice in choosing chemotherapy. As is the case with any drug treatment guideline, what is considered an appropriate chemotherapy regimen now may not be considered appropriate at a later time. Even drugs considered appropriate for indicated use have pros and cons and often there is more than one good option for treatment. It is important to acknowledge that although a selected protocol may have good evidence of response rates, there is no guarantee that the patient will achieve the desired response. Response rates to antineoplastic agents have improved greatly and with the development of new drugs, it is expected that these rates will improve even further. However, there are numerous factors that make it impossible to predict therapy outcomes for any one individual. The companion drug grid will help you better understand some of the advantages and disadvantages of these agents when used in your patients.

Platinum Complexes

Platinum-containing anti-cancer drugs react in the body, binding to DNA and causing the DNA strands to cross-link which ultimately triggers cells to die in a preprogrammed manner way. These agents, namely cisplatin, are well known for their emetogenic properties. It is recommended that prophylaxis for chemotherapy agents with a high emetic potential include a $5HT_3$ antagonist (i.e., ondanestron), corticosteroid, and neurokinin 1 receptor (NK_1) antagonist. NK_1 agonists are in a class of drug used to treat nausea and vomiting associated with chemotherapy. Aprepitant and fosaprepitant are NK_1 drugs and are discussed in the *Gastrointestinal Agents* chapter.

Platinum Complexes

Carboplatin
Cisplatin
Oxaliplatin

Retinoids

Retinoids are relatives of vitamin A. Retinoids control normal cell growth, cell differentiation (the normal process of making cells different from each other), and cell death during embryonic development and in certain tissues later in life. The effects of retinoids on cells are controlled by receptors on the nucleus of each cell (nuclear receptors). Retinoids are relatively new types of anti-cancer drugs and have been used alone and in combination to treat a variety of cancers.

Retinoids

Bexarotene
Tretinoin

Spindle Poisons (from Plants)

A spindle poison is an agent that disrupts cell division by affecting the protein threads that connect certain regions within the chromosomes, known as spindles. These agents are also known as spindle toxins, known for effectively ceasing the production of new cells by interrupting cell division. Two specific families of spindle poisons exist: vinca alkaloids and taxanes. Vinca alkaloids work by causing the inhibition of the polymerization of tubulin into microtubules, eventually resulting in cell death. In contrast, taxanes interrupt the mitotic cell cycle by stabilizing microtubules against depolymerization. Edema can be a side effect related to administration of these agents. Dexamethasone administered prior to docetaxel infusion will prevent (or reduce) fluid retention. The companion drug grid will provide additional detail about the specific limitations of each of these agents listed.

Spindle Poisons (from Plants)

Taxanes

Cabazitaxel
Docetaxel
Paclitaxel

Vinca Alkaloids

Vinblastine
Vincristine
Vinorelbine

Miscellaneous Antineoplastic Agents

Arsenic trioxide
Bortezomib
Carfilzomib
Dabrafenib
Denileukin
Eribulin
Idelalisib
Interferon alfa
Ixabepilone
Lenalidomide
Olaparib
Omacetaxine
Peginterferon alfa
Pomalidomide
Trametinib
Ziv-aflibercept

Case Studies and Conclusions

RG is a 52-year-old female with stage IV non-small cell lung cancer. She is negative for the EGFR mutation. Her doctor wishes to start her on a regimen of cisplatin + pemetrexed.

1. What is the emetic potential of this regimen?
   a. High
   b. Moderate
   c. Low
   d. Minimal

Answer A is correct. Cisplatin is associated with a high emetic potential (the frequency of nausea/vomiting is more than 90% if antiemetics are not given as pretreatment).

2. Which antiemetics should be given to RG as prophylaxis for acute chemotherapy-induced nausea and vomiting?
   a. Zofran (ondansetron) + dexamethasone + aprepitant
   b. Zofran (ondansetron) + dexamethasone
   c. Dexamethasone + aprepitant
   d. Compazine + lorazepam

Answer A is correct. It is recommended that prophylaxis for chemotherapy agents with a high emetic potential include a $5HT_3$ antagonist (such as ondansetron), corticosteroid, and NK_1 antagonist.

Four months later, RG's lung cancer has further metastasized to her bones. RG is started on cisplatin + docetaxel.

3. Premedication with dexamethasone starting 1 day prior to the docetaxel infusion is recommended to prevent which side effect?
    a. Fatigue
    b. Bone marrow suppression
    c. Fluid retention
    d. Peripheral neuropathy

Answer C is correct. Dexamethasone administered prior to docetaxel infusion will prevent (or reduce) fluid retention.

4. Vinblastine is a member of which class of chemotherapy agents?
    a. Taxanes
    b. Vinca alkaloids
    c. Anthracyclines
    d. Platinum agents

Answer B is correct. Vinblastine is a vinca alkaloid.

5. Vinca alkaloids can be fatal if administered by which route?
    a. Intravenous
    b. Intrathecal
    c. Intramuscular
    d. Subcutaneous

Answer B is correct. Intrathecal administration of vinca alkaloids can result death.

RG has received several cycles of chemo and developed pancytopenia.

6. Which of the following agents is not likely to have caused this side effect?
    a. Vincristine
    b. Vinblastine
    c. Docetaxel
    d. Vinorelbine

Answer A is correct. Vincristine is the least likely culprit in causing pancytopenia.

Tips from the Field

Patient Assessment

All patients should have a general assessment at baseline and throughout their treatment according to treatment protocol requirements, including but not limited to (refer to companion drug grid for other agent-specific recommendations):

1. Allergy and drug reaction history.
2. Laboratory results; if blood parameters are abnormal notify provider, evaluate and take appropriate action.
3. Baseline observations specific to the treatment protocol including performance status. (Scales and criteria are available for use to assess how a patient's disease is progressing, how the disease affects the daily living abilities of the patient, and to determine appropriate treatment and prognosis.)
4. Evaluate results of pulmonary, renal, and hepatic function tests prior to and at regular intervals during treatment.
5. Weight, height, body surface area (BSA), and psychosocial status screening

Additional Factors to Consider

1. Many antineoplastic agents are high-alert medications—drugs that bear a heightened risk of causing significant patient harm when they are used in error. Although mistakes may or may not be more common with these drugs, the consequences are often more devastating to patients.
2. Many of these agents are also on the National Institute for Occupational Safety and Health (NIOSH) hazardous drug list. Observe and exercise usual cautions for handling, preparing, and administering cytotoxic drugs. Use of double gloving is suggested as contact with skin can cause burning and pigmentation changes. If the agent contacts the skin or mucosa, immediately wash the skin or mucosa thoroughly with soap and water.
3. The following recommendations are not all-inclusive, but do list important safety components for handling chemotherapy. Chemotherapy agents should be prepared in a ventilated biologic safety cabinet, which serves to both protect the personnel involved in the drug's preparation and protect the product from contamination. Those who are preparing and administering chemotherapy should wear personal protective equipment (PPE), including gloves, a long-sleeved gown with a closed front, closed footwear, and protective glasses or goggles. To prevent inadvertent ingestion, eating and drinking in the area of where chemotherapy is prepared should be prohibited. Cytotoxic waste and materials related to preparation and administration should be disposed of in a designated waste bin; this container should be clearly labeled and the lid tightly closed at all times. After providers who have handled chemotherapy remove their protective gowns or gloves, they should discard this protective equipment in the appropriate waste container and promptly wash their hands. In addition to these safety precautions, it is recommended that providers participate in a medical surveillance program that includes physical examinations and laboratory tests to monitor for any abnormalities or changes.
4. Different toxicities associated with specific antineoplastic agents are considered to be related to the part of the nerve structure that is damaged and are often dose dependent. Some neuropathies are temporary while others are permanent.
5. Most antineoplastic agents have potential emetic side effects (potential to cause nausea and vomiting). The emetic potential of each agent varies and is often based on patient specific factors. For patients experiencing nausea associated with cancer chemotherapy (CINV), consider eating smaller, more frequent meals, preferably at room temperature whenever possible. The nausea can be acute (less than 24 hours after chemo), delayed at times greater than 24 hours, anticipatory based on conditioned response to prior episodes, breakthrough (despite prophylaxis with antiemetic) or refractory with poor response to multiple antiemetic regimens.
6. Tumor lysis syndrome (TLS) is a group of metabolic abnormalities that can occur as a complication during the treatment of cancer, most commonly after the treatment of lymphomas and leukemias. Appropriate measures (e.g., aggressive hydration) must be taken to prevent or alleviate severe electrolyte imbalances and renal toxicity during and following chemotherapy administration in patients with large, chemosensitive tumors. Hyperkalemia, hyperphosphatemia, hyperuricemia, hypocalcemia, and decreased urine output may be indicative of TLS.
7. Consider non-hematologic toxicities that can include serum creatinine 2mg/dl or greater, SGPT or total bilirubin 2-times or greater than the upper limit of normal, and active or uncontrolled infection.
8. The suggested maximum tolerated doses (MTD) for chemo is dependent on performance status, other chemotherapy agents or radiation given in combination, and disease state. Therefore, dosing may vary from protocol to protocol. If questions arise, clinicians should consult the appropriate references to verify the dose. The manufacturer may also recommend maximum biologic doses, and some of these are expressed as cumulative maximum lifetime doses.
9. Temporary interruption of therapy and/or a dose reduction may be necessary in patients who develop toxicity. Consider discontinuing treatment if a response has not occurred or if patients experience unacceptable levels of toxicity.

10. Many antineoplastic regimens are dosed based on body surface area (BSA = m^2). For agents that require dose based on BSA, use care to ensure that dose is based on BSA and not body weight (i.e., mg/kg). Use appropriate mathematical equations to ensure accurate BSA calculations (and double check your math carefully).
11. These agents have myelosuppressive effects that have the potential to suppress immunity. Therefore, exposure to potential illness, including but not limited to administration of live vaccines, should be avoided. Refer to PI for vaccination recommendations. These myelosuppressive effects can also increase the risk of bleeding; therefore, dental work or other procedures should be delayed until blood counts have returned to normal. Patients, especially those with dental disease, should be instructed in proper oral hygiene, including cautious use of regular toothbrushes, dental floss, and toothpicks.
12. Antineoplastic agents are available in numerous administration forms. Some agents may require reconstitution prior to use. Refer to PI for product dilution and storage specifications and remember that compounded chemo has beyond use dates that must be monitored.
13. Some agents are severe vesicants. Extravasation of antineoplastic infusions should be avoided. If possible, avoid veins over joints or in extremities with compromised venous or lymphatic circulation. Administration in small vessels or repeated injections into the same vein may result in venous sclerosis. Patients should be closely monitored during IV infusions for signs and symptoms of extravasation, such as poor blood return, burning, stinging, or necrosis.
14. Generally, if extravasation occurs, the infusion should be stopped and the tubing should be removed. Attempt to aspirate the drug prior to removing the needle. Elevate the affected area and treat with ice packs. As this can be a progressive injury, appropriate long-term follow-up is required.

Tammie Lee and Jacque

Bibliography

American Geriatrics Society. 2015 updated Beers criteria for potentially inappropriate medication use in older adults. *J Am Geriatric Soc.* 2015; 63:2227-2246.

ChemoCare. How do doctors decide which chemotherapy drugs to give? http://chemocare.com/chemotherapy/what-is-chemotherapy/how-do-doctors-decide-which-chemotherapy-drugs-to-give.aspx. Accessed January 20, 2017.

Does A, Thiel T. Rediscovering Biology, Molecular to Global Perspectives. Unit 8: Cell Biology & Cancer. https://www.learner.org/courses/biology/textbook/cancer/cancer_3.html

Fu CH, Sakamoto KM. PEG-asparaginase. *Expert Opin Pharmacother.* 2007; 8:1977-1984.

Gerber DE. Targeted therapies: a new generation of cancer treatments. *Am Fam Physician.* 2008;77(3):311-319. http://www.aafp.org/afp/2008/0201/p311.html. Accessed June 10, 2016.

Luqmani YA. Mechanisms of drug resistance in cancer chemotherapy. *Med Princ Pract.* 2005;14(suppl 1):35-48. http://www.karger.com/Article/Pdf/86183. Accessed October 3, 2016.

McEvoy GK, ed. *AHFS: Drug Information.* Bethesda, MD: American Society of Health-System Pharmacists; 2016.

Medina PJ, Shord SS. Cancer treatment and chemotherapy. In: DiPiro JT, Talbert RL, Yee GC, Matzke GR, Wells BG, Posey LM, eds. *Pharmacotherapy: A Pathophysiologic Approach.* 8th ed. New York, NY: McGraw-Hill; 2011: 2085-2120.

National Center for Biotechnology Information. PubChem Compound Database; CID=5311, http://pubchem.ncbi.nlm.nih.gov/compound/Vorinostat#section=Top. Accessed October 3 2016.

National Institute for Occupational Safety and Health. NIOSH alert: preventing occupational Exposures to Antineoplastic and Other Hazardous Drugs in Healthcare Settings. Department of Health and Human Services, Centers for Disease Control and Prevention, National Institute for Occupational Safety and Health. 2004. http://www.cdc.gov/niosh/docs/2004-165/pdfs/2004-165.pdf. October 3, 2016.

Ropero S, Esteller M. The role of histone deacetylases (HDACs) in human cancer. *Molecular Oncology.* 2007; 1(1):19-25. http://www.sciencedirect.com/science/article/pii/S1574789107000026

Symbols

- ▲ Renal impairment: Dose adjustment is recommended.
- □ Hepatic impairment: Dose adjustment is recommended.
- ■ Black box warning exists for this drug.
- QT QTc prolongation effects have been reported.
- 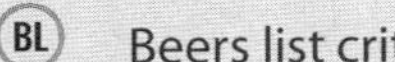 BL Beers list criteria (avoid in elderly).
- PD FDA-approved pediatric doses are available.
- GD FDA-approved geriatric doses are available.
-  See primary body system.

Antineoplastic Agents

Universal prescribing alerts:

- Known serious hypersensitivity to the specific drug or any other component of product/formulation selected warrants a contraindication for use.
- Adverse reactions associated with the use of some **antineoplastic agents** include dizziness, drowsiness, vertigo, or fatigue; these drugs may also impair the ability to perform tasks requiring mental alertness. Caution should always be recommended when using any new drug for the first time, when there is a dose change, and with continued use of known offending agents.
- Doses expressed are for the usual adult dosage ranges only. "Geriatric doses" are assumed to be the same as the adult doses unless otherwise noted with a symbol. Where FDA approved geriatric or pediatric dosing is available, a symbol will guide the reader to additional prescribing references. Please refer to real-time prescribing references for these age-specific doses.
- Use of antineoplastic agents in pregnancy is based on weighing clinical risk versus benefit; safety concerns are not represented in this grid. Refer to the package insert (PI) for more information. Clinicians should continue to provide education about the reproductive risks of any medication and offer risk-reduction strategies (which may include contraceptive use) to women of childbearing age and understand that these reproductive risks may also extend to males. Other medications may decrease the effectiveness of oral contraceptives. When necessary, an alternative means of birth control should be explored.
- Brand names are provided for those agents still available on the market. Due to the ever-changing product availability, refer to Food and Drug Administration (FDA) resources to confirm the actual brands available. This drug summary is intended for educational purposes only. Prescribing decisions should be based on real-time comprehensive drug databases that are updated on a regular basis.
- Generally, use of antineoplastic agents continues until the disease progression target is achieved, the patient is no longer responsive to treatment, or there is unacceptable toxicity. These agents may suppress immunity and may cause increased risk of fatal opportunistic infections.

Antibiotic Agents

Universal prescribing alerts:

- Antineoplastic agent doses are diagnosis dependent and regimens are individualized based on the patient's clinical status. Illustrative doses are provided as an educational tool and doses will vary from protocol to protocol. Clinicians should consult the appropriate references to verify the correct dose based on patient specific characteristics and clinical needs. The suggested maximum tolerated dose is often dependent on performance status, concomitant chemotherapy agents and/or radiation given in combination, as well as other concurrent disease states.

Drug Name	FDA-Approved Indications	Adult Dosage Range	Precautions and Clinical Pearls
Generic Name Bleomycin **Brand Name** Blenoxane ▲ ■ (PD)	Head and neck cancers Hodgkin's lymphoma Malignant pleural effusion Testicular cancer	**Usual parenteral dose for Hodgkin's lymphoma:** Single agent: IV/IM/SQ: 5 to 20 units/m^2 (0.25 to 0.5 unit/kg) administered 1 or 2 times per week Maximum lifetime cumulative dose = 400 mg Part of ABVD (doxorubicin, vinblastine, and dacarbazine): IV: 10 units/m^2	• Evaluate results of pulmonary function tests prior to and at regular intervals during treatment • Patients may experience skin or nail discoloration, weight loss, lack of appetite, alopecia, or asthenia • Initial test dose is recommended prior to scheduled use • Hepatotoxicity • Renal toxicity • Older adults may be more sensitive and require adjusted dosing (no specific recommendations are reported by manufacturer) Associated with: • Severe idiosyncratic reactions consisting of hypotension, mental confusion, fever, chills, and wheezing have been reported in 1% of lymphoma patients treated with bleomycin • Occurrence of pulmonary fibrosis is the most severe toxicity • Requires experienced clinician who is knowledgeable in the use of chemotherapy agents
Generic Name Dactinomycin **Brand Name** Cosmegen ■	**Common indications for use:** Wilms' tumor Ewing's sarcoma Metastatic testicular tumors Gestational trophoblastic neoplasm Regional perfusion of locally recurrent or locoregional solid tumors	**Usual parenteral dose for Wilms' tumor and Ewing's sarcoma:** IV: 15 mcg/kg per day for 5 days or IV: 400 to 600 mcg/m^2 per day for 5 days Maximum tolerated doses generally noted to be: IV:15 mcg/kg per day or 400 to 600 mcg/m^2 per day for 5 days or 45 mcg/kg IV as a single dose.	• High emetic potential; antiemetics are recommended to prevent nausea and vomiting • Hepatotoxicity; may cause hepatic sinusoidal obstruction syndrome • Use caution to prevent inadvertent exposure to this medication • Assess results of hematology, renal, and hepatic function test on a regular basis throughout therapy • Refer to PI for additional indications • Begin at the low end of the dosing range due to increased risk of myelosuppression Associated with: • Extravasation caution: extremely corrosive to soft tissues; recommended for IV administration only • Requires experienced clinician who is knowledgeable in the use of chemotherapy agents

Generic Name Mitomycin **Brand Name** Mutamycin ■	**Common indications for use:** Adenocarcinoma of stomach or pancreas	**Usual parenteral dose for the treatment of pancreatic cancer:** IV: 20 mg/m^2 every 6 to 8 weeks	• Pulmonary toxicity • Monitor complete blood count (CBC) with differential; serum creatinine; pulmonary function tests; monitor for signs and symptoms of hemolytic-uremic syndrome (HUS) • Infusion site must be closely monitored to prevent extravasation; mitomycin is a potent vesicant • Mitomycin regimens include other chemotherapy agents • Evaluate hydration and nutritional status • Monitor renal function; avoid use in patients with severe renal impairment (i.e., serum creatinine greater than 1.7 mg/dL or creatinine clearance [CrCL] less than 30 mL/min) Contraindications: • Patients with thrombocytopenia, coagulopathy, or an increase in risk of bleeding due to other causes Associated with: • Requires experienced clinician who is knowledgeable in the use of chemotherapy agents and specialized care setting • Bone marrow suppression (thrombocytopenia and leukopenia) is common and may be severe and/or contribute to infections • Hemolytic-uremic syndrome

Antimetabolite Agents

Folate Antagonists

Drug Name	FDA-Approved Indications	Adult Dosage Range	Precautions and Clinical Pearls
Generic Name Methotrexate **Brand Name** Rheumatrex Trexall	**Common indications for use:** ALL. Meningeal leukemia Trophoblastic neoplasms Breast cancer	Dose varies with indication for use and patient's clinical response **Illustrative dose for ALL:** Orally or IM:	• Use with caution (or avoid) in patients with conditions such as renal impairment, peptic ulcer disease, ulcerative colitis, pericardial or pleural effusion, hepatic impairment, or bone marrow suppression • Provide close monitoring of CBC with differential, liver function tests, and pulmonary function • Monitor renal function; may affect dosing • Monitor for acute neurotoxicity signs including drowsiness, blurred vision, and headaches

Drug Name	FDA-Approved Indications	Adult Dosage Range	Precautions and Clinical Pearls
Otrexup Rasuvo ▲ ■ (PD) (GD)	Advanced non-Hodgkin's lymphoma	3.3 mg/m^2 daily for 4 to 6 weeks or until remission occurs; followed by twice weekly maintenance therapy with a total weekly dose of 30 mg/m^2 orally or IM	• Refer to PI for additional indications • May cause sun sensitivity; protect skin when exposed Associated with: • May cause renal damage leading to acute renal failure, especially with high-dose methotrexate • Bone marrow suppression • Severe and potentially fatal dermatologic reactions • Acute and potentially fatal chronic hepatotoxicity • Gastrointestinal toxicity • Tumor lysis syndrome has been reported • Requires experienced clinician who is knowledgeable in the use of chemotherapy agents • When given concurrently with radiation therapy may increase the risk of soft tissue necrosis and bone necrosis
Generic Name Pemetrexed **Brand Name** Alimta ▲ ■	**Common indications for use:** Mesothelioma NSCLC, nonsquamous	Dose varies with indication for use and patient's clinical response **Illustrative parenteral dose for malignant pleural mesothelioma:** IV: 500 mg/m^2 on day 1 of each 21-day cycle (in combination with cisplatin) 500 mg/m^2 on day 1 of each 21-day cycle (as a single agent)	• Bone marrow suppression: may cause anemia, neutropenia, thrombocytopenia, or pancytopenia; frequent laboratory monitoring is necessary • Cutaneous reactions may occur; reduce dose by half of previous dose if patient develops grade 3 or 4 mucositis • Corticosteroids may be used to reduce cutaneous reactions • Gastrointestinal toxicity may occur • Hepatotoxicity has been observed with monotherapy and in association with other chemotherapy • Premedication with oral folic acid and vitamin B_{12} IM is required to reduce the severity of hematologic and gastrointestinal (GI) toxicities • Do not substitute oral vitamin B_{12} for IM • Monitor CBC with differential and platelets before each dose • Maintenance or second-line treatments require specific cycles; refer to PI for guidance

Drug Name	FDA-Approved Indications	Adult Dosage Range	Precautions and Clinical Pearls
Generic Name Pralatrexate **Brand Name** Folotyn ▲ ■	Relapsed or refractory peripheral T-cell lymphoma (PTCL)	**Usual parenteral dose**: IV: 30 mg/m^2 once weekly for 6 weeks of a 7-week treatment cycle; continue until disease progression or unacceptable toxicity	• Bone marrow suppression • Severe and potentially fatal dermatologic reactions, including skin exfoliation, ulceration, and toxic epidermal necrolysis (TEN) • Tumor lysis syndrome has been reported • Hepatotoxicity and liver function test abnormalities have been reported • Monitor CBC with differential (baseline and weekly) and serum chemistries, including renal and liver function tests • Use with caution and monitor in the presence of renal or hepatic impairment
Purine Antagonists			
Drug Name	**FDA-Approved Indications**	**Adult Dosage Range**	**Precautions and Clinical Pearls**
Generic Name Cladribine **Brand Name** Leustatin (DSC) ▲ ■ ■	Treatment of active hairy cell leukemia	**Usual parenteral dose**: IV: 0.09 mg/kg per day continuous infusion for 7 days for 1 cycle	• Monitor CBC with differential (particularly during the first 4 to 8 weeks post treatment) • Monitor for fever and signs and symptoms of neurotoxicity • Monitor for myelosuppression, cardiac changes, and renal failure regularly during therapy and following therapy Associated with: • Dose-dependent myelosuppression (neutropenia, anemia, and thrombocytopenia) • Serious, dose-related neurologic toxicity (including irreversible paraparesis and quadriparesis) • Acute nephrotoxicity (e.g., acidosis, anuria, increased serum creatinine), particularly when administered with other nephrotoxic agents • Requires experienced clinician who is knowledgeable in the use of chemotherapy agents

Drug Name	FDA-Approved Indications	Adult Dosage Range	Precautions and Clinical Pearls
Generic Name Clofarabine **Brand Name** Clolar ▲ ■ (PD)	ALL Treatment of relapsed or refractory ALL	**Usual parenteral dose**: IV: 52 mg/m^2 per day on days 1 through 5; repeat every 2 to 6 weeks Subsequent cycles should begin no sooner than 14 days from day 1 of the previous cycle	• Serious and fatal cases of Stevens-Johnson syndrome (SJS) and TEN • Drugs with known renal or hepatic toxicity should be avoided • Monitor cardiac function, CBC, platelets, and renal/hepatic function closely • Monitor for signs of potential systemic inflammatory response syndrome (SIRS), capillary leak syndrome, and organ dysfunction (e.g., tachypnea, tachycardia, hypotension, pulmonary edema) • Maintain adequate hydration with IV fluids during drug-administration periods • Severe myelosuppression should be anticipated; monitor labs and provide supportive therapy as needed (generally dose dependent and reversible) • See age-specific recommendations in the PI
Generic Name Fludarabine **Brand Name** Fludara Oforta ▲ ■	B-cell CLL	**Usual parenteral dose**: IV: 25 mg/m^2 per day for 5 days every 28 days	• Monitor CBC with differential, platelet count, aspartate transaminase (AST), alanine transaminase (ALT), serum creatinine, serum albumin, and uric acid • Monitor for signs of infection and neurotoxicity • Use caution in the presence of infection, fever, or history of opportunistic infection; renal insufficiency; hematologic disorders; central nervous system (CNS) disorders; or peripheral neuropathy Associated with: • Severe bone marrow suppression • Severe neurologic toxicity (delayed blindness, coma, death); similar neurotoxicity (agitation, coma, confusion, seizure) • Drug interactions may require dose adjustments or avoidance of certain drug combinations or avoidance of certain drug combinations. • Life-threatening autoimmune effects, including hemolytic anemia, autoimmune thrombocytopenia/thrombocytopenic purpura (ITP) • Requires experienced clinician who is knowledgeable in the use of chemotherapy agents

Generic Name Mercaptopurine **Brand Name** Purixan Purinethol (DSC) ▲	ALL (as part of a combination chemotherapy regimen)	**Usual oral dose:** Maintenance: 1.5 to 2.5 mg/kg once daily (50 to 75 mg/m^2 once daily); continue based on blood counts	• Bone marrow suppression: dose-related leukopenia, thrombocytopenia, and anemia • Associated with the development of lymphoma and other malignancies • Monitor CBC with differential, bone marrow exam, liver function tests, and bilirubin • Assess hepatic function; jaundice, ascites, and encephalopathy are possible: hepatotoxicity reported • Monitor nutritional status and renal status • Monitor for dehydration, myelosuppression, anemia, and leukopenia on a regular basis • Initiate treatment at the low end of the recommended dose range
Generic Name Nelarabine **Brand Name** Arranon ■ (PD)	T-cell acute lymphoblastic leukemia/lymphoma following at least 2 chemotherapy regimens	**Usual parenteral dose**: IV: 1500 mg/m^2 per dose on days 1, 3, and 5; repeat every 21 days	• Assess CBC and renal and hepatic function; dose adjustment for impairment is not available • Demyelination and ascending peripheral neuropathies similar to Guillain-Barré syndrome have been reported • Tumor lysis syndrome (TLS) may occur as a consequence of leukemia treatment Associated with: • Severe neurologic events, including mental status changes, severe somnolence, seizures, and peripheral neuropathy. Monitor for neurotoxicity (somnolence, confusion, convulsions, hypoesthesia, paresthesia, peripheral neuropathy), diarrhea, nausea, vomiting, gastrointestinal pain, dehydration, anemia, neutropenia, thrombocytopenia, and edema at beginning of therapy and regularly throughout the course of treatment
Generic Name Pentostatin **Brand Name** Nipent ▲ ■	Hairy cell leukemia	**Usual parenteral dose**: IV: 4 mg/m^2 every 2 weeks	• Monitor CBC with differential and platelet count, peripheral blood smears, liver function, serum uric acid, renal function, bone marrow evaluation, and signs and symptoms of pulmonary and CNS toxicity • Severe CNS, liver, pulmonary, and renal toxicities have occurred • Use caution in the presence of renal insufficiency, fever, infection, or renal dysfunction Associated with: • Requires experienced clinician who is knowledgeable in the use of chemotherapy agents • Drug interactions may require dose adjustment or avoidance of certain drug combinations

Drug Name	FDA-Approved Indications	Adult Dosage Range	Precautions and Clinical Pearls
Generic Name Thioguanine **Brand Name** Tabloid	Acute myelogenous (nonlymphocytic) leukemia (AML)	**Usual oral dose:** 100 mg/m^2 every 12 hours for 5 to 10 days, usually in combination with cytarabine Single agent: 2 to 2.5 mg/kg per day, which can be increased to 3 mg/kg per day in the absence of serious toxicity	• Monitor for myelosuppression, nausea, vomiting, anorexia, malaise, and hepatotoxicity weekly when beginning therapy, then monthly or sooner if clinically indicated • Myelosuppression (anemia, leukopenia, and/or thrombocytopenia); infection (due to leukopenia) and/or bleeding (due to thrombocytopenia) have been reported • Long-term continuous therapy or maintenance treatment is associated with a high risk for hepatotoxicity. Use with caution in patients with hepatic impairment • Secondary malignancies: potentially carcinogenic

Pyrimidine Antagonists

Drug Name	FDA-Approved Indications	Adult Dosage Range	Precautions and Clinical Pearls
Generic Name Azacitidine **Brand Name** Vidaza	Myelodysplastic syndromes (MDS)	**Usual parenteral dose**: IV/SQ: 75 mg/m^2 per day for 7 days every 4 weeks	• Bone marrow suppression: neutropenia, thrombocytopenia, and anemia are common • Gastrointestinal toxicity: moderate emetic potential • Injection-site reactions • Monitor liver function tests, electrolytes, CBC with differential and platelets, renal function (blood urea nitrogen [BUN] and serum creatinine) at baseline, prior to each cycle, and more frequently if indicated • Use with caution in the presence of hepatic or renal impairment (dose adjustment may be required) • Monitor for nausea/vomiting and for injection-site reactions • Pretreatment with an antiemetic recommended to reduce nausea and vomiting • Tumor lysis syndrome has been reported
Generic Name Capecitabine **Brand Name** Xeloda	Metastatic breast cancer resistant to paclitaxel and anthracyclines Metastatic colorectal cancer	**Usual oral dose:** 1250 mg/m^2 twice daily for 2 weeks, every 21 days	• Bone marrow suppression may occur; hematologic toxicity is more common when used in combination therapy • Cardiotoxicity including myocardial infarction, ischemia, angina, dysrhythmias, cardiac arrest, cardiac failure, sudden death, ECG changes, and cardiomyopathy • Evaluate renal and hepatic function and CBC with differential at baseline and regularly during therapy • Monitor for diarrhea, dehydration, hand-foot syndrome, SJS, TEN, stomatitis, and cardiotoxicity Associated with: • Drug interactions may require dose adjustments or avoidance of certain drug combinations or avoidance of certain drug combinations

Generic Name Cytarabine **Brand Name** Cytosar U ▲ ■	Acute myeloid leukemia (AML) ALL Chronic myeloid leukemia (CML) Meningeal leukemia	**Usual parenteral dose for AML:** IV: 100 mg/m^2 to 200 mg/m^2 per day continuous infusion for 7 days	• Cytarabine (ARA-C) syndrome is characterized by fever, myalgia, bone pain, chest pain (occasionally), maculopapular rash, conjunctivitis, and malaise • Monitor CBC, uric acid, and liver and renal function; white blood cells (WBC) nadir is reached in 7 to 10 days; platelets (PLT) nadir is reached in 12 to 15 days • Assess for signs and symptoms of infection • Monitor for ocular pain, conjunctivitis, signs of GI bleed, and CNS toxicity • Can be administered by intrathecal route with specific instructions provided by the manufacturer; refer to PI Associated with: • Myelosuppression (leukopenia, thrombocytopenia and anemia) • Gastrointestinal toxicities (less serious): nausea, vomiting, diarrhea, abdominal pain, oral ulcerations, and hepatic dysfunction • Hepatotoxicity • Requires experienced clinician who is knowledgeable in the use of chemotherapy agents and specialized care setting
Generic Name Decitabine **Brand Name** Dacogen	Myelodysplastic syndromes (MDS)	**Usual parenteral dose**: 3-day regimen: IV: 15 mg/m^2 infusion over 3 hours, repeated every 8 hours for 3 days; repeat every 6 weeks 5-day regimen: IV: 20 mg/m^2 infusion over 1 hour daily for 5 days, repeat every 4 weeks	• It is recommended that patients be treated for a minimum of 4 cycles; however, a complete response may take longer than 4 cycles • Myelosuppression and worsening neutropenia are more common in the first two treatment cycles and may not correlate with progression of underlying MDS. Bone marrow suppression: neutropenia, thrombocytopenia, anemia, and neutropenic fever have been reported • Hematologic toxicity may require dosage adjustment • Monitor for infection • Monitor CBC with differential and platelets, liver enzymes, and serum creatinine • Use with caution in the presence of renal and hepatic impairment • Premedication with an antiemetic is recommended • Monitor for worsening neutropenia, thrombocytopenia, anemia, pulmonary edema, gastrointestinal disturbance, CNS changes, hyperglycemia, and infection prior to each cycle and periodically as indicated during therapy • Advise patients with diabetes to monitor serum glucose closely; may cause hyperglycemia

Drug Name	FDA-Approved Indications	Adult Dosage Range	Precautions and Clinical Pearls
Generic Name Floxuridine **Brand Name** FUDR ■	Colorectal cancer, hepatic metastases Palliative management of hepatic metastases of colorectal cancer	**Usual parenteral dose**: Intra-arterial: 0.1 to 0.6 mg/kg per day as a continuous infusion; continue until intolerable toxicity occurs	• Bone marrow suppression: may cause severe hematologic toxicity (anemia, leukopenia, and thrombocytopenia) • Cardiovascular toxicity: myocardial ischemia • May cause gastrointestinal toxicity. • Bleeding may occur; discontinue if hemorrhage occurs • Monitor CBC with differential and platelet count; liver function; signs and symptoms of stomatitis/esophagopharyngitis, gastrointestinal ulceration/bleeding, hemorrhage, vomiting, and diarrhea • Use with caution in patients with impaired liver or kidney function • Monitor for CNS changes and acute gastrointestinal reactions • Teach patient or caregiver to use and care for the implantable pump; drug is administered into hepatic artery. • Drug interactions may require dose adjustments or avoidance of certain drug combinations or avoidance of certain drug combinations Associated with: • Risk of severe toxicity, patients should be hospitalized for their first course of floxuridine therapy • Requires experienced clinician who is knowledgeable in the use of chemotherapy agents and specialized care setting
Generic Name Fluorouracil **Brand Name** Adrucil ■	Breast cancer Colon cancer Rectal cancer Pancreatic cancer Stomach (gastric) cancer	Dose is based on indication for use and patient's clinical response. Various protocols exist. The manufacturer recommends a maximum 5-FU dose of 800 mg per day IV; however, higher doses are routinely given. Higher doses are more safely given as continuous infusion versus bolus dosing which can result in severe toxicity or fatalities due to hemorrhagic colitis or bone marrow suppression.	• Often described as "5-FU" • Palmar–plantar erythrodysesthesia (hand–foot syndrome) has been associated with use; symptoms include a tingling sensation, which may progress to pain, and then to symmetrical swelling and erythema with tenderness • Inform prescriber if intractable vomiting or diarrhea occurs. Discontinue if the patient experiences intractable vomiting, diarrhea, precipitous fall in leukocyte or platelet counts, myocardial ischemia, hemorrhage, gastrointestinal ulcer or bleeding, stomatitis, or esophagopharyngitis • Monitor lab tests, CBC, and renal and hepatic function throughout therapy; avoid in patients if elevated serum bilirubin greater than 5 mg/dL • Instruct patients to report any signs of chest pain; assess for EKG changes or elevated cardiac enzymes • Assess cardiovascular, respiratory, and renal function prior to each infusion and on a regular basis • Teach the patient about the importance of adequate hydration • Drug interactions may require dose adjustments or avoidance of certain drug combinations

		By continuous infusion, higher daily doses (i.e., 1 or 2 g per day) have been given successfully with less hematologic toxicity.	Contraindications: • Patients with patients with potentially serious infections and/or bone marrow suppression • Patients with dihydropyrimidine dehydrogenase (DPD) deficiency; they are at significant risk of toxicity • Malnourished patients Associated with: • Requires experienced clinician who is knowledgeable in the use of chemotherapy agents and specialized care setting
Generic Name Gemcitabine **Brand Name** Gemzar	Breast cancer NSCLC Ovarian cancer Pancreatic cancer	Dose is based on the indication for use and the patient's clinical response **Illustrative parenteral dose for NSCLC:** IV: 1000 mg/m^2 over 30 minutes on days 1, 8, and 15; repeat cycle every 28 days	• May cause bone marrow suppression (neutropenia, thrombocytopenia, and anemia) • Capillary leak syndrome may have serious consequences • Hemolytic-uremic syndrome has been reported; may lead to renal failure and dialysis (including death) • Posterior reversible encephalopathy syndrome (PRES) • Pulmonary toxicity, including adult respiratory distress syndrome, interstitial pneumonitis, pulmonary edema, and pulmonary fibrosis • Monitor hepatic and renal function and use with caution in the presence of renal or hepatic impairment; serious hepatotoxicity has been reported • Assess CBC with differential and platelet count prior to each dose • Monitor for fever, CNS changes, rash, gastrointestinal upset, myelosuppression, anemia, dyspnea, and infection prior to each treatment and on a regular basis
Generic Name Hydroxyurea **Brand Name** Droxia Hydrea ▲ ■	Refractory CML Management of locally advanced squamous cell head and neck cancer Management of sickle cell anemia	Dose based on indication for use, patient's clinical response, and ideal or actual body weight, whichever is less (per manufacturer) **Illustrative oral dose for antineoplastic uses (CML, head and neck cancer):** 20 to 30 mg/kg once per day as a single dose; continue therapy if a response is observed after 6 weeks of therapy	• Vasculitic ulcerations and gangrene have been reported • Self-limiting macrocytosis/megaloblastic erythropoiesis may be seen early in treatment • Specific criteria are required for use if the patient has sickle cell anemia • Assess results of CBC; myelosuppression could be life threatening; interruption of therapy recommended for specific blood cell count thresholds; refer to PI • Monitor for CNS changes, gastrointestinal upset, hepatotoxicity, cutaneous toxicity, and peripheral neuropathy • Teach proper use and safe handling of medication Associated with: • Severe myelosuppression • Hydroxyurea is carcinogenic; monitor patients for additional malignancies • Advise sun protection

DNA Agents

DNA Alkylating Agents: Nitrosoureas

Universal prescribing alerts:

- Long-term use of nitrosoureas may be associated with development of secondary malignancies.

Drug Name	FDA-Approved Indications	Adult Dosage Range	Precautions and Clinical Pearls
Generic Name Carmustine **Brand Name** BiCNU Gliadel ■	**Common indications for use:** Brain tumors Hodgkin's disease Multiple myeloma Non-Hodgkin's lymphoma	**Usual parenteral dose for brain tumors:** IV: 150 to 200 mg/m^2 every 6 weeks or 75 to 100 mg/m^2 per day for 2 days every 6 weeks	• Hematologic toxicity generally is delayed; monitor blood counts for at least 6 weeks following treatment • Myelosuppression is cumulative • Wafer implant: brain edema has been reported in patients with newly diagnosed glioma • Administer antiemetic prior to therapy • Infusion site should be monitored closely to prevent extravasation • For bone marrow transplant (BMT) high-dose infusion: patient must be monitored closely during and following infusion; fluid and vasopressor support should be available • Assess results of hematology, pulmonary, hepatic, and renal function tests at baseline and periodically during therapy • Pulmonary function should be assessed for extended periods following high doses or BMT doses Associated with: • Bone marrow suppression, primarily thrombocytopenia and leukopenia • Dose-related pulmonary toxicity; delayed onset of pulmonary fibrosis may occur years after treatment • Requires experienced clinician who is knowledgeable in the use of chemotherapy agents
Generic Name Lomustine **Brand Name** Gleostine CeeNU (DSC) ■	Brain tumors Hodgkin's lymphoma	Dose is based on indication for use and patient's clinical response **Illustrative oral dose for brain tumors:** 130 mg/m^2 once every 6 weeks; reduce dose to 100 mg/m^2 once every 6 weeks in patients with compromised bone marrow function	• Do not administer courses more frequently than every 6 weeks due to delayed myelotoxicity • Patients can develop delayed-onset pulmonary fibrosis; monitor for pulmonary symptoms during and after treatment. May cause delayed pulmonary toxicity (infiltrates and/or fibrosis) • Evaluate hematologic, hepatic, pulmonary, and renal status at baseline and periodically throughout therapy, and for at least 6 weeks after a dose • Reversible hepatotoxicity has been reported. • Monitor for symptoms of abnormal bleeding and signs of infection • Instruct the patient to notify the physician of fever, chills, sore throat, bleeding or bruising, shortness of breath, swelling of feet or lower legs, or yellowing of eyes and skin

			• Drug interactions may require dose adjustments or avoidance of certain drug combinations or avoidance of certain drug combinations • Instruct the patient that the dose may be made up of two or more different shapes and colors of capsules in the dispensed container • Inform patients that only one lomustine dose should be taken no sooner than every 6 weeks Associated with: • Bone marrow suppression, particularly thrombocytopenia and leukopenia • Potential for overdose or poisoning; fatal toxicity has been reported with lomustine overdose. Do not prescribe, dispense, or administer more than one dose at a time.
Generic Name Streptozocin **Brand Name** Zanosar ■	Metastatic islet cell carcinoma of the pancreas	**Usual parenteral dose**: IV: 500 mg/m^2 per day for 5 consecutive days every 6 weeks until maximum benefit is achieved or unacceptable toxicity occurs	• Antiemetic should be administered prior to therapy (emetic potential is 100%) • Infusion site should be monitored closely to prevent extravasation • Monitor for nephrotoxicity/renal dysfunction (input and output [I & O], hematuria, edema, BUN), hepatotoxicity (jaundice, fatigue, liver function tests [LFTs]), hypoglycemia, and diarrhea (dehydration) on a regular basis • Caution patients with diabetes to monitor glucose levels closely; may precipitate hypoglycemia • Select the dose cautiously, beginning at the lower end of the dosing range Associated with: • Hematologic toxicity • May cause severe nausea and vomiting and diarrhea • Liver dysfunction • Renal toxicity is dose related and cumulative; may be severe or fatal • Streptozocin is mutagenic; parenteral use is tumorigenic and carcinogenic in animals • Requires experienced clinician who is knowledgeable in the use of chemotherapy agents and specialized care setting

DNA Cross-linking/Alkylating Agents

Universal prescribing alerts:

- All chemotherapeutic agents (including cross-linking alkylating agents) may require temporary interruption of therapy and a dosage reduction may be necessary in patients who develop toxicity or intolerable side effects, including but not limited to, blood counts that fall below threshold values. Refer to each agent's package insert (PI) for greater details.

Drug Name	FDA-Approved Indications	Adult Dosage Range	Precautions and Clinical Pearls
Generic Name Altretamine **Brand Name** Hexalen ■ GD	Recurrent ovarian cancer	**Usual oral dose:** 260 mg/m^2 per day in 4 divided doses for 14 to 21 days of a 28-day cycle	• Use with caution in patients previously treated with other myelosuppressive drugs or with preexisting neurotoxicity • Monitor for neuropathy, gastrointestinal upset, and anemia • Monitor CBC with differential (before each cycle and regularly during treatment); perform neurologic examination (before each cycle and regularly during treatment) • Antiemetics are recommended to prevent nausea and vomiting • Temporary discontinuation may be required if side effects become intolerable and/or if blood counts fall below threshold; refer to PI Contraindications: • Patients with preexisting severe neurotoxicity and/or bone marrow suppression Associated with: • Bone marrow suppression: peripheral blood counts should be done routinely before each cycle and during treatment • Neurotoxicity: neurologic examinations should be done routinely before each cycle and during treatment
Generic Name Bendamustine **Brand Name** Treanda Bendeka	CLL Non-Hodgkin's lymphoma	Dose is based on indication for use and patient's clinical response **Illustrative parenteral dose for CLL:** IV: 100 mg/m^2 infusion over 30 minutes (Treanda) on days 1 and 2 of a 28-day treatment cycle, for up to 6 cycles	• Myelosuppression (neutropenia, thrombocytopenia, and anemia) • Rash, toxic skin reactions and bullous exanthema have been reported with monotherapy and with combination therapy • Different formulations have different administration rates; refer to PI • Tumor lysis syndrome (usually occurring in the first treatment cycle) • Use with caution in the presence of hepatic or renal impairment. Not recommended in presence of severe impairment • Infusion site must be monitored closely to avoid extravasation. • Monitor infusion reactions, including skin reactions; can occur with first or subsequent cycles and may require premedication or discontinuation • Drug interactions may require dose adjustments or avoidance of certain drug combinations
Generic Name Busulfan **Brand Name** Busulfex Myleran ■ PD	CML	**Illustrative oral dose:** **For treatment of CML in chronic stage:** 4 to 8 mg per day	• Hematopoietic progenitor cell transplantation is required to prevent potentially fatal complications from prolonged myelosuppression due to IV busulfan • Cardiac tamponade has been reported in certain age-specific populations with thalassemia treated with high-dose oral busulfan; refer to PI • Hepatic sinusoidal obstruction syndrome has been reported • Identify any history of seizures, recent myelosuppressive therapy, and/or radiation treatment • Dosing for obese patients should be based on adjusted ideal body weight. • Hematopoietic stem cell transplantation (HSCT): phenytoin or clonazepam may be ordered prophylactically during and for at least 48 hours following completion of busulfan therapy to reduce the risk of seizures if the patient is predisposed to seizures

			• Assess CBC with differential, platelet count, and LFTs • Monitor for adverse pulmonary or hematologic effects during therapy and for several months following therapy • Start with lowest recommended doses Associated with: • Severe and prolonged bone marrow suppression • Potential for secondary malignancy
Generic Name Chlorambucil **Brand Name** Leukeran ■	CLL Hodgkin's lymphoma Non-Hodgkin's lymphomas	Dose is based on indication for use and patient's clinical response **Illustrative oral dose for CLL:** 0.1 mg/kg per day for 3 to 6 weeks or 0.4 mg/kg pulsed doses administered intermittently, biweekly, or monthly	• Use with caution in the presence of seizure disorder or bone marrow suppression • Seizures have been observed with use; patients with a history of nephrotic syndrome and high pulse doses are at higher risk of seizures • Monitor for hematologic myelosuppression, hypersensitivity rash, drug fever, seizures, gastrointestinal upset, and hepatotoxicity Associated with: • Severe bone marrow suppression • May be mutagenic and carcinogenic
Generic Name Cyclophosphamide **Brand Name** Cytoxan ▲ QT BL PD	**Common indications for use:** ALL Acute myelocytic leukemia (AML) CLL CML	Dose is based on indication for use and patient's clinical response **Illustrative parenteral dose for breast cancer:** IV: 500 to 1000 mg/m^2 on day 1; additional doses and drug combinations based on selected regimen (refer to PI)	• Leukopenia, neutropenia, thrombocytopenia, and anemia have been reported • Cardiotoxicity has been reported (some fatal) • Monitor for infections; immunosuppression and serious infections may occur • Use is associated with the development of hemorrhagic cystitis, pyelitis, ureteritis, and hematuria • Monitor the IV site for signs of extravasation • Assess results of urinalysis, BUN, and serum creatinine to evaluate for nephrotoxicity. Monitor renal function to ensure appropriate doses are used • Monitor CBC with differential and platelet count to identify myelosuppression • Monitor for hemorrhagic cystitis and renal tubular necrosis, especially when high doses are given • Teach patients about the importance of adequate hydration, especially patients who are taking oral tablets • Teach patients about the importance of follow-up to monitor for secondary malignancies

Drug Name	FDA-Approved Indications	Adult Dosage Range	Precautions and Clinical Pearls
	Hodgkin's and non-Hodgkin's lymphoma Ovarian cancer Breast cancer	Oral: 100 to 200 mg/m^2 per day for 4 to 14 days.	• Drug interactions may require dose adjustments or avoidance of certain drug combinations • Specific recommendations for patients undergoing dialysis. Contraindications: • Patients with bladder or other urinary tract obstruction
Generic Name Dacarbazine **Brand Name** DTIC-Dome ■ (PD) (GD)	Malignant melanoma Hodgkin's lymphoma	Dose is based on indication for use and patient's clinical response **Illustrative parenteral dose for metastatic melanoma:** IV: 250 mg/m^2 per dose on days 1 to 5; repeat every 3 weeks	• Anaphylaxis may occur following dacarbazine administration • Use with caution and monitor for toxicity in the presence of renal or hepatic impairment • Premedicate patients with an antiemetic (emetic potential is moderately high) • Patients must be monitored closely for anaphylactic reaction; emergency treatment should be available • Monitor the infusion site closely; extravasation can cause severe cellulitis or tissue necrosis • Assess the results of the CBC with differential and LFTs prior to each treatment and throughout therapy • Drug interactions may require dose adjustments or avoidance of certain drug combinations Associated with: • Bone marrow suppression is a common toxicity • May be carcinogenic • Hepatotoxicity with hepatocellular necrosis and hepatic vein thrombosis has been reported • Requires experienced clinician who is knowledgeable in the use of chemotherapy agents and specialized care setting
Generic Name Estramustine **Brand Name** Emcyt	Prostate cancer: palliative treatment of progressive and/or metastatic prostate cancer	**Usual oral dose:** 14 mg/kg per day in 3 or 4 divided doses	• Allergic reactions and angioedema, including airway involvement • Elevated blood pressure or congestive heart disease may occur • Estrogenic effects may decrease testosterone levels; may cause gynecomastia and/or impotence • Peripheral edema (new onset or exacerbation) or congestive heart disease may occur • Use with caution in the presence of renal or hepatic impairment, metabolic disease, seizure disorders, or migraine history • Assess serum calcium levels and LFTs • Monitor for hypertension, CNS changes, and thromboembolism on a regular basis • Caution patients with diabetes to monitor glucose carefully; glucose tolerance may be decreased Contraindications: • Patients with active thromboembolic disease, stroke, or thrombophlebitis unless benefit outweighs risk

Generic Name Ifosfamide **Brand Name** Ifex ▲ ■	Germ cell testicular cancer	**Usual parenteral dose as part of combination chemotherapy and with mesna:** IV: 1200 mg to 2000 mg/m^2 per day for 5 days every 3 weeks or after hematologic recovery	• To prevent bladder toxicity, maintain adequate hydration for 72 hours prior to infusion to minimize risk of hemorrhagic cystitis • Obtain baseline urinalysis prior to each dose and throughout therapy to evaluate for hematuria • Premedicate patients with an appropriate antiemetic prior to each infusion • Monitor for CNS depression or psychoses • Obtain CBC with differential; myelosuppression may be dose limiting • Monitor liver function and renal function tests • Evaluate for signs and symptoms of pulmonary toxicity • Drug interactions may require dose adjustments or avoidance of certain drug combinations Contraindications: • Patients with severe bone marrow suppression Associated with: • Severe bone marrow suppression • CNS toxicity, which may be severe, resulting in encephalopathy and death: monitor for CNS toxicity; discontinue for encephalopathy • Hemorrhagic cystitis • Severe nephrotoxicity, resulting in renal failure
Generic Name Mechlorethamine **Brand Name** Mustargen ■ ■	**Common indications for use:** Palliative treatment of Hodgkin's lymphoma Palliative treatment of effusions from metastatic carcinomas	Dose is based on indication for use and patient's clinical response **Illustrative parenteral dose for Hodgkin's lymphoma:** IV: 0.2 mg/kg or 6 mg/m^2 as a single dose day 1 or as a dose on days 1 and 8 of regimen	• May cause lymphopenia, leukopenia, granulocytopenia, thrombocytopenia and anemia • Monitor for bone marrow suppression, infection, and bleeding • Educate patients about lifelong monitoring for secondary cancers • Avoid administration of live vaccines • If extravasation occurs, promptly manage it by infiltrating the area (specific dilution instructions available in PI), followed by dry cold compresses for 6 to 12 hours Associated with: • Need for special handling; highly toxic; refer to PI • Requires experienced clinician who is knowledgeable in the use of chemotherapy agents and specialized care setting • Mechlorethamine is a potent vesicant; extravasation results in painful inflammation with induration and sloughing

Drug Name	FDA-Approved Indications	Adult Dosage Range	Precautions and Clinical Pearls
Generic Name Melphalan **Brand Name** Alkeran Evomela ▲ (QT)	Multiple myeloma Ovarian carcinoma	Dose is based on indication for use and patient's clinical response **Illustrative oral dose for multiple myeloma (palliative):** 6 mg once daily for 2 to 3 weeks initially, followed by up to 4 weeks of rest, then a maintenance dose of 2 mg daily as hematologic recovery begins Parenteral therapy is available for whom oral therapy is not appropriate. Dose and administration route is specific to indication for use; refer to PI Maximum IV dose: 100 mg/m^2 for 2 consecutive days (Evomela)	• Assess hematologic parameters at baseline and at regular intervals • IV: Follow administration specifics and monitor infusion site carefully to prevent extravasation • Monitor for pulmonary toxicity, gastrointestinal upset, myelosuppression (leukopenia), diarrhea, and hypersensitivity reaction on a regular basis • Use caution and begin at the lower end of the dosing range Associated with: • Bone marrow suppression is common; may be severe and result in infection or bleeding • Hypersensitivity reactions (including anaphylaxis) have occurred in approximately 2% of patients receiving IV melphalan • Produces chromosomal abnormalities and is leukemogenic and potentially mutagenic • May result in secondary malignancy • Requires experienced clinician who is knowledgeable in the use of chemotherapy agents and specialized care setting
Generic Name Procarbazine **Brand Name** Matulane ■ (PD)	Hodgkin's lymphoma	**Illustrative oral dose:** 100 mg/m^2 on days 1 to 7 every 21 days (in combination with bleomycin, etoposide, doxorubicin, cyclophosphamide, vincristine, and prednisone), for 8 cycles	• Bone marrow suppression: hematologic toxicity (leukopenia and thrombocytopenia) may occur 2 to 8 weeks after treatment initiation • Monitor for neurotoxicity, nausea and vomiting, pneumonitis, arthralgia, and paresthesia • Withhold treatment for CNS toxicity; use of CNS depressants increases the risk of adverse reactions • May cause hemolysis or the presence of Heinz inclusion bodies in erythrocytes • Emetic potential is high; an antiemetic is generally required • Reduced dosage may be necessary with renal and hepatic impairment; no specific doses recommendations are available • Instruct patients about dietary and alcohol cautions (procarbazine has some monoamine oxidase [MAO] inhibitory effects and can result in life-threatening hypertension when combined with tyramine; its use with alcohol may cause a disulfiram-like reaction)

			Contraindications: • Patients with severe bone marrow suppression Associated with: • Requires experienced clinician who is knowledgeable in the use of chemotherapy agents and specialized care setting
Generic Name Temozolomide **Brand Name** Temodar ▲ ■ (GD)	Anaplastic astrocytoma Glioblastoma multiforme	Dose is based on indication for use and patient's clinical response **Illustrative oral dose for glioblastoma multiforme:** 75 mg/m^2 per day for 42 days with focal radiotherapy Dose may be administered IV	• Myelosuppression may occur • Do not open capsules; avoid drug exposure from inhalation or inadvertent skin and mucous membrane contact; thoroughly rinse affected area as per PI • Monitor renal function; changes in function may affect dose • Monitor liver function tests at baseline, halfway through the first cycle, prior to each subsequent cycle, and at 2 to 4 weeks after the last dose. Hepatotoxicity has been reported; may be severe or fatal • *Pneumocystis jirovecii* pneumonia (PCP) may occur; the risk is increased in patients receiving steroids or on longer dosing regimens • Monitor CBC with differential and platelets prior to each cycle, and weekly during the glioma concomitant-phase treatment • Monitor for CNS effects, gastrointestinal disturbance, myelosuppression, opportunistic infection, vision disturbance, and cough on a regular basis • Female patients and older adults (i.e., patients 70 years of age and older) are more likely to experience severe myelosuppression
Generic Name Thiotepa	Bladder cancer Breast cancer Ovarian cancer Effusions	Dose is based on indication for use and patient's clinical response **Illustrative parenteral dose for ovarian and breast cancer:** IV: 0.3 to 0.4 mg/kg every 1 to 4 weeks	• May be mutagenic • Myelosuppression commonly occurs; use with caution in patients with bone marrow damage • Potentially carcinogenic; myelodysplastic syndrome and AML have been reported • Use with caution in the presence of hepatic or renal impairment and compromised bone marrow reserve • Monitor for myelosuppression, leukopenia, dysuria, bleeding, and infection • Teach patients about the importance of adequate hydration • Drug interactions may require dose adjustments or avoidance of certain drug combinations • When using for intravesical instillation (in which the drug is directly inserted into the bladder through a catheter): retention for 2 hours once weekly for 4 weeks is required

Enzymes

Drug Name	FDA-Approved Indications	Adult Dosage Range	Precautions and Clinical Pearls
Generic Name Asparaginase (*Erwinia chrysanthemi*) **Brand Name** Erwinaze	ALL	Dose based on indication for use and patient's clinical response **Illustrative parenteral dose:** As a substitute for asparaginase (*E. coli*): IM/IV: 25,000 units/m^2 for each scheduled asparaginase dose	• Serious hypersensitivity reactions (grade 3 and 4); anaphylaxis and pancreatitis have been reported • Glucose intolerance can occur during therapy and in many cases, is irreversible and may require treatment • Monitor CBC with differential, amylase, liver enzymes, blood glucose, and coagulation parameters; for IV administration, consider monitoring nadir serum asparaginase activity (NSAA) levels • Monitor for symptoms of hypersensitivity, pancreatitis, thrombosis, or hemorrhage • Be prepared to handle potential adverse events such as severe hypersensitivity reactions, hyperglycemia, pancreatitis, and thrombosis • May also be used as a substitute for pegaspargase; refer to specific dosing and schedule guidance in the PI
Generic Name Pegaspargase **Brand Name** Oncaspar	ALL For use in patients with hypersensitivity to native forms of L-asparaginase First-line agent as part of multi-agent chemotherapeutic regimen	**Usual parenteral dose**: IM/IV: 2500 units/m^2 do not administer more frequently than every 14 days	• Anaphylaxis and serious allergic reactions may occur • Increased prothrombin time, increased partial thromboplastin time, and hypofibrinogenemia may occur • Tumor lysis syndrome has been reported • Altered liver function tests and decreased serum albumin, plasma fibrinogen) may occur • Monitor CBC with differential, platelets, amylase/lipase, liver function tests, fibrinogen, prothrombin time (PT), partial thromboplastin time (PTT), renal function tests, urine glucose, blood glucose, and triglycerides • Monitor vital signs during administration • Monitor for onset of abdominal pain; observe for allergic reaction and signs and symptoms of thrombosis or bleeding • Monitor for GI disturbance, thrombotic events, pancreatitis, depression of clotting factors, glucose intolerance, and hypotension • IV is preferred to IM administration; reduced chance of reduced adverse effects including hematoma Contraindications: • Patients with past or current pancreatitis • Patients who have had prior severe reactions to the drug including but not limited to significant hemorrhagic events

Histone Deacetylase Inhibitors

Drug Name	FDA-Approved Indications	Adult Dosage Range	Precautions and Clinical Pearls
Generic Name Belinostat **Brand Name** Beleodaq	Peripheral T-cell lymphoma (relapsed or refractory)	**Usual parenteral dose**: IV: 1000 mg/m^2 daily on days 1 to 5 every 21 days until disease progression or unacceptable toxicity	• Bone marrow suppression (e.g., thrombocytopenia) • Gastrointestinal toxicity • Reduced UGT1A1 activity (dose adjustment may be necessary in certain ethnic populations) • Monitor CBC with platelets (thrombocytopenia), electrolytes, hepatic/renal function tests, and for infection prior to first dose of cycle and throughout therapy as necessary; ANC and platelets must be evaluated prior to each cycle • Premedicate patients with antiemetics and/or antidiarrheals • Monitor for tumor lysis syndrome and signs and symptoms of GI toxicity • Drug interactions may require dose adjustments or avoidance of certain drug combinations
Generic Name Panobinostat **Brand Name** Farydak ■ ■ QT	Multiple myeloma	**Usual oral dose:** 20 mg once every other day for 3 doses each week during weeks 1 and 2 of a 21-day treatment cycle (e.g., Monday, Wednesday, and Friday of weeks 1 and 2 only; rest during week 3) for up to 8 cycles (along with bortezomib and dexamethasone)	• Bone marrow suppression; severe thrombocytopenia, neutropenia, and anemia have occurred; hemorrhage has been reported • Hepatotoxicity (elevation in LFTs and bilirubin); avoid use in patients with severe hepatic impairment • Infection, including severe infections • Consider pretreatment with antiemetics to prevent nausea and vomiting • Administer at the same time on scheduled days, without regard to food • Swallow the capsule whole with a cup of water; do not open, crush, or chew the capsule • Drug interactions may require dose adjustments or avoidance of certain drug combinations • Avoid consuming star fruit, pomegranate, and grapefruit with the treatment • Monitor CBC and platelets (prior to initiation, then weekly or as clinically indicated), electrolytes (especially potassium and magnesium), and LFTs • Monitor hydration status and for GI toxicity, signs and symptoms of hemorrhage and/or infection, and cardiovascular events • Avoid direct skin or mucous membrane contact with the powder inside the capsule; if contact occurs, wash thoroughly • Treatment may continue (the same schedule for panobinostat; the bortezomib and dexamethasone schedules are modified) for an additional 8 cycles in patients experiencing clinical benefit and acceptable toxicity • Total duration of therapy may be up to 16 cycles (48 weeks) • Determine QTc prior to the start of therapy and verify that QTc is less than 450 prior to initiation • Baseline absolute neutrophil count (ANC) should be at least 1500/mm^3 and platelets at least 100,000/mm^3 prior to treatment

Drug Name	FDA-Approved Indications	Adult Dosage Range	Precautions and Clinical Pearls
			Associated with: • Severe and fatal cardiac ischemic events, severe arrhythmias, QTc and EKG changes • Severe diarrhea
Generic Name Romidepsin **Brand Name** Istodax QT	Cutaneous T-cell lymphoma Peripheral T-cell lymphoma	Dose is based on indication for use and patient's clinical response **Illustrative parenteral dose for cutaneous T-cell lymphoma:** IV: 14mg/m^2 on days 1, 8, and 15 of a 28-day treatment cycle	• Anemia, leukopenia, neutropenia, lymphopenia, and thrombocytopenia may occur • Serious infections (occasionally fatal) have been reported, including pneumonia, sepsis, and viral reactivation • QTc prolongation has been observed • Obtain ECG and renal function tests prior to administering the drug to determine QT interval, potassium level, and magnesium level are normal • Monitor for tumor lysis syndrome after the drug is administered • Obtain the patient's current medications list, as concurrent use of diuretics may contribute to electrolyte imbalances • Drug interactions may require dose adjustment or avoidance of certain drug combinations
Generic Name Vorinostat **Brand Name** Zolinza ■ QT	Cutaneous T-cell lymphoma	**Usual oral dose:** 400 mg once daily until disease progression or unacceptable toxicity	• Dose-related anemia and thrombocytopenia may occur • May cause dizziness or fatigue • QTc prolongation has been observed • Monitor CBC with differential and serum chemistries, including calcium, magnesium, potassium, glucose, and creatinine • Use with caution in the presence of mild to moderate hepatic impairment; contraindicated in patients with severe impairment • Electrolyte abnormalities should be corrected prior to treatment • Use care to avoid accidental exposure of skin or mucous membranes to the powder within capsules; do not open or crush capsules; if such contact occurs, rinse area thoroughly • Drug interactions may require dose adjustment • Caution patients with diabetes to monitor serum glucose closely

Hormone/Hormone Modifiers

Drug Name	FDA-Approved Indications	Adult Dosage Range	Precautions and Clinical Pearls
Generic Name Abiraterone **Brand Name** Zytiga ■	Prostate cancer: metastatic, castration-resistant prostate cancer	**Usual oral dose:** 1000 mg once daily with prednisone 5 mg every 12 hours	• Concurrent infection, stress, or interruption of daily corticosteroids is associated with reports of adrenocortical insufficiency • Increased mineralocorticoids due to hepatic inhibition may result in hypertension, hypokalemia, and fluid retention • Significant increases in liver enzymes have been reported

			• Use with caution in patients with cardiovascular disease, recent myocardial infarction (MI), or ventricular arrhythmia; may cause hypertension, hypokalemia, and fluid retention • Not recommended for patients with severe hepatic impairment • Monitor for signs and symptoms of adrenocorticoid insufficiency • Drug interactions may require dose adjustments or avoidance of certain drug combinations
Generic Name Aldesleukin **Brand Name** Proleukin ■	Melanoma, metastatic Renal cell cancer, metastatic	Dose is based on indication for use and patient's clinical response **Illustrative parenteral dose for metastatic melanoma:** IV: 600,000 international units/kg every 8 hours, for a maximum of 14 doses 9-day rest period recommended prior to administration of additional doses.	• Monitor the infusion site for extravasation • Monitor vital signs; cardiac, respiratory, and CNS status; and fluid balance • Monitor for signs of systemic sepsis and changes in mental status • Laboratory reports should be assessed daily prior to beginning the infusion and for 2 hours following the infusion Contraindications: • Patients significant CNS impairment, cardiac disease, pulmonary disease, renal disease, hepatic disease, abnormal pulmonary function tests, and/or organ transplant Associated with: • Capillary leak syndrome, characterized by vascular tone loss and extravasation of plasma proteins and fluid into the extravascular space • Withhold treatment for patients developing moderate to severe lethargy or somnolence • Impaired neutrophil function is associated with treatment • Requires experienced clinician who is knowledgeable in the use of chemotherapy agents and specialized care setting
Generic Name Anastrozole **Brand Name** Arimidex	Breast cancer	Dose is based on indication for use and patient's clinical response **Illustrative oral dose for breast cancer, advanced:** 1 mg once daily	• Monitor bone mineral density, total cholesterol, and LDL cholesterol • Associated with a reduction in bone mineral density (BMD): decreases (from baseline) in total hip and lumbar spine BMD • Elevated total cholesterol levels (especially increases in low-density lipoprotein [LDL] cholesterol) have been reported in patients • Use caution in patients with preexisting cardiac disease and/or hepatic impairment • Drug interactions may require dose adjustments or avoidance of certain drug combinations

Drug Name	FDA-Approved Indications	Adult Dosage Range	Precautions and Clinical Pearls
Generic Name Bicalutamide **Brand Name** Casodex	Prostate cancer, metastatic	**Usual oral dose:** 50 mg once daily	• Anemia may occur with testosterone suppression • Rare cases of death or hospitalization due to hepatitis have been reported in post-marketing surveillance • ILD has been reported in rare cases • Use with caution in the presence of hepatic impairment • Assess the LFT results at baseline and periodically throughout therapy • Advise patients with diabetes to monitor their glucose levels closely; may induce hyperglycemia • Drug interactions may require dose adjustments or avoidance of certain drug combinations • The manufacturer lists females as a contraindicated population for use
Generic Name Degarelix **Brand Name** Firmagon QT	Prostate cancer, advanced	**Usual parenteral dose**: SQ initial dose: 240 mg administered as two 120-mg (3-mL) injections SQ maintenance dose: 80 mg administered as one (4-mL) injection every 28 days	• Decreased bone mineral density • Supplemental calcium and vitamin D may reduce risk of osteoporosis due to androgen deprivation • Use with caution in the presence of, or in patients with a history of, cardiovascular disease; minimize cardiovascular risk factors • Androgen deprivation therapy may prolong the QT interval • Hypersensitivity reactions (including anaphylaxis, urticaria, and angioedema) have been reported • Evaluate prostate-specific antigen (PSA) and serum testosterone levels, LFTs, electrolytes, and bone density on a regular basis during therapy • Double check the vial strength to ensure accuracy prior to administering; there are multiple dosage strengths available and these formulations are not interchangeable
Generic Name Enzalutamide **Brand Name** Xtandi	Metastatic prostate cancer (castration resistant)	**Usual oral dose:** 160 mg once daily	• Seizures are possible (but rare); use with caution in patients with seizure disorder or other predisposing factors • Monitor cardiac function and for signs and symptoms of posterior reversible encephalopathy syndrome (PRES) • May increase the risk for cardiovascular disease (CVD) (e.g., increase blood pressure or worsen preexisting hypertension) • Administer without regard to food; swallow capsules whole • Monitor for signs and symptoms of seizure, loss of consciousness, dizziness, hallucinations, and peripheral edema, at baseline and periodically • Monitor CBC (risk of neutropenia), LFTs, and blood pressure

			• Perform additional international normalized ration (INR) monitoring (if patient is on warfarin) • Drug interactions may require dose adjustments or avoidance of certain drug combinations • Not indicated for use in females
Generic Name Exemestane **Brand Name** Aromasin	Breast cancer	**Usual oral dose:** 25 mg once daily	• Obtain a bone density exam and vitamin D level before initiating therapy • Leads to a reduction in bone mineral density over time • Grade 3 or 4 lymphopenia has been observed • Use with caution in patients with liver and kidney disease or uncontrolled hypertension • Elevations of AST, ALT, alkaline phosphatase, and gamma glutamyl transferase more than 5 times the upper limit of normal (ULN) have been observed • Do not use in premenopausal women • Monitor for new or unusual bone pain or swelling of the face, lips, or throat • Drug interactions may require dose adjustments or avoidance of certain drug combinations
Generic Name Flutamide **Brand Name** Eulexin ■	Prostate cancer	**Usual oral dose:** 250 mg 3 times daily	• Elevated serum transaminase levels, jaundice, hepatic encephalopathy, and acute hepatic failure have been reported • Assess serum transaminase levels prior to and periodically during therapy • Monitor for galactorrhea, CNS changes, ataxia, anorexia, vomiting, lacrimation, anemia and potential for hepatic impairment on a regular basis • Monitoring of methemoglobin concentrations should be considered in patients predisposed to metabolite accumulation (i.e., smokers, G6PD deficiency, etc.); refer to PI • Teach patients to report chest pain, respiratory difficulty, abdominal pain, and signs of liver dysfunction • Drug interactions may require dose adjustments or avoidance of certain drug combinations Contraindications: • Patients with severe hepatic impairment Associated with: • Hospitalization and death (rare) due to liver failure

Drug Name	FDA-Approved Indications	Adult Dosage Range	Precautions and Clinical Pearls
Generic Name Fulvestrant **Brand Name** Faslodex	Treatment of hormone-receptor–positive metastatic breast cancer	**Usual parenteral dose**: IM initial: 500 mg on days 1, 15, and 29 IM maintenance: 500 mg once monthly	• Hypersensitivity reactions, including urticaria and angioedema, have been reported • Use with caution in patients with a history of bleeding disorders (including thrombocytopenia) and patients on anticoagulant therapy • Use with caution in the presence of hepatic impairment • Monitor for thromboembolism, vasodilation, edema, gastrointestinal disturbances, dyspnea, and pain on a regular basis throughout therapy • Drug interactions may require dose adjustments or avoidance of certain drug combinations
Generic Name Goserelin **Brand Name** Zoladex QT	Breast cancer, advanced Endometrial thinning Endometriosis Prostate cancer, advanced	Dose is based on indication for use and patient's clinical response **Illustrative parenteral dose for males with prostate cancer (advanced):** SQ: 28-day implant: 3.6 mg every 28 days SQ: 12-week implant: 10.8 mg every 12 weeks	• Decreased bone density • Hypercalcemia has been reported in prostate and breast cancer patients with bone metastases • Hyperglycemia has been reported in males and may manifest as diabetes or worsening of preexisting diabetes; monitor patients for development of diabetes; manage cardiovascular risk factors • Monitor blood glucose and HbA_{1c} (periodically), bone mineral density, serum calcium, and cholesterol/lipids; monitor for signs and symptoms of abdominal hemorrhage following injection • Refer to PI to verify specific administration location (i.e., into the upper abdominal wall) • Drug interactions may require dose adjustments or avoidance of certain drug combinations
Generic Name Histrelin **Brand Name** Supprelin LA Vantas PD	**Common indication for use:** Palliative treatment of advanced prostate cancer	Dose is based on indication for use, product formulation selected, and patient's clinical response **Illustrative parenteral dose for prostate cancer (advanced):** SQ: 50 mg implant, surgically inserted every 12 months	• Transient increases in estradiol serum levels (female) or testosterone levels (female and male) may occur • Androgen-deprivation therapy (ADT) may increase the risk for cardiovascular disease (including MI) and hyperglycemia which may manifest as diabetes or worsening of preexisting diabetes • Monitor for and manage cardiovascular risk factors • Evaluate the results of laboratory tests after insertion and then periodically thereafter • CPP: assess luteinizing hormone (LH), follicle-stimulating hormone (FSH), estradiol, or testosterone, height, and bone age; monitor for clinical evidence of suppression of CPP manifestations • Monitor serum testosterone levels, prostate-specific antigen, and bone mineral density • Monitor for weakness, paresthesias, and urinary tract obstruction

Generic Name Letrozole **Brand Name** Femara GD	Breast cancer (postmenopausal women)	**Usual oral dose:** 2.5 mg once daily	• May cause dizziness, fatigue, and somnolence • May cause decreases in bone mineral density • May increase total serum cholesterol • Monitor periodically during therapy: CBC; thyroid function tests; serum electrolytes, cholesterol, transaminases, and creatinine; blood pressure; bone density • For use in postmenopausal women only • Monitor for hypertension, pain, gastrointestinal upset, and hot flashes on a regular basis • Monitor renal and hepatic function; use with caution in patients with severe impairment
Generic Name Leuprolide **Brand Name** Eligard Lupron Depot Lupron Depot-Ped QT PD	**Common indications for use:** Endometriosis Advanced prostate cancer Uterine leiomyomata (fibroids)	Dose is based on indication for use, product formulation selected, and patient's clinical response **Illustrative parenteral dose for prostate cancer (advanced):** IM: 7.5 mg depot monthly	• Androgen-deprivation therapy may increase the risk for cardiovascular disease • Spinal cord compression has been reported when leuprolide is used for prostate cancer • Assess carefully for use-related cautions prior to beginning therapy • If self-administered, teach the patient or caregiver about proper storage, injection technique, and syringe/needle disposal • Monitor patients for development of diabetes; manage cardiovascular risk factors; diabetes and worsening of glycemic control have been reported • Multiple regimens and formulations are available (including SQ) • Seizures have been reported; carefully weigh risks versus benefits when deciding on treatment options • Drug interactions may require dose adjustments or avoidance of certain drug combinations
Generic Name Megestrol **Brand Name** Megace ES Megace BL	Breast cancer Endometrial cancer	Dose is based on indication for use and patient's clinical response **Illustrative oral dose for breast cancer (advanced):** 40 mg 4 times daily	• May suppress the hypothalamic–pituitary–adrenal (HPA) axis during chronic administration • Cushing syndrome has been reported with long-term use • Monitor for hypertension, CNS changes (confusion, insomnia), rash, changes in menses, gastrointestinal upset, jaundice, and thrombophlebitis regularly during therapy • Hyperglycemia which may manifest as diabetes or worsening of preexisting diabetes has been reported • Appetite stimulating effects may be beneficial • Use with caution in patients with renal and/or hepatic impairment as well as those with history of thromboembolic disease

Drug Name	FDA-Approved Indications	Adult Dosage Range	Precautions and Clinical Pearls
Generic Name Mitotane **Brand Name** Lysodren ■	Treatment of inoperable adrenocortical carcinoma	**Usual oral dose:** Initial: 2 to 6 g daily in 3 to 4 divided doses, then increase incrementally to 9 to 10 g daily in 3 to 4 divided doses	• CNS adverse effects may include lethargy, sedation, and vertigo • Use with caution in patients with kidney, or heart disease; diabetes; gout; or heart failure • Drug accumulation may occur in patients with liver disease; use with caution with these patients • Dosed to desirable serum concentrations; refer to PI • Evaluate for CNS changes, such as depression or somnolence • Drug may be initiated while the patient is in the hospital to titrate the tolerated daily dosing • Primary action of mitotane is through adrenal suppression • Drug interactions may require dose adjustments or avoidance of certain drug combinations Associated with: • Temporary shock or severe trauma upon discontinuation of mitotane • Requires experienced clinician who is knowledgeable in the use of agents and specialized care setting
Generic Name Nilutamide **Brand Name** Nilandron ■	Treatment of metastatic prostate cancer	**Usual oral dose:** 300 mg once daily for 30 days, followed by 150 mg once daily	• Hepatitis and marked increases in liver enzymes have been observed • Avoid use in patients with hepatic impairment • Evaluate results of chest x-rays (baseline) and laboratory tests (baseline and at regular intervals) • Monitor for signs of interstitial pneumonitis (dyspnea, chest pain, cough, fever), hepatitis, and visual changes (impaired dark adaptation) • Teach patients about orthostatic precautions • Drug interactions may require dose adjustments or avoidance of certain drug combinations Associated with: • Interstitial pneumonitis; Asian patients may be at higher risk
Generic Name Tamoxifen **Brand Name** Soltamox ■ QT	Breast cancer Breast cancer prevention	**Usual oral dose for breast cancer treatment:** 20 to 40 mg per day in divided doses twice daily for at least 5 years	• Thrombocytopenia and/or leukopenia • Monitor for thromboembolism, flushing, fluid retention, hot flashes, vaginal bleeding or discharge, constipation, rash, and mood changes • Teach patients about the importance of periodic ophthalmic evaluations, annual gynecologic exams and mammograms with long-term use • May cause metabolic changes • Increased incidence of uterine or endometrial cancers (some fatal)

			Associated with: • Drug interactions may require dose adjustments or avoidance of certain drug combinations • Serious and life-threatening events (some fatal), including stroke and pulmonary emboli
Generic Name Toremifene **Brand Name** Fareston ■ (QT)	Breast cancer (metastatic)	**Usual oral dose:** 60 mg once daily	• Leukopenia and thrombocytopenia • Endometrial hyperplasia • Obtain ECG (baseline and periodically during treatment) in patients at risk for QT prolongation • In patients with bone metastases, monitor closely for hypercalcemia during the first few weeks of treatment • Drug interactions may require dose adjustments or avoidance of certain drug combinations (includes agents recommended for IM administration) • Monitor for thromboembolism, MI, edema, hypercalcemia, endometriosis, nausea, vomiting, and vision changes • Hepatic impairment increases risk of toxicity Associated with: • Prolongation of the QT interval
Generic Name Triptorelin **Brand Name** Trelstar (QT)	Advanced prostate cancer	**Usual parenteral dose**: IM: 3.75 mg once every 4 weeks or IM: 11.25 mg once every 12 weeks or IM: 22.5 mg once every 24 weeks	• Use with caution in patients with risk factors for decreased bone mineral density • Hyperglycemia and an increased risk of developing diabetes have been reported with therapy • Monitor for signs and symptoms of emerging cardiovascular disease • Monitor serum testosterone levels, prostate-specific antigen, glucose and HbA_{1c} (periodically), and bone density • Hypersensitivity reactions, including angioedema, anaphylaxis, and anaphylactic shock, have (rarely) occurred • Be alert to the potential onset of spinal cord compression, diabetes, or cardiovascular disease • Monitor renal and hepatic function; may affect dosing

Immunosuppressant Agents

Drug Name	FDA-Approved Indications	Adult Dosage Range	Precautions and Clinical Pearls
Generic Name Everolimus **Brand Name** Afinitor Disperz Zortress ■ ■	**Vary with product selected:** Breast cancer, advanced Pancreatic neuroendocrine tumors (PNET) Renal angiomyolipoma with tuberous sclerosis complex (TSC) Renal cell carcinoma, advanced Subependymal giant cell astrocytoma Kidney transplant rejection prophylaxis	**Usual oral dose for breast cancer:** 10 mg once daily	• Decreases in hemoglobin, neutrophils, platelets, and lymphocytes have been reported • Increased risk of secondary malignancies, including lymphoma or skin cancers; chronic monitoring is required for detection • Patients with hepatic impairment may need a reduced dose and careful monitoring of hepatic lab tests Associated with: • An increased risk of renal arterial and venous thrombosis has been reported • Everolimus has immunosuppressant properties that may result in secondary malignancy, infection and associated mortality • Increased risk of nephrotoxicity • Drug interactions may require dose adjustments or avoidance of certain drug combinations • Immunosuppressant use may result in the development of malignancy, including lymphoma and skin cancer
Generic Name Temsirolimus **Brand Name** Torisel ■	Advanced renal cell carcinoma (RCC)	**Usual parenteral dose**: IV: 25 mg once weekly; continue until unacceptable toxicity occurs or the therapeutic endpoint is achieved	• Angioneurotic edema has been reported • Increases in serum glucose commonly occur during treatment • Use with caution in patients with hyperlipidemia; may increase serum lipids • Premedicate patients with an antihistamine prior to beginning the infusion • Monitor patients closely for anaphylaxis, dyspnea, flushing, and chest pain during and following each infusion • Monitor for hypersensitivity, altered glucose control, opportunistic infections or impaired wound healing, ILD bowel perforations, and renal failure • Drug interactions may require dose adjustment or avoidance of certain drug combinations

Monoclonal Antibodies

Drug Name	FDA-Approved Indications	Adult Dosage Range	Precautions and Clinical Pearls
Generic Name Ado-trastuzumab emtansine **Brand Name** Kadcyla ■	Metastatic breast cancer, HER2+	**Usual parenteral dose**: IV: 3.6 mg/kg every 3 weeks until disease progression target is achieved or unacceptable toxicity (maximum of 3.6 mg/kg)	• Bone marrow suppression (e.g., thrombocytopenia) • Local reactions due to extravasation • Hemorrhage • Peripheral neuropathy • Pulmonary toxicity

			Monitoring: • Thrombocytopenia (higher incidence in patients of Asian ancestry), bilirubin, and LFTs • Do not confuse ado-trastuzumab emtansine with trastuzumab; they are not interchangeable • Assess for GI tolerance • Assess cardiac function regularly • Drug interactions may require dose adjustments or avoidance of certain drug combinations Associated with: • Cardiotoxicity, possibly resulting in a reduced left ventricular ejection fraction (LVEF) • Hepatotoxicity
Generic Name Alemtuzumab **Brand Name** Campath Lemtrada ■	B-cell CLL Multiple sclerosis (Lemtrada)	Dose is based on indication for use, product formulation selected, and patient's clinical response **Illustrative parenteral dosing for B-CLL:** IV Campath: Gradually escalate to a maintenance dose of 30 mg 3 times weekly on alternate days, for a total duration of therapy of up to 12 weeks	• Dose escalation should be gradual and occur over 3 to 7 days • Premedicate with acetaminophen and an oral antihistamine • Evaluate the patient's response on a frequent basis throughout treatment; dosage adjustments may be necessary • Monitor for Graves' disease Contraindications: • HIV infection Specific formulations of this agent are associated with: • Patients must be monitored closely for infusion reactions; appropriate medications for the treatment of hypersensitivity reactions should be available • Serious and fatal cytopenias (including pancytopenia, bone marrow hypoplasia, autoimmune hemolytic anemia, and autoimmune idiopathic thrombocytopenia) • Serious and potentially fatal infections (bacterial, viral, fungal, and protozoan) • Sometimes fatal autoimmune conditions, such as immune thrombocytopenia and antiglomerular basement membrane disease • Increased risk of malignancies, including thyroid cancer, melanoma, and lymphoproliferative disorders • Requires experienced clinician who is knowledgeable in the use of chemotherapy agents

Drug Name	FDA-Approved Indications	Adult Dosage Range	Precautions and Clinical Pearls
Generic Name Bevacizumab **Brand Name** Avastin	Cervical cancer Colorectal cancer Glioblastoma multiforme NSCLC, nonsquamous Ovarian cancer Renal cell carcinoma, metastatic	Dose is based on indication for use and patient's clinical response **Illustrative parenteral dosing for colorectal cancer (metastatic):** IV: 5 mg/kg every 2 weeks	• Regimens generally contain other antineoplastic agents (i.e., 5-fluorouracil) • Assess patients for abdominal pain, nausea, fever, vomiting, constipation, and bleeding • Evaluate for arterial thromboembolism, cardiovascular disease, and CNS metastases prior to beginning treatment • Regularly monitor blood pressure (may cause hypertension), CBC, and urine for proteinuria • Assess for serious bleeding, nephrotic syndrome, encephalopathy, and heart failure Associated with: • GI perforation (sometimes fatal) has occurred • Severe or fatal hemorrhage, including hemoptysis, gastrointestinal bleeding, CNS hemorrhage, epistaxis, and vaginal bleeding, has been reported • The incidence of wound healing and surgical complications, including serious and fatal events, is increased in patients who have received bevacizumab
Generic Name Brentuximab **Brand Name** Adcetris ▲ ■ ■	Hodgkin's lymphoma	**Usual parenteral dose**: IV: 1.8 mg/kg infused over 30 minutes (maximum of 180 mg); repeat every 3 weeks	• SJS and TEN have been reported; advise patients to report symptoms of these conditions • Prolonged, severe neutropenia may occur • Side effects may include fatigue, diarrhea, nausea, vomiting, anemia, thrombocytopenia, upper respiratory tract infection, cough, pyrexia, and rash • Monitor CBC prior to each treatment • Drug interactions may require dose adjustment or avoidance of certain drug combinations Associated with: • Progressive multifocal leukoencephalopathy (PML) and death; tell patients to report symptoms of peripheral neuropathy or PML
Generic Name Cetuximab **Brand Name** Erbitux ■ (GD)	Colorectal cancer, metastatic Head and neck cancer	Dose is based on indication for use and patient's clinical response **Illustrative parenteral dose for head and neck squamous cell cancer:** IV: Initial loading dose: 400 mg/m^2; infuse over 120 minutes Maintenance dose: 250 mg/m^2; infuse over 60 minutes, weekly	• Hypomagnesemia is common • Premedication with antihistamines is recommended • Monitor patients closely for airway obstruction, hives, and hypotension during and for 1 hour following infusion • Instruct patients to report skin reactions, cough, dyspnea, gastrointestinal upset, and opportunistic infection • Monitor for skin reactions and signs of dermatologic toxicities; avoid sun exposure • Monitor serum electrolytes, including magnesium, potassium, and calcium, during and after therapy Associated with: • Cardiopulmonary arrest and/or sudden death • Serious infusion reactions

Generic Name Ibritumomab **Brand Name** Zevalin ■ ■	Non-Hodgkin's lymphoma	Specific dosing recommendations are based on patient's clinical status and treatment plan **Illustrative parenteral dose:** Within 4 hours of completion of the rituximab infusion Platelet count 150,000 cells/mm^3 or greater: IV: Inject 0.4 mCi/kg (14.8 MBq/kg) actual body weight over 10 minutes; maximum dose: 32 mCi (1184 MBq) Maximum dose: the prescribed, measured, and administered dose of Y-90 ibritumomab must not exceed 32 mCi (1184 MBq), regardless of the patient's body weight	• Monitor patients closely during each infusion • Monitor effects on the hematologic system and assess for infections • Monitor blood counts after therapy; expect delayed nadir periods with myelosuppression • Maintain radiation precautions for body fluids up to 7 days after therapy • Drug interactions may require dose adjustments or avoidance of certain drug combinations • Initiate the ibritumomab therapeutic regimen following recovery of platelet counts to 150,000/mm^3 or greater at least 6 weeks, but no more than 12 weeks, following the last dose of first-line chemotherapy • Refer to PI for dose regimens for platelet counts less than 150,000/mm^3 Associated with: • Delayed, prolonged, and severe cytopenias (thrombocytopenia and neutropenia) • Severe cutaneous and mucocutaneous skin reactions, including blisters or peeling of skin in the mouth or nose • Serious fatal infusion reactions may occur with the rituximab component of the therapeutic regimen
Generic Name Ipilimumab **Brand Name** Yervoy ■ ■	Treatment of unresectable or metastatic melanoma	**Usual parenteral dose for metastatic melanoma (single agent):** IV: 3 mg/kg every 3 weeks for 4 doses	• Severe, life-threatening or fatal hepatotoxicity • Monitor liver function for signs of hepatotoxicity • Monitor serum chemistries prior to each dose • Monitor for signs of hypophysitis, adrenal insufficiency, and thyroid disorders • Monitor thyroid-stimulating hormone (TSH), free T_4, and cortisol levels • Monitor for signs and symptoms of enterocolitis • Monitor for signs of motor or sensory neuropathy (unilateral or bilateral weakness, sensory changes, or paresthesia) • Monitor for ocular toxicity at baseline, then at 4 to 8 weeks with further evaluations as clinically indicated

Drug Name	FDA-Approved Indications	Adult Dosage Range	Precautions and Clinical Pearls
			Associated with: • Severe and fatal immune-mediated adverse effects due to T-cell activation and proliferation (include severe diarrhea, hepatitis, etc.); refer to PI • Can result in severe and fatal immune-mediated neuropathies, including Guillain-Barre syndrome. • Severe or life-threatening endocrine disorders (hypopituitarism, adrenal insufficiency, hypogonadism, and hypothyroidism) • Severe and sometimes fatal serious rash or dermatitis. Monitor for rash and pruritus
Generic Name Nivolumab **Brand Name** Opdivo	**Common indications for use:** Hodgkin's lymphoma Unresectable or metastatic melanoma Metastatic NSCLC Clear cell (advanced) renal cell cancer	**Usual parenteral dose for Hodgkin's lymphoma:** IV: 3 mg/kg once every 2 weeks until disease progression target is achieved or unacceptable toxicity occurs	• Dermatologic toxicity (e.g., immune-mediated rash) • GI toxicity; diarrhea and colitis are common • Hepatotoxicity; elevated LFTs, alkaline phosphatase (ALP), and bilirubin • Nephrotoxicity (e.g., elevated SCr) • Thyroid disorders (e.g., elevated TSH); hyperthyroidism or hypothyroidism) • Other immune-mediated toxicities • Monitor hepatic, renal, and thyroid functions (baseline and periodically); blood glucose • Monitor for signs and symptoms of adrenal insufficiency, hypophysitis, thyroid disorders, colitis, pneumonitis, rash, and encephalitis • Monitor for infusion reactions
Generic Name Obinutuzumab **Brand Name** Gazyva ■ GD	**Common indications for use:** CLL Follicular lymphoma	Dose is based on indication for use and patient's clinical response **Illustrative parenteral dose for CLL:** IV: Cycle 1: 100 mg on day 1, followed by 900 mg on day 2, followed by 1000 mg weekly for 2 doses (days 8 and 15) Cycles 2–6: 1000 mg on day 1 every 28 days for 5 doses	• Bone marrow suppression (e.g., severe & life-threatening neutropenia; thrombocytopenia) • Cardiovascular effects • Infection (e.g., bacterial, fungal, and new or reactivated viral infections); do not administer to patients with an active infection • Infusion reactions; may be severe • Premedication with acetaminophen (APAP), an antihistamine, and a glucocorticoid may be required to prevent infusion reactions • Tumor lysis syndrome (e.g., hyperkalemia, hypocalcemia, hyperphosphatemia) • Increased risk of hypotension and hemorrhagic events • Administration of live virus vaccines during treatment is not recommended • In patients with severe neutropenia lasting more than 1 week, antimicrobial prophylaxis is strongly recommended; antiviral and antifungal prophylaxis should be considered

			• Use with caution in patients with preexisting cardiac or pulmonary conditions and chronic or recurring infections • Screen all patients for hepatitis B virus (HBV) infection prior to use and monitor during the course of therapy for HBV reactivation • Avoid administration of live vaccines during treatment • Assess patients' neurologic status for potential risk of PML; perform lab tests (e.g., uric acid level) to evaluate for TLS with high tumor burden; monitor for hemorrhage • Monitor CBC (i.e., neutropenia), renal function, and electrolytes • Most common side effects are low blood cell counts, fever, cough, and muscle and joint pain • Other therapeutic interventions may be administered in combination with bendamustine • Patients with stable disease, complete response, or partial response after 6 cycles of combination therapy should continue on obinutuzumab monotherapy for 2 years Associated with: • Hepatitis B reactivation may occur and may result in fulminant hepatitis, hepatic failure, and death • PML resulting in death may occur
Generic Name Ofatumumab **Brand Name** Arzerra ■	CLL, previously untreated, or refractory	**Usual parenteral dose previously untreated:** IV: Cycle 1 (cycle is 28 days): 300 mg on day 1, followed by 1000 mg on day 8	• Assess risk for tumor lysis syndrome • Monitor patients closely for infusion reactions, which are most likely to occur with the first two treatments • May premedicate patients if reactions occur • Monitor CBC with differential and metabolic panel • More aggressive regimens are available for refractory cases; refer to PI Associated with: • Hepatitis B reactivation (HBV) reactivation with fulminant hepatitis, hepatic failure, and death; perform hepatitis B screening prior to prescribing therapy; may cause reactivation of HBV • PML resulting in death may occur

Drug Name	FDA-Approved Indications	Adult Dosage Range	Precautions and Clinical Pearls
Generic Name Panitumumab **Brand Name** Vectibix ■	Colorectal cancer, metastatic	**Usual parenteral dose**: IV: 6 mg/kg every 14 days	• Magnesium and/or calcium depletion may occur during treatment • Pulmonary fibrosis and ILD have been observed • Monitor patients closely during and following infusion for infusion reactions • Infusion reactions may include dyspnea, shortness of breath, wheezing, chest tightness, or bronchospasm • Assess patients for *KRAS* wild-type genes • Monitor for severe skin reactions, peripheral edema, and gastrointestinal upset (pain, nausea, diarrhea, constipation, vomiting) at each infusion and throughout therapy. • Monitor electrolytes and replace calcium and magnesium as needed Associated with: • Dermatologic toxicities
Generic Name Pembrolizumab **Brand Name** Keytruda ■	Unresectable or metastatic melanoma Metastatic NSCLC	**Usual parenteral dose for malignant melanoma:** IV: 2 mg/kg once every 3 weeks until the disease progression target is achieved or unacceptable toxicity occurs	• Hyperglycemia • GI toxicity • Infusion-related reactions (e.g., pruritus, rash, fever) • Hypothyroidism and hyperthyroidism • Other immune-mediated toxicities • Monitor PD-L1 expression status in patients with NSCLC, LFTs (AST, ALT, and total bilirubin), renal function, thyroid function (baseline and periodically), and glucose • Monitor for immune-mediated adverse reactions: pneumonitis, nephritis, hypothyroidism or hyperthyroidism, colitis, hepatitis, and hypophysitis • Therapy may be withheld or permanently discontinued based on reaction severity; if it is resumed, corticosteroids should be administered
Generic Name Pertuzumab **Brand Name** Perjeta ■	Metastatic breast cancer (HER2+) Breast cancer (neoadjuvant treatment, HER2+)	Dose is based on indication for use and patient's clinical response **Illustrative parenteral dose for breast cancer, metastatic HER2+:** IV: 840 mg over 60 minutes, followed by a maintenance dose of 420 mg over 30 to 60 minutes every 3 weeks until the disease progression target is achieved or unacceptable toxicity occurs (in combination with trastuzumab and docetaxel)	• GI adverse events (e.g., diarrhea) • Hypersensitivity/infusion reactions • For early-stage breast cancer, the safety of treatment beyond 6 cycles has not been determined • Monitoring: determine HER2 status; used only in HER2+ patients • Use with caution in patients with heart failure; measure LVEF prior to beginning drug therapy; monitor for symptoms of heart failure such as edema, weight gain, and increased shortness of breath • Serious infusion reactions may be life threatening; have appropriate hypersensitivity reaction medications available at the bedside (discontinue infusion immediately)

			• Monitor CBC and metabolic panel • Alternative regimens are available that allow dosing of every 3 weeks for 3 to 6 cycles; may be administered as one of three regimens (refer to the manufacturer's labeling) • For combination regimens, pertuzumab and trastuzumab may be administered in any order; however, docetaxel should be given after these agents. Observe patients for 30 to 60 minutes after each pertuzumab infusion and before the subsequent infusions of trastuzumab or docetaxel. Associated with: • Cardiac failure (clinical and subclinical) manifesting as decreased LVEF and heart failure; assess cardiac function at baseline and during treatment
Generic Name Ramucirumab **Brand Name** Cyramza ■ ■	Colorectal cancer (metastatic) Advanced or metastatic gastric cancer Metastatic NSCLC	Dose is based on indication for use and patient's clinical response **Illustrative parenteral dose for gastric cancer, advanced or metastatic:** IV: 8 mg/kg every 2 weeks as a single agent or in combination with paclitaxel; continue until disease progression target is achieved or unacceptable toxicity occurs	• Higher incidence of neutropenia and thrombocytopenia were observed when ramucirumab was combined with paclitaxel • May cause or worsen hypertension • Use with caution in patients with cardiovascular disease or hepatic impairment • Associated with proteinuria • Check for history of hypertension, bleeding disorders, and liver function impairment prior to prescribing • Monitor LFTs, urine protein, thyroid function, CBC, and blood pressure (baseline and routinely) • Monitor for signs and symptoms of infusion-related reactions, thromboembolic events, bleeding/hemorrhage, GI perforation, wound healing impairment, and reversible posterior leukoencephalopathy syndrome (RPLS) • Monitor for signs of MI, cerebrovascular accident (CVA), or ischemia • Premedicate patients prior to the infusion with an IV H_1 antagonist; for patients who experienced a grade 1 or 2 infusion reaction with a prior infusion, also provide premedication with dexamethasone (or equivalent) and acetaminophen Associated with: • Increased risk of GI perforation, a potentially fatal event • Increased risk of hemorrhage and GI hemorrhage, which may be severe or sometimes fatal • Impaired wound healing can occur, with antibodies inhibiting the VEGF pathway

Drug Name	FDA-Approved Indications	Adult Dosage Range	Precautions and Clinical Pearls
Generic Name Rituximab **Brand Name** Rituxan ■	**Common indications for use:** Treatment of CD20-positive non-Hodgkin's lymphomas (NHL) Treatment of CD20-positive CLL	Dose is based on indication for use and patient's clinical response **Illustrative parenteral dose for NHL:** IV infusion: 375 mg/m^2 once weekly for 4 or 8 doses	• Pretreatment with acetaminophen and diphenhydramine is recommended • In the event of a severe infusion reaction, the infusion should be stopped and the patient assessed • Monitor patients closely for abdominal pain (bowel obstruction and perforation), hypertension/hypotension, CNS changes, hyperglycemia/ hypoglycemia, and rash • Bowel obstruction and perforation can occur early in therapy Associated with: • Hepatitis B reactivation may occur with use and may result in fulminant hepatitis, hepatic failure, and death • Severe infusion-related reactions • Severe and sometimes fatal mucocutaneous reactions • PML due to John Cunningham (JC) virus infection
Generic Name Siltuximab **Brand Name** Sylvant (GD)	Castleman disease (HIV negative and human herpesvirus-8 [HHV-8] negative)	**Usual parenteral dose**: IV: 11 mg/kg over 1 hour every 3 weeks until treatment failure	• GI perforation • May result in elevated hemoglobin levels • May mask signs and symptoms of infection • Monitor CBC with differential; signs and symptoms of infusion-related, allergic, or anaphylactic reaction; signs and symptoms of infection and GI perforation • Drug interactions may require dose adjustments or avoidance of certain drug combinations • Do not administer live vaccines to patients receiving siltuximab • Severe infusion reactions have been reported
Generic Name Trastuzumab **Brand Name** Herceptin ■	Breast cancer, adjuvant treatment Breast cancer, metastatic Gastric cancer, metastatic	Dose is based on indication for use and patient's clinical response **Illustrative parenteral dose for breast cancer, metastatic, HER2+:** Initial loading dose: 4 mg/kg infused over 90 minutes Maintenance dose: 2 mg/kg infused over 30 minutes weekly until disease progression target is achieved or adverse effects become dangerous or intolerable	• Assess cardiac function prior to deciding on therapy • Assess for signs of an infusion reaction during infusion • Monitor for signs and symptoms of heart failure • Evaluate baseline LVEF prior to first dose and periodically throughout course of treatment Associated with: • Symptomatic and asymptomatic reductions in LVEF and heart failure • Infusion reactions (including death) have been associated with use • May cause serious pulmonary toxicity

Tyrosine Kinase Inhibitors

Drug Name	FDA-Approved Indications	Adult Dosage Range	Precautions and Clinical Pearls
Generic Name Afatinib **Brand Name** Gilotrif ▲ ■ GD	NSCLC (metastatic EGFR mutation–positive and metastatic squamous) EGFR exon 19 deletions or exon 21 (L858R) substitution mutations	**Usual oral dose:** 40 mg once daily until disease progression target is achieved or unacceptable toxicity occurs	• Cardiovascular toxicity • Severe diarrhea, stomatitis, and cutaneous reactions are common • Hepatotoxicity: closely monitor afatinib use in patients with hepatic impairment, including LFTs • Ocular toxicity • Paronychia (infection around nails) • Pulmonary toxicity has been reported. Asian patients appear to be at higher risk • Afatinib should not be used in combination with vinorelbine for the treatment of HER2+ metastatic breast cancer; associated with increased mortality • Monitor patients with a history of heart, lung, kidney, or liver disease and with visual problems (e.g., keratitis, contact wearer) • Take at least 1 hour before or 2 hours after a meal
Generic Name Axitinib **Brand Name** Inlyta ■ GD	Renal cell carcinoma (advanced)	**Usual oral dose:** Initial: 5 mg twice daily	• Gastrointestinal perforation and fistulas (including fatality) have been reported • May cause hypertension • Use is associated with proteinuria • Arterial thrombotic events (cerebrovascular accident, MI, retinal artery occlusion, and transient ischemic attack) have been reported, with fatalities • Carefully assess increases in the patient's blood pressure throughout the course of therapy • Control hypertension; it must be well controlled before initiating therapy • Monitor renal, hepatic, and thyroid function • Obtain urinalysis at baseline and periodically throughout treatment • Drug interactions may require dose adjustments or avoidance of certain drug combinations
Generic Name Bosutinib ▲ ■ QT	Chronic myelogenous leukemia (CML)	**Usual oral dose:** 500 mg once daily; continue until the disease progression target is achieved or unacceptable toxicity occurs	• Bone density changes • Bone marrow suppression • Fluid retention and edema • GI toxicity: GI side effects are common • Use with caution in patients with hepatic and renal impairment; hepatotoxicity has been reported • Hypersensitivity reactions have been reported • GI medications can affect the absorption • Give with food; do not crush or break tablets

Drug Name	FDA-Approved Indications	Adult Dosage Range	Precautions and Clinical Pearls
			• Monitor CBC and platelets, LFTs, renal function, diarrhea episodes, and fluid/edema status (e.g., weight gain) • Monitor for signs of infections • Monitor patients at risk for bleeding episodes; use with caution in patients with significant cardiovascular disease or history of pancreatitis • Drug interactions may require dose adjustments or avoidance of certain drug combinations; avoid consumption of grapefruit juice during therapy
Generic Name Cabozantinib **Brand Name** Cometriq Cabometyx ■ ■	Metastatic medullary thyroid cancer	**Usual oral dose for thyroid cancer:** 140 mg capsules once daily until disease progression target is achieved or unacceptable toxicity occurs	• Palmar–plantar erythrodysesthesia (PPES) and hypertension • Thromboembolic events • Cabometyx tablets and Cometriq capsules are not interchangeable • Administer on an empty stomach (1 hour before or 2 hours after eating) • Swallow whole; do not open capsules • Avoid consumption of grapefruit and grapefruit juice throughout therapy • Monitor renal and liver function, CBC and platelets, electrolytes, and blood pressure • Monitor for perforations, fistulas, signs and symptoms of bleeding, PPES, RPLS, venous thromboembolism (VTE), proteinuria, osteonecrosis of jaw, wound healing complications, diarrhea, and stomatitis • Drug interactions may require dose adjustments or avoidance of certain drug combinations • Use is not recommended in patients with moderate to severe hepatic impairment Associated with: • Hemorrhage • GI perforations and fistulas
Generic Name Ceritinib **Brand Name** Zykadia ■ QT	Metastatic NSCLC (ALK-positive)	**Usual oral dose:** 750 mg once daily; continue until disease progression target is achieved or unacceptable toxicity occurs	• Bradycardia; if possible, avoid concurrent medication use with additive effects • GI side effects occur in the majority of patients • Hepatotoxicity (e.g., increased LFTs); use with caution in patients with hepatic impairment • QTc prolongation and pancreatic enzyme elevations • ILD • Antiemetics may be needed to prevent nausea and vomiting

			• Administer on an empty stomach (at least 2 hours before or 2 hours after a meal) • Drug interactions may require dose adjustments or avoidance of certain drug combinations; avoid consumption of grapefruit and grapefruit juice • Drugs affecting gastric pH may have an effect on ceritinib's absorption • Monitor anaplastic lymphoma kinase (ALK) positivity; CBC; renal, liver, and cardiac (QTc interval) function; lipase and amylase; electrolytes; vital signs (heart rate, blood pressure); and signs and symptoms of GI or pulmonary toxicity and pancreatitis • Monitor blood glucose and optimize use of glycemic control drugs; may cause hyperglycemia
Generic Name Crizotinib **Brand Name** Xalkori ■ QT	NSCLC, metastatic	**Usual oral dose:** 250 mg twice daily; continue treatment until disease progression target is achieved or unacceptable toxicity occurs	• Symptomatic bradycardia may occur, in which heart rate less than 50 beats per minute • Fatalities due to crizotinib-induced hepatotoxicity have been reported • Pancreatitis has been reported • Severe, life-threatening, and potentially fatal ILD and pneumonitis have been reported • Monitor for hepatotoxicity, ocular toxicities, pneumonitis, and QT prolongation • Monitor EKGs regularly; reassess the dose if QTc prolongation occurs • Monitor CBC with differential and liver function tests • Drug interactions may require dose adjustments or avoidance of certain drug combinations
Generic Name Dasatinib **Brand Name** Sprycel QT	ALL CML	Dose is based on indication for use and patient's clinical response **Illustrative oral dose for CML:** 140 mg once daily until the disease progression target is achieved or unacceptable toxicity occurs	• Severe dose-related bone marrow suppression (thrombocytopenia, neutropenia, anemia) • Cardiac ischemic events, cardiac fluid retention–related events, and conduction abnormalities (arrhythmia and palpitations) • Tumor lysis syndrome has been reported • May cause fluid retention, including pleural and pericardial effusions, pulmonary hypertension, and generalized or superficial edema • May prolong QT interval • Assess CBC, LFTs, electrolytes, and weight and fluid status on a regular basis • Monitor for gastrointestinal disturbance, hemorrhage, anemia, and respiratory or CNS changes • Drug interactions may require dose adjustments or avoidance of certain drug combinations

Drug Name	FDA-Approved Indications	Adult Dosage Range	Precautions and Clinical Pearls
Generic Name Erlotinib **Brand Name** Tarceva ■	NSCLC Pancreatic cancer	**Usual oral dose:** 150 mg once daily until disease progression target is achieved or unacceptable toxicity occurs	• Bullous, blistering, or exfoliating skin conditions, SJS or TEN • Hepatic failure and hepatorenal syndrome • Ensure patient is well hydrated • Use with caution in the presence or with risk of cardiovascular disease, renal impairment, or hepatic impairment. • Assess LFTs; monitor more frequently with worsening liver function • Monitor for gastrointestinal perforation, diarrhea, ocular reactions, severe skin reactions, and ILD (including fever, etc.) • Treatment adjustments may be necessary with severe renal toxicities • Drug interactions may require dose adjustments or avoidance of certain drug combinations • Smokers will experience lower serum concentrations and reduced effectiveness of drug; encourage cessation
Generic Name Gefitinib **Brand Name** Iressa	First-line treatment of metastatic NSCLC	**Usual oral dose:** 250 mg once daily until disease progression target is achieved or unacceptable toxicity occurs	• Skin reactions occur in nearly half of patients taking gefitinib • Diarrhea occurs in approximately one-third of patients • Increases in ALT, AST, and bilirubin, including grade 3 or higher toxicity • Monitor for EGFR-mutation status, liver function tests, BUN, creatinine, electrolytes, and INR or prothrombin time • Avoid in patients with hepatic impairment • Monitor for signs and symptoms of dermatologic toxicity, gastrointestinal perforation, ocular toxicity, and pulmonary toxicity • Assess results of liver function tests on a regular basis • Drug interactions may require dose adjustments or avoidance of certain drug combinations
Generic Name Ibrutinib **Brand Name** Imbruvica ■ (GD)	**Common indications for use:** CLL Mantle cell lymphoma Waldenström macroglobulinemia	Dose is based on indication for use and patient's clinical response	• Cardiovascular effects (e.g., atrial fibrillation and atrial flutter, particularly in patients with cardiac risk factors) • CNS effects (e.g., dizziness, fatigue) • Diarrhea • Hematologic effects (e.g., lymphocytosis upon initiation) • Hemorrhage, hypertension, and infections • Second primary malignancies • Tumor lysis syndrome has been reported

		Illustrative oral dose for CLL: 420 mg once daily until disease progression target is achieved or unacceptable toxicity occurs	• Use with caution in patients with hepatic and renal impairment; avoid use in patients with moderate to severe hepatic impairment • Waldenström macroglobulinemia: hyperviscosity may require plasmapheresis prior to or during ibrutinib treatment • Administer with water at approximately the same time every day; swallow capsules whole • Maintain adequate hydration during treatment • Drug interactions may require dose adjustments or avoidance of certain drug combinations; avoid consumption of grapefruit and Seville oranges during therapy • Monitor CBC and LFTs (monthly or as clinically necessary), renal and hepatic function, and uric acid levels; increased uric acid levels and serum creatinine (SCr) have been reported • Monitor for signs and symptoms of bleeding, infections, second primary malignancies, TLS, PML, and atrial fibrillation; perform an ECG prior to therapy initiation and during therapy (patient specific) • Assess the patient's vaccination record; consider bringing the patient up-to-date on vaccinations prior to initiating therapy
Generic Name Imatinib **Brand Name** Gleevec ▲ ■	ALL Aggressive systemic mastocytosis CML Dermatofibrosarcoma protuberans: GI stromal tumors Hypereosinophilic syndrome and/or chronic eosinophilic leukemia: myelodysplastic/ myeloproliferative diseases	Dose is based on indication for use and patient's clinical response **Usual oral dose for ALL:** 600 mg once per day until disease progression target is achieved or unacceptable toxicity occurs	• May cause bone marrow suppression (anemia, neutropenia, and thrombocytopenia) • Severe heart failure (HF) and left ventricular dysfunction (LVD) have been reported • Often associated with fluid retention, weight gain, and edema; monitor renal function • Evaluate CBC, serum electrolytes, LFTs, thyroid function tests (TFTs), and renal function tests on a regular basis • Contains iron; patients with hemochromatosis may not be appropriate candidates for therapy • Monitor for symptoms of hypothermia, which can be preceded by mild thyrotoxicosis, tachycardia, heat intolerance, frequent bowel movements, and eyelid retraction/lag • Monitor weight and fluid status • Monitor for hemorrhage, paresthesia, and respiratory or CNS changes • Treatment may be continued until disease progression or unacceptable toxicity occurs; the optimal duration of therapy for CML in complete remission has not been determined • Drug interactions may require dose adjustments or avoidance of certain drug combinations

Drug Name	FDA-Approved Indications	Adult Dosage Range	Precautions and Clinical Pearls
Generic Name Lapatinib **Brand Name** Tykerb QT	Breast cancer	Dose is based on indication for use and patient's clinical response **Illustrative oral dose for breast cancer, metastatic, HER2+ (hormonal therapy indicated):** 1500 mg once daily	• Diarrhea is common • Decreases in LVEF have been reported • Evaluate CBC, LFTs, electrolytes, and LVEF at baseline and on a regular basis • Monitor ECG for cardiac changes, especially when the patient has a history or increased risk of QTc prolongation; QTc prolongation has been observed • Evaluate for gastrointestinal disturbances; adjust treatment for significant diarrhea • Monitor for ILD and pneumonitis • Drug interactions may require dose adjustments or avoidance of certain drug combinations Associated with: • Hepatotoxicity (ALT or AST more than 3 times ULN and total bilirubin more than 2 times ULN) has been reported with lapatinib
Generic Name Lenvatinib **Brand Name** Lenvima QT	**Common indication for use:** Differentiated thyroid cancer	**Usual oral dose for thyroid cancer:** 24 mg once daily until disease progression target is achieved or unacceptable toxicity occurs	• Monitor for signs and symptoms of cardiac decompensation, arterial thrombosis, GI perforation/fistula, hemorrhagic events, RPLS, and toxicities • Cardiac effects (e.g., hypertension, pulmonary edema) and thromboembolic events have been reported • Increased TSH, GI toxicity, and hypocalcemia • Hemorrhage (e.g., epistaxis) • Hepatotoxicity (e.g., increased LFTs) • Palmar–plantar erythrodysesthesia • Renal toxicity (e.g., proteinuria); maintain adequate hydration • Antiemetics are recommended to prevent nausea and vomiting • Administer at the same time each day, without regard to meals • Monitor LFTs (every 2 weeks for 2 months and at least monthly), renal function, electrolytes and calcium; TSH, urine protein level, BP (prior to initiation and regularly), and EKG (patient specific) • Drug interactions may require dose adjustments or avoidance of certain drug combinations

Generic Name Nilotinib **Brand Name** Tasigna ■ ■ QT	Chronic myelogenous leukemia (CML)	Dose is based on indication for use and patient's clinical response **Illustrative oral dose for CML Ph+, newly diagnosed in chronic phase:** 300 mg twice daily until disease progression target is achieved or unacceptable toxicity occurs	• Take on empty stomach • Tumor lysis syndrome has been reported • Electrolyte abnormalities may occur during treatment • Fluid retention, including pleural and pericardial effusions, ascites, and pulmonary edema, has been reported • May cause hepatotoxicity, including dose-limiting elevations in bilirubin, transaminases, and alkaline phosphatase; monitor liver function • Evaluate CBC, electrolytes, LFTs, and serum lipase at baseline and on a regular basis • Monitor for myelosuppression, cardiac changes, gastrointestinal disturbance, and hyperglycemia • Monitor for symptoms of hypothyroidism • Monitor pulmonary status • Capsules should be swallowed intact and whole; if the whole capsule cannot be swallowed, the capsule contents may be dispersed in 1 teaspoon of applesauce; the mixture must be consumed within 15 minutes; do not store for future use • Drug interactions may require dose adjustments or avoidance of certain drug combinations Associated with: • Prolonged QT interval
Generic Name Pazopanib **Brand Name** Votrient ■ ■ QT	Renal cell carcinoma, advanced (RCC) Soft-tissue sarcoma, advanced	Dose is based on indication for use and patient's clinical response **Illustrative oral dose for advanced RCC:** 800 mg once daily until disease progression target is achieved or unacceptable toxicity occurs	• Take on empty stomach • May cause or worsen hypertension • ILD/pneumonitis has been reported with therapy • QTc prolongation, including torsades de pointes, has been observed • Monitor liver function tests at baseline; at weeks 3, 5, 7, and 9; at months 3 and 4; and as clinically necessary, then periodically after month 4 • Monitor for hypertension, gastrointestinal perforation, diarrhea, hyperglycemia/hypoglycemia, and cardiac changes; dose adjustments may be necessary • Drug interactions may require dose adjustments or avoidance of certain drug combinations Associated with: • Severe and fatal hepatotoxicity (transaminase and bilirubin elevations) in studies

Drug Name	FDA-Approved Indications	Adult Dosage Range	Precautions and Clinical Pearls
Generic Name Ponatinib **Brand Name** Iclusig ■ ■	ALL CML	Dose is based on indication for use and patient's clinical response **Illustrative oral dose for ALL:** 45 mg once daily	• Cardiac arrhythmias • Bone marrow suppression • Fluid retention/edema • Hemorrhage (e.g., cerebral and GI) • Hypertension development or worsening • Peripheral neuropathy • Treatment-related lipase elevations • Administer without regard to food • Must swallow tablets whole; do not crush or dissolve • Drug interactions may require dose adjustments or avoidance of certain drug combinations; avoid consumption of grapefruit juice • Use with caution in patients with a history of blood clots, hypertension, diabetes mellitus, alcohol use, pancreatitis, or hypercholesteremia • Closely assess heart function prior to initiating therapy; monitor for arrhythmias; routinely assess vital signs • Elderly patients may not tolerate treatment well; more likely to experience side effects • Ocular exams should be performed at baseline and periodically • Avoid use in patients with moderate to severe hepatic impairment • Monitor CBC, metabolic panel, uric acid, and LFTs • Monitor for signs and symptoms of GI perforation/fistula, hemorrhage, edema, neuropathy, wound healing impairment, and TLS • Consider discontinuing therapy if no response has occurred by 3 months of therapy Associated with: • Serious heart failure or left ventricular dysfunction, including fatalities • Liver failure and death resulting from ponatinib-induced hepatotoxicity • Arterial and venous thrombosis and occlusions
Generic Name Regorafenib **Brand Name** Stivarga ■ ■	Metastatic colorectal cancer GI stromal tumors	**Usual oral dose:** 160 mg once daily for the first 21 days of each 28-day cycle; continue until disease progression target is achieved or unacceptable toxicity occurs	• Increased incidence of hemorrhage • Take at the same time each day; swallow tablets whole with water after a low-fat meal • Drug interactions may require dose adjustments or avoidance of certain drug combinations; avoid consumption of grapefruit juice • Monitor blood pressure closely, especially during the first 6 weeks of therapy; may cause elevated blood pressure

			• Monitor CBC, platelets, and electrolytes • Severe hepatic failure may occur • Obtain LFTs at baseline and regularly during therapy • Monitor for signs and symptoms of RPLS and hand–foot skin reaction; palmar–plantar erythrodysesthesia and skin rash are common; Asian patients may be at higher risk • Hold medication for 2 weeks prior to surgery to allow proper wound healing • Monitor for bleeding, signs and symptoms of GI perforation/fistula, and cardiac ischemia or infarction Associated with: • Severe and sometimes fatal hepatotoxicity • Monitor hepatic function at baseline and during treatment; use is not recommended in patients with severe hepatic impairment
Generic Name Ruxolitinib **Brand Name** Jakafi	Myelofibrosis Polycythemia vera	Dose is based on indication for use and patient's clinical response **Illustrative oral dose for polycythemia vera:** Initial dose: 10 mg twice daily	• Use with caution in patients with a history of bradycardia, conduction disturbances, ischemic heart disease, or heart failure • Hematologic toxicities, including thrombocytopenia, anemia, and neutropenia, may occur • Non-melanoma skin cancers (basal cell, squamous cell, and Merkel cell carcinoma) have been reported • Monitor CBC before and during therapy • Drug dosing depends on the platelet count • Hypercholesterolemia (e.g., elevated total cholesterol, elevated low-density lipoprotein [LDL] cholesterol) and hypertriglyceridemia have been reported • Instruct patients to report shortness of breath, painful skin rashes, or blisters • Drug interactions may require dose adjustments or avoidance of certain drug combinations
Generic Name Sorafenib **Brand Name** Nexavar QT	Hepatocellular cancer Renal cell cancer, advanced Thyroid cancer, differentiated	**Usual oral dose:** 400 mg twice daily; continue until the patient no longer experiences any clinical benefit or unacceptable toxicity occurs	• Increased risk of bleeding • May cause cardiac ischemia or infarction • Monitor for signs and symptoms of gastrointestinal perforation, including black tarry stools, severe abdominal pain, and bloody diarrhea • Dermatologic toxicities (i.e., SJS, TEN, etc.) reported • Use with caution in patients with a history of hypertension, chest pain, MI, irregular heart rhythm, or kidney or liver disease • Monitor for symptoms of hypothyroidism • Monitor CBC, metabolic panel, and TSH • Drug interactions may require dose adjustments or avoidance of certain drug combinations

Drug Name	FDA-Approved Indications	Adult Dosage Range	Precautions and Clinical Pearls
Generic Name Sunitinib **Brand Name** Sutent ■ QT	GI stromal tumor (GIST) Pancreatic neuroendocrine tumors, advanced Renal cell carcinoma, advanced	Dose is based on indication for use and patient's clinical response **Illustrative oral dose for GIST:** 50 mg once daily for 4 weeks of a 6-week treatment cycle	• QTc prolongation and torsades de pointes • Proteinuria and nephrotic syndrome; fatal renal failure reported • Monitor for symptoms of hypothyroidism and adrenal insufficiency • Monitor for bleeding (especially GI) • Routine labs and blood pressure need to be monitored throughout the course of therapy • Swallow capsules whole • Monitor for thrombolic side effects in addition to hypertension, MI, and congestive heart failure (CHF) • Cutaneous effects include palmar–plantar erythema and rash • Drug interactions may require dose adjustments or avoidance of certain drug combinations Associated with: • Hepatotoxicity, which may be severe or fatal
Generic Name Vandetanib **Brand Name** Caprelsa ▲ ■ ■ QT	Thyroid cancer	**Usual oral dose:** 300 mg once daily; continue treatment until the patient no longer experiences a clinical benefit or unacceptable toxicity occurs	• Diarrhea has been reported with use; may cause electrolyte imbalances • Serious and sometimes fatal hemorrhagic events have been reported with use • Monitor ECG and potassium and magnesium concentrations • Evaluate CBC with differential for low white blood cells and thrombocytopenia • Drug interactions may require dose adjustments or avoidance of certain drug combinations; avoid concomitant use with drugs that cause QT prolongation Associated with: • Prolonged QT interval; do not use in patients predisposed to QT prolongation • Torsades de pointes • Sudden death
Generic Name Vemurafenib **Brand Name** Zelboraf QT	Treatment of unresectable or metastatic malignant melanoma	**Usual oral dose:** 960 mg every 12 hours; continue until disease progression target is achieved or unacceptable toxicity occurs	• Liver injury has been reported with use; may cause functional impairments such as coagulopathy or other organ dysfunction • Cutaneous squamous cell carcinomas (cuSCC), keratoacanthomas, and melanoma have been reported • QT prolongation (dose dependent) has been observed • Confirm that the patient is *BRAF* mutation positive prior to beginning treatment with vemurafenib • Regular ECGs are required to evaluate for QT prolongation • Routine dermatologic exams prior to beginning therapy and every 2 months are essential • Instruct patients on photosensitivity precautions • Severe skin reactions that require attention include a red or purple rash, which may cause peeling or blistering in the face or trunk area • Drug interactions may require dose adjustments or avoidance of certain drug combinations

Generic Name Vismodegib **Brand Name** Erivedge ■	Basal cell carcinoma, metastatic or locally advanced	**Usual oral dose:** 150 mg once daily until disease progression target is achieved or unacceptable toxicity occurs	• Amenorrhea • Blood donation not recommended; refer to PI for complete details

Topoisomerase Inhibitors

Anthracyclines

Universal prescribing alerts:

- These agents are severe vesicants. Intramuscular administration and subcutaneous administration are to be avoided due to severe skin and tissue necrosis.
- These agents are associated with cardiotoxicity, with the risk of this side effect increasing with higher cumulative lifetime doses.

Drug Name	FDA-Approved Indications	Adult Dosage Range	Precautions and Clinical Pearls
Generic Name Daunorubicin **Brand Name** Cerubidine ▲ ■ ■ (PD) (GD)	Acute lymphocytic leukemia (ALL) AML	Dose is based on indication for use and patient's clinical response **Illustrative parenteral dose for ALL:** IV: 45 mg/m^2 on days 1, 2, and 3 Repeat doses and schedule are based on overall treatment plan; refer to PI	• Dosage reductions are recommended in patients with hepatic or renal impairment • Assess CBC with differential, LFTs, renal function, uric acid levels, cardiac function (ECG, ECHO/ejection fraction, multigated acquisition [MUGA] scan) • Infusion site must be closely monitored; extravasation can cause severe cellulitis or tissue necrosis • Assess for tachycardia, cough, dyspnea, and gastrointestinal upset prior to each infusion and throughout therapy Associated with: • Severe bone marrow suppression, when used at therapeutic doses • Potent vesicant; if extravasation occurs, severe local tissue damage leading to ulceration, necrosis, and pain may occur. IM and SQ administration is contraindicated • Cumulative, dose-related myocardial toxicity; may lead to heart failure • Dose adjustments and careful monitoring if renal and hepatic impairment • Requires experienced clinician who is knowledgeable in the use of chemotherapy agents and specialized care setting

Drug Name	FDA-Approved Indications	Adult Dosage Range	Precautions and Clinical Pearls
Generic Name Doxorubicin **Brand Name** Adriamycin	**Common indications for use:** Breast cancer Metastatic cancers or disseminated neoplastic conditions	Dose is based on indication for use and patient's clinical response **Illustrative parenteral dose for breast cancer:** IV: 60 mg/m^2 on day 1 of a 21-day cycle	• Assess cardiac function prior to beginning therapy and periodically during therapy • Give patients antiemetics to help prevent nausea and vomiting • Infusion site must be closely monitored • Drug interactions may require dose adjustments or avoidance of certain drug combinations Associated with: • Severe myelosuppression • Cumulative, dose-related, myocardial toxicity • Vesicant; if extravasation occurs, severe local tissue damage leading to tissue injury, blistering, ulceration, and necrosis may occur; IM and SQ administration should be avoided • Secondary acute myelogenous leukemia and myelodysplastic syndrome have been reported • Initiate routine surveillance for secondary malignancies • Requires experienced clinician who is knowledgeable in the use of chemotherapy agents and specialized care setting
Generic Name Epirubicin **Brand Name** Ellence	Breast cancer, adjuvant treatment	**Usual parenteral dose**: IV: 120 mg/m^2 per 3- or 4-week treatment cycle Given along with other chemotherapeutic agents	• Myocardial toxicity, including fatal heart failure, may occur • Use with caution in the presence of hepatic or renal impairment; evaluate for impairments at baseline and during treatment • Premedication with an antiemetic may be useful • Monitor for acute nausea and vomiting, anemia, infection, bleeding, and cardiotoxicity • Teach patients about the importance of adequate hydration Associated with: • Severe myelosuppression, including leukopenia, thrombocytopenia, and anemia • For IV administration only; if extravasation occurs, severe local tissue damage and necrosis may occur; IM and SQ administration is contraindicated. • Treatment with anthracyclines (including epirubicin) may increase the risk of secondary AML • Requires experienced clinician who is knowledgeable in the use of chemotherapy agents and specialized care setting

Generic Name Idarubicin **Brand Name** Idamycin PFS ■ ■ (GD)	ALL Acute promyelocytic leukemia (APL)	**Usual parenteral dose for APL:** IV: 12 mg/m^2 per day for 3 days Regimen may include combinations with other chemotherpeutic agents	• Infusion site must be closely monitored; extravasation can cause severe cellulitis or tissue necrosis • Monitor for cardiac toxicity, myelosuppression, and peripheral neuropathy frequently during therapy Associated with: • Severe myelosuppression, when used at therapeutic doses • Vesicant; may cause severe local tissue damage and necrosis if extravasation occurs; IM and SQ administration should be avoided • Myocardial toxicity and heart failure • Cautious use in hepatic disease • Caution in renal impairment, dose reduction may be required; no specific recommendations available • Requires experienced clinician who is knowledgeable in the use of chemotherapy agents and specialized care setting
Generic Name Valrubicin **Brand Name** Valstar	Bladder cancer	**Usual intravesical dose:** 800 mg once weekly (retain for 2 hours) for 6 weeks	• Symptoms of irritable bladder may occur during instillation and retention, and for a brief time after voiding • Red-tinged urine may occur in the first 24 hours after instillation • Use caution to prevent inadvertent exposure to this medication • Assess the patient's response during and following instillation: genitourinary (frequency, urgency, incontinence, dysuria, bladder spasm or pain, hematuria, urinary tract infection [UTI]) rash, nausea, vomiting, myalgia, hyperglycemia Contraindications: • Patients with active UTI • Patients with bladder perforation
Camptothecins			
Drug Name	**FDA-Approved Indications**	**Adult Dosage Range**	**Precautions and Clinical Pearls**
Generic Name Irinotecan **Brand Name** Camptosar ■ (GD)	Colorectal cancer (metastatic)	**Usual parenteral dose**: IV: Weekly regimen: 125 mg/m^2 over 90 minutes on days 1, 8, 15, and 22 of a 6-week treatment cycle Regimen may additional chemotherapeutic agents (i.e., bolus 5-FU/leucovorin)	• Fatal cases of interstitial pulmonary disease (IPD)–like events have been reported • Use caution and closely monitor use in patients with increased risk of neutropenia, patients with history of pelvic or abdominal radiation, and elderly patients with comorbid conditions • Premedicate patients with an antiemetic (moderate emetic potential) • Assess CBC with differential and platelet count • Monitor for neutropenia, immediate or delayed diarrhea (can be fatal), sepsis, mucositis, and stomatitis • Drug interactions may require dose adjustments or avoidance of certain drug combinations Associated with: • Severe myelosuppression • Severe diarrhea may be dose limiting and potentially fatal

Drug Name	FDA-Approved Indications	Adult Dosage Range	Precautions and Clinical Pearls
Generic Name Topotecan **Brand Name** Hycamtin	Cervical cancer, recurrent or resistant Ovarian cancer, metastatic Small cell lung cancer, relapsed	Dose is based on indication for use and patient's clinical response **Illustrative parenteral dose for cervical cancer:** IV: 0.75 mg/m^2 per day for 3 days (in combination with cisplatin on day 1 only) every 21 days	• Monitor for diarrhea symptoms and hydration status • ILD (with fatalities) has been reported. Monitor for symptoms of lung disease • Topotecan-induced neutropenia may lead to typhlitis (neutropenic enterocolitis) • Monitor CBC with differential and platelet count, renal function tests, and bilirubin • Evaluate renal function (I & O, edema) and monitor for signs of myelosuppression, gastrointestinal disturbance, and dyspnea prior to each infusion and on a regular basis when the oral formulation is used • Administrate with adequate hydration • Irritant; avoid extravasation Associated with: • Severe myelosuppression

Podophyllotoxins

Drug Name	FDA-Approved Indications	Adult Dosage Range	Precautions and Clinical Pearls
Generic Name Etoposide **Brand Name** Toposar VePesid	Small cell lung cancer (oral and IV) Testicular cancer (IV)	Dose is based on indication for use and patient's clinical response **Illustrative parenteral dose for small cell lung cancer (combination chemotherapy):** IV: 35 mg/m^2 per day for 4 days, up to 50 mg/m^2 per day for 5 days every 3 to 4 weeks	• Hypotension may occur with rapid administration • Secondary acute leukemias have been reported • Monitor CBC with differential, liver function (bilirubin, ALT, AST), albumin, renal function, and vital signs (blood pressure) • Monitor for signs of an infusion reaction • Monitor patients closely for anaphylactic reaction • Assess renal and hepatic function prior to each treatment and on a regular basis • Drug interactions may require dose adjustments or avoidance of certain drug combinations Associated with: • Severe dose-limiting and dose-related myelosuppression with resulting infection or bleeding • Requires experienced clinician who is knowledgeable in the use of chemotherapy agents

Generic Name Mitoxantrone **Brand Name** Novantrone ■ ■	**Common indications for use:** Initial treatment of acute nonlymphocytic leukemias AML Treatment of advanced hormone-refractory prostate cancer	Dose is based on indication for use and patient's clinical response **Illustrative parenteral dose for AML induction:** 12 mg/m^2 once daily for 3 days Combination chemotherapy	• Monitor for cardiotoxicity, hypersensitivity reactions, myelosuppression, gastrointestinal upset, and opportunistic infections with each dose and throughout therapy • Usually should not be administered if baseline neutrophil count less than 1500 cells/mm^3 • For IV administration only; may cause severe local tissue damage if extravasation occurs Associated with: • Myocardial toxicity and potentially fatal heart failure • Increased risk of developing secondary acute myelogenous leukemia in patients with cancer and in patients with multiple sclerosis • Requires experienced clinician who is knowledgeable in the use of chemotherapy agents • Infusion site must be monitored closely to prevent extravasation • Intrathecal administration is not recommended and should be avoided
Generic Name Teniposide **Brand Name** Vumon (DSC) ■ (PD)	ALL, refractory	**Usual parenteral dose**: IV: 165 mg/m^2 per dose on days 1, 4, 8, and 11 of alternating consolidation cycles	• Hypotension may occur with rapid infusion • Acute CNS depression, hypotension, and metabolic acidosis have been reported • Premedication with corticosteroids and antiemetics is recommended • Infusion site should be closely monitored to prevent extravasation • Monitor for mucositis, diarrhea, myelosuppression, and neutropenia prior to each infusion and throughout therapy • Drug interactions may require dose adjustments or avoidance of certain drug combinations • Designated an orphan drug by the FDA for refractory ALL in certain age-specific populations; refer to PI for additional details • Tumor lysis syndrome has been reported Associated with: • Severe myelosuppression resulting in infection or bleeding • Hypersensitivity reactions, including anaphylaxis-like reactions • Requires experienced clinician who is knowledgeable in the use of chemotherapy agents and specialized care setting

Other Antineoplastic Agents

Platinum Complexes

Drug Name	FDA-Approved Indications	Adult Dosage Range	Precautions and Clinical Pearls
Generic Name Carboplatin **Brand Name** Paraplatin ▲ ■ (BL)	Ovarian cancer	**Usual parenteral dose**: IV: 360 mg/m^2 every 4 weeks	• Assess the patient's allergy history prior to therapy and note specific cautions for use (e.g., bone marrow suppression and impaired renal function) • Assess hematology, electrolytes, and renal and hepatic function tests prior to treatment and on a regular basis during therapy • Specific recommendations for patients undergoing dialysis • Monitor for nausea and vomiting, ototoxicity, bone marrow depression, anemia, bleeding, and peripheral neuropathy • Use the Calvert formula to calculate dosing for elderly patients; refer to PI Associated with: • Bone marrow suppression, which may be severe, is dose related; may result in infection • Anaphylactic-like reactions • Vomiting • Requires experienced clinician who is knowledgeable in the use of chemotherapy agents and specialized care setting
Generic Name Cisplatin **Brand Name** Platinol ▲ ■ (BL)	**Common indications for use:** Bladder cancer, advanced Ovarian cancer, metastatic Testicular cancer, metastatic	Dose is based on indication for use and patient's clinical response **Illustrative parenteral dose for testicular cancer (metastatic):** IV: 20 mg/m^2 per day for 5 days repeated every 3 weeks Combination chemotherapy	• Patients should be vigorously hydrated prior to and for 24 hours following infusion • Cisplatin is highly emetogenic; antiemetics should be administered prior to each treatment and as needed between infusions • Monitor for acute or chronic renal failure; peripheral neuropathy and ototoxicity may be irreversible • Teach patients about the importance of adequate hydration; assess urine output for adequacy Associated with: • Myelosuppression: a major dose-related toxicity • Nausea and vomiting: dose-related toxicities • Anaphylactic-like reactions • Cumulative renal toxicity associated with cisplatin is severe; contraindicated with preexisting renal disease • Ototoxicity; contraindicated in patients with preexisting hearing impairment • Requires experienced clinician who is knowledgeable in the use of chemotherapy agents and specialized care setting

Drug Name	FDA-Approved Indications	Adult Dosage Range	Precautions and Clinical Pearls
Generic Name Oxaliplatin **Brand Name** Eloxatin ▲ ■ (QT)	Colon cancer Colorectal cancer, advanced	Dose is based on indication for use and patient's clinical response **Illustrative parenteral dose for advanced colorectal cancer:** IV: 85 mg/m^2 every 2 weeks Combination chemotherapy	• Associated with a moderate emetic potential • Hepatotoxicity (including rare cases of hepatitis and hepatic failure) • Monitor for pulmonary or hepatic toxicity, neuropathy, GI disturbance, anemia, chest pain, and thromboembolism • Monitor for signs of GI or other bleeding • Monitor blood counts, platelets, and coagulation studies • Monitor for swelling, numbness, pain, and tingling or burning in the hands and feet • Monitor for dehydration secondary to diarrhea Associated with: • Anaphylactic/anaphylactoid reactions
Retinoids			
Drug Name	FDA-Approved Indications	Adult Dosage Range	Precautions and Clinical Pearls
Generic Name Bexarotene **Brand Name** Targretin ■	**Common indications for use:** Cutaneous T-cell lymphoma, refractory	**Usual oral dose:** Initial: 300 mg/m^2 once daily	• Take with food • Avoid sun exposure; photosensitivity reported • Dose-related elevations in ALT, AST, and bilirubin • Rapid suppression of TSH levels • Leukopenia has been reported • Induces significant lipid abnormalities in the majority of patients; pancreatitis has been reported • Monitor lipid panel, LFTs, thyroid function, and CBC prior to and during therapy and blood glucose if the patient has diabetes • Monitor for CNS and cardiovascular effects, opportunistic infection, visual abnormalities, and hypoglycemia • Contact with the medication can harm the skin; wash with soap and water immediately • Drug interactions may require dose adjustments or avoidance of certain drug combinations

Drug Name	FDA-Approved Indications	Adult Dosage Range	Precautions and Clinical Pearls
Generic Name Tretinoin **Brand Name** Vesanoid ■ (PD) (GD)	**Common indications for use:** Induction of remission in patients with APL Acne vulgaris	Dose varies with indication for use and patient's clinical status **Usual oral dose for APL:** 45 mg/m^2 per day in 2 equally divided doses	• Retinoids have been associated with pseudotumor cerebri (benign intracranial hypertension) • Perform bone marrow cytology to confirm t(15;17) translocation or the presence of the PML/RARα fusion protein • Patients will require close monitoring of their cardiac, CNS, and respiratory status on a frequent basis during therapy • Details concerning dosing in combination regimens should also be consulted • Drug interactions may require dose adjustments or avoidance of certain drug combinations Associated with: • Many patients with APL treated with tretinoin will experience "APL differentiation syndrome" • Many patients will develop rapidly evolving leukocytosis • Requires experienced clinician who is knowledgeable in the use of chemotherapy agents and specialized care setting
Spindle Poisons (from Plants)			
Taxanes			
Drug Name	FDA-Approved Indications	Adult Dosage Range	Precautions and Clinical Pearls
Generic Name Cabazitaxel **Brand Name** Jevtana ■ ■	Prostate cancer (metastatic)	**Usual parenteral dose**: IV: 25 mg/m^2 once every 3 weeks	• Nausea, vomiting, and diarrhea may occur • Premedicate the patient 30 minutes prior to each dose (antihistamine, corticosteroid, and H_2 antagonist) • Monitor for hypersensitivity, hypotension, myelosuppression, and GI irritation (including severe diarrhea), GI bleeding (and perforation) prior to, during, and between each infusion • Renal failure has been reported; ensure patient maintains adequate hydration Associated with: • Deaths due to neutropenia • Severe hypersensitivity reactions, including generalized rash, erythema, hypotension, and bronchospasm (confirm past reaction and allergy history)
Generic Name Docetaxel **Brand Name** Docefrez Taxotere ■ ■	Breast cancer NSCLC Prostate cancer	Dose is based on indication for use and patient's clinical response	• Severe hypersensitivity reactions have been reported; premedication with dexamethasone may be advisable for 3 days starting one day before infusion; this will help lessen potential fluid retention/edema • Drug interactions may require dose adjustments or avoidance of certain drug combinations • Formulations may contain ethanol; may impair one's ability to drive or operate machinery

		Illustrative parenteral dose for breast cancer: IV infusion: 60 to 100 mg/m^2 every 3 weeks	• Monitor patients continuously during infusion; dosing adjustments may be necessary • Monitor for neutropenia, severe fluid retention, pleural effusion, opportunistic infections, and anemia prior to each infusion and on a regular basis • Patients must have an adequate threshold ANC to receive therapy; refer to PI Associated with: • Severe fluid retention, characterized by pleural effusion (requiring immediate drainage), ascites, peripheral edema (poorly tolerated), dyspnea at rest, cardiac tamponade, generalized edema, and weight gain • Severe hypersensitivity reactions, characterized by generalized rash/erythema, hypotension, bronchospasms, and anaphylaxis; confirm past reaction and allergy history • Avoid in hepatic disease; fatal toxicity has been reported despite dose adjustments • Increased mortality reported in certain individuals
Generic Name Paclitaxel **Brand Name** Taxol ■ ■	Breast cancer Kaposi sarcoma (AIDS related) NSCLC Ovarian cancer	Dose is based on indication for use and patient's clinical response **Illustrative parenteral dose for breast cancer:** IV: 175 mg/m^2 over 3 hours every 3 weeks	• Assess patients carefully for cautious-use indications and contraindications • Infusion site must be monitored closely to avoid extravasation • Monitor for hypersensitivity reaction, cardiovascular abnormalities, sensory neuropathy, myelosuppression, and GI irritation prior to, during, and between each infusion • Formulations may contain ethanol; may impair one's ability to drive or operate machinery • Drug interactions may require dose adjustments or avoidance of certain drug combinations Associated with: • Bone marrow suppression (primarily neutropenia); may be severe or result in infection • Anaphylaxis and severe hypersensitivity reactions (dyspnea requiring bronchodilators, hypotension requiring treatment, angioedema, and/or generalized urticaria); confirm past reaction and allergy history • Requires experienced clinician who is knowledgeable in the use of chemotherapy agents and specialized care setting

Vinca Alkaloids			
Drug Name	FDA-Approved Indications	Adult Dosage Range	Precautions and Clinical Pearls
Generic Name Vinblastine **Brand Name** Velban ■ ■	**Common indications for use:** Breast cancer Hodgkin's lymphoma Histiocytic lymphoma Mycosis fungoides Testicular cancer Kaposi sarcoma	**Usual parenteral dose for breast cancer:** IV: 4.5 mg/m^2 on day 1 of every 21 days Combination chemotherapy with doxorubicin and thiotepa.	• Acute shortness of breath and severe bronchospasm • Obtain liver function tests prior to therapy; dosage adjustments may be needed • Premedication with an antiemetic is advisable • Monitor for syndrome of inappropriate antidiuretic hormone secretion (SIADH), bone marrow suppression, leukopenia, hypertension, gastrointestinal disturbance, myalgia, depression, neurotoxicity, and paresthesia throughout therapy • Drug interactions may require dose adjustments or avoidance of certain drug combinations Associated with: • Bone marrow suppression; leukopenia commonly occurs; granulocytopenia may be severe with higher doses • Vesicant; ensure proper catheter or needle position prior to (and during) infusion; monitor infusion site; IM and SQ administration should be avoided • Requires experienced clinician who is knowledgeable in the use of chemotherapy agents • Fatal if administered intrathecally; for IV use only
Generic Name Vincristine **Brand Name** Oncovin, Vincasar PFS ■ ■ (BL) (PD)	Treatment of ALL Hodgkin's lymphoma Non-Hodgkin's lymphomas Wilms' tumor Neuroblastoma Rhabdomyosarcoma	**Usual parenteral dose**: IV: 1.4 mg/m^2 every week (maximum: 2 mg per dose)	• Premedication with an antiemetic is advisable • May cause severe constipation, paralytic ileus, intestinal obstruction, necrosis, and perforation • Assess CNS status (motor difficulties, seizure, depression), neuromuscular status (myalgia, peripheral neuropathy, jaw pain, cramping), and photophobia throughout therapy; alterations in mental status such as depression, confusion, or insomnia reported • Drug interactions may require dose adjustments or avoidance of certain drug combinations Associated with: • Vesicant; ensure proper catheter or needle position prior to (and during) infusion; monitor infusion site; IM and SQ administration should be avoided • Requires experienced clinician who is knowledgeable in the use of chemotherapy agents • Fatal if administered intrathecally; for IV use only

Generic Name Vinorelbine **Brand Name** Navelbine ■ ■	Treatment of NSCLC	**Usual parenteral dose**: Single-agent therapy: 30 mg/m^2 every 7 days until disease progression target is achieved or unacceptable toxicity occurs	• May cause severe constipation, paralytic ileus, intestinal obstruction, necrosis, and perforation • Premedication with an antiemetic is advisable • Monitor for peripheral neuropathy • Drug interactions may require dose adjustments or avoidance of certain drug combinations • Assess pulmonary status and liver function prior to each infusion and throughout therapy • Vesicant; ensure proper catheter or needle position prior to (and during) infusion; monitor infusion site; IM and SQ administration should be avoided • If dispensed in a syringe, should be labeled "for IV use only" Associated with: • Severe bone marrow suppression (including granulocytopenia) reported

Miscellaneous Antineoplastic Agents

Drug Name	FDA-Approved Indications	Adult Dosage Range	Precautions and Clinical Pearls
Generic Name Arsenic trioxide **Brand Name** Trisenox ■ QT	APL	Dose is based on indication for use and patient's clinical response **Illustrative parenteral dose for APL, relapsed or refractory:** IV induction: 0.15 mg/kg once daily until bone marrow remission occurs Consolidation: starting 3 to 6 weeks after completion of induction therapy	• Monitor electrolytes (potassium, calcium, and magnesium), CBC with differential, serum creatinine, hepatic function, blood glucose, and coagulation parameters • Assess cardiac and electrolyte status at beginning of and periodically during therapy • Monitor renal and hepatic function. Dose adjustments may be necessary with impairment; however, no specific recommendations are available • Monitor for secondary malignancy Associated with: • APL differentiation syndrome, which is characterized by dyspnea, fever, weight gain, pulmonary infiltrates, and pleural or pericardial effusions, with or without leukocytosis • May prolong the QT interval and lead to torsades de pointes or complete AV block

Drug Name	FDA-Approved Indications	Adult Dosage Range	Precautions and Clinical Pearls
Generic Name Bortezomib **Brand Name** Velcade ■ QT	Mantle cell lymphoma (MCL) Multiple myeloma	Dose is based on indication for use and patient's clinical response **Illustrative parenteral dose for mantle cell lymphoma MCL:** IV:1.3 mg/m^2 per dose on days 1, 4, 8, and 11 of a 21-day treatment cycle, for 6 cycles Combination chemotherapy May also administer SQ	• Hematologic toxicity, including severe neutropenia and thrombocytopenia; monitor for bleeding • Evaluate patients who develop new or worsening cardiopulmonary symptoms • Has been associated with the development or exacerbation of heart failure and decreased LVEF • Nausea, vomiting, diarrhea, and constipation • Assess CBC with differential and platelets, liver function tests, and blood glucose levels • Watch for signs of tumor lysis syndrome (elevated uric acid, potassium, and phosphate; hypocalcemia; acute renal failure) and worsening cardiac function, particularly heart failure • Monitor for peripheral neuropathy, postural hypotension, dehydration, and infections • Specific recommendations for patients undergoing dialysis; refer to PI • Drug interactions may require dose adjustment Associated with: • Warning to not administer intrathecally; may result in fatality.
Generic Name Carfilzomib **Brand Name** Kyprolis ▲ ■ GD	Relapsed/refractory multiple myeloma	Dose is calculated based on body surface area (BSA), cycle number, and number of agents used **Illustrative parenteral dose for a single cycle:** IV: 20 mg/m^2 over 10 minutes on days 1 and 2 Refer to PI for additional cycles and regimen details	• Bone marrow suppression • Cardiovascular effects (e.g., cardiac failure, edema) • Increased LFTs • Hypertension • Tumor lysis syndrome has been reported • Serious and potentially fatal bleeding reported • Pulmonary toxicities (e.g., dyspnea, pneumonia, pulmonary edema) • Renal toxicity (e.g., renal failure) has been reported • Vials contain the excipient cyclodextrin, which may accumulate in patients with renal insufficiency; clinical significance is uncertain • Thromboembolic events; thromboprophylaxis is recommended with combination therapy (patient specific) • Provide adequate hydration prior to therapy • Monitor CBC and platelets; potassium levels during treatment; electrolytes; alkaline phosphatase; renal, cardiac, and pulmonary function; LFTs; and blood pressure • Monitor for signs and symptoms of infusion-related reactions, thrombotic thrombocytopenic purpura (TTP)/hemolytic-uremic syndrome (HUS), peripheral neuropathy, VTE events, and evidence of volume overload • Hydration, premedication with dexamethasone, combination with lenalidomide, and/or thromboprophylaxis may be required before and after therapy

Generic Name Dabrafenib **Brand Name** Tafinlar QT	Metastatic or unresectable melanoma (with *BRAF* V600E or *BRAF* V600K mutation)	Dose is based on indication for use and patient's clinical response **Illustrative oral dose for melanoma, metastatic or unresectable (with *BRAF* V600E mutation):** 150 mg twice daily (approximately every 12 hours) until disease progression target is achieved or unacceptable toxicity occurs (single-agent therapy)	• Monitor CBC, blood glucose, LVEF, and electrolytes • Monitor for signs and symptoms of hemorrhage, VTE, hemolytic anemia, and interstitial lung disease • Cardiomyopathy, rash, palmar–plantar syndrome, and hyperglycemia may occur • Transient loss of vision and blurred vision • VTE (deep vein thrombosis and pulmonary embolism) may occur when used in combination with trametinib • Drugs affecting gastric pH may decrease bioavailability • Use with caution in patients with glucose-6-phosphate dehydrogenase (G6PD) deficiency; may be at risk for hemolytic anemia • Administer at least 1 hour before or 2 hours after a meal; doses should be approximately 12 hours apart • Do not open, crush, or break capsules • When administered in combination with trametinib, take once-daily dose at the same time each day with either the morning or evening dose of dabrafeni • Use with caution in patients with liver or kidney disease, hypertension, heart failure, or autoimmune conditions such as Crohn's disease or ulcerative colitis • Assess for hepatotoxicity • Patients may be at risk for new skin cancers; monitor skin for changes (e.g., moles, new warts) • Assess for stomach pain, unusual bleeding, or diarrhea • Serious side effects include rash, chills, fever reaction, changes in urination, renal failure, visual changes, and hand–foot syndrome • Drug interactions may require dose adjustments or avoidance of certain drug combinations
Generic Name Denileukin **Brand Name** Ontak ■	Cutaneous T-cell lymphoma	**Usual parenteral dose**: IV: 9 or 18 mcg/kg daily for 5 consecutive days; repeat every 21 days	• Perform CBCs, blood chemistries, and renal and hepatic function tests prior to initiation of therapy and at weekly intervals during therapy • Monitor weight, edema, blood pressure, and serum albumin Associated with: • Risk of severe and/or fatal capillary leak syndrome; monitor patients with cardiac disease • Severe infusion related reactions (and fatalities) have been reported • Visual impairment has been reported with use • Requires experienced clinician who is knowledgeable in the use of chemotherapy agents

Drug Name	FDA-Approved Indications	Adult Dosage Range	Precautions and Clinical Pearls
Generic Name Eribulin **Brand Name** Halaven ▲ ■ QT	**Common indications for use:** Breast cancer (metastatic)	**Usual parental dose**: IV: 1.4 mg/m^2 per dose on days 1 and 8 of a 21-day treatment cycle	• Hematologic toxicity, including severe neutropenia • Peripheral neuropathy commonly occurs and is the most frequent toxicity leading to discontinuation; assess for peripheral neuropathy prior to giving each dose • Perform CBC with differential prior to giving each dose • Monitor renal and liver function tests and serum electrolytes, including potassium and magnesium • Monitor ECG in patients with heart failure, bradyarrhythmia, use of concomitant medications known to prolong the QT interval, and electrolyte abnormalities • Drug interactions may require dose adjustments or avoidance of certain drug combinations
Generic Name Idelalisib **Brand Name** Zydelig ■ ■	CLL Follicular B-cell non-Hodgkin's lymphoma Small lymphocytic lymphoma (All relapsed treatment)	**Usual oral dose for CLL:** 150 mg twice daily; continue until disease progression target has been achieved or unacceptable toxicity occurs Combination chemotherapy with rituximab is used for CLL	• Bone marrow suppression • Drug interactions may require dose adjustments or avoidance of certain drug combinations • Administer without regard to food; swallow tablets whole • Monitor CBC (particularly for neutropenia) and LFTs (every 2 weeks for first 3 months) • Monitor for signs/symptoms of diarrhea/colitis, intestinal perforation, pneumonitis, dermatologic toxicity, infection, and hypersensitivity reactions • Assess the patient's vaccination records; consider bringing the patient up-to-date prior to initiating therapy Associated with: • Serious hepatotoxicity • Severe diarrhea/colitis • Pneumonitis • Intestinal perforation • Serious infusion-related reactions
Generic Name Interferon alfa 2b **Brand Name** Intron A ■ GD	**Common indications for use:** AIDS-related Kaposi sarcoma Condylomata acuminate Follicular lymphoma	Dose is based on indication for use and patient's clinical response	• Causes bone marrow suppression, including potentially severe cytopenias and, very rarely, aplastic anemia • Patients with preexisting cardiac abnormalities or in advanced stages of cancer should have ECGs taken before and during treatment • Monitor for neuropsychiatric changes, especially depression, suicidal or homicidal ideation, psychosis, or mania; decreased pulmonary function; and ophthalmic changes • Immediately evaluate any reported changes in vision • Drug interactions may require dose adjustments or avoidance of certain drug combinations

	Hairy cell leukemia Malignant melanoma	**Illustrative parenteral dose for hairy cell leukemia:** IM or SQ: 2 million international units/m^2 3 times per week for up to 6 months	Associated with: • Avoid use in severe hepatic impairment or disease; contraindicated • Caution in those with cardiac or pulmonary disease • Severe neuropsychiatric adverse events • Myelosuppressive effects increase the risk of infection and bleeding • Fatal or life-threatening autoimmune disorders
Generic Name Ixabepilone **Brand Name** Ixempra ■ ■ (GD)	Breast cancer: metastatic or locally advanced	**Usual parenteral dose**: IV: 40 mg/m^2 per dose over 3 hours every 3 weeks Combination chemotherapy	• Peripheral (sensory and motor) neuropathy occurs commonly • Premedication with H_1 and H_2 antagonists is recommended 1 hour before infusion • Monitor patients closely for hypersensitivity reaction (rash, flushing, bronchospasm) • In case of adverse infusion reactions, the infusion should be stopped and the prescriber notified • Monitor for hypersensitivity, hypotension, myelosuppression, peripheral neuropathy, and gastrointestinal upset prior to, during, and between each infusion • Drug interactions may require dose adjustments or avoidance of certain drug combinations • Formulations may contain ethanol; may impair one's ability to drive or operate machinery Contraindications: • Patient with neutropenia or thrombocytopenia. Dose-dependent myelosuppression, particularly neutropenia, may occur Associated with: • Contraindication for use in hepatic disease
Generic Name Lenalidomide **Brand Name** Revlimid ▲ ■	MCL Multiple myeloma Myelodysplastic syndromes	Dose is based on indication for use and patient's clinical response **Illustrative oral dose for MCL:** 25 mg once daily for 21 days of a 28-day treatment cycle	• May cause dizziness or fatigue • Use with caution in patients with a history of clotting disorders, pulmonary embolism, or kidney, heart, or liver disease • Monitor CBC with differential, LFTs, and renal function tests • Select dose carefully and closely monitor renal function • May increase patients' risk of clots; monitor for signs of thrombosis or thromboembolism • Monitor for hypothyroidism • Monitor for neutropenia, thrombocytopenia, and electrolyte imbalances Associated with: • Hematologic toxicity (neutropenia and thrombocytopenia); interrupt therapy based on manufacturer's recommendation; refer to PI • Significantly increased risk for arterial and venous thromboembolic events

Drug Name	FDA-Approved Indications	Adult Dosage Range	Precautions and Clinical Pearls
Generic Name Olaparib **Brand Name** Lynparza ▲	Advanced ovarian cancer	**Usual oral dose:** 400 mg twice daily until disease progression target is achieved or unacceptable toxicity occurs	• Bone marrow suppression (e.g., anemia, neutropenia) • Antiemetics are recommended to prevent nausea and vomiting; moderate emetic potential • Secondary malignancy (MDS/AML)— rare • Swallow capsule whole; do not chew or open • Drug interactions may require dose adjustments or avoidance of certain drug combinations; avoid consumption of grapefruit and Seville oranges • Monitor CBC at baseline and monthly, or until hematologic toxicity recovery • Monitor for signs and symptoms of AML, MDS, and pneumonitis • Administer only to patients with deleterious or suspected deleterious germline *BRCA* mutations, as detected by an approved test
Generic Name Omacetaxine **Brand Name** Synribo	CML (chronic or accelerated phase)	**Usual parenteral dose:** Induction: SQ: 1.25 mg/m^2 twice daily for 14 consecutive days of a 28-day treatment cycle; continue until hematologic response is achieved. Continue until no longer achieving clinical treatment benefit	• Monitor CBC and platelets weekly during induction and the initial maintenance cycles, then as clinically indicated • Bone marrow suppression: neutropenia, thrombocytopenia, and anemia are common; hemorrhage has been reported • Monitor for signs and symptoms of infection, fever, and bleeding • Drug interactions may require dose adjustments or avoidance of certain drug combinations • May induce glucose intolerance or cause hyperglycemia; avoid use in patients with poorly controlled diabetes; monitor blood glucose • Administer subcutaneously at approximately 12-hour intervals • If home administration is performed, advise the patient and caregiver on proper handling, storage, administration, disposal, and cleanup of spillage. Avoid skin and eye contact • The maintenance regimen (twice daily for 7 consecutive days of a 28-day treatment cycle)
Generic Name Peginterferon alfa 2b **Brand Name** Peg-Intron Peg-Intron Redipen Sylatron ▲ ■ (PD)	Chronic hepatitis C (CHC) Melanoma (Sylatron)	**Usual parenteral dose for melanoma:** SQ: Initial: 6 mcg/kg per week for 8 doses Maintenance: 3 mcg/kg per week for up to 5 years	• Bone marrow suppression • Flu-like symptoms commonly seen • Use with caution in patients with thyroid disorders and in elderly patients • Peripheral neuropathy has been reported when used in combination with telbivudine • Due to differences in dosage, patients should not change brands of interferon • Monitor TSH (baseline and periodically), CBC and platelets, LFTs (weeks 2 and 8, 2 and 3 months, then every 6 months), renal function, triglycerides, glucose and HbA_{1c} (patients with diabetes mellitus)

			• Perform baseline eye examination and ECG (patient specific) • Monitor for vision changes, ischemic disorders, autoimmune disease development, and pulmonary function (e.g., shortness of breath), signs and symptoms of colitis and pancreatitis, hypersensitivity reactions, and opportunistic infections • Drug interactions may require dose adjustments or avoidance of certain drug combinations • Premedicate the patient with acetaminophen (500 to 1000 mg orally) 30 minutes prior to the first dose and as needed for subsequent doses thereafter Contraindications: • Hepatic decompensation or autoimmune hepatitis hemoglobinopathies (e.g., thalassemia major, sickle cell anemia) • Renal dysfunction (creatinine clearance [CrCl] less than 50 mL/min) • Patients developing signs or symptoms of severe skin reactions or severe hypersensitivity must discontinue therapy. Associated with: • May cause or aggravate severe depression or other neuropsychiatric adverse events (including suicide/ideation) in patients with and without history of psychiatric conditions; evaluate mental status for psychiatric symptoms • May cause or exacerbate autoimmune disorder, infectious disorders, and ischemic and hemorrhagic cerebrovascular events • Combination with ribavabirin may cause hemolytic anemia, genotoxicity, and mutagenicity; may possibly be carcinogenic • Tachycardia has been observed; use with caution in patients with active or past cardiovascular disease (MI)
Generic Name Pomalidomide **Brand Name** Pomalyst ▲ ■ ■	Relapsed and/or refractory multiple myeloma	**Usual oral dose:** 4 mg once daily on days 1 to 21 of 28-day cycles (in combination with dexamethasone); continue until disease progression target is achieved or unacceptable toxicity occurs	• Available through risk evaluation and mitigation strategy (REMS) program • Bone marrow suppression; neutropenia, anemia, and thrombocytopenia are common • Tumor lysis syndrome has been reported • CNS effects (e.g., dizziness, confusion) • Peripheral and sensory neuropathy • Avoid use in patients with renal or hepatic impairment • Swallow capsules whole; do not break or open capsules • Administer on an empty stomach with water, at least 2 hours before or 2 hours after a meal • Drug interactions may require dose adjustments or avoidance of certain drug combinations

Drug Name	FDA-Approved Indications	Adult Dosage Range	Precautions and Clinical Pearls
			• Confirm smoking status: cigarette smoking may reduce systemic exposure and efficacy • Assess for signs and symptoms of hepatotoxicity, thromboembolism, bone marrow suppression, and neuropathy • Monitor CBC and platelets weekly for first 8 weeks and then monthly or as clinically needed; perform renal and liver function tests monthly • Confirm ANC values meet required threshold prior to dosing; refer to PI Associated with: • Venous and arterial thromboembolic events such as DVT, pulmonary embolism, MI, and stroke have occurred • Thromboprophylaxis is recommended • Requires experienced clinician who is knowledgeable in the use of this agent
Generic Name Trametinib **Brand Name** Mekinist QT	Metastatic or unresectable melanoma	**Usual oral dose:** 2 mg once daily (either as a single agent or in combination with dabrafenib); continue until disease progression target is achieved or unacceptable toxicity occurs	• Use with caution in patients with a history of hypertension, heart disease/failure, liver or kidney disease, or bleeding problems; hemorrhage reported • Left ventricular dysfunction or decreased LVEF. Evaluate heart function prior to and throughout therapy • Monitor CBC, comprehensive metabolic panel (CMP), and serum albumin • Monitor for signs and symptoms of pulmonary or dermatologic toxicity, changes in blood pressure and diarrhea • Rash and acneiform rash are common • New onset of cough could indicate progressive lung disease • Administer at least 1 hour before or 2 hours after a meal • Certain chemotherapy combinations result in greater potential adverse effects (i.e., febrile reactions, fever, and hyperglycemia may occur when combined with dabrafenib); refer to PI • Monitor vision for changes • Drug interactions may require dose adjustments or avoidance of certain drug combinations

Generic Name Ziv-aflibercept **Brand Name** Zaltrap ■	Metastatic colorectal cancer	**Usual parenteral dose:** IV: 4 mg/kg every 2 weeks (in combination with leucovorin, fluorouracil, and irinotecan [FOLFIRI]); continue until disease progression target is achieved or unacceptable toxicity occurs	• Bone marrow suppression: high incidence of neutropenia; leukopenia and thrombocytopenia • Increased risk of hypertension • Proteinuria and nephrotic syndrome reported • Diarrhea, weakness, weight loss, and dehydration • Monitor CBC with differential, urine protein, and blood pressure • Monitor for signs and symptoms of hemorrhage or GI perforation • Drug needs to be stopped well before surgery is performed Associated with: • Severe or fatal GI perforation • Severe and occasionally fatal hemorrhage, including GI bleeding • Wound healing impairment

Chapter 4

Autonomic Agents

Author: **Tammie Lee Demler, PharmD, BS Pharm, MBA, RPh, BCPP**

Editor: **Claudia Lee, RPh, MD**

Learning Objectives

- Identify current pharmacologic agents that are appropriate for each condition/diagnosis.
- Recommend optimal pharmacologic interventions based on patient-specific characteristics.
- Provide appropriate patient-specific counseling points and optimal overall medication management.

Key Terms: parasympathetic (cholinergic) agents, anticholinergic agents, antiparkinsonian agents, antimuscarinic agents, antispasmodic agents, sympathomimetic (adrenergic) agents, alpha-adrenergic agonists, beta-adrenergic agonists, non-selective beta-adrenergic agonists, selective beta-adrenergic agonists, alpha- and beta-adrenergic agonists, sympatholytic (adrenergic blocking) agents, alpha-adrenergic blocking agents, nonselective alpha-adrenergic blocking agents, selective alpha-adrenergic blocking agents, beta-adrenergic blocking agents, nonselective beta-adrenergic blocking agents, selective beta-adrenergic blocking agents, skeletal muscle relaxants, centrally acting skeletal muscle relaxants, direct-acting skeletal muscle relaxants, GABA derivative skeletal muscle relaxants, neuromuscular blocking agents, miscellaneous skeletal muscle relaxant agents, miscellaneous autonomic agents

Overview of Autonomic Agents

The variety of vital functions that are regulated by the nervous system has led to the development of a class of drugs with a significant number of important therapeutic uses. The central nervous system (CNS) is divided into two distinct pathways based on the presence of parasympathetic (cholinergic/muscarinic) versus sympathetic (adrenergic) receptors. Autonomic drugs generally produce either excitation or inhibition of certain types of smooth muscle, such as those found in the blood vessels of organs and glands and in the skin and mucous membranes. These drugs may also lead to metabolic and endocrine changes that include, but are not limited to, increased hepatic glycogenolysis and modulation of the secretion of insulin and other hormones. Respiration, gastrointestinal motility, and muscular movements are also influenced by drugs that impact the autonomic system.

Many of the agents within the autonomic drug class have either little or no action when administered orally, and the degree of their action and the intensity of their pharmacologic effects vary significantly when the drugs are administered intramuscularly, intravenously, or are inhaled into the lungs. The response to autonomic agents depends on the density and proportion of receptors available, but is also balanced by the body's reaction to reflex homeostatic adjustments coordinated by the baroreceptor system. Clinicians must be mindful that patients with comorbid medical illness or advancing age will exhibit altered reaction and reflex mechanisms and, therefore, may be subject to exaggerated or unexpected adverse drug reactions or impaired intended therapeutic effects of autonomic drugs.

Autonomic drugs are used for a number of indications that include blood pressure reduction, respiratory bronchodilation, and allergic reactions/anaphylaxis. Autonomic agents are frequently selected for use in patients experiencing cardiac arrest and who are in need of cardiopulmonary resuscitation. In addition, they are routinely used in topical form for vasoconstriction and to shrink mucous membranes. Interest in the use of these agents for patients with congestive heart failure has been increasing, and although the responses of certain receptors are often less robust in a failing heart, there may be future consideration for new roles for agents within this class.

4.1 Autonomic-Parasympathomimetic (Cholinergic) Agents

Drugs within this therapeutic category are agents that imitate or influence the action of the neurotransmitter acetylcholine. Muscarinic acetylcholine receptors in the peripheral nervous system are found with the highest density within the CNS, the hippocampus, cortex, and thalamus. Acetylcholine (ACh) is the neurotransmitter responsible for stimulating muscarinic receptors; thus it is described as having "cholinergic" activity. Acetylcholine is the primary neurotransmitter of nerve signals within the peripheral nervous system and it is quickly broken down by the enzymes acetylcholinesterase (AChE) and plasma butyrylcholinesterase, rendering it inactive. Drugs that mimic muscarinic agonists are generally able to provide longer actions systemically owing to chemical manipulations involving congeners (relative "like" substances) of ACh or natural alkaloids that stimulate both nicotinic and muscarinic receptors. The action of ACh is highly variable, but can be generally described as activity influencing parasympathetic nerves in the sweat glands, skeletal muscle with somatic innervation, and smooth muscle in blood vessels and other cardiac tissue. Dilation of blood vessels, increased bodily secretions, and decreased heart rate are all associated with the actions of acetylcholine and are responsible for the adverse-effect profile, as well as the beneficial therapeutic effects, of a drug within this therapeutic category.

The properties of muscarinic receptors vary. Five such receptors have been identified, designated as M1 through M5. Although specific muscarinic receptor subtypes have been identified, the development of selective agonists and antagonists for these subtypes has been a challenge because currently recognized agents have a broad spectrum of activity at most of these receptors.

Drugs influencing ACh are responsible for respiratory bronchoconstriction and secretion as well as urinary effects, with their stimulating actions causing detrusor muscle contraction, increased voiding pressure, and ureteral peristalsis. Gastrointestinal (GI) actions that result from exposure to ACh include, but are not limited to, increased secretions. For this reason, caution should be used when considering the use of these agents in patients with peptic ulcer disease, as acetylcholinesterase inhibitors can increase stomach acid.

Both the bladder and GI effects are thought to be mediated by multiple muscarinic receptor subtypes. ACh stimulates secretions from other glands, including the lacrimal, nasopharyngeal, salivary, and sweat glands. Endogenous and exogenous ACh has limited ability to cross the blood-brain barrier; however, muscarinic agonists that are formulated to enter into the CNS play an important role in cognitive function, motor control, appetite regulation, nociception, seizure threshold, and other processes.

Due to their intrinsic pharmacologic actions, cholinesterase inhibitors have vagotonic effects on the sinoatrial and atrioventricular nodes, leading to bradycardia and atrioventricular (AV) block, which may then exacerbate syncope or hypotensive events. All patients should be considered at risk for adverse cardiac effects when they take cholinesterase inhibitors, as bradycardia and heart block have occurred in patients without previously diagnosed cardiac conduction abnormalities. These agents should be used with caution in patients with cardiac disease, such as sick sinus syndrome, severe cardiac arrhythmias, or cardiac conduction disturbances (e.g., sinoatrial block, AV block).

Acetylcholinesterase inhibitors are also likely to exaggerate the effects of neuromuscular blocking agents during anesthesia, resulting in potentially extended respiratory depression. Among other concerns, their use is not recommended in patients recovering from gastrointestinal surgery due to the effects on the GI tract resulting from the cholinergic actions of these drugs.

Autonomic-Parasympathomimetic (Cholinergic) Agents

Ambenonium
Bethanechol
Cevimeline
Donepezil

*Galantamine
Neostigmine
Physostigmine
Pyridostigmine
Rivastigmine

Case Studies and Conclusions

BP is a 72-year-old female with newly diagnosed mild-stage Alzheimer's disease (AD). Her daughter LS would like to know which of the acetylcholinesterase inhibitors her mother could take for the duration of her illness as it progresses.

1. Which agent is approved only for mild to moderate illness, but NOT severe illness?
   a. Donepezil
   b. Galantamine
   c. Rivastigmine
   d. Pyridostigmine

Answer B is correct. Of the three acetylcholinesterase inhibitors, only galantamine is approved only for mild to moderate illness, not for severe stages of AD.

LS would like to know more about the possible side effects of these acetylcholinesterase inhibitors.

2. What is the most common side effect that she should expect her mother to experience?
   a. Weight gain
   b. Tachycardia
   c. Seizure
   d. Diarrhea

Answer D is correct. Diarrhea is the most common side effect of acetylcholinesterase inhibitors among the options listed.

JR is a candidate for bethanechol therapy due to a recent diagnosis of neurogenic bladder.

1. Which concurrent medical illness would preclude use of bethanechol due to an absolute contraindication?
   a. COPD
   b. Hypertension
   c. Inflammatory bowel disease
   d. Orthostatic hypotension

Answer C is correct. Inflammatory bowel disease (especially severe conditions) is a contraindication to bethanechol use. The other conditions warrant caution, but do not present as potentially serious a concern (i.e., patients should avoid their use "if possible").

JR has read about this new medication and is worried about the potential for nausea and stomach upset.

2. What is a recommendation to reduce the potential for this adverse effect?
   a. Administer on an empty stomach 1 hour before a meal
   b. Administer on a full stomach 2 hours after a meal
   c. Administer without regard to meals, take just before bedtime
   d. Administer without regard to meals, take just upon awakening

Answer A is correct. Timing administration of bethanechol for 1 hour before a meal provides the necessary "empty stomach" condition to optimize this therapy and to reduce adverse GI side effects.

4.2 Autonomic-Anticholinergic Agents

The muscarinic receptor antagonists include natural, synthetic, and semisynthetic alkaloid derivatives. The antagonists that have been developed to mimic the action of the natural compounds exhibit greater selectivity (though not absolute) as well as different rates of onset and durations of action (some shorter, some longer). Muscarinic antagonists inhibit the action of ACh by preventing binding to parasympathetic and sympathetic cholinergic receptors. For this reason, this class of medications has been termed "anticholinergic" agents.

Decreased salivary and bronchial secretions and sweating, pupillary dilation, visual changes, increased heart rate, bronchodilation, inhibited urination, and decreased intestinal tone and motility are all typical effects seen with the administration of anticholinergic medications. Some antagonists of acetylcholine, such as trihexyphenidyl, exhibit additional inhibition of cholinergic stimuli at muscarinic receptors in the CNS and, to a lesser extent, in smooth muscle. This multiple receptor site action allows for additional direct antispasmodic actions on smooth muscle, as well as the typical antisecretory, mydriatic, and positive chronotropic activities seen with these agents.

Autonomic-anticholinergic agents have been used to reduce GI hypermotility. However, caution must be exercised when they are used in patients with gastroesophageal reflux disease (GERD) or hiatal hernia associated with reflux esophagitis, because the decreased gastric motility and relaxation of the lower esophageal sphincter can promote gastric retention and aggravate reflux in these patients. The anticholinergic effects of drugs in this class can also cause increased intraocular pressure, so they should be used with extreme caution in patients with open-angle glaucoma. Their use may cause patients to complain of dry eyes and discomfort when using contact lenses, often requiring additional lubricating drops or leading to discontinuation of the use of lenses while on these medications. Older male patients may exhibit exacerbations of symptoms of benign prostatic hypertrophy due to worsening urinary retention. Anticholinergic drugs may exacerbate symptoms associated with dementia and may cause tachycardia, increasing adverse risks for patients with cardiac disease. The total anticholinergic side effect burden increases when multiple concurrent medications with the same side effects are co-administered and can lead to increased toxicity.

While receptor selectivity has been difficult to target, some synthetic and semisynthetic muscarinic receptor antagonist derivatives have exhibited a greater degree of selectivity for subtypes of muscarinic receptors. Examples of such agents include homatropine and tropicamide, which both have a shorter duration of action than atropine, and methscopolamine, ipratropium, and tiotropium, which do not readily cross the blood–brain barrier or other membranes. The synthetic derivatives possessing some degree of M3 receptor selectivity include the newer agents darifenacin and solifenacin.

Antiparkinsonian Agents

Benztropine (*see also the Antiparkinsonian Agents in the Central Nervous System Agents chapter*)
Diphenhydramine (*see also the First-Generation Antihistamine Agents section in the Antihistamine Agents chapter*)
Trihexyphenidyl (*see also the Antiparkinsonian Agents in the Central Nervous System Agents chapter*)

Antimuscarinic and Antispasmodic Agents

Like other anticholinergic medications, antimuscarinic agents can cause blurred vision, drowsiness, or dizziness. For this reason, patients should use caution when driving or operating machinery until they determine the side effects of the drug. Due to the potential to increase heart rate and to potentiate arrhythmias, some patients may experience ischemia when using these agents. Antimuscarinic agents should be used with caution in patients with known cardiac disease or in other comorbid disease states that could be worsened with tachycardia.

Drugs associated with anticholinergic effects, including antimuscarinic agents, should be used cautiously in patients with renal compromise because decreased elimination can result in extended and exaggerated side effects of these drugs. Additionally, the systemic antimuscarinic effects of atropine may precipitate or complicate urinary retention, especially in patients with BPH or urinary obstruction due to higher risk of serious adverse effects.

Short-acting antimuscarinic antagonists (SAMAs) have generally been used along with short-acting β_2 agonists (SABAs) as the backbone of therapy for a number of respiratory illnesses, including chronic obstructive pulmonary disease (COPD). Although COPD and asthma are different inflammatory processes that produce different kinds of bronchoconstriction, both diseases can have serious consequences if not managed adequately. COPD involves a significant cholinergic component, so antimuscarinics can be as effective in inhibiting bronchoconstriction as SABAs are at reversing it.

Antimuscarinic agents have also been used as augmentation therapy in treatment of irritable bowel disease and peptic ulcer disease. However, their adverse effects limit their use and only a limited number of well-controlled studies have been published to support their use in most conditions. Consequently, these agents have been replaced by other medications that are more effective or cause fewer adverse effects. A careful review of individual agents listed on the companion drug grid is warranted for a more comprehensive understanding of the unique characteristics of each drug and will help you to prepare to answer the case studies at the end of each section.

Antimuscarinic and Antispasmodic Agents

Aclidinium
Atropine
Belladonna
Dicyclomine
Glycopyrrolate
Hyoscyamine
Ipratropium
Methscopolamine
Propantheline
Scopolamine
Tiotropium
Umeclidinium

Case Studies and Conclusions

JP is a 55-year-old college professor who has been a 2-pack-per-day smoker for the last 20 years. He presents to the clinic today with a new diagnosis of COPD and a prescription for tiotropium capsule inhalation (Spiriva Handihaler). He is also seeking information on smoking cessation. JP has no other medical comorbidities, but his primary care provider stated that his renal function is "lower" than she would like it to be.

1. Which adverse effects from tiotropium might JP experience in light of his impaired renal function as compared to his peers with normal/adequate renal function?
    a. Renal failure
    b. Increased anticholinergic effects
    c. Elevated liver function tests (LFTs)
    d. syndrome of inappropriate antidiuretic hormone secretion (SIADH)

Answer B is correct. Tiotropium is primarily eliminated in the urine, so patients with moderate to severe renal impairment (creatinine clearance [CrCl] less than 60 mL per minute) may be at an increased risk of anticholinergic-induced events.

One month after initiating tiotropium therapy, JP returns to clinic and describes having used this medication to control one of his "breathing attacks," only to have his family call 911 because he was unable to catch his breath. He denies any swelling of his lips or tongue during the events.

2. What would be the most reasonable approach in discussing future recommendations for JP so that he can have more successful treatment and symptom control in the future?
    a. Discontinue tiotropium, because he must be allergic to it.
    b. The lactose in tiotropium causes this reaction in everyone.
    c. Tiotropium is not intended to be a rescue intervention.
    d. Seek a diagnostic reevaluation.

Answer C is correct. Tiotropium is not intended for rescue therapy of acute bronchospasm attacks. Although immediate hypersensitivity reactions (including swelling of the lips, tongue, or throat) may occur after its administration, JP has been taking his tiotropium only "as needed," which is likely the reason for his shortness of breath.

JP describes a "less robust" improvement in his COPD than he expected with the start of tiotropium a month ago.

3. What do you advise?
   a. Tiotropium may take up to 8 weeks to see the full effect.
   b. He must be using the product incorrectly.
   c. His COPD may be too severe for this medication to be effective.
   d. He may be a candidate for a lung transplant.

Answer A is correct. Tiotropium may take up to 8 weeks to see the full effect. Given that this patient has been having "some relief," though not as "robust" as he would expect, continuation would be warranted to see if he can achieve his optimal therapeutic goals.

CS is a 25-year-old waitress who is experiencing irritable bowel disease. She has received a prescription for dicyclomine 10 mg capsules to be taken 4 times daily for 30 days. She has not begun taking her medication yet and asks you if you have any "recommendations" for her as a clinician.

1. What would you advise CS regarding her new medication?
   a. This type of medication takes time to build up in her system before it works.
   b. She should request an increased dose after a few days if the medication does not work.
   c. She should expect immediate results with complete symptom resolution.
   d. Data indicate that this medication works best if used longer than 2 weeks.

Answer B is correct. For optimal control of symptoms, the manufacturer recommends a dose increase up to 40 mg taken 4 times per day for the first week, and if symptoms do not improve within 2 weeks or significant adverse effects develop during treatment, drug discontinuation should be considered.

CS tells you that the pharmacist indicated that this drug carries a universal prescribing alert relative to its anticholinergic side effects.

2. What would you describe as one of the elements of this universal prescribing alert?
   a. This class of medications may decrease the effectiveness of birth control pills.
   b. This class of medications may cause ovarian benign hyperplasia.
   c. This class of medications may cause wakefulness and insomnia.
   d. This class of medications may alter her ability to regulate her body temperature.

Answer D is correct. Anticholinergic medications impair the body's natural ability to sweat and decrease an elevated body temperature. Generally, these agents are sedating. They also cause complications for male patients who are predisposed to benign prostatic hypertrophy. They are not known to interfere with the efficacy of oral contraceptives.

4.3 Autonomic-Sympathomimetic Adrenergic Agents

Sympathomimetic amines are adrenergic receptor agonists that produce sympathomimetic-stimulant-like effects that facilitate the release, block the transport (or reuptake), decrease metabolism or "imitate" the actions of norepinephrine (NE), a hormone that is associated with sympathetic neurons. Some medications (such as ephedrine) may directly activate the release of NE while also indirectly causing a release of NE; thus, they are classified as "mixed-acting" sympathomimetic drugs. Other agents are described as either direct or indirect acting. These agents can be used to treat cardiac arrest and low blood pressure among other conditions.

While autonomic-sympathomimetic agents are indicated for use in patients with open-angle glaucoma, they can exacerbate closed-angle glaucoma and, therefore, are contraindicated in patients with this condition. Other contraindications include severe hypertension and ventricular tachycardia, including arrhythmias associated with tachycardia. These agents are also contraindicated in patients with thyrotoxicosis, including hyperthyroidism. The FDA labeling of autonomic-sympathomimetic agents carry black box warnings with which clinicians should become familiar.

Autonomic-sympathomimetic agents, particularly when administered parenterally, should be avoided in patients with severe cardiac disease (such as coronary artery disease, angina, and myocardial infarction) or with bradycardia or AV block. Further caution is warranted in patients with uncontrolled hypertension due to the increased likelihood of adverse cardiac events. Even ophthalmic or nasal formulations can complicate these preexisting conditions, so they should also be used with caution in patients with known or suspected cardiac disease. This caution is extended to patients with cerebrovascular disease and history of or increased risk for stroke. Severe tissue necrosis due to vasoconstriction of small blood vessels has been reported with autonomic-sympathomimetic agents, so caution in patients with extensive peripheral vascular disease is warranted to avoid excessive vasoconstriction or ischemia of vital organs.

These agents should also be used with caution in men with symptomatic, benign prostatic hypertrophy, due to the potential for urinary retention. Sympathomimetic autonomic agents may also stimulate insulin production, increase glycogenolysis in the liver, and complicate the management of diabetes mellitus.

Alpha-Adrenergic Agonists

Midodrine
Phenylephrine
Clonidine (*see also the Hypotensive Agents section in the Cardiovascular Agents chapter*)
Guanabenz (*see also the Hypotensive Agents section in the Cardiovascular Agents chapter*)
Methyldopa (*see also the Hypotensive Agents section in the Cardiovascular Agents chapter*)

Beta-Adrenergic Agonists

Beta-adrenergic drugs may exhibit a strong inotropic effect that alters or changes the strength of muscular contraction of the heart and, therefore, are potentially harmful in the presence of a severe mechanical obstruction such as idiopathic hypertrophic subaortic stenosis. In patients with this condition, the presence of narrow aortic valves increases the demand on the left ventricle to pump harder in order to force blood through these valves, resulting in enlargement of the left ventricle, contributing to increased risk of heart failure. Certain medications in this category can be used with caution to treat patients with cardiac diseases including acute myocardial infarction, unstable angina, and severe coronary artery disease. The inotropic and chronotropic effects of drugs within this class may increase cardiac oxygen demand due to the increased muscle activity.

Use these agents with caution in patients with occlusive vascular disease such as atherosclerosis, peripheral vascular disease, or Raynaud's disease, as well as in patients with preexisting vascular damage because of the risk of vasoconstriction and subsequently decreased circulation to the extremities associated with some of these drugs (such as dopamine).

Nonselective Beta-Adrenergic Agonists

Isoproterenol

Selective Beta$_1$-Adrenergic Agonists

Dobutamine
Dopamine

Selective Beta$_2$-Adrenergic Agonists

These medications are further subdivided into short-acting and long-acting beta$_2$ receptor agonists (SABA and LABA), which are generally administered by oral inhalation via metered-dose inhaler (MDI) or nebulizer for patients with a variety of respiratory conditions. The LABAs are indicated for maintenance treatment, whereas SABAs may be used for rescue therapy if the patient experiences breakthrough shortness of breath. All LABAs are contraindicated for monotherapy treatment of asthma. Thus, if LABAs are prescribed for patients with asthma, they must be used concurrently with a medication indicated for use to control asthma (i.e., inhaled corticosteroid [ICS]).

Some of these agents (including certain LABAs) can be used to prevent exercise-induced bronchospasm (EIB). When used for EIB, the dose should be administered at least 15 minutes before exercise, with additional doses taken only according to the manufacturer's directions and not in excess of the Food and Drug Administration's (FDA) total daily recommended maximum dose. Patients who are on scheduled SABA/LABA maintenance therapy should not use additional doses to prevent EIB. If maintenance dosing or dosing prior to exercise with SABA/LABA therapy does not control EIB, then other appropriate treatment for EIB should be considered; this would include avoiding the use of LABAs alone without another long-acting controller medication because of the increased rate of serious adverse events such as asthma-related mortality, exacerbations requiring hospitalization, increased costs, and morbidity. Controller agents generally used concurrently with LABAs include ICSs, which are typically added as first-line adjuncts to SABAs; however, exact guidance regarding the addition of a LABA to the EIB treatment regimen is not available.

Inhaled formulations are preferred over oral (swallowed) bronchodilators for many respiratory conditions, including COPD. Given that many of these products are administered via oral inhalation, it is important that clinicians provide education on proper technique to optimize the drug therapy.

Selective Beta$_2$-Adrenergic Agonists

Albuterol/levalbuterol
Arformoterol
Formoterol
Indacaterol
Metaproterenol
Olodaterol
Salmeterol
Terbutaline
Vilanterol

Alpha-and Beta-Adrenergic Agonists

These agents are well known for their vasoconstricting properties. From a therapeutic standpoint, this effect may be beneficial in decreasing anaphylaxis as well as when used for an intervention for hypotension and shock. The class-related side effects are mainly attributable to this vasoconstriction. Caution should be observed to avoid extravasation during intravenous administration, as peripheral ischemia, tissue necrosis, and gangrene in the surrounding area can occur due to vasoconstriction. These agents must also be used with caution in patients with cardiovascular disease, diabetes, prostatic hyperplasia, seizures, thyroid dysfunction, and unstable motor symptoms due to their cardiovascular effects.

Alpha-and Beta-Adrenergic Agonists

Droxidopa
Ephedrine
Epinephrine
Norephinephrine
Pseudoephedrine

Case Studies and Conclusions

SD is a 25-year-old male who has recently been diagnosed with asthma and has read that he should not be receiving a "LABA." He would like to discuss this issue further with his primary care provider.

1. What would you advise him?
   a. LABAs are appropriate to use when combined with corticosteroids.
   b. LABAs used as monotherapy are dangerous only if you overuse them.
   c. LABAs can be replaced with a once-daily SABA if the patient prefers.
   d. LABA monotherapy is dangerous only if the patient has severe asthma.

Answer A is correct. LABAs are appropriate when used in combination with other asthma control agents. Monotherapy with LABAs presents safety risks across the spectrum of care, not just when overused and not only in cases of severe asthma.

SABAs cannot be interchanged with LABAs on the same schedule. SABAs are short acting, so they need more frequent dosing than LABAs.

2. Which of the following medications would be considered a "LABA"?
   a. Albuterol
   b. Metaproteronol
   c. Salmeterol
   d. Isoproterenol

Answer C is correct. The rest of the options are SABAs.

DP is a 30-year-old female patient who would like to try to use a LABA for exercise-induced bronchospasm prior to dance class. She has a friend who uses formoterol for his asthma.

1. What would you advise this patient relative to her request?
   a. LABAs are not appropriate for EIB under any condition.
   b. Use formoterol 15 minutes prior to exercise.
   c. Add formoterol for EIB as an extra dose to the twice-daily scheduled dose.
   d. Use LABA intervention only if EIB occurs, not as prevention.

Answer B is correct. The formoterol package insert (PI) specifically recommends use prior to EIB, but the dose should not be "added" to the regular scheduled dose (it should not exceed the maximum daily dose [MDD]). Formoterol has an EIB indication, so not all LABAs are considered "inappropriate" for use in preventing bronchospasm; using any LABA as rescue, however, is inappropriate and dangerous.

DP has metabolic syndrome that results in abnormally high lipids, elevated blood glucose (she has diabetes), and obesity.

2. Which of these metabolic panels could be complicated by the use of LABAs such as formoterol?
   a. Hyperlipidemia
   b. Hyperglycemia
   c. Obesity
   d. All of these elements

Answer B is correct. LABAs and beta$_2$-adrenergic agonists as a class can cause an increase in blood glucose. The other answers are not associated with the use of LABAs.

4.4 Autonomic-Sympatholytic (Adrenergic Blocking) Agents

Autonomic-sympatholytic agents are associated with cardiac-stimulating effects, which in turn increase myocardial oxygen demand. Reflex tachycardia can be expected with their use and may exacerbate angina. For this reason, these agents are contraindicated in patients with acute myocardial infarction, a history of myocardial infarction, coronary insufficiency, angina, or any evidence of coronary artery disease.

Some drugs within this class may also have histamine-like effects and can stimulate gastric acid secretion, thereby complicating peptic ulcer disease.

Alpha Adrenergic Blocking Agents

Nonselective Alpha-Adrenergic Blocking Agents

Dihydroergotamine
Ergoloid mesylates
Ergotamine
Phenoxybenzamine
Phentolamine

Nonselective Alpha$_1$-Adrenergic Blocking Agents

Doxazosin (*see also the Adrenergic Agents section in the Cardiovascular Agents chapter*)
Prazosin (*see also the Adrenergic Agents section in the Cardiovascular Agents chapter*)
Terazosin (*see also the Adrenergic Agents section in the Cardiovascular Agents chapter*)

Selective Alpha$_1$-Adrenergic Blocking Agents

Alfuzosin
Silodosin
Tamsulosin
Carvedilol (*see also the Adrenergic Agents section in the Cardiovascular Agents chapter*)
Labetalol (*see also the Adrenergic Agents section in the Cardiovascular Agents chapter*)

Beta-Adrenergic Blocking Agents

Nonselective Beta-Adrenergic Blocking Agents

Carvedilol (*see also the Adrenergic Agents section in the Cardiovascular Agents chapter*)
Labetalol (*see also the Adrenergic Agents section in the Cardiovascular Agents chapter*)
Nadolol (*see also the Adrenergic Agents section in the Cardiovascular Agents chapter*)
Nebivolol (*see also the Adrenergic Agents section in the Cardiovascular Agents chapter*)
Pindolol (*see also the Adrenergic Agents section in the Cardiovascular Agents chapter*)
Propranolol (*see also the Adrenergic Agents section in the Cardiovascular Agents chapter*)
Stalol (*see also the Adrenergic Agents section in the Cardiovascular Agents chapter*)
Timolol (*see also the Adrenergic Agents section in the Cardiovascular Agents chapter*)

Selective Beta-Adrenergic Blocking Agents

Acebutolol (*see also the Adrenergic Agents section in the Cardiovascular Agents chapter*)
Atenolol (*see also the Adrenergic Agents section in the Cardiovascular Agents chapter*)
Betaxolol (*see also the Adrenergic Agents section in the Cardiovascular Agents chapter*)
Bisoprolol (*see also the Adrenergic Agents section in the Cardiovascular Agents chapter*)
Esmolol (*see also the Adrenergic Agents section in the Cardiovascular Agents chapter*)
Metoprolol (*see also the Adrenergic Agents section in the Cardiovascular Agents chapter*)

Case Studies and Conclusions

TC is a 35-year-old mortgage broker who presents to clinic today after a long-standing history of migraine headaches that seems to be worsening with stress at work. He reports he was just evaluated by a neurologist to rule out anything "more serious" and was cleared with normal findings after magnetic resonance imaging (MRI) and neurology workup. He was told that he was unable to use a "triptan" because he is on Zoloft 100 mg daily for depression.

1. Why was TC told he could not take a triptan?
    a. Triptans do not work well for patients who are depressed.
    b. Triptans may increase the risk of serotonin syndrome.
    c. Antidepressants block the triptan receptor.
    d. All of these are true.

Answer B is correct. Triptans (e.g., sumatriptan) exert an influence on serotonin that can cumulatively add increased risk of serotonin syndrome while a patient is taking a serotonin reuptake inhibitor (SSRI) such as sertraline (Zoloft). Triptans work just as well for depressed patients and do not block receptors for antidepressant treatment.

TC would like to take ergotamine because his mother takes this medication and has good results with it.

2. Which dosing recommendation would you make for TC for an ergotamine regimen?
   a. 2 mg at first sign of migraine, then 2 mg every 30 minutes if needed
   b. Maximum 6 mg per day, 10 mg per week
   c. Take only "as needed," as ergotamine is not meant for scheduled administration
   d. All of these are true.

Answer D is correct. All of these recommendations are correct.

JP is a 65-year-old male who presents to clinic today with a chief complaint of urgency and feelings of always "having to go to the bathroom." He is otherwise medically healthy and is on no other medication except a multiple daily vitamin.

1. If it is determined that this patient has benign prostatic hypertrophy and is prescribed tamsulosin, which advice would you provide to optimize his medication therapy?
   a. Take in the morning so his sleep is not disturbed
   b. Time the dose so it is taken a half-hour after a meal
   c. Open the capsules and mix them in yogurt
   d. May cause hypertension, so monitor his blood pressure

Answer B is correct. The patient should time dose so it is taken 30 minutes after the same meal daily. It is best to avoid morning administration, especially given that the hypotensive effects occur within the first 4 to 8 hours of taking the dose. Capsules cannot be opened or chewed.

A few weeks later, JP describes an "amazing" improvement after taking his tamsulosin. He even comments about an episode where he had an erection that lasted for more than 3 hours and said he would not need to ask for a prescription for Viagra.

2. What would you offer as a response?
   a. Tamsulosin can often take the place of Viagra and saves money.
   b. Tamsulosin can cause a medical emergency called priapism.
   c. Tamsulosin can improve depression and increase libido.
   d. All of these are true.

Answer B is correct. Although improvement of the patient's urinary symptoms is a good thing, the emergency of prolonged erections is not. Prolonged erections should be reported promptly, as priapism is a medical emergency that may not resolve without emergency intervention and may have significant negative physiologic consequences.

4.5 Skeletal Muscle Relaxants and Miscellaneous Autonomic Agents

Centrally Acting Skeletal Muscle Relaxants

The action of centrally acting skeletal muscle relaxants is associated with an interrupted communication of neurons within the CNS and not a direct effect on the muscle tissue. In addition to decreasing muscle tone and promoting relaxation, the CNS effects also include sedation, which in part is thought to be responsible for altered pain perception. Although overall evidence of comparable effectiveness of drugs within this class is lacking, GABA-derivative antispasmodic agents such as baclofen are known to be more effective when used for muscular spasm associated with multiple sclerosis as compared to those that relieve other musculoskeletal conditions.

Centrally Acting Skeletal Muscle Relaxants

Carisoprodol
Chlorzoxazone
*Cyclobenzaprine
Metaxalone
Methocarbamol
Tizanidine

Direct-Acting Skeletal Muscle Relaxants

Dantrolene

GABA-Derivative Skeletal Muscle Relaxants

*Baclofen

Neuromuscular Blocking Agents

Atracurium
Cisatracurium
Pancuronium
Rocuronium
Succinylcholine
Vecuronium

Miscellaneous Skeletal Muscle Relaxants

Orphenadrine

Miscellaneous Autonomic Agents

Nicotine is a substance found in tobacco smoke that is well known for its addictive properties. It is not known to be carcinogenic, nor is it associated with the smoking-related adverse effects attributed to the polycyclic aromatic hydrocarbons (PAH) and other chemicals found in cigarettes. The therapeutic use of nicotine replacement has been widely accepted as a mainstay in smoking cessation, allowing the individual the opportunity to have a "controlled withdrawal" from nicotine and a more successful attempt to stay smoke free. Nicotine agonists, such as varenicline, have become increasingly more popular as an alternative aid for smoking cessation although there has been some recent focus on the potential neuropsychiatric side effects reported with their use.

Miscellaneous Autonomic Agents

Nicotine
Varenicline

Case Studies and Conclusions

LL is a 55-year-old female who is diagnosed with early-stage lung cancer that appears to be responsive to treatment. She would like to begin a smoking cessation regimen to finally "quit" once and for all.

1. Which of the following nicotine-replacement formulations is NOT dosed according to when the first cigarette of the day is smoked?
   a. Gum
   b. Lozenge
   c. Inhaler
   d. Patch

Answer D is correct. Lozenge strength is determined according to when the first cigarette of the day is smoked (if more than 30 minutes after waking up, use 2 mg lozenge; if less than 30 minutes, use 4 mg lozenge). The gum and inhaler are also dosed based on time to first cigarette smoked (starting doses may also include the total number of cigarettes smoked per day). The nicotine patch is dosed based on the total number of cigarettes smoked within 24 hours.

2. Given that LL smokes roughly half a pack per day, which strength of gum would you order for her?

   a. 2 mg gum
   b. 4 mg gum
   c. 6 mg gum
   d. No gum

Answer A is correct. The patient should use 2 pieces of gum if smoking less than 25 cigarettes per day and 4 pieces of gum if smoking 25 or more cigarettes per day. Gum is still an appropriate replacement for this patient if she agrees to it.

A 70-year-old family member calls to ask your professional advice about using varenicline (Chantix) for smoking cessation. She has heard a lot of good and bad things about this drug, but wants to hear what you have to say before talking to her physician.

1. What would you advise your family member about the proper way to use varenicline?

   a. Patients must stop smoking for 1 week prior to the quit date so nicotine is cleared from the body.
   b. Therapy is limited to 12 weeks, so patients must be serious about quitting before starting varenicline.
   c. Patients must get a prescription before the quit date and start the drug 1 week before that quit date.
   d. This patient is too old to take varenicline, so she should use nicotine patches.

Answer C is correct. The varenicline regimen must be established at least 1 week prior to the quit date (some patients require a longer baseline prior to the quit date—refer to the PI). Varenicline engages the nicotine receptors so that even if the patient smokes, he or she will not experience the same degree of reward.

Tips from the Field

Metered-Dose Inhalers

1. Instruct the patient on proper inhalation technique according to the product's directions.
2. Prior to first use (and if not used again for a few days or longer), "priming" is often required.
3. The patient should exhale slowly and fully, and then close the lips around the end of the mouthpiece and inhale slowly, breathing deeply through the mouth, while pressing the dose-release button and continuing to breathe in slowly for as long as possible.
4. The patient should hold the breath for 10 seconds or for as long as comfortable.
5. The mouthpiece (and all other parts as recommended by the manufacturer) should be cleaned with a damp cloth or tissue at least once a week (or more frequently).
6. The inhaler contains a certain number of inhalation doses (products vary significantly regarding this number). Some products have dose indicators showing approximately how much medicine is left. Many inhalers have "beyond use dates" that require discarding the remaining product, even if the inhaler is not empty.

Smoking Cessation

1. Recognize that tobacco use disorder is a chronic disease and thus patients who are nicotine dependent may have remission and relapse. Be patient, encourage, and motivate.

2. Continue to remind your patients of the overall health benefits of quitting, including both short- and long-term gains.

3. Provide resources to your patients, including nicotine-replacement options. There are many "quit" support programs that may even offer free nicotine replacement.

4. During every episode of care, inquire about nicotine use, counsel about the need to quit, evaluate the willingness of the patient to quit, offer support to assist your patient along the entire spectrum of cessation, and arrange for follow-ups that will help identify problems, challenges, and to celebrate successes, no matter how small they may seem.

Tammie Lee and Jacque

Bibliography

American Geriatrics Society. 2015 updated Beers criteria for potentially inappropriate medication use in older adults. *J Am Geriatr Soc.* 2015;63:2227-2246.

Chantix (varenicline) package insert. New York, NY: Pfizer Labs; October 2014.

Clinical Pharmacology (online database). Tampa, FL: Gold Standard, Inc.; 2013.

McEvoy GK, ed. *AHFS: Drug Information.* Bethesda, MD: American Society of Health-System Pharmacists; 2016.

MD Anderson Cancer Center. Using nicotine-replacement and other therapies. http://www2.mdanderson.org/app/team/en/mod3_print.cfm. Accessed January 20, 2017.

Parsons JP, Hallstrand TS, Mastronarde JG, et al. An official American Thoracic Society clinical practice guideline: exercise-induced bronchoconstriction. *Am J Respir Crit Care Med.* 2013;187:1016-1027.

PDR. Atropine sulfate: drug summary. http://www.pdr.net/drug-summary/Atropine-Sulfate-Injection-atropine-sulfate-684. Accessed January 20, 2017.

Reeves RR, Pinkofsky HB, Carter OS. Carisoprodol: a drug of continuing abuse. *J Am Osteopath Assoc.* 1997;97:723-724.

U.S. Food and Drug Administration (FDA). FDA drug safety communication: safety review update of Chantix (varenicline) and risk of neuropsychiatric adverse events. 2011. http://www.fda.gov/Drugs/DrugSafety/ucm276737.htm. Accessed October 24, 2011.

Symbols

- ▲ Renal impairment: Dose adjustment is recommended.
- ▢ Hepatic impairment: Dose adjustment is recommended.
- ■ Black box warning exists for this drug.
- (QT) QTc prolongation effects have been reported.
- (BL) Beers list criteria (avoid in elderly).
- (PD) FDA-approved pediatric doses are available.
- (GD) FDA-approved geriatric doses are available.
- 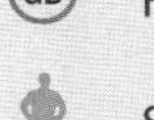 See primary body system.

Autonomic Agents

Universal prescribing alerts:

- Known serious hypersensitivity to the specific drug or any other component of the product/formulation selected warrants a contraindication for use.
- Adverse reactions associated with the use of some **autonomic agents** include dizziness, drowsiness, vertigo, or fatigue; these agents may also impair the ability to perform tasks requiring mental alertness. Caution should always be recommended when using any new drug for the first time, when there is a dose change, and for continued use of known offending agents.
- Doses expressed are for usual adult dosage ranges only. "Geriatric doses" are assumed to be the same as adult doses unless otherwise noted with a symbol. Where pediatric dosing is available, a symbol will guide the reader to additional prescribing references. Refer to real-time prescribing references for these age-specific doses.
- Use of autonomic agents in pregnancy is based on weighing clinical risk versus benefit; safety concerns are not represented in this grid. Refer to the package insert (PI) for more information. Clinicians should continue to provide education about the reproductive risks of any medication and offer risk-reduction strategies (which may include contraceptive use) to women of childbearing age and understand that these reproductive risks may also extend to males. Other medications may decrease the effectiveness of oral contraceptives. When necessary, an alternative means of birth control should be explored.
- Brand names are provided for those agents still available on the market. Due to ever-changing product availability, refer to Food and Drug Administration (FDA) resources to confirm the actual brands available. This drug summary is intended for educational purposes only. Prescribing decisions should be based on real-time comprehensive drug databases that are updated on a regular basis.

Autonomic-Parasympathomimetic (Cholinergic) Agents

Drug Name	FDA-Approved Indication	Adult Dosage Range	Precautions and Clinical Pearls
Generic Name Ambenonium **Brand Name** Mytelase	Myasthenia gravis	Dose depends on the response and clinical status of the patient **Usual oral dose:** Initial: 5 mg 3 or 4 times daily; dose may be increased gradually Usual maintenance: 15 to 100 mg daily	• Drug interactions may require dose adjustment or avoidance of certain drug combinations • Ganglionic blocking agents (e.g., mecamylamine, guanadrel, guanethidine) and routine use of atropine sulfate are contraindicated for use with ambenonium • Use with caution in patients with mechanical gastrointestinal (GI) obstruction (or ileus) or urinary tract obstruction (due to muscarinic effects) • Use with caution in patients with asthma, owing to cholinergic stimulation • Use with caution in patients with Parkinson's disease • Very narrow therapeutic index (overdose may occur with little or no warning)

Drug Name	FDA-Approved Indication	Adult Dosage Range	Precautions and Clinical Pearls

Generic Name
Bethanechol
 	
Brand Name
Urecholine
	Neurogenic bladder
	
	Urinary retention postoperatively or nonobstructive postpartum and treatment of atonic neurogenic bladder
		Usual oral dose for acute postoperative/postpartum non-obstructive urinary retention:
		Initial: 5 to 10 mg; may be repeated hourly for effective response or cumulative dose of 50 mg is given
		
		Usual parenteral dose (urinary retention as above):
		SQ: 5 mg 3 to 4 times per day as needed
			• Administer on an empty stomach to minimize nausea/vomiting (1 hour before or 2 hours after a meal)
			• Do not administer IM or IV
			• Flushing and warmth of the skin (particularly about the face), diaphoresis, and bronchospasm are among the numerous side effects reported with use
			• Use precautions and/or avoid use in patients with:
			  • Chronic obstructive pulmonary disease (COPD)
			  • Hypertension
			  • Ileus
			  • Orthostatic hypotension
			  • Syncope (use caution when driving or operating machinery)
			Contraindications:
			• Asthma
			• Bradycardia or hypotension (pronounced), vasomotor instability
			• Coronary artery disease (CAD)
			• Gastrointestinal or genitourinary (GU) tract, bladder obstruction (or recent surgery)
			• Inflammatory bowel disease (including spastic GI disturbances)
			• Hyperthyroidism
			• Parkinsonism
			• Peptic ulcer disease (PUD)
			• Peritonitis
			• Seizure disorder (epilepsy) or seizure

Generic Name Cevimeline **Brand Name** Evoxac	Xerostomia associated with Sjögren's syndrome	**Usual oral dose:** 30 mg 3 times per day	• May administer with food to lessen GI upset • Excessive sweating in elderly patients may lead to dehydration • May cause decreased visual acuity and impaired depth perception; use with caution when driving or operating machinery especially at night, and in patients with miosis • Use with caution in patients with choledocholithiasis (gallstones in the bile duct) or nephrolithiasis (kidney stones); may induce smooth muscle spasms precipitating cholangitis, cholecystitis, or biliary obstruction in susceptible patients • Use with caution and under close medical supervision in patients with controlled COPD, bronchitis, or asthma

			• Use with caution in patients with cardiovascular disease (especially those with angina or history of myocardial infarction [MI]) or in patients with cardiac arrhythmia; cevimeline may alter cardiac conduction and/or heart rate Contraindications: • Uncontrolled asthma • Narrow-angle glaucoma • Iritis
Generic Name Donepezil **Brand Name** Aricept QT BL	Alzheimer's disease dementia (mild to severe)	**Usual oral dose for mild to moderate dementia:** 5 mg once daily; may increase to 10 mg once daily after 4 to 6 weeks Moderate to severe dementia requires higher doses; refer to PI	• Available in orally disintegrating tablets • May cause anorexia or weight loss • May cause diarrhea, nausea, and vomiting that are transient and often dose related • Rare cases of neuroleptic malignant syndrome (NMS) have been reported; must evaluate patients and may need to discontinue donepezil if symptoms of NMS emerge • Rare cases of rhabdomyolysis have been reported within a few months of initiating the therapy; monitor creatine phosphokinase (CPK) levels and signs and symptoms such as muscle pain, malaise, fever, and dark urine • Use with caution in patients with peptic ulcer disease • Use with caution in patients with underlying cardiac conduction abnormality, respiratory disease, seizure disorder, and urinary tract obstruction
Generic Name Galantamine **Brand Name** Razadyne ▲ ■ QT BL	Alzheimer's disease dementia (mild to severe)	**Usual oral dose for mild to moderate dementia:** Immediate release (IR including liquid formulations): Initial: 4 mg twice daily with food If this dose is well tolerated after a minimum of 4 weeks, the dose may be increased to 8 mg twice daily A subsequent increase to 12 mg twice daily may be considered after at least 4 weeks of the previous dose, if well tolerated	• If treatment is interrupted for more than 3 days and then reinitiated, reinitiate therapy with the lowest dose (i.e., 4 mg twice daily) and slowly retitrate to the current dose • Patients should be maintained on their highest well-tolerated dose to achieve maximum benefit • Nausea, diarrhea, and vomiting are the most common side effects (greater than 10% incidence), and may be dose related; take with food and fluids to decrease risk (ensure adequate fluid intake during treatment) • Many dose formulations are available; use caution when ordering • Oral solution dosage should be diluted according to the manufacturer's recommendations immediately prior to administration • All patients should be considered at risk for adverse cardiac effects • Use with caution in patients with peptic ulcer disease, pulmonary disease • May induce or exacerbate urinary tract obstruction and/or bladder obstruction • Avoid in patients with severe renal or hepatic impairment

Drug Name	FDA-Approved Indication	Adult Dosage Range	Precautions and Clinical Pearls
		Alternatively: Extended release (ER): Initial: 8 mg once daily in the morning with food After a minimum of 4 weeks, the dose may be increased to the recommended initial maintenance dosage of 16 mg once daily A subsequent increase to 24 mg once daily may be considered after at least 4 weeks of the previous dose, if well tolerated	• Use should be discontinued at the first appearance of a skin rash, unless the rash is clearly not drug related; if signs or symptoms suggest a serious skin reaction, use of this drug should not be resumed and alternative therapy should be considered
Generic Name Neostigmine **Brand Name** Bloxiverz ▲ (BL)	Postoperative nonobstructive abdominal distension (adynamic ileus) Myasthenia gravis Postoperative bladder distension and urinary retention Reversal of nondepolarizing muscle relaxants	**Illustrative doses for adynamic ileus:** IM or SQ: 0.5 mg Need for repeat dosage depends on patient's response; refer to PI	• Bradycardia, hypotension, and dysrhythmia may occur with IV use; risk is increased with cardiovascular disease and myasthenia gravis • Overdose results in cholinergic crisis, characterized by extreme muscle paralysis, extreme muscle weakness, and potentially fatal respiratory paralysis • Large doses of neostigmine administered to reverse minimal neuromuscular blocking agent blockade can result in neuromuscular dysfunction • Use with caution in patients with cardiovascular disease, pulmonary disease (may cause bronchospasm), hyperthyroidism, myasthenia gravis, peptic ulcer disease, seizure disorder, and vagotonia • Elderly patients may require dose reductions, but no specific dosing is currently recommended • Oral dosing is still available for reference in some databases, although there are no commercially available oral dose formulations in the United States Contraindications: • Peritonitis • Mechanical obstruction of intestinal or urinary tract • Hypersensitivity reactions have been reported; have atropine and epinephrine ready to treat hypersensitivity reactions; review patient's allergy and past reaction history

Generic Name Physostigmine (PD) (BL)	Reversal of toxic anticholinergic effect Treatment of open-angle glaucoma	**Usual parenteral dose:** IM/IV: 0.5 to 2 mg; may repeat every 10 to 30 minutes until response occurs **Ophthalmic solution for open-angle glaucoma:** 0.25% to 0.5% solution: 1 or 2 drops into each eye up to 4 times daily or ointment applied 1 to 3 times daily	• Avoid in patients with closed-angle glaucoma; worsens blockage of aqueous humor outflow and increases intraocular pressure • Discontinue if excessive cholinergic activity occurs • When administering IV, administer no faster than 1 mg per minute to prevent adverse effects associated with too-rapid administration • Avoid in patients with asthma (can cause bronchcoconstriction) and cardiovascular disease • Use with caution in patients with hypotension and bradycardia (increased vagal tone will worsen these conditions) • May cause alter insulin requirements for patients with diabetes • Use with caution (or avoid) in patients peptic ulcer disease and/or seizures Contraindications: • Gastrointestinal/ileus or urinary obstruction
Generic Name Pyridostigmine **Brand** Mestinol Regonol (PD)	Myasthenia gravis Reversal of neuromuscular blockade Pretreatment for Soman nerve gas exposure	Different dose formulations are available (including solution/syrup) **Illustrative oral dose for myasthenia gravis:** Immediate release (IR): 600 mg given in 5 to 6 divided doses per day Sustained release: 180 to 540 mg once or twice daily (separated by no less than 6 hours) **Illustrative parenteral dose for treatment of myasthenia gravis:** IV/IM: 2mg every 2 to 3 hours; IV must be administered slowly Dosing for Soman nerve gas exposure requires specific protocol	• Highly individualized dosage ranges • Discontinue if excessive cholinergic activity occurs, such as excessive salivation, urinary or fecal incontinence, or vomiting • Muscle weakness may be a symptom of myasthenic crisis • Failure of patients to show clinical improvement may reflect underdosage or overdosage (which may result in a life-threatening cholinergic crisis) • Use with caution in patients with cardiovascular disease, as this drug may cause bradycardia or arrhythmias • Use with caution in patients with asthma, COPD, glaucoma, peptic ulcer disease, seizures, or renal impairment • Electrolyte imbalances associated with adrenal cortical insufficiency may enhance or inhibit neuromuscular blockade • No specific dosage adjustment is required for renal impairment, but lower initial doses may be required due to prolonged elimination in renal impairment; titrate dose to effect • IV infusions used for reversal of neuromuscular blockade should be administered only by trained clinicians familiar with the use of these agents (dosing specific to reversal protocol) Contraindications: • Gastrointestinal/ileus or urinary obstruction

Drug Name	FDA-Approved Indication	Adult Dosage Range	Precautions and Clinical Pearls
Generic Name Rivastigmine **Brand Name** Exelon (BL)	Mild to moderate and severe Alzheimer's disease Alzheimer's dementia Mild to moderate Parkinson's disease dementia (PDD)	**Usual oral dose for Alzheimer's disease:** 1.5 mg twice daily; may increase by 3 mg daily up to 6 mg twice daily **Transdermal patch:** Apply 4.6 mg per 24 hours once daily; if well tolerated, titrate up to 9.5 mg per 24 hours Continue as long as therapeutically beneficial; if needed, may increase to 13.3 mg per 24 hours (maximum dose) Dose titrations should occur at no less than 2-week intervals for oral regimens and 4 weeks for transdermal regimens Refer to specific dose strategies when converting to transdermal patch If medication is interrupted (i.e., a few days missed), the dose should be evaluated for restarting at the same, lower, or initial dose based on the formulation and the patient's individualized needs	• Available in oral and transdermal formulations; specific dose forms are indicated for varying degrees of severity of illness, so confirm the correct form prior to use • Take with food • Allergic dermatitis have been reported with transdermal (TD) formulations; discontinue TD therapy if intense local reactions occur • Significant nausea, vomiting, diarrhea or weight loss, and decreased appetite have been reported; occur frequently in women during titration phase; monitor weight during therapy • Cigarette smoking will decrease serum concentrations by roughly 25% • Use with caution in patients with cardiovascular disease (cardiac conduction abnormality), as this drug may cause bradycardia or arrhythmias • Use with caution in patients with asthma, COPD, glaucoma, or seizure • Use with caution in patients with peptic ulcer disease • Patients with hepatic and/or renal impairment may require lower doses; adjust the dose based on individual tolerability and therapeutic needs Contraindications: • Patients who may experience hypersensitivity reactions; review patient's allergy and past reaction history

Autonomic-Anticholinergic Agents

Antiparkinsonian Agents

Benztropine	Refer to the Central Nervous System Agents chapter.
Diphenhydramine	Refer to the Antihistamine Agents chapter.
Trihexyphenidyl	Refer to the Central Nervous System Agents chapter.

Antimuscarinic and Antispasmodic Agents

Universal prescribing alerts:

- Anticholinergic side effects are a class effect and should be considered to varying degree with all agents in this therapeutic category and others that share anticholinergic side effects (e.g., dry eyes, constipation, worsening of benign prostatic hyperplasia [BPH] and glaucoma). These anticholinergic effects are cumulative (exhibit increased intensity) when multiple agents with this same effect are used concomitantly.
- Use with caution in patients with narrow-angle glaucoma, myasthenia gravis, prostatic hyperplasia/GI or GU obstruction (and other conditions negatively affected by anticholinergic potentiating factors).
- Use with caution in hot weather and during exercise, as these agents reduce the body's ability to sweat and to thermoregulate.
- May cause drowsiness and blurred vision; use with caution while performing tasks that require mental alertness.
- Use with caution in patients with narrow-angle glaucoma, myasthenia gravis, or prostatic hyperplasia/bladder neck obstruction.
- Anticholinergic agents may alter heart rate, with the predominant clinical effect being tachycardia. This action may exacerbate undesirable side effects in patients with hyperthyroidism, hypertension, and underlying cardiac conditions.

Drug Name	FDA-Approved Indication	Adult Dosage Range	Precautions and Clinical Pearls
Generic Name Aclidinium (long-acting) **Brand Name** Tudorza Pressair	COPD	**Usual dose:** 400 mcg (1 actuation) twice daily; maximum daily dose (MDD): 800 mcg	• Rare paradoxical bronchospasms may occur • Immediate hypersensitivity reactions have been reported

Drug Name	FDA-Approved Indication	Adult Dosage Range	Precautions and Clinical Pearls
Generic Name Atropine (BL)	**Common indications for use:** inhibition of salivation and secretion (aspiration prophylaxis) Bradycardia Neuromuscular blockade reversal GI disorders resulting from cholinergic stimulation Induction of mydriasis	Both the usual and maximum dosages of atropine vary depending on the route of administration and indication for use Clinicians must evaluate the individual patient's response **Illustrative parenteral dose for sinus bradycardia:** 0.5 to 1 mg IV push; repeat if needed every 5 minutes up to 2 mg	• Subject to all the universal prescribing alerts for anticholinergic agents • Avoid use in patients with obstructive neuropathy • Avoid in patients with respiratory conditions; may thicken secretions and dryness (however, anticholinergics may also facilitate bronchodilation depending on dose and route; clinical judgment warranted) • Avoid use in conditions resulting in urinary retention or renal failure • Caution in GI disease or obstruction; decreases GI motility and may cause paralytic ileus • Caution in cardiac patients (especially during MI); may potentiate arrhythmias and may alter heart rate
Generic Name Belladonna (BL) (PD)	Moderate pain to severe pain associated with ureteral spasm (bladder spasm) not responsive to non-narcotic analgesics	**Illustrative dose:** 1 suppository rectally 1 to 2 times daily; maximum of 4 doses per day Currently available suppositories contain 16.2 mg belladonna extract with 30 mg powdered opium	• Subject to all the universal prescribing alerts for anticholinergic agents • Few dose formulations are still available; found in combination with other ingredients such as opium • Side effects: fatigue, dry mouth, constipation, vomiting, nausea • Report immediately: severe dizziness, fainting, confusion, tachycardia, vision changes, urinary retention, change in amount of urine passed, sensitivity to light • Precautions: CNS depression, adrenal insufficiency, biliary tract impairment, cardiovascular disease, drug abuse, increased intracranial pressure, prostatic hyperplasia, psychosis, thyroid dysfunction Contraindications: • Glaucoma • Severe renal or hepatic disease • Bronchial asthma • Respiratory depression • Convulsive disorders (seizures) • Acute alcoholism or delirium tremens
Generic Name Dicyclomine **Brand Name** Bentyl	Irritable bowel syndrome	**Usual oral dose:** 20 mg 4 times daily for 1 week; may increase to 40 mg 4 times daily for up to 2 weeks	• Subject to all the universal prescribing alerts for anticholinergic agents • Parenteral formulation for IM use only • Avoid long-term use in elderly patients • Effects of sedatives maybe potentiated with concurrent use • Use with caution in patients with hepatic or renal disease

		Alternative: IM: 20 mg every 4 to 6 hours for 1 to 2 days. Maximum 80 mg per day. Convert to oral therapy as soon as clinically appropriate.	• Increase dose up to 40 mg orally 4 times per day during the first week; if the dosage is not effective within 2 weeks of therapy, or if side effects develop that require doses less than 80 mg per day orally, the manufacturer recommends drug discontinuation • There are no studies on the safety of doses greater than 80 mg per day for periods longer than 2 weeks Contraindications: • Obstructive diseases of GI tract • Severe ulcerative colitis • Reflux esophagitis • Unstable cardiovascular status in acute hemorrhage (and shock) • Urinary tract obstruction • Glaucoma • Myasthenia gravis
Generic Name Glycopyrrolate **Brand Name** Cuvposa Glycate Robinul (BL) (PD)	**Common indications for use:** Inhibition of salivation and respiratory secretions preoperatively Bradycardia (specific) Chronic sialorrhea (drooling) COPD	Both the usual and maximum dosages depend on the indication and weight of the patient **Illustrative parenteral dose (preoperative):** IM: 4 mcg/kg 30 to 60 minutes before procedure **Usual oral dose for sialorrhea:** 1 mg twice per day **Usual inhaled dose for COPD:** 2 capsules per day (total of 31.2 mcg) via oral inhalation	• Subject to all the universal prescribing alerts for anticholinergic agents • Diarrhea may occur in patients with ileostomy and colostomy; discontinue if this occurs • Use with caution in patients with cardiovascular disease, hepatic impairment, renal impairment, hyperthyroidism, neuropathy, prostatic hyperplasia, or ulcerative colitis • Avoid in patients with dementia and other cognitive decline (use with caution in elderly patients) Contraindications: • GI or GU obstruction • Myasthenia gravis • Paralytic ileus • Intestinal atony in elderly and debilitated patients • Severe ulcerative colitis • Toxic megacolon complicating ulcerative colitis • Unstable cardiovascular status • Narrow-angle glaucoma • Acute hemorrhage (hemorrhagic shock) • Tachycardia • Oral dosage form: concomitant usage of oral potassium chloride

Drug Name	FDA-Approved Indication	Adult Dosage Range	Precautions and Clinical Pearls
Generic Name Hyoscyamine **Brand Name** Anaspaz Ed-Spaz Hyosyne Levbid Levsin NuLev Oscimin Symax (BL) (PD)	**Common indications for use:** Preanesthesia (aspiration prophylaxis) GI disorders (reduces secretion, hypermotility, and spasm in GI) Relaxation of GI tract for diagnostic procedures Bradycardia Urinary system disorder	Doses vary based on indication for use **Illustrative dosing to control gastric secretion or spasm:** Regular-release oral formulations, sublingual and orally dissolvable tablets: 0.125 to 0.25 mg every 4 hours or as needed Extended release: 0.375 to 0.75 mg every 12 hours or 0.375 mg every 8 hours. Maximum of 1.5 mg per day Maximum IV dose depends on indication **Illustrative parenteral dosing:** IV/IM/SQ: 0.25 to 0.5 mg (some patients respond to one dose, others require additional doses, refer to PI)	• Subject to all the universal prescribing alerts for anticholinergic agents • Additional dosage forms are available (elixir, concentrated drops) for special populations • Use with caution in patients with cardiovascular disease, hepatic impairment, renal impairment, hyperthyroidism, neuropathy, prostatic hyperplasia, ulcerative colitis • May cause increased heart rate and result in adverse effects for patients with unstable cardiovascular status (e.g., blood loss, hyperthyroidism, congestive heart failure [CHF]) • Prolonged use may cause dental caries, periodontal disease, oral candidiasis, or discomfort due to decreased salivation • Avoid long-term use in elderly patients Contraindications: • GI or GU obstruction • Glaucoma • Myasthenia gravis • Paralytic ileus • Toxic megacolon • Severe ulcerative colitis
Generic Name Ipratropium **Brand Name** Atrovent HFA Atrovent (nasal spray 0.03% or 0.06%) Ipratropium (oral inhalation)	Cold: symptomatic relief of rhinorrhea Allergic rhinitis Seasonal allergic rhinitis COPD	Depends on route of administration and indication for use **Nasal administration:** 2 sprays in each nostril 2 to 3 times (up to 4 times) per day depending on indication for use and product selected (42 mcg and 84 mcg nasal sprays available for dosing)	• Subject to all the universal prescribing alerts for anticholinergic agents • Limited days duration recommended based on formulation and indication for use • Rare paradoxical bronchospasms may occur; immediate hypersensitivity reactions have been reported • Inhalation/nebulizer can be used in conjunction with beta-adrenergic agonists based on the patient's medical condition and updated guideline recommendations • Nebulizer solution may be mixed with albuterol if mixed and used within an hour; refer to PI for detailed compatibility information • Geriatric and pediatric populations can use a spacer if using the MDI is difficult

		Maximum dose for oral inhalation: Usual: 2 sprays (17 mcg/spray) 3 to 4 times per day, not more often than every 4 hours; maximum 12 sprays (204 mcg) per day via MDI Nebulization: 500 mcg (1 ampule/vial) nebulized every 6 to 8 hours	
Generic Name Methscopolamine **Brand Name** Pamine	Adjunctive treatment of duodenal or gastric ulcer	**Usual oral dose:** 2.5 mg 30 minutes before meals and 2 to 5 mg at bedtime	• Subject to all the universal prescribing alerts for anticholinergic agents • Use with caution in patients with prostatic hyperplasia, ulcerative colitis, or other conditions negatively affected by anticholinergic potentiating factors • May cause drowsiness and blurred vision; use with caution while performing tasks that require mental alertness • Use with caution in patients with hepatic or renal impairment • May cause increased heart rate and result in adverse effects for patients with unstable cardiovascular status and cardiovascular disease (e.g., blood loss, hyperthyroidism, CHF) Contraindications: • GI or GU obstruction • Glaucoma • Myasthenia gravis • Paralytic ileus • Toxic megacolon • Severe ulcerative colitis • Patients with unstable cardiovascular status (i.e., hemorrhagic shock)
Generic Name Propantheline (BL) (GD)	Adjunctive treatment of duodenal or gastric ulcer	**Usual oral dose:** 15 mg 3 times daily before meals or food and 30 mg at bedtime	• Subject to all the universal prescribing alerts for anticholinergic agents • Use with caution in patients with prostatic hyperplasia, ulcerative colitis, or other conditions negatively affected by anticholinergic potentiating factors

Drug Name	FDA-Approved Indication	Adult Dosage Range	Precautions and Clinical Pearls
		Patients with mild symptoms (or older adults) may see benefit with a 7.5 mg dose	• May cause drowsiness and blurred vision; use with caution while performing tasks that require mental alertness • Use with caution in patients with hepatic or renal impairment • May cause increased heart rate and result in adverse effects for patients with unstable cardiovascular status and cardiovascular disease (e.g., blood loss, hyperthyroidism, CHF) Contraindications: • GI or GU obstruction • Glaucoma • Myasthenia gravis • Paralytic ileus • Toxic megacolon • Severe ulcerative colitis • Patients with unstable cardiovascular status (i.e., hemorrhagic shock)
Generic Name Scopolamine **Brand Name** Transderm-Scop (BL) (PD)	**Common indications for use:** **Transdermal:** Prevention of nausea and vomiting associated with: Motion sickness and recovery from anesthesia and surgery **IM injection:** Produce amnesia, sedation, tranquilization, and amnestic effects Decrease salivary and respiratory secretions **Ophthalmic:** Induction of mydriasis or cycloplegia and treatment of iritis or uveitis	**Usual transdermal dose for motion sickness:** Apply 1 patch (1.5 mg) behind the ear at least 4 hours before anticipated need (best 12 hours before); removal instructions are specific to the indication; may reapply once every 3 days Parenteral dose depends on indication **Illustrative parenteral dosing for nausea and vomiting:** IM/IV/SQ: 0.6 to 1 mg; may be repeated 3 to 4 times per day Maximum dose: 2.4 mg per day	• Subject to all the universal prescribing alerts for anticholinergic agents • Use with caution in patients with hepatic or renal impairment • May cause increased heart rate and result in adverse effects for patients with unstable cardiovascular status and cardiovascular disease (e.g., blood loss, hyperthyroidism, CHF) Contraindications: • GI or GU obstruction • Myasthenia gravis • Paralytic ileus • Toxic megacolon • Severe ulcerative colitis • Patients with unstable cardiovascular status (i.e., hemorrhagic shock) • Narrow-angle glaucoma

Generic Name Tiotropium **Brand Name** Spiriva (PD)	Asthma COPD	Maximum dose is indication and formulation specific **Usual inhalation dose for COPD:** 5 mcg per day (2 inhalations of **Respimat** 2.5 mcg per actuation) via oral inhalation **Usual inhalation dose of dry-powder Handihaler inhaler:** 18 mcg (2 inhalations from one powder capsule for dose) per day	• Subject to all the universal prescribing alerts for anticholinergic agents • Use with caution in patients with moderate to severe renal impairment and monitor closely; may be more sensitive to the anticholinergic effects • Administer at the same time each day • May use short-acting beta agonists for "rescue" treatment; tiotropium is not indicated for bronchospasm • May take 4 to 8 weeks to see full therapeutic effects • Use with caution in patients with hepatic or renal impairment Inhalation powder (Spiriva Handihaler): • Instruct patients not to swallow the capsules; cases of inadvertent oral administration have been reported to the FDA • Discard capsules that have been opened and not used immediately • Place a single capsule in the device; press the button to puncture the capsule • Must use the appropriate inhalation technique (should hear or feel the capsule vibrate within the inhaler for proper dosing) • The gelatin capsule might break into very small pieces that pass through the inhaler screen and reach the mouth or throat; advise patients that this is normal and not expected to cause harm • Do not use the Handihaler device for more than one person; clean it according to the package instructions Inhalation spray (Spiriva Respimat): • Instruct the patient on the proper inhalation technique according to the product directions • Prior to first use, must prime the unit (do not remove canister once inserted into the inhaler); repriming after days of non-use is required • Color-coded dose indicator shows approximately how much medicine is left • Discard 3 months after insertion of cartridge into inhaler Contraindications: • GI or GU obstruction • Glaucoma • Myasthenia gravis • Paralytic ileus • Toxic megacolon • Severe ulcerative colitis • Patients with unstable cardiovascular status (i.e., hemorrhagic shock)

Drug Name	FDA-Approved Indication	Adult Dosage Range	Precautions and Clinical Pearls
Generic Name Umeclidinium **Brand Name** Incruse Ellipta	COPD	**Usual dose:** Umeclidinium 62.5 mcg (1 inhalation) every 24 hours	• Subject to all the universal prescribing alerts for anticholinergic agents • Available in combination with other agents • Side effects: pharyngitis, rhinorrhea, muscle spasms, painful extremities, constipation, diarrhea, neck pain • Precautions: bronchospasm, cardiovascular disease, diabetes, glaucoma, hypokalemia, prostatic hyperplasia, bladder neck obstruction, seizure disorder, thyrotoxicosis

Autonomic-Sympathomimetic Adrenergic Agents

Alpha-Adrenergic Agonists

Drug Name	FDA-Approved Indication	Adult Dosage Range	Precautions and Clinical Pearls
Generic Name Midodrine ▲ ■ QT	Symptomatic orthostatic hypotension	**Usual oral dose:** 10 mg 3 times daily every 3 to 4 hours during daytime when the patient is upright	• May cause bradycardia due to vagal reflex; use with caution when administered with inotropes, and discontinue if signs of bradycardia occur • Use is not recommended in patients with initial supine elevated blood pressure • Use with caution in patients with diabetes • Drug interactions may require adjustment of dose or may require avoidance of certain drug combinations • Use with caution in patients with renal or hepatic impairment • Use only when benefits of this drug exceed potential risks and no safer treatment option exists Contraindications: • Cardiac disease • Acute renal failure • Urinary retention • Pheochromocytoma • Thyrotoxicosis • Persistent and excessive supine hypertension Associated with: • Severe and persistent systolic supine hypertension (especially when using doses of 20 mg or greater) • Emphasize importance of not administering within 4 hours of bedtime or after the evening meal to prevent supine hypertension during sleep

Generic Name			
Phenylephrine ■ QT BL	**Common indications for use:** Open-angle glaucoma Pupillary dilation (uveitis) Eye/ear/nose/throat (EENT) congestion Vasoconstriction (hemorrhoids) Critical care interventions: paroxysmal supraventricular tachycardia (PSVT), hypotension during anesthesia	Doses vary based on formulation, administration route, and indication for use **Illustrative parenteral dosing for prevention of hypotension or shock:** IM/SQ: 2 to 5 mg, repeated no more often than every 10 to 15 minutes. Maximum initial IM or SC dose is 5 mg **Usual oral dose for EENT congestion:** 10 to 20 mg per dose every 4 to 6 hours, up to 60 mg per day	• IV, oral, and topical dosage forms exist for specific indications for use; refer to PI for additional information • The same cautions exist with the ophthalmic, nasal, and topical rectal products, because they all may be absorbed systemically • Avoid use in patients with cerebrovascular disease (e.g., cerebral arteriosclerosis, aneurysm, intracranial bleeding, history of stroke) as this drug may increase the risk of cerebrovascular hemorrhage, especially with intravenous use • Use with caution in men with symptomatic, benign prostatic hypertrophy, due to the potential for urinary retention • Some formulations are contraindicated in patients with thyrotoxicosis, including hyperthyroidism, and should be given with caution to patients with diabetes mellitus • Avoid use as an adjunct to anesthesia in the fingers, toes, nose, and genitalia because it can cause severe tissue necrosis due to vasoconstriction of small blood vessels • Use with caution in patients with extensive peripheral vascular disease; can cause excessive vasoconstriction and ischemia to vital organs • Use with caution when administering to patients with hepatic and renal disease: larger doses may be needed in patients with hepatic disease; lower doses may be needed in patients with renal failure Contraindications: • Avoid use in patients with cardiac disease including coronary artery disease and arrhythmias (e.g., severe hypertension, atrial fibrillation, atrial flutter, ventricular fibrillation) • Thyrotoxicosis, including hyperthyroidism • Patients with closed-angle glaucoma; contraindicated for this use (ophthalmic solutions of phenylephrine indicated for open-angle glaucoma) Associated with: • Requires experienced clinician who is knowledgeable in the use of this agent
Clonidine	Refer to the Cardiovascular Agents chapter.		
Guanabenz	Refer to the Cardiovascular Agents chapter.		
Methyldopa	Refer to the Cardiovascular Agents chapter.		

Beta-Adrenergic Agonists			
Nonselective Beta-Adrenergic Agonists			
Drug Name	FDA-Approved Indication	Adult Dosage Range	Precautions and Clinical Pearls
Generic Name Isoproterenol **Brand Name** Isuprel QT	**Common indications for use:** For use in specific conditions associated with atrioventricular (AV) block or for treatment of Adams-Stokes syndrome Bradycardia	Dose depends on indication for therapy and patient response **Illustrative parenteral dosing for treatment of ventricular arrhythmias secondary to AV block:** IM/SQ: 0.2 mg initially; additional doses are based on route of administration, continued indication for use and patients clinical response	• Use with caution in patients with cardiovascular disease, diabetes, shock, or hyperthyroidism • Stimulates insulin production, may complicate diabetes management Contraindications: • Angina • Preexisting tachyarrhythmias (ventricular, atrial [flutter] and fibrillation) • Cardiac glycoside intoxication
Selective Beta$_1$-Adrenergic Agonists			
Drug Name	FDA-Approved Indication	Adult Dosage Range	Precautions and Clinical Pearls
Generic Name Dobutamine QT	Short-term inotropic management of patients with cardiac decompensation (low output states)	**Usual parenteral dose:** IV: 0.5 to 1 mcg/kg per minute as a continuous infusion, then titrated every few minutes (usual range 2 to 20 mcg/kg per minute titrated as needed depending on the severity of the patient's condition and indication for use)	• Arrhythmias have been reported; ensure that the ventricular rate is controlled prior to starting dobutamine and monitor closely; use with caution in patients with underlying cardiac conditions • Increase in blood pressure is common due to increased cardiac output • Tachycardia may be dose dependent • Correct electrolyte abnormalities to prevent arrhythmias • Patients with hypovolemia should receive adequate fluid resuscitation prior to administration of dobutamine • Use with caution in elderly patients; start at lower dosages (no specific recommendation available from FDA) • Use with caution in patients with renal impairment Contraindications: • Idiopathic hypertrophic subaortic stenosis

Generic Name Dopamine ■ QT PD	Adjunct treatment of shock Short-term treatment of severe, refractory heart failure	Dose depends on indication for use; and patient response **Illustrative dosing for heart failure:** 3 to 10 mcg/kg per minute as a continuous IV infusion Discontinuation schedule recommendations are specific to patient's age and clinical status	• May increase the patient's heart rate • Use with caution in patients with cardiovascular disease (especially post MI, angina, etc.) and in patients with pre-existing vascular damage or occlusive conditions • May cause decreased peripheral perfusion, leading to tissue necrosis and gangrene • Correct electrolyte abnormalities to prevent arrhythmias • Higher doses (greater than 20 mcg/kg per minute) may increase the risk of tachyarrhythmias and abrupt discontinuation may result in significant hypotension Contraindications: • Pheochromocytoma • Uncorrected tachyarrhythmias • Ventricular fibrillation Associated with: • Sloughing and necrosis in ischemic areas; infiltrate the area as soon as possible with normal saline containing phentolamine (refer to PI for proper emergency management)

Selective Beta$_2$-Adrenergic Agonists

Universal prescribing alerts:

- Recently a conversion to the propellant hydrofluoroalkane (HFA) has been made to avoid further depletion of the protective ozone layer in the atmosphere for the many products available for oral inhalation.
- Agents are subdivided into short-acting (SABA) and long-acting (LABA) agents. LABAs have been associated with an increased risk of severe asthma exacerbations and asthma-related deaths; thus the black box warning on their labels states that monotherapy is contraindicated when treating asthma.
- Avoid use with beta blockers, as these will negate the effects of the beta agonists.
- Beta agonists may cause EKG changes, blood pressure, heart rate elevation, elevated blood glucose, and CNS stimulation.
- Generally these agents should be avoided in any patient with increased risk of prolonged QTc.

Drug Name	FDA-Approved Indication	Adult Dosage Range	Precautions and Clinical Pearls
Generic Name Albuterol **Brand Name** ProAir Proventil Ventolin VoSpire QT PD	Acute bronchospasm (i.e., asthma exacerbation) Bronchospasm prophylaxis Exercise-induced bronchospasm	Dosing requirements vary based on indication for use **Illustrative dosing:** Inhaled MDI: 2 inhalations (90 mcg per actuation) every 4 to 6 hours as needed; maximum 12 puffs per day (inhaler)	• Available in combination products • Rare paradoxical bronchospasms may occur • Use with caution in patients with cardiovascular disease and diabetes • Use with caution in patients with glaucoma hyperthyroidism, hypokalemia, renal impairment, seizures, or any condition (including concurrent medications that cause the same adverse effect) that increases the risk of prolonged QTc

Drug Name	FDA-Approved Indication	Adult Dosage Range	Precautions and Clinical Pearls
		Dry powder inhalation (DPI) also available Oral immediate release tablets/syrup: 2 to 4 mg every 6 to 8 hours; maximum of 32 mg per day Alternatively: Oral extended release tablets: 4 to 8 mg every 12 hours Nebulized: 2.5 mg 3 to 4 times daily as needed; maximum 4 doses per day (nebulizer solution) for oral inhalation	• Usage of a spacer might benefit elderly patients and others that may experience difficulty using MDI • Regular, scheduled daily usage for long-term control of asthma is not recommended • For exercise-induced bronchospasm, use inhalations 5 minutes prior to exercise • Instruct patients on proper inhalation technique according to the product directions
Generic Name Arformoterol **Brand Name** Brovana ■ QT	COPD	**Usual dose:** Oral inhalation via nebulization: 15 mcg twice daily (MDD: 30 mcg)	• Use for maintenance therapy, not for acute bronchospasm; this drug is a LABA • Rare paradoxical bronchospasms may occur • Use with caution in patients with cardiovascular disease and diabetes • Drug interactions may require dose adjustments or avoidance of certain drug combinations • Use with caution in patients with glaucoma, hyperthyroidism, hypokalemia, renal impairment, or seizures • Tolerance may develop Contraindications: • Monotherapy of LABA is contraindicated Associated with: • LABAs have been associated with an increased risk of severe asthma exacerbations and asthma-related death

Generic Name Formoterol **Brand Name** Foradil Aerolizer powder for inhalation Perforomist nebulizer solution ■ QT PD	COPD Asthma: for maintenance treatment of asthma in **patients receiving optimal treatment** with anti-inflammatory asthma agents and who still require an inhaled beta-adrenergic bronchodilator on a regular schedule	**Usual dose for asthma in patients already on an optimal treatment:** Oral inhalation dosage dry powder inhalation Foradil Aerolizer: 12 mcg every 12 hours (MDD: 24 mcg) Maximum dose via nebulizer is 40 mcg per day	• Many formulations available; use caution when prescribing or administering • Rare paradoxical bronchospasms may occur • Highly selective LABA, not a treatment for acute episodes • Use with caution in patients with cardiovascular disease and diabetes • Use with caution in patients with glaucoma, hyperthyroidism, hypokalemia, renal impairment, seizures, or pheochromocytoma • If used for exercise-induced bronchospasm (EIB), inhale 12 mcg (contents of 1 capsule) via Aerolizer at least 15 minutes before exercise; do not repeat dose sooner than 12 hours • Patients already on this drug for scheduled maintenance should not take additional doses for EIB Contraindications: • Monotherapy of LABA is contraindicated Associated with: • LABAs have been associated with an increased risk of severe asthma exacerbations and asthma-related death
Generic Name Indacaterol **Brand Name** Arcapta Neohaler ■ QT	COPD	**Usual dose:** Inhalation: contents of 1 capsule (75 mcg) inhaled once daily	• Available in combination products • Rare paradoxical, life-threatening bronchospasms • Use with caution in patients with cardiovascular disease, diabetes, hyperthyroidism, hyperkalemia, or seizure disorders • Do not use for acute COPD episodes • Do not use with other LABAs; significant numbers of cardiovascular deaths have been reported with excessive sympathomimetic use Contraindications: • Monotherapy of LABA is contraindicated Associated with: • LABAs have been associated with an increased risk of severe asthma exacerbations and asthma-related death • The safety and efficacy have not been established in patients with asthma
Generic Name Metaproterenol QT	Bronchoconstriction in asthma and COPD	**Usual oral dose tablets/ syrup:** 20 mg 3 to 4 times per day MDD: 80 mg Oral inhalation maximum depends on the formulation used	• Many dose formulations available; use care when prescribing and administering • Not recommended in management of asthma because it causes excessive cardiac stimulation • Use with caution in patients with diabetes • Use with caution in patients with glaucoma, hyperthyroidism, hypokalemia, renal impairment, or seizures • Use with caution perioperatively due to its $beta_1$ effects

Drug Name	FDA-Approved Indication	Adult Dosage Range	Precautions and Clinical Pearls
Generic Name Olodaterol **Brand Name** Striverdi Respimat ■ QT	Chronic obstructive pulmonary disease (COPD)	**Usual dose:** 5 mcg per day via oral inhalation (i.e., 2 inhalations per day of Striverdi Respimat)	• May cause pharyngitis • Combination products are available • Do not use as monotherapy for treatment of asthma or for acute bronchospasm • Precautions: cardiovascular disease, diabetes, hyperthyroidism, hypokalemia, seizure disorders, or predisposing risks for QTc prolongation Associated with: • LABAs have been associated with an increased risk of severe asthma exacerbations and asthma-related death • The safety and efficacy in the treatment of asthma have not been established
Generic Name Salmeterol **Brand Name** Serevent Diskus PD QT	Asthma/bronchospasm COPD Exercise-induced bronchospasm	**Usual dose:** 50 mcg (1 inhalation) twice a day	• Do not use for acute bronchospasm • Combination products are available • May cause rhinitis, pharyngitis, cough, rhinorrhea • Precautions: bronchospasm, upper airway symptoms, cardiovascular disease, diabetes, hepatic impairment, hyperthyroidism, hypokalemia, seizures, and patients with predisposing risks for QTc prolongation Associated with: • LABAs have been associated with an increased risk of severe asthma exacerbations and asthma-related death • Should be used in patients with asthma only as adjuvant therapy in patients who are currently receiving but are not adequately controlled on a long-term asthma control medication (i.e., an inhaled corticosteroid)
Generic Name Terbutaline ▲ ■ QT PD	Acute bronchospasm or bronchospasm Prophylaxis in patients with asthma or COPD	**Usual oral dose:** 5 mg per dose every 6 hours up to 3 times daily If side effects occur, reduce dose to 2.5 mg per dose MDD: 15 mg **Illustrative parenteral dosing:** SQ: 0.25 mg per dose, repeat every 15 to 30 minutes; maximum of 0.5 mg within 4 hours	• Rare paradoxical, life-threatening bronchospasms • Use with caution in patients with cardiovascular disease, diabetes, hyperthyroidism, hyperkalemia, or seizure disorders • Avoid in patients predisposed to QTc prolongation

Generic Name Vilanterol **Brand Name** Breo Ellipta (combined with fluticasone) Anoro Ellipta (combined with umeclidinium) ■ QT	COPD	**Usual dose:** One oral inhalation of Anoro Ellipta 62.5/25 (62.5 mcg of umeclidinium and 25 mcg of vilanterol per inhalation) once daily	• Available only as combination with either fluticasone or umeclidinium • May cause pharyngitis, rhinorrhea, muscle spasms, painful extremities, constipation, diarrhea, neck pain • Precautions: bronchospasm, cardiovascular disease, diabetes, glaucoma, hypokalemia, prostatic hyperplasia, bladder neck obstruction, seizure disorder, thyrotoxicosis, high-risk QTc-prolonging agents • Not indicated for relief of acute bronchospasm or asthma; do not use other LABAs concurrently Contraindications: • Use as primary treatment of status asthmaticus or other acute episodes of COPD or asthma where intensive measures are required Associated with: • Increased risk of asthma-related death

Alpha- and Beta-Adrenergic Agonists

Drug Name	FDA-Approved Indication	Adult Dosage Range	Precautions and Clinical Pearls
Generic Name Droxidopa **Brand Name** Northera ■	Neurogenic orthostatic hypotension	**Usual dose:** Initial: 100 mg 3 times daily; titrate in increments of 100 mg 3 times a day every 24 to 48 hours; maximum of 1800 mg per day	• May cause nausea, syncope, urinary tract infection (UTI), falling, headache, dizziness, and hypertension • Report immediately: severe headache, severe dizziness, fainting, vision changes, or signs of neuroleptic malignant syndrome • Use with caution in patients with cardiovascular disease and renal impairment • Give the last dose no later than 3 hours prior to bedtime Associated with: • May cause or exacerbate supine hypertension; advise patients to elevate the head of bed when resting or sleeping • Monitor blood pressure in supine position and in recommended head-elevated sleeping position; reduce or discontinue if supine hypertension persists
Generic Name Ephedrine QT	Treatment of reversible acute bronchospasm in patients with asthma or COPD Anesthesia-induced hypertension	Dose varies based on patient's clinical condition, indication for use, administration route, and formulation of product selected	• May cause hypertension • Use with caution in patients with cardiovascular disease, diabetes, prostatic hyperplasia, seizures, thyroid dysfunction, and unstable motor symptoms • Use with caution in elderly patients • Avoid in patients with closed-angle glaucoma

Drug Name	FDA-Approved Indication	Adult Dosage Range	Precautions and Clinical Pearls
		Illustrative parenteral dosing for acute bronchospasm: IM/SQ: 12 to 25 mg; may give 50 mg; maximum of 150 mg per 24 hours	
Generic Name Epinephrine **Brand Name** EpiPen QT PD	**Common indications for use:** Anaphylaxis Hypotension/shock Mydriasis during intraocular surgery Treatment of bronchospasm associated with bronchial asthma	Dose varies based on patient's clinical condition, indication for use administration route, and formulation of product selected **Illustrative parenteral dosing for anaphylaxis:** SQ or IM: 0.3 to 0.5 mg may be repeated if necessary every 5 to 10 minutes	• May cause arrhythmias; use with caution in patients with cardiac disease • Pulmonary edema may occur • May cause decreased urine output due to renal blood vessel constriction • Use with caution in patients with diabetes, hypovolemia, Parkinson's disease, hypertension, or hyperthyroidism • There are specific strengths of injection solution for emergency resuscitation and for anaphylaxis; use care when prescribing and administering • Can induce arrhythmias and angina in patients predisposed (i.e., underlying cardiac or cerebrovascular disease) • Use with caution in elderly patients • Avoid in patients with closed-angle glaucoma • IV administration should be reserved for patients who are profoundly hypotensive or in cardiopulmonary arrest refractory to volume resuscitation and several epinephrine injections • IM route preferred over SQ if administered for anaphylaxis • Caution should be observed to avoid extravasation during intravenous administration, as peripheral ischemia, tissue necrosis, and gangrene in the surrounding area can occur due to vasoconstriction
Generic Name Norepinephrine **Brand Name** Levophed ■ QT	Treatment of acute hypotension, cardiogenic shock, or septic shock	**Illustrative parenteral dosing:** IV infusion: 8 to 12 mcg per minute; titrate to desired response Dosage range and maximum dose vary depending on clinical situation; usual maximum is 30 mcg per minute IV continuous infusion	Contraindications: • Hypotension from hypovolemia, except use as an emergency measure to maintain coronary or cerebral perfusion until volume can be replaced • Mesenteric or peripheral vascular thrombosis, unless it is life-saving procedure • Do not use during anesthesia with cyclopropane or halothane • Extravasation may occur; ensure proper needle or catheter placement prior to and during infusion Associated with: • Risk of extravasation; if it occurs, infiltrate the area with diluted phentolamine with a fine hypodermic needle (see the manufacturer's recommendations for further details)

Generic Name Pseudoephedrine **Brand Name** Sudafed (BL) (PD)	Symptomatic relief of nasal congestion	**Usual oral dose:** Immediate release (IR): 60 mg every 4 to 6 hours Extended release (ER): 120 mg every 12 hours or 240 mg every 24 hours MDD: 240 mg	• Combination products available (OTC) • Use with caution in patients with diabetes, prostatic hyperplasia, renal impairment, seizure disorder, or hyperthyroidism • Use with caution in elderly patients • When using for self-medication, if symptoms do not improve within 7 days or are accompanied by fever, notify healthcare provider • Discontinue and notify healthcare provider if dizziness, nervousness, or sleepiness occurs Contraindications: • Bronchitis • Closed-angle glaucoma • Coronary artery disease • Emphysema • Hypertension • Peptic ulcer disease • Urinary retention

Autonomic-Sympatholytic (Adrenergic Blocking) Agents

Alpha-Adrenergic Blocking Agents

Nonselective Alpha-Adrenergic Blocking Agents

Drug Name	FDA-Approved Indication	Adult Dosage Range	Precautions and Clinical Pearls
Generic Name Dihydroergotamine **Brand Name** DHE 45 Migranal ■ (PD)	Migraine headache with or without aura Treatment of cluster headache	**Usual parenteral dose:** IM/SQ: 1 mg at first sign of headache Can be repeated hourly; MDD: 3 mg; maximum dose per week: 6 pm IV: 1 mg at first sign of headache Can be repeated hourly; MDD: 2mg; maximum dose per week: 6 mg	• Ergoid alkaloids have been associated with fibrotic valve thickening • Vasospasms can occur • Can result in decreased blood flow, ECG changes, and hypertension • Cerebral hemorrhage, subarachnoid hemorrhage, and stroke have been reported following the injection • Ergot alkaloids may result in intense vasoconstriction, leading to peripheral vascular ischemia and possibly gangrene • Avoid use in elderly patients; if used, monitor cardiac and peripheral effects closely • Nasal spray may cause local irritation to the nose and throat Contraindications: • Uncontrolled hypertension • Ischemic heart disease • Angina pectoris • History of MI

Drug Name	FDA-Approved Indication	Adult Dosage Range	Precautions and Clinical Pearls
		Usual intranasal dose: 1 spray (0.5 mg) in each nostril Can be repeated every 15 minutes up to a total of 4 sprays Maximum dose per day: 3 mg or 6 sprays Maximum dose per week: 4 mg or 8 sprays	• Silent ischemia • Coronary artery spasm • Hemiplegic or basilar migraine • Peripheral vascular disease • Sepsis • Severe renal and hepatic dysfunction • Following vascular surgery • Concurrent use of ergot alkaloids Associated with: • Serious and life-threatening peripheral ischemia and vasoconstriction
Generic Name Ergoloid mesylates (BL)	Treatment of cerebrovascular insufficiency in progressive dementia	**Usual oral dose:** 1 mg 3 times daily, up to 9 mg per day Clinical improvement may require weeks of treatment after initiation	• Ergoid alkaloids have been associated with fibrotic valve thickening • Avoid in patients with hepatic impairment • Rare cases of pleural or retroperitoneal fibrosis have been reported with prolonged daily use • Avoid use in elderly patients • Caution in patients with hypotension or bradycardia • Available in a sublingual formulation Contraindications: • Acute or chronic psychosis, regardless of etiology
Generic Name Ergotamine **Brand Name** Ergomar ■	Migraine	**Usual dose:** Sublingual: 2 mg at first sign of migraine, then 2 mg every 30 minutes if needed; maximum of 6 mg per day, 10 mg per week	• Combination products are available • Use with caution (or avoid) in elderly patients • Do not crush or chew the tablets • Side effects: nausea and vomiting • Report immediately: angina, shortness of breath, bradycardia, tachycardia, arrhythmia, edema, severe dizziness, fainting, severe headache, muscle pain, muscle weakness, change in color of hands or feet from pale to blue or red, burning or numbness of hands or feet, or wounds on fingers or toes • Precautions: cardiac valvular fibrosis, cardiovascular effects, ergotism, pleural or retroperitoneal fibrosis • Discontinuation may result in rebound headaches after prolonged use • Drug interactions may require dose adjustments or avoidance of certain drug combinations

			Contraindications: • Peripheral vascular disease • Hepatic or renal impairment • Coronary artery disease • Hypertension • Sepsis • Dialysis Associated with: • Serious and life-threatening peripheral ischemia and vasoconstriction
Generic Name Phenoxybenzamine **Brand Name** Dibenzyline	Pheochromocytoma (associated hypertension and excessive sweating)	**Usual oral dose:** 10 mg twice daily; increase by 10 mg every other day until optimal blood pressure goal is achieved Usual range: 20 to 40 mg 2 to 3 times day	• Drug interactions may require dose adjustments or avoidance of certain drug combinations • Exaggerated hypotensive or tachycardia may occur • Discontinue if symptoms of severe hypotension or angina occur; avoid use in patients with cardiac conditions (e.g., coronary artery disease [CAD], CHF) • Reduced salivary flow may contribute to the development of dental disease • Use with caution in patients with atherosclerosis, renal impairment, or respiratory tract infections • Use with caution in elderly patients, as they are at higher risk of side effects • Long-term use is not recommended, as there are reports of cancer with such use in humans
Generic Name Phentolamine **Brand Name** Oraverse	**Common indications for use:** Management of norepinephrine extravasation (resulting from alpha-adrenergic effects) Diagnosis of pheochromocytoma (phentolamine blocking test) Hypertensive episodes associated with pheochromocytoma (prevention and management) Reversal of oral soft-tissue anesthesia	Dose varies based on indication for use and formulation of medication selected **Illustrative parenteral dose:** 5 to 10 mg (diluted as per manufacturer in specified amount of normal saline) injected into affected extravasation area within 12 hours	• Side effects: nausea, diarrhea, injection site pain, headache, itching • May stimulate gastric acid secretion • Report immediately: angina, tachycardia, arrhythmia, severe dizziness, syncope, severe headache, paresthesia of hands or feet • Precautions: cardiovascular effects Contraindications: • History of MI • Coronary insufficiency • Angina • Coronary artery disease

Nonselective Alpha$_1$-Adrenergic Blocking Agents			
Doxazosin	Refer to the Cardiovascular Agents chapter.		
Prazosin	Refer to the Cardiovascular Agents chapter.		
Terazosin	Refer to the Cardiovascular Agents chapter.		

Selective Alpha$_1$-Adrenergic Blocking Agents

Universal prescribing alert:

- Alpha adrenergic antagonists have been associated with priapism (persistent painful penile erection unrelated to sexual activity). Priapism, if not treated promptly, can result in irreversible damage to the erectile tissue. Patients who have an erection lasting greater than 4 hours, whether painful or not, should seek emergency medical attention.

Drug Name	FDA-Approved Indication	Adult Dosage Range	Precautions and Clinical Pearls
Generic Name Alfuzosin **Brand Name** Uroxatral	Benign prostatic hyperplasia	**Usual oral dose:** 10 mg once daily	• Take immediately following a meal to increase absorption • Do not crush or chew tablets • Side effects: headache, reduced strength or energy • Immediately report: severe dizziness, fainting, angina, priapism • Precautions: discontinue with severe or worsening angina, CNS depression, floppy iris syndrome, orthostatic hypotension, priapism, patients with history of tachyarrhythmia or myocardial ischemia, prostate cancer, QT prolongation, severe renal impairment • Drug interactions may require dose adjustments or avoidance of certain drug combinations • Generally well tolerated in elderly patients, as it is a uroselective alpha blocker Contraindications: • Hepatic impairment (moderate to severe)

Generic Name Silodosin **Brand Name** Rapaflo ▲	Benign prostatic hyperplasia	**Usual oral dose:** 8 mg once daily	• First-dose orthostatic hypotension may occur 4 to 8 hours after dosing • Administer with food • Capsules may be opened and sprinkled over applesauce and consumed within 5 minutes, followed by 8 ounces of water • Side effects: sexual dysfunction, orthostatic hypotension, headache, insomnia, weakness, nasal congestion, rhinorrhea, sinusitis • Report immediately: hepatic impairment, severe dizziness, syncope, angina, priapism • Precautions: floppy iris syndrome, orthostatic hypotension, concurrent use of phosphodiesterase type 5 (PDE-5) inhibitors, concurrent antihypertensive agents, mild to moderate hepatic impairment, prostate cancer, moderate renal impairment • Use with caution in elderly patients, as there is an increased risk of orthostatic hypotension • Discontinuation should be done with a gradual taper Contraindications: • Renal impairment (creatinine clearance [CrCl] less than 30 mL per minute) • Hepatic impairment (severe) • Drug interactions may require dose adjustment or avoidance of certain drug combinations
Generic Name Tamsulosin **Brand Name** Flomax	Benign prostatic hyperplasia	**Usual oral dose:** 0.4 mg once daily 30 minutes after same meal; may be increased to 0.8 mg once daily after 2 to 4 weeks; restart with 0.4 mg daily if interrupted for several days	• Significant first-dose orthostatic hypotension may occur; use caution • Administer 30 minutes after the same meal each day • Do not crush, chew, or open capsules • Drug interactions may require dose adjustments or avoidance of certain drug combinations • Side effects: headache, dizziness, sexual dysfunction, back pain, diarrhea, rhinitis, rhinorrhea, asthenia, infection, drowsiness, insomnia, weakness • Immediately report: severe dizziness, syncope, blurred vision, angina, tachycardia, chills, pharyngitis, dyspnea, priapism • Precautions: angina, floppy iris syndrome, orthostatic hypotension, syncope, concurrent priapism, prostate cancer • Use with caution in elderly patients, as there is an increased risk of orthostatic hypotension
Carvedilol	Refer to the Cardiovascular Agents chapter.		
Labetalol	Refer to the Cardiovascular Agents chapter.		

Beta-Adrenergic Blocking Agents	
Nonselective Beta-Adrenergic Blocking Agents	
Carvedilol	Refer to the Cardiovascular Agents chapter.
Labetalol	Refer to the Cardiovascular Agents chapter.
Nadolol	Refer to the Cardiovascular Agents chapter.
Nebivolol	Refer to the Cardiovascular Agents chapter.
Pindolol	Refer to the Cardiovascular Agents chapter.
Propranolol	Refer to the Cardiovascular Agents chapter.
Sotalol	Refer to the Cardiovascular Agents chapter.
Timolol	Refer to the Cardiovascular Agents chapter.
Selective Beta-Adrenergic Blocking Agents	
Acebutolol	Refer to the Cardiovascular Agents chapter.
Atenolol	Refer to the Cardiovascular Agents chapter.

Betaxolol	Refer to the Cardiovascular Agents chapter.
Bisoprolol	Refer to the Cardiovascular Agents chapter.
Esmolol	Refer to the Cardiovascular Agents chapter.
Metoprolol	Refer to the Cardiovascular Agents chapter.

Skeletal Muscle Relaxants and Miscellaneous Autonomic Agents

Centrally Acting Skeletal Muscle Relaxants

Universal prescribing alerts:

- These drugs cause CNS depression, so patients must be cautioned about performing activities that require mental alertness.

Drug Name	FDA-Approved Indication	Adult Dosage Range	Precautions and Clinical Pearls
Generic Name Carisoprodol **Brand Name** Soma (BL)	Acute musculoskeletal pain	**Usual oral:** 250 to 350 mg 3 times daily and at bedtime	• Use with caution in patients with history of seizures • Use with caution in patients with history of drug abuse; carisoprodol is a DEA-controlled substance • Use with caution in patients with hepatic and renal impairment • Exaggerated effects in may be seen in "poor metabolizers" (Asian patients may be at higher risk) • Increases the effects of sedatives and alcohol • Muscle relaxants are poorly tolerated in elderly patients; avoid their use in the elderly • Recommended for short-term use (2 to 3 weeks) • Abrupt discontinuation may lead to withdrawal symptoms Contraindications: • History of acute intermittent porphyria

Drug Name	FDA-Approved Indication	Adult Dosage Range	Precautions and Clinical Pearls
Generic Name Chlorzoxazone **Brand Name** Lorzone Parafon Forte DSC BL	Muscle pain associated with acute muscle conditions (spasms)	**Usual oral dose:** 250 to 500 mg 3 to 4 times daily; may increase up to 750 mg 3 to 4 times	• Rare episodes of hepatotoxicity have been reported (some fatal); discontinue if patient develops signs of fever, rash, anorexia, nausea, vomiting, fatigue, dark urine, elevated liver enzymes, or jaundice • Use extreme caution or avoid use in patients with renal or hepatic impairment • Muscle relaxants are poorly tolerated by elderly patients due to their potent anticholinergic effects
Generic Name Cyclobenzaprine **Brand Name** Flexeril Amrix Fexmid QT BL GD	Muscle spasms	**Usual oral dose:** Immediate release (IR): 5 mg 3 times daily; may increase to 10 mg if needed Extended release (ER): 15 mg once daily; some patients may require up to 30 mg once daily	• Use with caution in patients with angle-closure glaucoma, increased ocular pressure, or urinary frequency/urgency • Cyclobenzaprine shares the toxic potential of tricyclic antidepressants (TCAs) • Recommended for short-term use (2 to 3 weeks) • Muscle relaxants are poorly tolerated by elderly patients due to their potent anticholinergic effects; also, since there is risk of fatal hepatic toxicity, avoid their use in the elderly • Avoid use in patients with hepatic impairment • Increases sun sensitivity; use appropriate precautions Contraindications: • Hyperthyroidism • Congestive heart failure • Heart block or conduction disturbances • Acute recovery phase of MI
Generic Name Metaxalone **Brand Name** Skelaxin BL	Relief of acute and painful musculoskeletal conditions	**Usual oral dose:** 800 mg 3 to 4 times per day	• False positive Benedict's test results (urine glucose test) has been reported • Not recommended for geriatric use due to anticholinergic effects Contraindications: • Significant impaired hepatic or renal function • Drug-induced hemolytic anemia or other anemias
Generic Name Methocarbamol **Brand Name** Robaxin PD BL	Common indication for use: Muscle spasms associated with acute painful musculoskeletal conditions	**Usual oral dose:** 1.5 g 4 times per day, then decrease 4 to 4.5 g per day in 3 to 6 divided doses **Usual parenteral dose:** IV/IM 1 g every 8 hours for 3 days	• Anticholinergic effects • Avoid in patients with seizure • Extravasation during intravenous administration may result in thrombophlebitis, sloughing, and pain at the injection site; use extra care • Use with caution in patients with hepatic impairment Contraindications: • Renal impairment

Generic Name Tizanidine **Brand Name** Zanaflex ▲ QT BL	Muscle spasticity	**Usual oral dose:** Initiate at 2 mg up to 3 times daily (6- to 8-hour intervals); may increase in 2- to 4-mg increments per dose every 1 to 4 days (MDD: 36 mg)	• When discontinuing the drug, gradually taper doses by 2 to 4 mg daily • Avoid use in patients with hepatic impairment • May cause dizziness, xerostomia, fatigue, asthenia, hypotension, sedation, weakness, bradycardia, constipation, nausea, UTI, blurred vision, pharyngitis, rhinitis, and flulike symptoms • Report immediately: signs of hepatic impairment, signs of infection, severe dizziness, behavioral changes, bradycardia, difficulty moving, back pain • Drug interactions may require dose adjustments or avoidance of certain drug combinations • Precautions: hepatic effects, hypotension, syncope, sedation, CNS depression, hallucinations, QTc prolongation • Monitor liver function at baseline and 1 month after maximum dose achieved; monitor blood pressure and renal function

Direct-Acting Skeletal Muscle Relaxants

Drug Name	FDA-Approved Indication	Adult Dosage Range	Precautions and Clinical Pearls
Generic Name Dantrolene **Brand Name** Dantrium Revonto Ryanodex ■ GD	Spasticity Malignant hyperthermia	Dose varies with indication for use, formulation selected, and patient's clinical response **Illustrative oral dose:** 25 mg once daily for 7 days; increase to 25 mg 3 times per day for 7 days, then 50 mg 3 times per day for 7 days, then 100 mg 3 times per day (MDD: 400 mg) **Illustrative parenteral dose for malignant hyperthermia:** 2.5 mg/kg continuously until symptoms subside or cumulative dose of 10 mg/kg is reached	• IV administration is formulation specific: refer to PI for guidance • May cause fatigue, flushing, nausea, vomiting, change in voice, drowsiness, headache, rash or itching, kidney stones, abdominal pain, or change in urination • Immediately report: signs of liver problems, signs of infection, loss of strength or energy, shortness of breath, excessive weight gain, swelling of arms or legs, angina, tachycardia, blood in urine, black tarry stools, vomiting blood, change in thoughts, depression, severe abdominal pain, urinary retention, seizures, severe headache, bruising, bleeding, vision changes, severe dizziness, fainting, severe diarrhea, dysphagia, choking, change in speech, injection-site pain • Drug interactions may require dose adjustments or avoidance of certain drug combinations • Precautions: CNS depression, hepatotoxicity, muscle weakness, photosensitivity, cardiovascular disease, hepatic disease, respiratory disease • Avoid extravasation of injectable dantrolene; the pH is high, and tissue necrosis is possible Associated with: • Oral formulation has potential for hepatotoxicity

GABA-Derivative Skeletal Muscle Relaxants			
Drug Name	**FDA-Approved Indication**	**Adult Dosage Range**	**Precautions and Clinical Pearls**
Generic Name Baclofen **Brand Name** Gablofen Lioresal (GD)	Common indication for use: Spasticity	Dose varies with indication for use, formulation selected, and patient's clinical response **Illustrative oral dose:** 5 mg 3 times daily; may increase by 5 mg per dose every 3 days; do not exceed 80 mg daily **Illustrative intrathecal dose:** Initiate with 50 mcg for 1 dose with 4- to 8-hour observation	• Gradual dose reduction over 1 to 2 weeks is recommended • Use with caution in patients with renal impairment, as it is primarily renally eliminated • Drug interactions may require dose adjustments • Precautions: CNS depression, ovarian cysts, urinary retention, gastrointestinal disorders, infections, psychiatric disease, renal impairment, respiratory disease, seizure disorder • May cause: drowsiness, confusions, hypotonia, hyperglycemia, headache, nausea, vomiting, hypotension, peripheral edema, convulsions, insomnia, paresthesia, speech disturbance, altered thinking, itching, constipation, xerostomia, diarrhea, urinary retention, urinary frequency, impotence, back pain, weakness, pneumonia • Additional intrathecal doses may be administered based on the specific protocol; refer to the PI; baseline and ongoing lab values are required • Not indicated for all spastic conditions (i.e., not recommended in patients with trauma-induced cerebral lesions, cerebral palsy, intracranial bleeding, parkinsonism, or a prior stroke or cerebrovascular accident) Associated with: • Abrupt withdrawal of intrathecal baclofen has resulted in severe sequelae, leading to organ failure and death • Not for intravenous administration, intramuscular administration, subcutaneous administration, or epidural administration

Neuromuscular Blocking Agents (NMBA)

Universal prescribing alert:

- Certain conditions may potentiate the pharmacological actions of nondepolarizing neuromuscular blockers and may increase the risk of prolonged neuromuscular block. These states include, but are not limited to, dehydration, electrolyte imbalance (hypokalemia, hypocalcemia, hyponatremia, or hypermagnesemia), and severe acid/base imbalance (respiratory acidosis or metabolic alkalosis). Severe acid/base imbalance may alter a patient's sensitivity to neuromuscular blocking agents (NMBAs) respiratory acidosis may enhance neuromuscular blockade and metabolic alkalosis may counteract it. Dehydration and hypothermia can also increase a patient's sensitivity to NMBAs.
- NMBAs can cause respiratory paralysis as a result of respiratory depression and therefore should be used with caution in patients with pulmonary disease such as chronic obstructive pulmonary disease (COPD).
- Patients with conditions that impair neuromuscular function can experience prolonged or exaggerated neuromuscular block with nondepolarizing agents. These conditions include myasthenia gravis, among others; refer to PI prior to use.
- Patients with history of malignant hyperthermia (MH) should be treated with NMBAs with great caution; malignant hyperthermia can develop in patients receiving general anesthesia.
- NMBAs stimulate histamine release. The degree of release is agent specific, but all should be used with caution in any condition such as asthma in which a significant release of histamine may be contraindicated.
- Obese patients require special care; refer to PI for each product for details.

Drug Name	FDA-Approved Indication	Adult Dosage Range	Precautions and Clinical Pearls
Generic Name Atracurium ■ (PD)	Neuromuscular blockade: adjunct to general anesthesia Facilitate endotracheal intubation Provide skeletal muscle relaxation during surgery or ventilation	Dose varies with indication for use, formulation selected, and patient's clinical response **Illustrative parenteral dose:** IV: 0.4 to 0.5 mg/kg, then 0.08 to 0.1 mg/kg administered 20 to 45 minutes after initial dose; repeat dose at 15- to 25-minute intervals if needed	• Rare anaphylaxis reactions have been reported with use • May cause bradycardia; may not have a significant effect on heart rate • Resistance may occur in burn and immobilized patients • Conditions that may antagonize neuromuscular blockade include respiratory alkalosis, hypercalcemia, demyelinating lesions, peripheral neuropathies, denervation, and muscle trauma • Electrolyte abnormalities such as severe hypocalcemia, severe hypokalemia, neuromuscular disease, metabolic acidosis, and myasthenia gravis may potentiate neuromuscular blockade • Drug interactions may require adjustments in dose or avoidance of certain drug combinations • Maintenance of an adequate airway and respiratory support are critical • Initial dose should be reduced in patients with significant cardiovascular disease or history of elevated histamine release Associated with: • Respiratory depression and insufficiency; requires experienced clinician who is knowledgeable in the use of this agent and specialized care setting
Generic Name Cisatracurium **Brand Name** Nimbex (PD)	Neuromuscular blockade: adjunct to general anesthesia Facilitate endotracheal intubation Provide skeletal muscle relaxation during surgery or ventilation	Dose varies with indication for use and patient's clinical response **Illustrative initial parenteral dose:** IV: 0.15 to 0.2 mg/kg, then repeat doses as per recommendations in PI (individualize dose)	• Rare anaphylaxis reactions have been reported with use • Drug interactions may require dose adjustments or avoidance of certain drug combinations • May cause severe bradycardia (though rare) • Resistance may occur in burn and immobilized patients • Conditions that may antagonize neuromuscular blockade include respiratory alkalosis, hypercalcemia, demyelinating lesions, peripheral neuropathies, denervation, and muscle trauma • Electrolyte abnormalities such as severe hypocalcemia, severe hypokalemia, neuromuscular disease, metabolic acidosis, and myasthenia gravis may potentiate neuromuscular blockade • Maintenance of an adequate airway and respiratory support are critical • Initial dose may be reduced in patients with significant cardiac disease
Generic Name Pancuronium Pancuronium bromide ■	Facilitate endotracheal intubation Provide skeletal muscle relaxation during surgery or ventilation	Dose varies with indication for use and patient's clinical response	• Rare anaphylaxis reactions have been reported; verify allergy and past reaction history • May produce tachycardia secondary to vagolytic activity and sympathetic stimulation • Resistance may occur in burn and immobilized patients

Drug Name	FDA-Approved Indication	Adult Dosage Range	Precautions and Clinical Pearls
	Mechanical ventilation of ICU patients	**Illustrative parenteral dose:** IV: 40 to 100 mcg/kg initially followed by incremental doses of 10 mcg/kg at 25 to 60 minute intervals as needed to maintain muscle relaxation during prolonged surgery	• Conditions that may antagonize neuromuscular blockade include respiratory alkalosis, hypercalcemia, demyelinating lesions, peripheral neuropathies, and denervation, muscle trauma • Electrolyte abnormalities such as severe hypocalcemia, severe hypokalemia, neuromuscular disease, metabolic acidosis, and myasthenia gravis may potentiate neuromuscular blockade • Maintenance of an adequate airway and respiratory support are critical • Classified as long-acting NMBA; its muscular blockade will be prolonged in patients with renal dysfunction • Some protocols recommend use after an initial dose of succinylcholine for intubation • Use with caution in patients with renal and hepatic impairment Associated with: • Respiratory depression and insufficiency; requires experienced clinician who is knowledgeable in the use of this agent and specialized care setting
Generic Name Rocuronium **Brand Name** Zemuron (PD)	Facilitate endotracheal intubation Provide skeletal muscle relaxation during rapid sequence intubation Mechanical ventilation of ICU patients	Dose varies with indication for use and patient's clinical response **Illustrative parenteral dose for endotracheal intubation:** IV: Initially 0.45 to 0.6 mg/kg; maximum effects typically noted within 3 to 4 minutes and last up to 22 to 30 minutes	• Dosing protocols allow use of ideal body weight (IBW) for obese patients; refer to PI • Some patients (i.e., older adults) may experience prolonged recovery of neuromuscular function after administration • Resistance may occur in burn and immobilized patients • Conditions that may antagonize neuromuscular blockade include respiratory alkalosis, hypercalcemia, demyelinating lesions, peripheral neuropathies, denervation, and muscle trauma • Electrolyte abnormalities such as severe hypocalcemia, severe hypokalemia, neuromuscular disease, metabolic acidosis, and myasthenia gravis may potentiate neuromuscular blockade • Use with caution in patients with pulmonary hypertension, respiratory disease, or valvular heart disease • If extravasation occurs, local irritation may ensue; discontinue administration immediately, and restart in another vein • Drug interactions may require dose adjustment or avoidance of certain drug combinations • Use with caution in patients with hepatic impairment Associated with: • Rare anaphylaxis reactions have been reported; review patient's allergy and past reaction history • Respiratory depression and insufficiency; requires experienced clinician who is knowledgeable in the use of this agent and specialized care setting

Generic Name Succinylcholine **Brand Name** Anectin Quelicin Quelicin 1000 ■ (PD)	Facilitate endotracheal intubation Provide skeletal muscle relaxation during surgery or ventilation Mechanical ventilation of ICU patients	Dose varies with indication for use and patient's clinical response **Illustrative parenteral dose for neuromuscular blockade during short procedures:** IV: Average dose is 0.6 mg/kg (range 0.3 to 1.1 mg/kg) administered over 10 to 30 seconds Alternatively may give: IM: 3 to 4 mg/kg (MDD: 150 mg)	• Dosing protocols allow use of total body weight (TBW) for obese patients; refer to PI • Rare anaphylaxis reactions have been reported • Risk of bradycardia may be increased with second dose; pretreating with atropine may reduce the risk • Use with caution in patients with increased intraocular pressure, intracranial pressure, or gastric pressure • Use with caution in patients with fractures or muscle spasms • Electrolyte abnormalities such as severe hypocalcemia, severe hypokalemia, neuromuscular disease, metabolic acidosis, and myasthenia gravis may potentiate neuromuscular blockade • Use with extreme caution in patients with hyperkalemia Contraindications: • Personal of familial history of malignant hyperthermia • Skeletal muscle myopathies • Acute phase of injury following major burns • Multiple trauma • Extensive denervation of skeletal muscle • Upper motor neuron injury Associated with: • Rare reports of acute rhabdomyolysis with hyperkalemia followed by ventricular dysrhythmias, cardiac arrest, and death after administration have occurred • Respiratory depression and insufficiency; requires experienced clinician who is knowledgeable in the use of this agent and specialized care setting
Generic Name Vecuronium **Brand Name** Norcuron ■	Facilitate endotracheal intubation Provide skeletal muscle relaxation during surgery or ventilation Mechanical ventilation of ICU patients	Dose varies with indication for use and patient's clinical response **Illustrative parenteral dose:** IV: 0.08 to 0.1 mg/kg	• Drug interactions may require dose adjustment or avoidance of certain drug combinations • Dose must be considered based on the type of anesthesia used (inhalation anesthesia or balanced anesthesia) • Protocol allows for use of IBW for obese patients • Some patients may experience delayed recovery of neuromuscular function after administration • Electrolyte abnormalities such as severe hypocalcemia, severe hypokalemia, neuromuscular disease, metabolic acidosis, and myasthenia gravis may potentiate neuromuscular blockade • Duration of action may be prolonged in patients with renal and hepatic impairment

Drug Name	FDA-Approved Indication	Adult Dosage Range	Precautions and Clinical Pearls
			• Use with caution in patients with cardiac disease or with slower circulation • Resistance may occur in burn and immobilized patients Associated with: • Respiratory depression and insufficiency; requires experienced clinician who is knowledgeable in the use of this agent and specialized care setting • Rare anaphylaxis reactions have been reported; review patients allergy and past reaction history
Miscellaneous Skeletal Muscle Relaxants			
Universal prescribing alerts: • These agents cause CNS depression, so patients must be cautioned about performing activities that require mental alertness.			
Drug Name	FDA-Approved Indication	Adult Dosage Range	Precautions and Clinical Pearls
Generic Name Orphenadrine **Brand Name** Norflex (BL)	Muscle spasms associated with acute painful musculoskeletal conditions	**Usual oral dose:** 100 mg twice daily **Usual parenteral dose:** IM/IV: 60 mg every 12 hours	• Use with caution in patients with cardiovascular disease such as heart failure, cardiac decompensation, coronary insufficiency, tachycardia, or cardiac arrhythmia • Use with caution in patients with history of drug abuse or acute alcoholism, owing to potential for abuse • Use with caution in patients with renal and/or hepatic impairment • Effects of sedatives and ethanol may be potentiated • Muscle relaxants are poorly tolerated by elderly patients due to their potent anticholinergic effects, and their efficacy in elderly patients is questionable • Avoid in patients who have conditions that could be worsened with the use of anticholinergic medications Contraindications: • Glaucoma • GI obstruction • Stenosing peptic ulcer • Prostatic hypertrophy • Bladder neck obstruction • Cardiospasms • Myasthenia gravis

Miscellaneous Autonomic Drugs			
Drug Name	**FDA-Approved Indication**	**Adult Dosage Range**	**Precautions and Clinical Pearls**
Generic Name Nicotine **Brand Name** Commit Nicoderm CQ Nicolrelief Nicorette Mini Nicorette Refill Nicorette Starter Kit Nicorette Nicotrol Nicotrol NS Thrive	Smoking cessation	Dose varies with indication for use, formulation selected, and patient's clinical response (illustrative dosing provided below) **Nicotine gum:** Every 1 to 2 hours for 6 weeks, then 4 to 8 hours for 3 weeks (MDD: 24 pieces) **Nicotine inhaler:** 6 to 16 cartridges daily; taper frequency of use over 6 to 12 weeks; can use for up to 6 months **Nicotine nasal spray:** 1 dose = 2 sprays (1 spray in each nostril); give 1 to 2 doses per hour; can use for up to 3 to 6 months (MDD: 40 doses) **Nicotine patch:** 14 mg for 6 weeks, then 7 mg for 2 weeks (if patient smokes less than 10 cigarettes per day; refer to PI for details) **Nicotine lozenge:** 1 lozenge every 1 to 2 hours for 6 weeks, then 1 lozenge every 2 to 4 hours for 3 weeks, then 1 lozenge every 4 to 8 hours for 3 weeks (MDD: 20 lozenges)	• If patient smokes fewer than 25 cigarettes per day, use 2 mg gum; if patient smokes more than 25 cigarettes per day, use 4 mg gum • Chew gum and "park" until peppery taste is gone • A 21-mg patch available for patients who smoke more than 10 cigarettes per day • Lozenge strength is determined by when the first cigarette of the day is smoked: more than 30 minutes after waking up, use 2 mg lozenge; less than 30 minutes, use 4 mg lozenge • Use with caution in patients with cardiovascular disease, as products increase blood pressure and heart rate • Discontinue if irregular heartbeat or palpitations occur • Avoid use during the immediate post–myocardial infarction period, in patients with serious arrhythmia, and in patients with severe or worsening angina • Use with caution in insulin-dependent diabetic patients • Use with caution in patients with peptic ulcer disease, hepatic impairment, hyperthyroidism, pheochromocytoma, or renal impairment • Inhaler: use with caution in patients with asthma and COPD; bronchospasm has been reported • Nasal spray is not recommended for patients with chronic nasal disorders such as allergy, rhinitis, nasal polyps, or sinusitis • Vivid dreams or sleep disturbances may occur with the transdermal patch • Remove the patch at bedtime and apply a new patch in the morning • In elderly patients, body aches, dizziness, and asthenia are frequently reported • The reversal of increased liver metabolism caused by cigarette smoking will not be mitigated with the use of nicotine replacement; evaluate medication therapy for need to proactively reduce dose

Drug Name	FDA-Approved Indication	Adult Dosage Range	Precautions and Clinical Pearls
Generic Name Varenicline **Brand Name** Chantix Chantix Continuing Month Pack Chantix Starting Month Pack ▲ ■	Smoking cessation	**Usual dose:** Initial: 0.5 mg daily days 1 to 3; 0.5 mg twice daily days 4 to 7 Maintenance (starting day 8): 1 mg twice daily for 11 weeks	• Start varenicline 1 week before QUIT date; patients must consider setting the quit date before starting varenicline • If the patient successfully quits smoking at the end of 12 weeks, may continue therapy for another 12 weeks to help maintain success • If patients could not quit after the treatment but are still motivated to quit, they should be encouraged to make another attempt with varenicline once the contributing factors for failure have been dealt with • May cause CNS depression, which may impair physical and mental abilities; use caution while performing tasks that require mental alertness • Dose-dependent nausea has been reported, which can be transient or persistent • Discontinue treatment if patients experience behavioral or mood changes • Angioedema and serious rashes have been reported; seek immediate medical care • Use with caution in patients with renal impairment; for specific recommendations for patients undergoing dialysis; refer to PI • Seizures can occur in the first month of therapy; weigh the risks against the benefits before initiating therapy • The reversal of increased liver metabolism caused by cigarette smoking will not be mitigated with the use of nicotine replacement; evaluate medication therapy for need to proactively reduce dose Contraindications: • Hypersensitivity or skin reactions to varenicline or any component of the formulation Associated with: • Neuropsychiatric events including, but not limited to, depression, suicidal ideation, suicide attempt, and completed suicide have been reported in patients taking varenicline • All patients taking varenicline should be observed and monitored for neuropsychiatric events and behavioral changes; FDA review for potential removal of black box warning for serious neuropsychiatric symptoms reported during use is pending

Chapter 5

Blood Formation, Coagulation, and Thrombosis Agents

Author: **Steven E. Pass, PharmD, FCCM, FCCP, FASHP, BCPS**

Co-authors: **Lauren Adams, PharmD, BCPS and Stephy Kuriakose, PharmD, BCPS**

Editor: **Krystal L. Edwards, PharmD, FCCP, BCPS**

Learning Objectives

- Identify current pharmacologic agents that are appropriate for blood formation, coagulation, and thrombosis.
- Recommend optimal pharmacologic interventions based on patient-specific characteristics.
- Provide appropriate patient-specific counseling points and optimal overall medication management.

Key Terms: antianemia agents, iron preparations, antithrombotic agents, anticoagulant agents, coumarin derivatives, direct thrombin inhibitors, direct factor Xa inhibitors, heparins, platelet-reducing agents, platelet-aggregation inhibitors, thrombolytic agents, hematopoietic agents, hemorrheologic agents, antihemorrhagic agents, hemostatics

Overview of Blood Formation, Coagulation, and Thrombosis Agents

Hemostasis is the physiological mechanism by which clots are formed to control bleeding from an injured blood vessel and to maintain the integrity of the circulatory system. Injury to organs and disruption of blood vessels can lead to internal and/or external bleeding. Depending on the total volume lost, this blood loss can be detrimental to human life. Because blood is the primary oxygen-transporting mechanism in our body, its loss can lead to hypoxia, hypotension, and an acute drop in hemoglobin and hematocrit. The initial mechanism of hemostasis is vasoconstriction, which decreases blood flow to the area of injury. Secondary mechanisms, involving activation of platelets and formation of thrombin, follow rapidly and are localized to decrease blood loss.

The endothelial lining of blood vessels contains collagen and tissue factors that are not exposed to blood under normal conditions. When a vessel is punctured, however, these subendothelial elements are exposed to blood, which in turn triggers the coagulation cascade as well as platelet activation and aggregation. Depending on whether the source of injury is internal or external to the vasculature, the intrinsic or extrinsic coagulation pathway will be activated. The extrinsic pathway, which is activated by exposed tissue factor at the site of injury, is the primary physiological process leading to thrombin production. The driving force of the clotting cascade is the sequential activation of a series of proenzymes to active enzymes, resulting in a sequential thrombin amplification process. Activated thrombin induces the production of fibrin, which helps with clot stabilization.

The coagulation system is essential to maintaining hemostasis within the body. When the blood vessels are injured and a bleed or bruise occurs, the platelets and coagulation cascade are activated to stop the bleed and repair the vessel. Without coagulation, even a minor injury could result in a catastrophic blood loss and, in the worst case scenario, lead to mortality. Conversely, when clots form in places they are not needed, it can be a medical emergency. Patients with hypercoagulation disorders, for example, form blood clots without any injury triggering the formation; these blood clots may then partially or totally occlude the blood vessels, causing ischemic damage. In these patients, therapeutic anticoagulants are indicated to allow for their blood to be thinner than the blood in the average person, thereby preventing the formation of clots when they are not necessary. Likewise, patients who have had grafts or stents placed, or those with abnormal heart rhythms such as atrial fibrillation, are more likely to develop clots.

The clotting cascade consists of the intrinsic and extrinsic pathways, which merge to form the common pathway. Each pathway consists of clotting factors that are activated during the progression down the clotting cascade. The intrinsic pathway factors include XII, XIIa, XI, XIa, IX, IXa, VIII, and X; the extrinsic pathway factors include VIIa and tissue factor. The common pathway factors include X, Xa, XIII, XIIIa, prothrombin (factor II), thrombin, fibrinogen (factor I), and fibrin. Ultimately, the intrinsic and extrinsic pathways merge at factor X. The activation of factor X to factor Xa allows for prothrombin to be converted to thrombin, and finally fibrinogen to be converted to fibrin, which then forms a cross-linked fibrin clot.

Anticoagulant drugs target specific clotting factors throughout the coagulation cascade to prevent clot formation. Warfarin inhibits factors II, XII, IX, and X, while the mechanisms of action for the newer oral anticoagulants, now termed direct oral anticoagulants (DOACs), vary. Apixaban, edoxaban, and rivaroxaban inhibit factor Xa, while dabigatran is a direct thrombin inhibitor.

The parenteral anticoagulants also vary in terms of their mechanism of action. Heparin primarily inhibits factor II by inactivating thrombin, which in turn prevents the conversion of fibrinogen to fibrin. The low-molecular-weight heparins (enoxaparin and dalteparin) and fondaparinux inhibit factor Xa, and argatroban is a direct thrombin inhibitor.

Some anticoagulants are considered maintenance therapy, such as warfarin and the DOACs. Others are administered parenterally for short-term initial therapy after the clotting event has occurred—for example, enoxaparin, heparin, dalteparin, and fondaparinux. Warfarin typically does not produce any therapeutic effects until 5–7 days after the first dose, due to the biologic half-lives of the factors that it inhibits (II, VII, IX, and X). Factor II has the longest half-life (50–80 hours) of these clotting factors; therefore, parenteral therapeutic anticoagulation is required to bridge the patient to the use of the oral formulation alone. Parenteral formulations may also be used for prophylaxis, typically being administered at lower doses in patients who are at high risk for developing a clot due to various risk factors.

The human body also has counter-regulatory mechanisms to balance the coagulation process, which rely on the release of the tissue plasminogen activator (tPA) enzyme from the vascular endothelial cells. This enzyme aids the conversion of inactive plasminogen on the surface of fibrin clots to a fibrinolytic protease called plasmin, which then promotes the hydrolysis of the cross-linked fibrin polymers. Other factors such as nitric oxide (NO), prostacyclin, antithrombin, tissue factor pathway inhibitor (TFPI), and activated protein C and protein S also play vital roles in terminating the coagulation process.

Under normal conditions, the thrombin-stimulated fibrin clot formation and plasmin-induced clot lysis are carefully regulated to maintain hemostasis within the body. When pathologic processes overwhelm the regulatory mechanisms of hemostasis, thrombin production can become unregulated, leading to thrombosis. Thrombosis can be responsible for detrimental events associated with increased morbidity and mortality, including myocardial infarction and stroke, venous thromboembolic disorders, and pulmonary embolism (PE). Thrombolytic agents such as recombinant human tissue plasminogen activators and streptokinase help dissolve blood clots by binding to the surface of fibrin molecules and activating fibrin-bound plasminogen. These agents have great utility if given quickly and appropriately to patients presenting with an acute ischemic event. They are considered high-risk therapy options, however, as they significantly increase the risk for bleeding; thus thrombolytic agents should be administered only after careful patient evaluation and with close monitoring.

Antiplatelet agents act by inhibiting platelet function at various receptors so as to prevent platelet activation, aggregation, and clot formation. Aspirin inhibits thromboxane, which leads to decreased platelet function. P2Y12 inhibitors such as clopidogrel, ticagrelor, and prasugrel, as well as phosphodiesterase inhibitors such as dipyridamole and cilostazol, prevent platelet aggregation. The final class of antiplatelet agents are the glycoprotein IIb/IIIa inhibitors, which are typically used in advanced cardiac procedures and further prevent the formation of cross-links between platelets. These antiplatelet agents can be used in combination—for example, after myocardial infarction or stroke, or after placement of stents to prevent platelet aggregation and total or partial vessel occlusion. Antiplatelet agents differ from anticoagulants in that they do not inhibit clotting factors in the coagulation cascade, but rather work specifically on receptors on the platelets to prevent platelet aggregation and clot formation.

Platelets contain a transporter protein that allows for the uptake of serotonin into the platelet. When a platelet becomes activated, serotonin is released and stimulates platelet aggregation. Selective serotonin reuptake inhibitors (SSRIs) block this transporter. Thus, when platelets are activated, SSRIs cause some inhibition of platelet aggregation, leading to a slight increase in bleeding risk. When use of SSRIs is coupled with use of anticoagulant or antiplatelet agents, it is important to be aware of this increased risk of bleeding and to educate the patient about the signs and symptoms of bleeding and bruising.

According to World Health Organization (WHO) guidelines, anemia is defined as a hemoglobin level of less than 13 g/dL in males, and less than 12 g/dL in females, which results in a decreased oxygen-carrying capacity of the blood. The causes of anemia are multifactorial, but center on three major issues: (1) blood loss, (2) inadequate production of red blood cells, or (3) increased destruction of red blood cells. There are three functional classifications of anemia—hypoproliferative, maturation disorders, and hemorrhage and hemolysis—and the type that is present determines the proper therapy.

- Hypoproliferative anemias—the most common type—include anemias of iron deficiency, inflammation, renal disease, malignancies, and hypometabolic states. Their treatment includes blood transfusions, iron replacement therapy, and erythropoietin.
- Maturation disorders include cytoplasmic defects and nuclear maturation defects. Cytoplasmic defects include thalassemia and sideroblastic anemia. More commonly known as megaloblastic anemias, nuclear maturation defects often involve folate or cyanocobalamin (vitamin B_{12}) deficiencies, but may also be associated with medication use (antifolate or chemotherapeutic agents).
- Hemorrhage and hemolysis include blood loss, intravascular hemolysis, autoimmune diseases, hemoglobinopathy, and metabolic defects. Their treatment includes strategies such as blood transfusions, immunosuppressant agents (e.g., corticosteroids, rituximab), plasma exchange, splenectomy, and stem cell transplantation.

5.1 Antianemia Agents

The antianemia class of medications is the cornerstone of anemia management. As noted earlier, anemia is classified into three main categories: hypoproliferative, maturation disorders, and hemorrhage/hemolysis. The choice of treatment is based on these general categories, although there can be some overlap.

Iron-deficiency anemia is the most common type of anemia, and iron replacement using oral iron products is the preferred therapy. Ferrous sulfate is the most commonly used product, but each variant has advantages and disadvantages based on its tolerance and adverse-effect profile. The most common adverse effects are flushing and gastrointestinal ([GI] nausea, constipation) effects. The intravenous iron products are typically reserved for those patients who cannot tolerate oral dosing and are associated with significant infusion-related reactions.

Erythropoietin-stimulating agents are used in patients who have deficiencies in red blood cell (RBC) production, such as chronic renal insufficiency or anemia of chronic disease. These patients require close monitoring, and should not receive therapy if their hemoglobin (Hgb) level is higher than 11 g/dL; in the United States, the labeling for erythropoietin-stimulating agents carry a black box warning to this effect.

Antianemia Agents

Darbepoetin alfa (*see also the Hematopoietic Agents section*)
Epoetin alfa (*see also the Hematopoietic Agents section*)

Iron Preparations

It is difficult to diagnose anemia because iron deficiency is not the only possible cause of this condition. Even when iron deficiency is identified, the monitoring of hemoglobin, total iron, iron binding capacity, and percent saturation must be evaluated at baseline and then ongoing to ensure optimal clinical improvement. Oral iron replacement can represent a number of challenges, including, but not limited to, the degree of stomach irritation and other GI adverse effects. Patients must be educated to not take antacids at the same time as their iron supplement because iron absorption is reduced significantly with increased pH (less acidic). Extending empathetic understanding of the possible side effects and demonstrating willingness to modify or change the therapy to improve patient comfort is key to effective iron replacement. Taking iron supplements with small non-dairy based snacks, or even changing the formulation of iron (available in numerous formulations that vary in the amount of elemental iron they contain, their absorption from the GI tract, and their stomach-irritating potential) may represent opportunities to improve patient acceptance and adherence. There are occasions when oral iron is not a viable option and parenteral iron replacement becomes necessary. Serious hypersensitivity reactions, including anaphylactic-type reactions (some fatal), may occur, even in patients who previously tolerated parenteral iron so caution is advised.

Iron Preparations

Ferric carboxymaltose
Ferumoxytol
Iron dextran
Iron preparations, oral
Iron sucrose
Sodium ferric gluconate

Case Studies and Conclusions

Todd is a 52-year-old male with a past medical history of gastroesophageal reflux disease (GERD) and hypertension who was recently diagnosed with iron-deficiency anemia. After discussion with his physician, he agrees to try adjusting his diet to include more iron. After several months, there is no improvement in Todd's condition. His primary care physician prescribes an initial dose of ferrous sulfate 325 mg by mouth twice daily.

1. Which important factors should be considered prior to Todd initiating ferrous sulfate therapy?
    a. Todd's use of antacids
    b. Todd's use of acetaminophen
    c. Todd's consumption of meat
    d. Todd's consumption of fat

Answer A is correct. The absorption of oral iron formulations is decreased by medications that increase the pH of the stomach. With Todd's history of GERD, it would be important to find out if he is currently on medications to relieve his symptoms, as proton-pump inhibitors, histamine-2 receptor antagonists, and antacids may reduce the absorption of oral iron products.

After two weeks of taking ferrous sulfate, Todd returns to the clinic with complaints of stomach upset, and no longer wants to stay on this medication.

2. Which options does this patient have for therapy?
    a. Stop the iron replacement, as the anemia should resolve naturally
    b. Stop the iron replacement and begin vitamin B_{12} therapy
    c. Continue the iron replacement, but take it with a small snack or meal
    d. Continue the iron replacement, but take it with an antacid

Answer C is correct. GI adverse effects are common with oral iron therapy. Although it is recommended to take doses on an empty stomach, patients may experience fewer GI effects if they take the doses with a small snack or meal. Other options to consider include taking lower doses at more frequent intervals.

3. Which monitoring is needed for iron replacement therapy?

   a. GI irritation
   b. Constipation
   c. Diarrhea
   d. Hemoglobin
   e. All of these are correct.

Answer E is correct. Todd should be monitored closely for all adverse effects, including GI irritation, nausea, vomiting, diarrhea, and constipation. His laboratory levels, such as hemoglobin, total iron, iron-binding capacity, and percent saturation, should be monitored for clinical improvement.

Mary is a 63-year-old female with end-stage renal disease who is receiving hemodialysis three days each week. She has anemia associated with chronic kidney disease (CKD), and has been taking polysaccharide iron complex 150 mg by mouth daily, along with ascorbic acid 1000 mg by mouth twice daily. After 6 months of treatment, her symptoms are not improving, and the decision is made to initiate intravenous iron therapy with iron dextran.

1. Which factors should be considered prior to initiating iron dextran therapy for this patient?

   a. Black box warning for QTc prolongation
   b. Black box warning for dementia-related psychosis
   c. Black box warning for anaphylactic reactions
   d. Black box warning for bowel obstruction

Answer C is correct. The labeling for iron dextran carries a black box warning about anaphylactic reactions. While this medication may be an appropriate option, it should be administered under the supervision of medical personnel (it is typically given during hemodialysis).

2. How should the first dose of iron dextran be administered to Mary?

   a. Partial oral test dose
   b. Partial parenteral test dose
   c. Full dose via Z-track technique
   d. Full dose subcutaneously

Answer B is correct. Dosing should begin with a 0.5 mL test dose to monitor for anaphylactic reactions. Caution should be used, as anaphylactic reactions may occur during the test dose, and successful administration of the test dose does not rule out the possibility of anaphylactic reactions during the regular dose.

3. Are there other intravenous iron options?

   a. Ferumoxytol
   b. Iron sucrose
   c. Sodium ferric gluconate
   d. All of these are alternatives.

Answer D is correct. Ferumoxytol, iron sucrose, and sodium ferric gluconate are alternative options to iron dextran. Each of these products carries a risk of significant infusion-type reactions, but may be better tolerated by patients.

5.2 Antithrombotic Agents

Anticoagulant Agents

Anticoagulants are a large class of medications that act at various steps of the coagulation cascade to prevent blood from clotting. The coagulation cascade comprises the intrinsic and extrinsic pathways, both of which involve several clotting factors. These clotting factors are activated in a stepwise manner before ultimately combining in the common pathway. In the common pathway, the activation of factor X results in prothrombin's conversion to thrombin followed by fibrinogen's conversion to fibrin, forming a stable clot.

Several classes of anticoagulants are available, including the vitamin K antagonists, heparins, and novel oral anticoagulants. Coumadin is a vitamin K antagonist that works by inhibiting factors II, VII, IX, and X. Some of its disadvantages compared with newer agents such as DOACs are the need for frequent international normalized ratio (INR) monitoring, longer half-life, drug–drug interactions, drug–food interactions, and possibly increased risk of bleeding. However, unlike the DOACs, excessive warfarin effects can be reversed relatively easily with the administration of vitamin K (phytonadione) or skipping a scheduled dose of the anticoagulant. DOACs are divided into two classes, direct thrombin inhibitors and anti-Xa inhibitors. Dabigatran is a direct thrombin inhibitor that acts by preventing the conversion of prothrombin to thrombin. The anti-Xa inhibitors, which include rivaroxaban and apixaban, target the first step of the common pathway, where the intrinsic and extrinsic pathways combine. Rivaroxaban and apixaban dosing regimens are significantly impacted by renal function and creatinine clearance, thus establishing a baseline renal function, with continued monitoring, are key to safe and effective medication use. Additionally, if patients are currently anticoagulated and are in need of transition or addition of a DOAC, it is important to note that rivaroxaban can be started when the INR is less than 3, but apixaban and dabigatran therapy cannot be initiated until the INR is less than 2. Heparin and low-molecular-weight heparins are short-acting anticoagulants that are used in the initial period of anticoagulation as well as to bridge patients to a therapeutic level of warfarin.

Anticoagulant Agents

Coumarin Derivatives

Warfarin

Direct Thrombin Inhibitors

Argatroban
Bivalirudin
Dabigatran
Desirudin

Direct Factor Xa Inhibitors

Apixaban
Edoxaban
Fondaparinux
Rivaroxaban

Heparins

Dalteparin
Enoxaparin
Heparin

Miscellaneous Anticoagulant Agents

Antithrombin III (Human)
Antithrombin alfa
Protein C (Human)

Antiplatelet Agents

Antiplatelet medications are used to stop platelet aggregation, thereby preventing formation of a blood clot. Platelets are sent to a site of injury in the body to prevent excess bleeding. Unfortunately, when patients experience a heart attack or a stroke, the platelets can aggregate and occlude a vessel, causing increased damage from ischemia. During a heart attack or stroke, a cholesterol plaque typically ruptures in an artery, causing platelets to aggregate at the site and leading to partial or total occlusion of the vessel. Likewise, when stents are placed in arteries, they can promote platelet aggregation and potential occlusion of the vessel.

Antiplatelet medications have several mechanisms of action, including cyclooxygenase (COX) inhibition, adenosine diphosphate (ADP) antagonism, phosphodiesterase inhibition, and glycoprotein (GP) IIb/IIIa inhibition. As there are several mechanisms of platelet inhibition, it is often appropriate in practice to use more than one medication to inhibit platelet activation and aggregation.

Aspirin inhibits platelet cyclooxygenase, thereby preventing the generation of thromboxane A_2, which is a mediator that causes platelet activation and aggregation. The thienopyridines such as clopidogrel and prasugrel block the P2Y12 receptor, where adenosine diphosphate acts to inhibit adenylate cyclase and cause platelet aggregation. Dipyridamole and cilostazol are phosphodiesterase inhibitors that inhibit adenosine uptake and cyclic GMP phosphodiesterase activity, thereby decreasing platelets' ability to aggregate. There are many clinical conditions that warrant a combination of P2Y12 agents along with aspirin. In some cases, aspirin may be required indefinitely while the P2Y12 agent therapy may have a limited therapeutic duration (i.e., 12 months). In cases where immediate intervention is warranted, loading doses of P2Y12 (i.e., clopidogrel 300 or 600 mg) along with non-enteric coated aspirin can be administered.

The glycoprotein IIb/IIIa inhibitors are typically parenteral agents used by cardiologists during percutaneous coronary interventions (PCIs). The GP IIb/IIIa receptors are located in the final common pathway for platelet aggregation, and inhibition of these receptors results in inability of platelets to cross-link and form clots.

Platelet-Reducing Agents

Anagrelide

Platelet-Aggregation Inhibitors

Abciximab
Cangrelor
Cilostazol
Clopidogrel
Eptifibatide
Prasugrel
Ticagrelor
Ticlopidine
Tirofiban
Aspirin (*see also the Analgesics and Antipyretics section in the Central Nervous System Agents chapter*)
Dipyridamole (*see also the Vasodilating Agents section in the Cardiovascular Agents chapter*)

Thrombolytic Agents

Thrombolytics, also known as fibrinolytics, are agents used to dissolve blood clots. These medications activate plasminogen on the surface of fibrin clots, which in turn activates a proteolytic enzyme called plasmin that is capable of breaking cross-links between fibrin molecules and disrupting the structural integrity of blood clots. The most common indications for thrombolytic therapy include ischemic cerebrovascular events and ST-segment elevation myocardial infarction (STEMI).

There are two major classes of fibrinolytic drugs: tissue plasminogen activator (tPA) and streptokinase (SK). Alteplase, tenecteplase, and reteplase are tissue plasminogen activators and bind primarily to clot-associated fibrin. Streptokinase is a nonspecific agent that can bind to both circulating and noncirculating plasminogen, and therefore has been a less favorable agent for thrombolytic therapy and is no longer used in the United States. Patients who present for treatment later than 3 hours from the initial cerebrovascular event or STEMI (or 4-hour window with additional exclusion criteria) are not candidates for thrombolytic therapy, so the quicker clinicians can intervene, the more likely it is they can use these life-saving agents. There are many dosing options for these agents, however an illustrative dose could be: loading dose of alteplase at 0.09 mg/kg bolus (10% of 0.9 mg/kg) with 0.81 mg/kg (90% of the 0.9 mg/kg) given as a continuous infusion over 60 minutes.

Contraindications to the use of thrombolytics include active internal bleeding, history of cerebrovascular accident, recent intracranial/intraspinal surgery or trauma, intracranial neoplasm, arteriovenous malformation or aneurysm, and severe uncontrolled hypertension. Common side effects seen with these agents include bleeding and reperfusion arrhythmias. Healthcare providers should cautiously monitor all potential bleeding sites and discontinue the thrombolytic therapy if bleeding occurs.

Thrombolytic Agents

Alteplase
Reteplase
Tenecteplase

Case Studies and Conclusions

DB is a 65-year-old male whose significant past medical history includes coronary artery disease (CAD), diabetes, hypertension, hyperlipidemia, congestive heart failure (CHF), and multiple deep venous thromboses (DVTs). His most recent DVT occurred 2 months ago during a hospital stay for a CHF exacerbation. For the past year, DB has been receiving warfarin 5 mg daily for treatment of his DVTs, with a goal INR of 2–3. Recently he has not been able to make it to clinic for frequent lab draws, and wants to try other options for treatment of his DVTs as he "cannot keep this level in range." His current lab data are as follows: CBC: WNL, BMP: WNL, Ht: 70 in., Wt: 90 kg.

1. Which alternative options can be pursued for DB's DVT treatment?
   a. Rivaroxaban 15 mg twice daily for 21 days, then 20 mg daily
   b. Apixaban 100 mg twice daily for 7 days, then 50 mg twice daily
   c. Dabigatran 150 mg daily
   d. All of these are appropriate treatment options.

Answer A is correct. Appropriate alternative options include rivaroxaban 15 mg twice daily for 21 days, then 20 mg daily with food; apixaban 10 mg twice daily for 7 days, then 5 mg twice daily; or dabigatran 150 mg twice daily.

2. If DB's creatinine clearance (CrCl) decreased to less than 30 mL per minute, which treatment options would be available?
   a. Apixaban 10 mg daily for 7 days, then 5 mg daily
   b. Apixaban 10 mg twice daily for 7 days, then 5 mg twice daily
   c. Apixaban 100 mg daily for 7 days, then 50 mg daily
   d. Apixaban 100 mg twice daily for 7 days, then 5 mg twice daily

Answer B is correct.

3. DB's INR is currently 2.8. Which DOAC agent could DB start today?
   a. Apixaban
   b. Dabigatran
   c. Rivaroxaban
   d. Warfarin

Answer C is correct. Rivaroxaban can be started when the INR is less than 3. With apixaban and dabigatran, therapy cannot begin until the INR is less than 2.

A 45-year-old female with atrial fibrillation is seen in the anticoagulation clinic for a routine INR check. She states that she has been taking her warfarin 5 mg by mouth daily as directed, and mentions that she is getting over a recent flu-like illness. Her INR today is 4.1 (the desired range is 2–3).

1. What are the most common complications of an elevated INR with warfarin therapy?
   a. Increased hematocrit
   b. Decreased hemoglobin
   c. Increased white blood cell (WBC)/absolute neutrophil count (ANC)
   d. Decreased platelets

Answer B is correct. Signs and symptoms of bleeding secondary to an elevated INR include increased bruising, gum bleeding, melena, blood in the stool (hematochezia), and decreased hemoglobin or hematocrit. Patients should be assessed to determine whether bleeding exists and for potential indications for warfarin reversal.

2. What are some possible reasons for this patient's elevated INR?
   a. Increased vitamin K intake
   b. Decreased vitamin K intake
   c. Increased potassium intake
   d. Decreased potassium intake

Answer B is correct. Possible explanations include a change in diet (inconsistent intake of vitamin K–rich foods) due to her illness. The patient's medication history should be reviewed to see if she was prescribed an antibiotic that interacts with warfarin (i.e., levofloxacin, moxifloxacin, clarithromycin).

3. What is the best course of action for this patient?
   a. Prescribe a lower dose of warfarin until the INR improves
   b. Do not give (hold) the dose of warfarin until the INR improves
   c. Seek a nutrition consult for future warfarin success
   d. All of these are appropriate.

Answer D is correct. The patient should either hold her warfarin dose or be prescribed a lower dose (2.5 mg) until her INR decreases to the desired range, and then be reassessed for dosage changes. She should return to clinic in 5–7 days for follow-up.

HR is a 59-year-old man who presents to the emergency department for new-onset left-sided weakness that began 7 hours ago. He has a history of hypertension, diabetes, and coronary artery disease. His medication list includes metoprolol 50 mg per day twice daily, hydrochlorothiazide 25 mg per day orally, and aspirin 325 mg per day orally. His vital signs include blood pressure (BP) 158/92 mm Hg, heart rate 82 beats per minute, respiratory rate 16 breaths per minute, and temperature 38°C.

1. What is your opinion on treating this patient with thrombolytic therapy for a myocardial infarction?
   a. He is a candidate for thrombolytics.
   b. He is not a candidate for thrombolytics.
   c. There is not enough information to determine whether thrombolytics are appropriate.

Answer B is correct. The patient is presenting outside the 3-hour window (or 4-hour window with additional exclusion criteria) and is not a candidate for thrombolytic therapy.

2. What are the contraindications for administration of thrombolytic therapy?
   a. Blood glucose concentration > 200 mg/dL
   b. Decreased blood pressure (systolic < 105 mm Hg or diastolic < 90 mm Hg)
   c. Abnormally low aPTT (lower than the lower limit of normal)
   d. History of previous intracranial hemorrhage

Answer D is correct. History of previous intracranial hemorrhage is just one of the contraindications for thrombolytic therapy. Additional contraindications include the following:

- Significant head trauma or prior stroke in previous 3 months
- Symptoms suggestive of subarachnoid hemorrhage
- Intracranial neoplasm, arteriovenous malformation, or aneurysm
- Recent intracranial or intraspinal surgery
- Elevated blood pressure (systolic > 185 mm Hg or diastolic > 110 mm Hg)
- Active internal bleeding
- Blood glucose concentration < 50 mg/dL
- Acute bleeding diathesis
- Heparin received within 48 hours, resulting in abnormally elevated activated partial thromboplastin time (aPTT) greater than the upper limit of normal
- Current use of anticoagulant with INR > 1.7 or PT > 15 seconds
- Current use of direct thrombin inhibitors or direct factor Xa inhibitors with elevated sensitive laboratory tests
- Presence of multilobar infarction (hypodensity more than one-third of the cerebral hemisphere)

3. What is the dosing recommendation for alteplase (tPA) in ischemic stroke?
   a. Loading dose: 0.09 mg/kg
   b. Loading dose: 0.9 mg/kg
   c. Loading dose: 9 mg/kg
   d. Loading dose: 90 mg/kg

Answer A is correct. The loading dose for tPA is 0.09 mg/kg (10% of 0.9 mg/kg dose) as an IV bolus over 1 minute, followed by 0.81 mg/kg (90% of 0.9 mg/kg dose) as a continuous infusion over 60 minutes. The maximum daily dose is 90 mg.

A 76-year-old Hispanic male who weighs 78 kg presents to the hospital. He is an active smoker who has a history of hypertension, insomnia, and chronic obstructive pulmonary disease (COPD). Two weeks ago, he began to experience substernal chest pain and dyspnea on exertion, with the pain radiating to his right arm and being associated with nausea and diaphoresis. He has had more frequent episodes recently, and yesterday had four to five episodes that were relieved with rest. Today he had 8/10 chest pain and went to the emergency department of a rural community hospital within 2 hours later. He was acutely dyspneic and had ongoing pain. Vital signs include HR 42 beats per minute (sinus bradycardia) and BP 104/48 mm Hg. Laboratory results include SCr 2.5 mg/dL and troponin 1.5 mcg/L (less than 0.1 mcg/L). His ECG shows a 3-mm ST-segment elevation. Aspirin, ticagrelor, morphine, and sublingual nitroglycerin were given in the emergency department. The nearest hospital with a catheterization laboratory facility is 2.5 hours away.

1. **The treatment team assesses this patient for treatment with tenecteplase and asks for your opinion. What do you tell them?**
   a. He can be treated with thrombolytics.
   b. He should not be treated with thrombolytics.

Answer A is correct. Because the patient is 2.5 hours away from a catheterization laboratory, he can be treated with thrombolytics. The goal for the medical contact to thrombolytic administration time is 30 minutes. STEMI is due to ischemia from a complete occlusion, and thrombolytics can help relieve some of the occlusions.

2. **Which dose of tenecteplase would be appropriate for this patient?**
   a. Administer a single weight-based bolus over 5 seconds
   b. Administer a weight-based dose by continuous infusion
   c. Administer the standard (non-weight-based) bolus STAT
   d. Administer the standard (non-weight-based) dose by continuous infusion

Answer A is correct. Administer a single weight-based bolus over 5 seconds based on the following guidelines:

Weight < 60 kg: 30 mg
Weight ≥ 60 to < 70 kg: 35 mg
Weight ≥ 70 to < 80 kg: 40 mg
Weight ≥ 80 to < 90 kg: 45 mg
Weight ≥ 90 kg: 50 mg

3. **What are some ways to monitor for signs of bleeding following administration of tPA?**
   a. Hematuria
   b. Tachycardia
   c. Hypotension
   d. All of these are correct.

Answer D is correct. Monitor for physical signs of bleeding (hematuria, GI bleeding, gingival bleeding), complete blood count (CBC), partial thromboplastin time (PTT), signs of hemorrhagic shock including tachycardia, hypotension, and so on.

JD is a 72-year-old male whose past medical history is significant for hypertension, hyperlipidemia, COPD, anxiety, post-traumatic stress disorder (PTSD), diabetes mellitus (DM), and psoriasis. He presents to the emergency room with crushing chest pain that radiates to his jaw and down his left arm. His stat labs in the emergency department reveal elevated troponins, and his EKG is positive for T-wave inversions. He was taken to the catheterization lab and had two drug-eluting stents placed in his coronary arteries. JD is admitted to the telemetry unit and started on metoprolol tartrate, lisinopril, and atorvastatin. The physician wants to put the patient on an antiplatelet regimen.

1. Which antiplatelet regimen should JD receive for outpatient therapy after his stent placements?

   a. Warfarin
   b. Apixaban
   c. Dabigatran
   d. Clopidogrel

Answer D is correct. Aspirin and either clopidogrel, prasugrel, or ticagrelor are options for post-stent antiplatelet therapy. The other agents listed here are anticoagulants.

2. How long should this patient receive antiplatelet therapy?

   a. 30 days
   b. 60 days
   c. 6 months
   d. 12 months

Answer D is correct. Aspirin should be given indefinitely and the P2Y12 agent (clopidogrel, prasugrel, or ticagrelor) for at least 12 months.

RK is a 66-year-old, 70-kg woman with a history of myocardial infarction (MI), migraines, hyperlipidemia, and diabetes mellitus. She presents with sweating, nausea, vomiting, and shortness of breath, followed by a bandlike upper-chest pain (8/10) radiating to her left arm. The EKG showed ST-segment depression in multiple leads and hyperdynamic T waves and positive cardiac enzymes. Her BP is 153/92 mm Hg, and all labs are normal; her serum creatinine (SCr) is 1.3 mg/dL. The patient is diagnosed with non-ST-segment elevation myocardial infarction (NSTEMI).

1. Which dose and route of ASA is appropriate for this patient?

   a. Rectal suppository ASA 160 mg
   b. Enteric-coated ASA 325 mg × 2
   c. Non-enteric-coated ASA 325 mg × 1
   d. Non-enteric-coated ASA 81 mg × 1

Answer C is correct. The patient should chew and swallow a single dose of non-enteric-coated aspirin, 162–325 mg. Clopidogrel may be given if the patient has aspirin allergy or GI intolerance.

2. What is the dose of clopidogrel for initiation and maintenance for RK?

   a. Loading dose of 3 mg, followed by 7.5 mg once daily for up to 1 year
   b. Loading dose of 30 mg, followed by 75 mg once daily for up to 1 year
   c. Loading dose of 300 mg, followed by 75 mg once daily for up to 1 month
   d. Loading dose of 300 mg, followed by 75 mg once daily for up to 1 year

Answer D is correct.

3. Given that patients are often started on acid suppressants such as a proton-pump inhibitor (PPI) for primary prophylaxis after GI bleeding during anticoagulation therapy, what is the concern for initiating this patient on pantoprazole?

   a. The drugs' interaction may exaggerate the effects of clopidogrel.
   b. The drugs' interaction may decrease the effects of clopidogrel.
   c. Pantoprazole has been associated with increased bleeding.
   d. Pantoprazole has been associated with decreased bleeding.

Answer B is correct. Pantoprazole is a hepatic enzyme inhibitor and may decrease serum concentrations of the active metabolite of clopidogrel. Due to the possible risk for impaired clopidogrel effectiveness, clinicians should carefully consider the need for proton-pump inhibitor therapy in patients receiving clopidogrel. Other acid-lowering therapies do not appear to interact with this medication.

AL, a 67-year-old Caucasian male, presents to the emergency department with complaints of abdominal pain, nausea, and dark tarry stools for the last 2 days. HE has a history of an MI 8 months ago and he received percutaneous coronary intervention (PCI) for it. His home medications include lisinopril 20 mg daily, metformin 500 mg twice daily, ticagrelor 90 mg twice daily, and naproxen 500 mg every 12 hours as needed. The patient has been adherent with all of these medications until yesterday, when the pain and nausea became too severe for AL to swallow.

1. What is the primary problem for this patient?
   a. Uncontrolled diabetes
   b. Uncontrolled pain
   c. Uncontrolled bleeding
   d. Uncontrolled blood pressure

Answer C is correct. AL is likely experiencing an upper GI bleed. The melenic stools are a result of RBC being digested down the GI tract.

2. Which medication(s) could have been the major cause for his GI bleed?
   a. Naproxen
   b. Metformin
   c. Lisinopril
   d. Acetaminophen

Answer A is correct. Ticagrelor and naproxen could be causative agents. All antiplatelet agents and anticoagulants increase the risk for bleeding within the body, and this risk is further increased when multiple medications with high bleeding risks are administered together.

5.3 Hematopoietic Agents

The hematopoietic agents are used for a variety of disorders to stimulate production of red blood cells, white blood cells, or platelets. As a class, these agents require specific attention to dosing and monitoring, which may vary based on factors such as the underlying disease state, the patient's actual or ideal body weight, laboratory values, and timing of chemotherapy. As most of these agents are dosed intravenously (IV) or subcutaneously (SC), it is also important to understand rates of administration and diluent requirements. Due to these issues, most of these agents will be administered under a strict, disease-state-specific protocol with close clinical monitoring. The most significant adverse reactions associated with these agents are infusion related reactions, which can be significant (e.g., hypotension, bradycardia).

Hematopoietic Agents

Darbepoetin alfa
Eltrombopag
Epoetin alfa
Filgrastim
Oprelvekin
Pegfilgrastim
Plerixafor
Romiplostim
Sargramostim

Case Studies and Conclusions

KD is a 63-year-old, 77-kg male with a history of diabetes mellitus type 2, hypertension, and end-stage renal disease. He is dependent on hemodialysis, and he receives dialysis every Monday, Wednesday, and Friday. Over the past 6 months, he has become more fatigued overall, and tires much more easily during his daily activities. Therapy was initiated with oral ferrous sulfate 325 mg 3 times daily, but KD's symptoms have not improved. Over the last two weeks, his hemoglobin and hematocrit levels have been low, and he has required two blood transfusions (one each week) after the Wednesday dialysis sessions. His nephrologist is initiating erythropoietin 8000 units subcutaneously every Wednesday.

1. Which factor(s) is (are) critical to consider prior to initiation of erythropoietin therapy?

   a. Other potential causes of anemia
   b. The patient's ability to come to clinic for injections
   c. Whether the patient has diabetes
   d. All of these are critical factors.

Answer A is correct. Prior to initiation of erythropoietin therapy, a full anemia workup should be completed to rule out other sources of potential blood loss or causes. For anemia associated with CKD, a hemoglobin level of less than 10 g/dL should be confirmed prior to initiation of erythropoietin. These injections are frequently administered at home, so travel to the clinic may not be necessary. Comorbid illnesses such as diabetes, though important, do not represent a critical factor when considering initiation of this medication.

2. Which monitoring is required for erythropoietin therapy?

   a. Rash
   b. Blood pressure
   c. Pruritus
   d. All of these are correct.

Answer D is correct. Patients should be monitored for adverse effects such as hypertension, fever, headache, pruritus, and rash. Hemoglobin levels should be monitored weekly, but dose increases should occur only every 4 weeks. If the hemoglobin level increases to more than 11 g/dL, erythropoietin should be discontinued.

Although the medication is effective, KD stops taking the erythropoietin due to its cost (his insurance plan prefers the use of darbepoetin).

3. How could he be transitioned over to this alternative agent?

   a. These products are not similar, so they are not interchangeable.
   b. These products are interchangeable at equal doses and schedules.
   c. Refer to the darbepoetin package labeling for the conversion strategy.
   d. Erythropoietin 80 units once weekly converts to darbepoetin 25 mg once weekly.

Answer C is correct. The efficacies of erythropoietin and darbepoetin are similar, and it is common that one agent may be preferred over the other by an insurance formulary. The darbepoetin package labeling includes a guide for conversion, and erythropoietin 8000 units once weekly would convert to darbepoetin 25 mcg once weekly.

A 55-year-old, 68-kg female is being treated for acute myeloid leukemia (AML) and has just completed her induction chemotherapy. The plan is for her to receive a second course, if needed, after assessment of response from the induction. Due to concern about the potential for chemotherapy-induced neutropenia, the decision is made to treat the patient with a hematopoietic growth factor.

1. Which monitoring is required for hematopoietic growth factor therapy?

   a. Chest pain
   b. Skin rash
   c. Headache
   d. All of these are correct.

Answer D is correct. The two agents most commonly used in the setting of AML are filgrastim and sargramostim. Both need to be monitored during the dose infusion for adverse reactions such as headache, chest pain, skin rash, and dyspnea. More severe effects associated with sargramostim include respiratory distress, syncope, tachycardia, and hypotension.

2. Which other important factors should be considered for filgrastim therapy?

   a. Doses should be administered slowly by continuous IV over 24 hours.
   b. Doses must be administered after 48 hours have elapsed since the chemotherapy dose.
   c. Doses should be administered only when the patient's ANC is greater than 10,000/mm^3.
   d. Doses should be administered as a 15- to 30-minute IV infusion.

Answer D is correct. There are three formulations of filgrastim, but only two are labeled for dose increases in AML. If the patient requires dose adjustment, only the Neupogen or Zarxio formulations should be used. All doses should be administered as a 15- to 30-minute IV infusion, should not be given more than 24 hours before or after chemotherapy, and should be discontinued if the ANC is greater than 10,000/mm^3.

5.4 Hemorrheologic Agents

Hemorrheologic agents decrease the viscosity of blood to improve its flow properties. Pentoxifylline (Trental) is an oral blood viscosity-reducing agent that enhances peripheral tissue oxygenation. By increasing erythrocyte flexibility and platelet disaggregation, pentoxifylline decreases blood thickness and increases blood flow. It is commonly used to improve function and symptoms in patients experiencing intermittent claudication due to chronic occlusive arterial disease of the limbs. Pentoxifylline is often taken three times a day with meals to alleviate its GI side effects.

Dextran is a complex branched polysaccharide that has plasma-expanding properties. It causes hemodilution by decreasing platelet adhesions and factor VIII activity. The use of this agent requires cautious monitoring due to dextran's serious side effects, which may include anaphylaxis, hypervolemia, renal failure, and a bleeding diathesis. These side effects may be overlooked because they could easily be attributed to the condition for which the drug is being given. Dextran administration should be cautious, starting with smaller bolus volumes of 500 to 1000 mL (Dextran 40) with evaluation of patient's volume status, including but not limited to, blood pressure, heart rate, renal function, and urine output before giving additional bolus doses.

Hemorrheologic agents should be avoided in patients with history of severe hemorrhage or other bleeding disorders.

Hemorrheologic Agents

Pentoxifylline •

Dextran 40 (*see also the Replacement and Removal Agents section in the Electrolytic, Caloric, and Water Balance Agents chapter*)

Case Studies and Conclusions

JT is a 47-year-old female who presents to the emergency department with a chief complaint of vomiting up blood. She is diagnosed with severe GI bleed. On physical exam, her skin is cold and clammy. She is unable to recall her home medication or any recent activity. Her blood pressure is 80/72 mm Hg, heart rate is 123 beats per minute, and respiratory rate is 22. The patient is in a state of hemorrhagic shock. There is a delay in the blood bank's response, so that administration of blood is currently not an option. The physician is considering using dextran 40 to treat JT.

1. How much dextran 40 should be administered?
   a. 50–100 mL of dextran 40 infusion
   b. 500–1000 mL of dextran 40 infusion
   c. 50–100 mL of dextran 10 infusion
   d. 500–1000 mL of dextran 10 infusion

Answer B is correct. Start with 500–1000 mL of dextran 40 infusion. Assess the patient's volume status after the infusion to determine whether additional bolus doses are necessary.

2. What are the monitoring parameters to evaluate this patient's volume status?
   a. Blood pressure
   b. Heart rate
   c. Renal function
   d. All of these are correct.

Answer D is correct. Blood pressure, heart rate, capillary refill time, oral mucosa, coagulation parameters, renal function, and urine output should be monitored to determine volume status.

After 1 hour, JT begins to develop a rash around her cheeks, which then quickly spreads throughout the body. JT's blood pressure soon drops to 61/70 mm Hg, and her respiratory rate is now 30. The physician is paged and when he arrives at the bedside, JT seems to be covered with hives and hyperventilating.

3. What might be the cause of JT's current state?
   a. Neuroleptic malignant syndrome
   b. Serotonin syndrome
   c. Eosinophilia and systemic syndrome
   d. Allergic reaction

Answer D is correct. JT most likely developed an allergic reaction to the dextran 40. The infusion must be discontinued, and this allergic reaction should be properly documented. Benadryl can be used to alleviate symptoms, and intubation might be necessary if the patient's respiratory distress continues.

PN is a 72-year-old Asian male who presents with a complaint of lower leg pain. His physician starts him on pentoxifylline 400 mg 3 times daily for the treatment of chronic lower limb ischemia due to peripheral artery disease. PN presents to the hospital for a follow-up visit a week later. A CBC and Chem 7 are ordered. The patient's platelets are 68 × 103/µL, and his CrCl is less than 20 mL per hour. At this point, it is realized that the patient has a history of CKD. Venous thromboembolism has been ruled out with an ultrasound. Vascular surgeons have also determined there is no indication for surgical intervention.

1. What is the mechanism of action for pentoxifylline?
   a. Increased blood viscosity
   b. Decreased blood viscosity
   c. Increased neutrophil activation
   d. All of these are correct.

Answer B is correct. Pentoxifylline lowers blood viscosity, increases erythrocyte flexibility, increases leukocyte deformability, and decreases neutrophil adhesion and activation.

5.5 Antihemorrhagic Agents

The use of hemostatic agents is an important tool for reversal of bleeding, especially bleeding related to the use of anticoagulant medications. These medications are administered in conjunction with blood products such as packed red blood cells, platelets, fresh frozen plasma, and/or cryoprecipitate. The U.S. Food and Drug Administration labeling of several hemostatic agents carries black box warnings for the risk of thromboembolic events, and each of these agents should be used under the advice of a physician. The most specific agents, such as specific clotting factors, may also require the intervention of a hematologist. The dosing is specific and based on calculations using actual or ideal body weight and the patient's current laboratory values. It is recommended that these calculations be double-checked for accuracy and to prevent medication errors. As most of these products are derived from human sources, patients should be monitored closely during their administration for infusion-related reactions, some of which may be severe (e.g., hypotension, bradycardia).

Antiheparin Agents

Protamine sulfate

Hemostatic Agents

Aminocaproic acid
Antihemophilic factor (human)
Antihemophilic factor (porcine)
Antihemophilic factor (recombinant)
Anti-inhibitor coagulant complex
Factor VIIa (recombinant)
Factor IX (human)
Factor IX complex (human)

Factor IX (recombinant)
Factor XIII (human)
Fibrinogen (human)
Prothrombin complex concentrate (human)
Thrombin alpha
Thrombin (bovine)
Thrombin (human)
Desmopressin (*see also the Pituitary Agents section in the Hormones and Synthetic Substitutes chapter*)

Case Studies and Conclusions

A patient is admitted to the emergency room with a subarachnoid hemorrhage after a fall off a ladder. His computed tomography (CT) scan reveals a bleed with midline shift, and neurosurgery plans to take him to the operating room for an evacuation. He is 69 inches tall and weighs 73 kg, and his labs indicate a hemoglobin level of 7 g/dL, a hematocrit of 24 g/dL, and an INR of 5.3. He is currently taking warfarin 5 mg by mouth daily for a DVT 2 months ago. The patient also states that he takes naproxen 200 mg every 8–12 hours for pain, and has been taking 3 doses per day for the last 5 days due to increased back pain. The ER physician wants to give an agent for reversal of warfarin, and asks for a recommendation.

1. Which agent is most appropriate for this patient's warfarin reversal?
   a. Vitamin K
   b. Fresh frozen plasma
   c. Prothrombin complex
   d. All of these are correct.

Answer D is correct. After administration of vitamin K and fresh frozen plasma, it would be appropriate to consider using prothrombin complex concentrate to reverse the INR due to the need for an emergent surgical procedure.

2. What else should be considered prior to prothrombin complex concentrate (PCC) administration?
   a. History of heparin-induced thrombocytopenia
   b. Hypersensitivity to blood products
   c. Signs of disseminated intravascular coagulation
   d. All of these are correct.

Answer D is correct. Due to the risk of thromboembolism, the decision to give PCC should be weighed against the risk of this potentially serious complication. The patient should be assessed for any history of heparin-induced thrombocytopenia, hypersensitivity to blood products, or signs of disseminated intravascular coagulation.

A patient is admitted to the emergency room with an acute upper GI bleed. Her labs on admission include a hemoglobin level of 6.3 g/dL and hematocrit of 21.5 g/dL. The patient is 64 inches tall and weighs 57 kg. The ER physician wants to administer a hemostatic agent due to the patient's history of hemophilia A.

1. Which agent is most appropriate for this patient?
   a. Vitamin K
   b. Recombinant factor VIIa
   c. Hemophilia complex
   d. All of these are correct.

Answer B is correct. There are numerous options for hemostatic agents, and the choice should be based on the indication and patient history. Potential options for treatment of hemophilia A include desmopressin, recombinant factor VIIa, and antihemophilic factor (recombinant, human, or porcine).

2. What else should be considered prior to factor VIII administration?
   a. The dose should be administered as STAT IM.
   b. The dose should be administered by slow IV infusion.
   c. The dose should be administered subcutaneously.
   d. All of these are appropriate options.

Answer B is correct. The dose should be administered by slow IV infusion no faster than 3 mL per minute, and the patient should be monitored for chest tightness and blurred vision.

Tips from the Field

Antianemia Agents

Remember with iron therapy:

1. Anemia should be reassessed after 6 months of iron replacement therapy. It takes time for the iron stores to replenish to a significant degree.
2. Do not crush or chew extended release formulations of any medication.
3. Iron may stain the tongue or teeth. It is recommended to drink liquid doses with a straw.
4. Oral liquid may be mixed to improve taste with plain chocolate syrup, fruit or vegetable juice (with no milk or dairy added), and whole portion consumed (with a straw) may help.
5. Administer with water or juice on an empty stomach.
6. Administer 2 hours before or 4 hours after antacid. Warn patients not to self-medicate with over-the-counter (OTC) "stomach remedies" that include H_2 blockers, such as Pepcid or Tagamet, or PPIs, such as Prilosec OTC.
7. Oral iron formulations are strong stomach irritants. Extending empathetic understanding of the possible side effects and demonstrating willingness to modify or change therapy to improve patient comfort is key to effective iron replacement.
8. Iron is available in numerous formulations that vary in the amount of elemental iron they contain, the amount of absorption expected, and the potential for stomach irritation.
9. For iron replacement, be familiar with the amount of elemental iron you are using:
   - Ferrous sulfate (20% elemental iron)
   - Ferrous gluconate (12% elemental iron)
   - Ferrous fumarate (33% elemental iron)
   - Polysaccharide-iron complex (100% elemental iron)
10. For parenteral replacement, reassure patients that test doses are meant to ensure their safety. Serious hypersensitivity reactions, including anaphylactic-type reactions (some fatal), have occurred, even in patients who tolerated previous doses. However, test doses can be a life-saving "litmus test." The parenteral formulations require close monitoring for hypersensitivity reactions and changes in blood pressure.
11. Proper storage of medication products is critical; if you obtain these from the pharmacy for later use, be familiar with how these are stored and what to do if there is a deviation from what is the recommended storage (i.e., left out of refrigerator).

12. The parenteral products administered via IM injection can be quite painful; therefore, excellent technique will improve patient acceptance and overall adherence to repeat injection schedules.

13. Although some patients may receive these antianemia products as a short-term therapy, other conditions—such as kidney disease—may require lifetime dosing schedules.

Anticoagulant Agents

1. Anticoagulation therapy represents a number of challenges to practitioners and clinicians.

2. Traditional anticoagulation with warfarin is still relevant and appropriate for many patients, however the newer DOACs may provide alternatives for patients who are not candidates or who prefer not to use warfarin.

3. The effects of warfarin are easily and predictably tracked with the INR blood test, whereas the DOACs are not.

4. The blood thinning effects of warfarin can be reversed with the administration either oral or parenteral vitamin K; however, the blood thinning effects of DOACs cannot be reversed with vitamin K. Current reversal options for DOACs are extremely limited and can only be administered parenterally in the hospital. Most DOACs are not reversible.

5. Keep vitamin K consistent in the diet—it should not be eliminated from the diet! Have a list of vitamin K–containing foods available for your patient. Generally, vitamin K is found in green leafy vegetables such as kale, spinach, and collard greens.

6. Mephyton (phytonadione) is another name for vitamin K and is not the same as K+, which is potassium.

7. Only 1 DOAC (Pradaxa) has a reversal agent available; however, this is not widely accessible as it must be administered in an acute care setting through parenteral administration.

8. The indications for use as well as duration of anticoagulation therapy become challenging and guidelines are subject to change frequently based on new emerging information and new drugs available on the market.

9. Combinations of the agents will be used and you must check guidelines regularly to ensure optimal treatment is being prescribed.

10. Clinician considerations include constant consideration of drug interactions, especially with patient's self-use of OTC medications.

11. When administering IM therapy, be aware that anticoagulated patients are more susceptible to the development of disfiguring, painful hematomas. Often IM therapy is not recommended for anticoagulated patients where safer alternatives exist.

12. It is important to note that while bleeding is the most common adverse effect experienced with anticoagulants and antiplatelet agents, nuisance bleeding (bruising, ecchymosis) is commonly encountered, especially if patients are on dual or combination therapy—and less significant nuisance bleeding events should not lead to therapy cessation. However, confirmation that a more serious bleeding condition (such as prolonged INR) should be ruled out first so the patient is not exposed to unnecessary risk of clot formation with discontinuation of anticoagulation therapy.

13. Patients should remember to ask about the need to discontinue anticoagulation before surgery and invasive procedures; this includes dental procedures as well.

14. Antiplatelet agents are different than anticoagulation agents, but when given together the risk of bleeding can increase.

15. There are appropriate and inappropriate combinations of anticoagulants and antiplatelet agents; refer to resources routinely and always inquire if you are in doubt.

Patients at Risk of Major Bleeding

1. The risk of major bleeding with warfarin therapy is increased during the drug initiation phase (or long-term treatment).

2. Patients who are 65 years of age or older are at risk of major bleeding.

3. The following patients are at risk of major bleeding: those with highly variable INRs and those with a history of cerebrovascular disease (e.g., stroke), GI bleeding, atrial fibrillation, or in the presence of serious comorbid conditions such as cardiac disease, malignancy (neoplastic disease), renal disease including renal impairment or renal failure, anemia or genetic polymorphisms that influence metabolism of this drug.

Conditions That Increase the Risk of Bleeding

1. Recent stroke; severe uncontrolled hypertension; infective endocarditis; advanced renal disease; dissecting aortic aneurysm; peptic ulcer disease; diverticulitis; inflammatory bowel disease; hemophilia; menstruation; hepatic disease (reduced vitamin K dependent clotting factors or vitamin K deficiency).

2. Recent major surgery or trauma, including eye, brain, or spinal cord surgery; lumbar puncture; spinal anesthesia; recent puncture of large vessels or organ biopsy; an anomaly of vessels or organs; or recent major bleeding (including intracranial bleeding, GI bleeding, intraocular bleeding, retroperitoneal bleeding, or pulmonary bleeding).

Tammie Lee and Jacque

Bibliography

Activase (alteplase) [prescribing information]. San Francisco, CA: Genentech; February 2015.

Adamson JW. Iron deficiency and other hypoproliferative anemias. In: Kasper D, Fauci A, Hauser S, Longo D, Jameson J, Loscalzo J, eds. *Harrison's Principles of Internal Medicine*. 19th ed. New York, NY: McGraw-Hill; 2015. http://accessmedicine.mhmedical.com/content.aspx?bookid=1130&Sectionid=79731112. Accessed January 5, 2016.

American College of Emergency Physicians, American Academy of Neurology. Clinical policy: use of intravenous tPA for the management of acute ischemic stroke in the emergency department. *Ann Emerg Med.* 2013;61(2):225-243.

American Geriatrics Society. 2015 updated Beers criteria for potentially inappropriate medication use in older adults. *J Am Geriatr Soc.* 2015;63:2227-2246.

Brass L. Thrombin and platelet activation. *Chest.* 2003;124(suppl):18S-25S.

Cesarman-Maus G, Hajjar K. Molecular mechanisms of fibrinolysis. *Br J Hematol.* 2005;129:307-321.

Cook K, Lyons WL. Anemias. In: DiPiro JT, Talbert RL, Yee GC, Matke GR, Wells BG, Posey LM, eds. *Pharmacotherapy: A Pathophysiologic Approach.* New York, NY: McGraw-Hill Education; 2014:1605-1624.

de Abajo FJ. Effects of selective serotonin reuptake inhibitors on platelet function: mechanisms, clinical outcomes and implications for use in elderly patients. *Drugs Aging.* 2011;28:345-367.

Fagan SC, Hess DC. Stroke. In: DiPiro JT, Talbert RL, Yee GC, Matke GR, Wells BG, Posey LM, eds. *Pharmacotherapy: A Pathophysiologic Approach.* 9th ed. New York, NY: McGraw-Hill; 2014: 279-289.

Furie B, Furie D. Mechanism of thrombus formation. *N Engl J Med.* 2008;359:938-949.

Hoffbrand A. Megaloblastic anemias. In: Kasper D, Fauci A, Hauser S, Longo D, Jameson J, Loscalzo J. eds. *Harrison's Principles of Internal Medicine.* 19th ed. New York, NY: McGraw-Hill; 2015. http://accessmedicine.mhmedical.com/content.aspx?sectionid=79731307&bookid=1130&Resultclick=2. Accessed January 5, 2016.

Hudson JQ, Wazny LD. Chronic kidney disease. In: DiPiro JT, Talbert RL, Yee GC, Matke GR, Wells BG, Posey LM, eds. *Pharmacotherapy: A Pathophysiologic Approach.* New York, NY: McGraw-Hill Education; 2014:633-663.

Jones C, Payne D, Hayes P. The antithrombotic effect of dextran-40 in man is due to enhanced fibrinolysis in vivo. *J Vascular Surg.* 2008;48(3):715-722.

Kidney Disease: Improving Global Outcomes. Clinical practice guidelines for anemia in chronic kidney disease. *Kidney Int Suppl.* 2012;2(4):279-355.

Luzzatto L. Hemolytic anemias and anemia due to acute blood loss. In: Kasper D, Fauci A, Hauser S, Longo D, Jameson J, Loscalzo J. eds. *Harrison's Principles of Internal Medicine.* 19th ed. New York, NY: McGraw-Hill; 2015. http://accessmedicine.mhmedical.com/content.aspx?bookid=1130&Sectionid=79731477. Accessed January 5, 2016.

Mannucci PM, Levi M. Prevention and treatment of major blood loss. *N Engl J Med.* 2007;356:2301-2311.

McEvoy GK, ed. AHFS: *Drug Information.* Bethesda, MD: American Society of Health-System Pharmacists; 2016.

Rasche H. Hemostasis and thrombosis: an overview. *Eur Heart J.* 2004;3(suppl):Q3-Q7.

Smith TJ, Khatcheressian J, Lyman GH, et al. 2006 update of recommendations for the use of white blood cell growth factors: an evidence-based clinical practice guideline. *J Clin Oncol.* 2006;24:3187-3205.

Srivastiva A, Brewer AK, Mauser-Bunschoten EP, et al. Guidelines for the treatment of hemophilia. *Hemophilia.* 2013;19(1):e1-e47.

Tiziani A. *Havard's Nursing Guide to Drugs.* 9th ed. Chatswood, Australia: Mosby Elsevier; 2013.

Trental [package insert]. Laval, Quebec: Sanofi-Aventis; 2007.

White H, Van de Werf F. Thrombolysis for acute myocardial infarction. *Circulation.* 1998;97:1632-1646.

Witt DM, Clark NP. Venous thromboembolism. In: DiPiro JT, Talbert RL, Yee GC, Matke GR, Wells BG, Posey LM, eds. *Pharmacotherapy: A Pathophysiologic Approach.* 9th ed. New York, NY: McGraw-Hill; 2014:245-278.

Symbols

Symbol	Meaning	Symbol	Meaning
▲	Renal impairment: Dose adjustment is recommended.	(BL)	Beers list criteria (avoid in elderly).
■ (gray)	Hepatic impairment: Dose adjustment is recommended.	(PD)	FDA-approved pediatric doses are available.
■	Black box warning exists for this drug.	(GD)	FDA-approved geriatric doses are available.
(QT)	QTc prolongation effects have been reported.	(figure)	See primary body system.

Blood Formation, Coagulation, and Thrombosis Agents

Universal prescribing alerts:

- Known serious hypersensitivity to the specific drug or any other component of the product/formulation selected warrants a contraindication to its use.
- Adverse reactions associated with the use of some **blood formation**, **coagulation**, and **thrombosis agents** include dizziness, drowsiness, vertigo, and fatigue; these agents may also impair the ability to perform tasks requiring mental alertness. Caution should always be recommended when using any new drug for the first time, when there is a dose change, and for continued use of known offending agents.
- Doses expressed are for usual adult dosage ranges only. "Geriatric doses" are assumed to be the same as the adult doses unless otherwise noted with a symbol. When pediatric dosing is available, a symbol will guide the reader to additional prescribing references. Refer to real-time prescribing references for these age-specific doses.
- Use of blood formation, coagulation and thrombosis agents in pregnancy is based on weighing clinical risk versus benefit; safety concerns are not represented in this grid. Refer to the package insert (PI) for more information. Clinicians should continue to provide education about the reproductive risks of any medication and offer risk-reduction strategies (which may include contraceptive use) to women of childbearing age and understand that these reproductive risks may also extend to males. Other medications may decrease the effectiveness of oral contraceptives. Where necessary, an alternative means of birth control should be explored.
- Brand names are provided for those agents still available on the market. Due to the ever-changing product availability, refer to Food and Drug Administration (FDA) resources to confirm the actual brands available. This drug summary is for educational purposes only. Prescribing decisions should be based on real-time comprehensive drug databases that are updated on a regular basis.

Antianemia Agents

Universal prescribing alerts:

- Erythropoiesis-stimulating agents (ESAs) increased the risk of serious cardiovascular events, myocardial infraction, stroke, venous thromboembolism, vascular access thrombosis, and mortality in clinical studies when administered to target hemoglobin levels greater than 11 g/dL.

Drug Name	FDA-Approved Indications	Adult Dosage Range	Precautions and Clinical Pearls
Darbepoetin alfa	Refer to Hematopoietic Agents section.		
Epoetin alfa	Refer to Hematopoietic Agents section.		

Iron Preparations

Universal prescribing alerts:

- Monitor patients for signs and symptoms of hypersensitivity reactions, including blood pressure and pulse during and for 30 minutes or longer (until clinically stable) following administration.
- Accidental exposure to excessive amounts of iron-containing products (i.e., overdose) is the leading cause of fatal poisoning in children and pets. Products that contain 30 mg or more of iron per dosage unit are packaged as individual unit-doses in order to limit the impact of accidental consumption. Patients must be educated to always store any iron-containing products out of the reach of children and pets and in case of accidental ingestion to call the poison control center immediately.
- Anaphylactic and other hypersensitivity reactions have occurred even in patients who tolerated test doses.

Drug Name	FDA-Approved Indications	Adult Dosage Range	Precautions and Clinical Pearls
Generic Name Ferric carboxymaltose **Brand Name** Injectafer	Iron-deficiency anemia with intolerance to oral iron or unsatisfactory response to oral iron Treatment of iron-deficiency anemia in adults with non-dialysis-dependent chronic kidney disease	**Usual parenteral dosing:** IV: for patients who weigh at least 50 kg: 750 mg on day 1, repeat dose after at least 7 days (max: 1500 mg)	• May cause hypophosphatemia, flushing, nausea, vomiting, hypertension • Avoid in hepatic impairment • Lower weight doses available, refer to PI • May repeat course if anemia recurs • Administer as slow IV push at 100 mg per minute or by IV infusion over 15 minutes • Monitor for hypertension during infusion
Generic Name Ferumoxytol **Brand Name** Feraheme ■	Iron-deficiency anemia in adults with chronic kidney disease	**Usual parenteral dose:** IV: 510 mg infused, followed by a second 510 mg infused 3 to 8 days after initial dose	• Administer as a slow IV infusion over at least 15 minutes • Avoid in chronic hepatic disease • Do not administer if patient has iron "overload" • Monitor for hypotension during infusion • May interfere with magnetic resonance imaging (MRI) for as long as 3 months after administration • Requires experienced clinician who is knowledgeable in the use of this agent Associated with: • Serious hypersensitivity reactions, including anaphylactic-type reactions (some fatal), may occur, even in patients who previously tolerated previous doses

Generic Name Iron dextran **Brand Name** Dexferrum (IV) Infed (IM) ■ (PD)	Iron-deficiency anemia Iron replacement therapy for blood loss	Total iron dextran dose (in mL) calculated based on clinical factors = 0.0442 × (desired hemoglobin – observed hemoglobin) × lean body weight (LBW) + (0.26 × LBW)	• Doses should be administered no faster than 50 mg per minute undiluted • Maximum undiluted daily dose is 100 mg • A test dose should be administered prior to the first therapeutic dose • Fatalities have occurred with the test dose • A history of drug allergy (including multiple drug allergies) and/or the concomitant use of an angiotensin-converting enzyme (ACE) inhibitor may increase the risk of anaphylactic-type reactions • Administration recommendation is product specific (IM or IV) • Do not administer during acute phase of infectious renal disease (see instructions for dialysis) Associated with: • Deaths associated with parenteral administration following anaphylactic-type reactions have been reported; use this agent only where resuscitation equipment and personnel are available
Generic Name Iron preparations (oral): Ferrous sulfate Ferrous gluconate Polysaccharide iron complex	Prevention and treatment of iron deficiency	Doses vary with indication for use, formulation selected, and patient's clinical response **Illustrative oral dosing for elemental iron:** Prevention: 60 mg daily Treatment: 100 to 200 mg daily in 2 to 3 divided doses	• US recommended dietary allowance (RDA) of iron varies based on age and sex • Should be reassessed after 6 months of therapy • Do not crush or chew extended-release formulations • Administer with water or juice on an empty stomach • Administer 2 hours before or 4 hours after antacid Contraindications: • Do not administer if patient has iron "overload" • Primary hemochromatosis • Peptic ulcer • Regional enteritis • Ulcerative colitis

Drug Name	FDA-Approved Indications	Adult Dosage Range	Precautions and Clinical Pearls
Generic Name Iron sucrose **Brand Name** Venofer (PD)	**Common indication for use:** Iron-deficiency anemia in CKD	**Illustrative doses are hemodialysis dependent:** IV: 100 mg during dialysis to cumulative dose of 1000 mg **Peritoneal dialysis:** IV: 300 mg on day 1 and day 14, then 400 mg on day 28 **Non-dialysis dependent:** IV: 100 mg for 5 doses within 14 days	• Significant hypotension • Patients with underlying cardiovascular disease may see exacerbation symptoms • Use with caution or avoid in patients with chronic hepatic disease • Do not administer if patient has iron "overload" • May administer doses less than 200 mg undiluted as a slow injection over 2 to 5 minutes or diluted over 15 minutes • Not recommended for IM or SQ administration • Administer 300 mg doses over 1.5 hours; administer 400 mg doses over 2.5 hours • Should be administered early in the hemodialysis session • Requires experienced clinician who is knowledgeable in the use of this agent and specialized care setting
Generic Name Sodium ferric gluconate **Brand Name** Ferrlecit	Iron-deficiency anemia, hemodialysis patients	**Illustrative parenteral dosing:** IV: 125 mg elemental iron in 100 mL normal saline (NS) (or undiluted) over 1 hour with each dialysis session	• Patients with underlying cardiovascular disease may see exacerbation symptoms • Use with caution or avoid in patients with chronic hepatic disease • Do not administer if patient has iron "overload" • Significant hypotension • Use with caution in elderly patients • Administer a test dose of 2 mL in 50 mL NS over 60 minutes • Monitor hemoglobin and hematocrit, serum ferritin, and iron saturation; vital signs; and signs and symptoms of hypersensitivity (monitor for at least 30 minutes following the end of administration and until clinically stable)

Antithrombotic Agents

Anticoagulant Agents

Coumarin Derivatives

Universal prescribing alerts:

- A contraindication for all these agents is active major bleeding.

Drug Name	FDA-Approved Indications	Adult Dosage Range	Precautions and Clinical Pearls
Generic Name Warfarin **Brand Name** Coumadin Jantoven ■ (GD)	**Common indications for use:** Treatment, prevent and prophylaxis of deep venous thrombosis (DVT) Thrombosis prophylaxis in atrial fibrillation Stroke prophylaxis in cardiomyopathy	Doses vary with indication for use, dosage formulation selected, and patient's clinical response **Illustrative dose:** Oral/IV: 2 to 5 mg per day **Usual maintenance dose:** Oral/IV: 2 to 10 mg daily Establish maintenance dose based on international normalized ratio (INR) results (goal INR varies with different indications)	• Monitor INR and bleeding risk • Large number of drug–drug interactions and drug–food interactions with vitamin K–containing foods • Doses are individualized based on the patient's clinical response and INR • Changes in dose do not equate to immediate changes in INR • Coumadin effects may be decreased (or reversed) with administration of vitamin K or by "holding" doses until INR returns to therapeutically desirable levels • Duration of therapy is indication dependent • Most common INR goal is 2–3 • Once INR is stable, monitor INR no less than every 4 to 6 weeks Associated with: • Major or fatal bleeding

Direct Thrombin Inhibitors

Universal prescribing alerts:

- A contraindication for all these agents is active major bleeding.

Drug Name	FDA-Approved Indications	Adult Dosage Range	Precautions and Clinical Pearls
Generic Name Argatroban □	**Common indications for use:** Heparin-induced thrombocytopenia (HIT) Percutaneous coronary intervention (PCI)	**Illustrative parenteral dose for treatment of DVT:** IV: 2 mcg/kg per minute	• Monitor hemoglobin, hematocrit, signs and symptoms of bleeding • Monitor aPPT before and 2 hours after start of therapy • Avoid in conditions associated with increased risk of bleeding; refer to Tips from the Field Contraindications: • Major bleeding

Drug Name	FDA-Approved Indications	Adult Dosage Range	Precautions and Clinical Pearls
Generic Name Bivalirudin **Brand Name** Angiomax ▲	**Common indications for use:** Percutaneous transluminal coronary angioplasty PCI HIT/heparin-induced thrombotic thrombocytopenia syndrome (HITTS)	**Usual parenteral dose for PCI in those at risk of HIT:** IV: 0.75 mg/kg bolus followed by 1.75 mg/kg per hour infusion for the remainder of the procedure	• Renal dose adjustment is needed for creatinine clearance (CrCl) less than 30 mL per minute • Avoid in conditions associated with increased risk of bleeding; refer to Tips from the Field • Monitor activated clotting time (ACT) or activated partial thromboplastin time (aPTT)
Generic Name Dabigatran **Brand Name** Pradaxa ▲ ■	**Common indications for use:** DVT Pulmonary embolism (PE) Atrial fibrillation	**Usual oral dose:** 150 mg twice daily	• Avoid abrupt discontinuation • Drug interactions may require dose adjustments or avoidance of certain drug combinations • Dyspepsia and increased risk of gastrointestinal (GI) bleeding • Do not open capsule or crush medication • Dabigatran therapy cannot begin until the INR is less than 2 Contraindications: • Mechanical prosthetic heart valves
Generic Name Desirudin **Brand Name** Iprivask ▲	**Common indications for use:** DVT prophylaxis	**Illustrative parenteral dosing:** SQ: 15 mg every 12 hours	• Monitor activated partial thromboplastin time (aPTT) Associated with: • Spinal hematoma: Consider the benefits and risks before neuraxial intervention (lumbar puncture, epidural, or spinal anesthesia)
Direct Factor Xa Inhibitors			
Universal prescribing alerts: • A contraindication for all these agents is active major bleeding.			

Drug Name	FDA-Approved Indications	Adult Dosage Range	Precautions and Clinical Pearls
Generic Name Apixaban **Brand Name** Eliquis ▲ ■ (GD)	**Common indications for use:** DVT PE Atrial fibrillation DVT prophylaxis-post hip and knee surgery	**Usual oral dose for DVT treatment:** 10 mg twice daily for 7 days, followed by 5 mg daily twice daily for at least 6 months	• Can be crushed and be given through an NG tube • Drug interactions may require dose adjustment or avoidance of certain drug combinations • Dosing strategies to convert from warfarin, to warfarin or to preferred agents are necessary and available; refer to PI • Use caution in renal impairment • Apixaban therapy cannot begin until INR is less than 2 Contraindications: • Active bleeding Associated with: • Premature discontinuation increases the risk of ischemic events; avoid abrupt discontinuation • Spinal/epidural hematomas
Generic Name Edoxaban **Brand Name** Savaysa ▲ ■ (BL)	**Common indications for use:** DVT PE Nonvalvular atrial fibrillation	**Usual oral dose:** 60 mg daily	• Avoid in severe renal impairment (i.e., CrCl less than 15 mL per minute) • Avoid in patients with moderate to severe hepatic impairment • Discontinue at least 24 hours prior to surgery and invasive procedures • Patients weighing 60 kg or less require half the usual dose Associated with: • Hemorrhage, abnormal hepatic function tests, and epistaxis • Reduced efficacy in patients with nonvalvular atrial fibrillation and CrCl greater than 95 mL per minute • Premature discontinuation increases the risk of ischemic events • Spinal/epidural hematomas
Generic Name Fondaparinux **Brand Name** Arixtra ▲ ■	**Common indications for use:** Acute DVT Acute PE DVT prophylaxis	Dose is based on weight **Usual parenteral dose for patients weighing 50 to 100 kg:** SQ: 7.5 mg daily	• Monitor complete blood count (CBC), platelet count, serum creatinine, and blood testing of stools • Patients weighing less than 50 kg or more than 100 kg require dose adjustments • Doses are administered subcutaneously Contraindications: • Severe renal impairment (i.e., CrCl less than 30 mL per minute) • Avoid in conditions associated with increased risk of bleeding; refer to Tips from the Field Associated with: • Spinal hematoma: Consider the benefits and risks before neuraxial intervention (lumbar puncture, epidural, or spinal anesthesia)

Drug Name	FDA-Approved Indications	Adult Dosage Range	Precautions and Clinical Pearls
Generic Name Rivaroxaban **Brand Name** Xarelto ▲ ■	**Common indications for use:** DVT prophylaxis and treatment PE prophylaxis and treatment Atrial fibrillation (Afib)	**Usual oral dose for stroke prevention in AFib:** 20 mg daily	• Must be given with a meal for absorption • Can be crushed and given through a nasogastric (NG) tube • Rivaroxaban can be started when the INR is less than 3 • Drug interactions may require dose adjustments or avoidance of certain drug combinations Contraindications: • Renal impairment (CrCl less than 30 mL per minute for DVT/PE and prophylaxis; CrCl less than 50 mL per minute in atrial fibrillation) Associated with: • Increased risk of thromboembolic events upon abrupt discontinuation • Spinal hematoma: Consider the benefits and risks before neuraxial intervention (lumbar puncture, epidural, or spinal anesthesia)

Heparins

Universal prescribing alerts:

- A contraindication for all these agents is active major bleeding.

Drug Name	FDA-Approved Indications	Adult Dosage Range	Precautions and Clinical Pearls
Generic Name Dalteparin **Brand Name** Fragmin	**Common indications for use:** Prophylaxis and treatment DVT PE Unstable angina	**Usual parenteral dose for treatment of DVT:** SQ: 200 IU/kg once daily for first month (maximum single dose: 18,000 IU), then 150 IU/kg once daily (maximum single dose: 18,000 IU) during months 2 to 6.	• Consists of smaller heparin molecules than unfractionated heparin (UFH), therefore considered low-molecular-weight heparin • Administer the prefilled syringe that contains the closest calculated dose • Use caution in renal impairment • Monitor CBC and platelet count Contraindications: • Active major bleeding and patients at risk of adverse effects (such as unstable angina or non-Q-wave MI) Associated with: • Spinal hematoma: Consider the benefits and risks before neuraxial intervention (lumbar puncture, epidural, or spinal anesthesia)

Generic Name Enoxaparin **Brand Name** Lovenox ▲ ■ (BL) (PD)	**Common indications for use:** Acute coronary syndromes DVT prophylaxis DVT	**Illustrative parenteral dose for DVT prophylaxis:** SQ: 30 mg every 12 hours **Alternatively may give:** 40 mg every 24 hours **DVT Treatment:** SQ: 1 mg/kg every 12 hours, up to 1.5 mg/kg per day	• Considered low-molecular-weight • Monitor platelets, occult blood, anti-factor Xa level, and serum creatinine • Dose and duration of treatment is indication specific • Specific recommendations for patients undergoing dialysis • Avoid in conditions associated with increased risk of bleeding; refer to Tips from the Field Associated with: • Spinal hematoma: Consider the benefits and risks before neuraxial intervention (lumbar puncture, epidural, or spinal anesthesia)
Generic Name Heparin (PD)	**Common indications for use:** Thromboprophylaxis DVT PE Line flushing	**Illustrative parenteral dose for prophylaxis:** IV bolus: 5000 units every 8 to 12 hours	• Monitor aPTT every 4 to 6 hours after treatment • Avoid in conditions associated with increased risk of bleeding; refer to Tips from the Field • Spinal hematoma: Consider the benefits and risks before neuraxial intervention (lumbar puncture, epidural, or spinal anesthesia)

Miscellaneous Anticoagulant Agents

Drug Name	FDA-Approved Indications	Adult Dosage Range	Precautions and Clinical Pearls
Generic Name Antithrombin alpha Antithrombin III **Brand Name** Thrombate ATryn	**Common indications for use:** Congenital antithrombin III deficiency	Dosing is individualized	• Thrombate III is derived from pooled human plasma; risk of transmission of viral illness • IM injections should not be administered to patients receiving this agent; may cause bleeding, bruising, or hematomas

Drug Name	FDA-Approved Indications	Adult Dosage Range	Precautions and Clinical Pearls
Generic Name Protein C concentrate (human) **Brand Name** Ceprotin	**Common indication for use:** Congenital protein C deficiency and related thrombosis treatment and prevention	**Usual parenteral dose:** IV initial: 100 to 120 international units/kg Subsequent 3 doses: 60 to 80 international units/kg every 6 hours Maintenance: 45 to 60 international units/kg every 12 hours	• HIT • Monitor C protein prior to and during therapy • Monitor signs and symptoms and bleeding • Sodium and fluid overload may occur; monitor patients who are at risk of potential adverse events (i.e., renal impairment) • May cause headache and bleeding

Antiplatelet Agents

Platelet-Reducing Agents

Drug Name	FDA-Approved Indications	Adult Dosage Range	Precautions and Clinical Pearls
Generic Name Anagrelide **Brand Name** Agrylin ■ QT PD	Thrombocytopenia	**Usual oral dose:** 0.5 mg 4 times per day or 1 mg 2 times per day MDD: 10 mg	• Avoid abrupt discontinuation • Use caution in renal impairment • Monitor platelet count, CBC with differential, liver function, BUN • May cause QTc prolongation, avoid in patients who are at risk and may be predisposed to adverse effects

Platelet-Aggregation Inhibitors

Universal prescribing alerts:

- A contraindication for all these agents is active major bleeding.
- Platelet aggregation inhibitors increase the risk of bleeding, especially in patients with predisposing conditions. Patients who are at increased risk (and in whom use of these agents is contraindicated) are patients with any of the following conditions: any evidence of active abnormal bleeding within the previous 30 days, acute pericarditis, intracranial aneurysm, intracranial mass, arteriovenous malformation, any coagulopathy or history of bleeding diathesis within 30 days, severe uncontrolled hypertension (SBP greater than 180 mmHg and/or DBP greater than 110 mmHg), recent (within 6 weeks) major surgery or trauma, history of stroke within 30 days or any history of hemorrhagic stroke, intracranial bleeding, or aortic dissection.

Drug Name	FDA-Approved Indications	Adult Dosage Range	Precautions and Clinical Pearls
Generic Name Abciximab **Brand Name** ReoPro	PCI Unstable angina (UA)/ST-segment elevation myocardial infarction (STEMI) unresponsive to conventional medical therapy with planned PCI within 24 hours	Dose varies with indication for use and patient's clinical status **Illustrative parenteral doses for PCI:** IV: 0.25 mg/kg bolus, then 0.125 mcg/kg per minute (max: 10 mcg per minute) for 12 hours	• Monitor prothrombin time, aPTT • May cause hypotension, chest pain, back pain, nausea, hemorrhage Contraindications: • Thrombocytopenia (less than 100,000 cells/μL) • Any condition that poses an increased risk of bleeding • Severe uncontrolled hypertension

Generic Name Cangrelor **Brand Name** Kengreal	Percutaneous coronary intervention (PCI)	**Usual parenteral dose:** IV: 30 mcg/kg prior to PCI, followed by 4 mcg/kg per minute infusion over 2 hours or the duration of the PCI	• May cause hemorrhage, dyspnea • Use caution in renal insufficiency • Administer bolus by rapid IV push • Begin infusion immediately after bolus • Reconstitute according to manufacturer's recommendations
Generic Name Cilostazol **Brand Name** Kengreal Pletal ■ QT	Intermittent claudication Peripheral vascular disease (PVD)	**Usual oral dose:** 100 mg twice daily	• Platelets and white blood cell (WBC) counts periodically • Administer 30 minutes before or 2 hours after meals on an empty stomach • May cause peripheral edema, palpitations, tachycardia and dizziness; use caution if history of cardiac disease • Use caution in renal and hepatic impairment • Drug interactions may require dose adjustments Associated with: • Contraindication for use in heart failure of any severity
Generic Name Clopidogrel **Brand Name** Plavix ■	UA/non-ST-segment elevation myocardial infarction (NSTEMI) STEMI Recent myocardial infarction, recent stroke, or established peripheral arterial disease	**Usual oral dose:** 75 mg daily	• Loading doses are necessary in some patients • Drug interactions may require dose adjustments; includes interaction with grapefruit juice • Monitor for signs of bleeding; monitor hemoglobin and hematocrit periodically Contraindications: • Peptic ulcer or active GI bleeding • Intracranial hemorrhage Associated with: • Diminished effect in patients identified as poor hepatic metabolizers; consider alternative treatment
Generic Name Eptifibatide **Brand Name** Integrilin ▲	Acute coronary syndrome PCI	**Illustrative parenteral dose:** IV: 180 mcg/kg bolus administered immediately before PCI, followed by 2 mcg/kg per minute continuous IV infusion	• Monitor coagulation parameters and signs and symptoms of excessive bleeding • Used in combination with aspirin (unless contraindicated) and heparin • Maximum doses are established based on patient's weight, refer to PI Contraindications: • Severe hypertension (greater than 200/110 mm Hg) • History of stroke within 30 days • Any active bleeding

Drug Name	FDA-Approved Indications	Adult Dosage Range	Precautions and Clinical Pearls
Generic Name Prasugrel **Brand Name** Effient ■	Acute coronary syndrome to be managed with PCI	**Usual oral dose:** 60 mg oral (loading) 10 mg daily (maintenance)	• Monitor hemoglobin and hematocrit periodically • Use is not recommended in patients older than 75 years • Asian patients and those weighing less than 60 kg may have higher concentration of active metabolite; use caution in this population (bleeding risk may be increased) • Use caution in renal impairment Contraindications: • Prior transient ischemic attack (TIA) or stroke Associated with: • Significant and sometimes fatal bleeding has been reported
Generic Name Ticagrelor **Brand Name** Brilinta ■	Acute coronary syndrome	**Usual oral dose:** 180 mg (loading) 90 mg twice daily (maintenance)	• Monitor for signs of bleeding, hemoglobin and hematocrit periodically, and renal function • Drug interactions may require dose adjustments • May cause dyspnea • May administer via NG tube • Avoid in severe hepatic impairment Contraindications: • History of intracranial hemorrhage Associated with: • Risk of bleeding, including significant and sometimes fatal bleeding • Plan to decrease the risk of bleeding, discontinue ticagrelor at least 5 days prior to any surgery when possible; do not start ticagrelor in patients planned to undergo urgent coronary artery bypass graft surgery (CABG)
Generic Name Ticlopidine ■ (BL)	Stroke prevention Coronary artery stenting	**Usual oral dose:** 250 mg twice daily	• Administer with food • Remind patients of the importance of good oral hygiene • Monitor clinical and hematologic status and signs of bleeding; perform CBC with differential every 2 weeks starting the second week through the third month of treatment or sooner if clinically indicated • Use caution in renal impairment Contraindications: • Hepatic disease or impairment Associated with: • Aplastic anemia, agranulocytosis and bone marrow suppression • Contraindicated in patients with blood dyscrasia • Increased total cholesterol and triglycerides • Diarrhea

Drug Name	FDA-Approved Indications	Adult Dosage Range	Precautions and Clinical Pearls
Generic Name Tirofiban **Brand Name** Aggrastat ▲	UA/STEMI	**Usual parenteral loading dose:** IV: 25 mcg/kg over 5 minutes or less **Usual parenteral maintenance dose:** IV: 0.15mcg/kg per minute continued for up to 18 hours	• Monitor platelet count (baseline; 6 hours after initiation and daily thereafter during therapy) • Venipuncture, arterial puncture, intramuscular injections, spinal or epidural procedures (e.g., spinal anesthesia, epidural anesthesia or lumbar puncture), use of urinary catheters, nasogastric tubes, and nasotracheal intubation should be minimized during use Contraindications: • Major surgical procedure • Severe physical trauma within the previous month
Aspirin	Refer to the Central Nervous System Agents chapter.		
Dipyridamole	Refer to the Cardiovascular Agents chapter.		

Thrombolytic Agents

Universal prescribing alerts:

- A contraindication for all these agents is active major bleeding.

Drug Name	FDA-Approved Indications	Adult Dosage Range	Precautions and Clinical Pearls
Generic Name Alteplase **Brand Name** Activase Catflo Activase (PD)	Acute ischemic stroke PE STEMI	Dosing is based on weight **Usual parenteral dose for treatment of ischemic stroke:** IV: 0.9 mg/kg (maximum daily dose [MDD]: 90 mg)	• Perform neurologic assessments every 15 minutes during infusion and every 30 minutes thereafter for the next 6 hours, then hourly until 24 hours after treatment • Administer within 3 hours of ischemic stroke • Use caution in renal and hepatic impairment Contraindications: • Recent stroke • Hypertension (HTN) • Fever • Bruising • Nausea and vomiting • Bleeding, hemorrhage, and genitourinary (GU) hemorrhage and factors predisposing patient to bleeding

Drug Name	FDA-Approved Indications	Adult Dosage Range	Precautions and Clinical Pearls
Generic Name Reteplase **Brand Name** Retavase Half-Kit [DSC] Retavase [DSC]	STEMI	**Usual parenteral dose:** IV: 10 units administered over 2 minutes, followed by a second dose 30 minutes later of 10 units over 2 minutes	• Withhold second dose if serious bleeding or anaphylaxis occurs • Use caution in renal and hepatic impairment • Monitoring: signs of bleeding (hematuria, GI bleeding, gingival bleeding); CBC and partial thromboplastin time (PTT); ECG Contraindications: • History of cerebrovascular accident • Recent (i.e., within 2 months) intracranial or intraspinal surgery or trauma • Intracranial neoplasm, arteriovenous malformations, or aneurysm • Known bleeding diathesis • Severe uncontrolled hypertension
Generic Name Tenecteplase **Brand Name** TNKase	STEMI	Dosing is based on weight IV: The recommended total dose should not exceed 50 mg and is based on weight **Illustrative dosing for patients weighing at least 60 kg but no more than 69 kg:** IV: 35 mg bolus over 5 seconds	• Monitor CBC, aPTT, signs and symptoms of bleeding, and ECG • Use caution in renal and hepatic impairment • Avoid IM injections within the first few hours of administration; hematomas are more likely Contraindications: • History of cerebrovascular accident • Recent (i.e., within 2 months) intracranial/intraspinal surgery or trauma • Intracranial neoplasm, arteriovenous malformation, or aneurysm • Bleeding tendency or predisposition • Severe uncontrolled hypertension

Hematopoietic Agents

Drug Name	FDA-Approved Indications	Adult Dosage Range	Precautions and Clinical Pearls
Generic Name Darbepoetin alfa **Brand Name** Aranesp	Anemia	Dosing is based on patient's clinical status: **Illustrative parenteral dosing:** Patient on dialysis: IV/SQ: Initial: 0.45 mcg/kg once weekly OR 0.75 mcg/kg once every 2 weeks	• Initiate therapy when Hgb less than 10 mg/dL • May cause hypertension, peripheral edema, edema, abdominal pain, dyspnea, cough • Monitor hemoglobin at least once per week until maintenance dose established and after dosage changes; do not increase dose more than once every 4 weeks • Evaluate history of hypertension or seizure and potential risk for thromboembolism prior beginning therapy • Epoetin alfa EPO conversion (in mcg per week) are available, refer to PI

		Patient not on dialysis: IV/SQ: Initial: 0.45 mcg/kg once every 4 weeks	• Must be enrolled in the erythropoiesis-stimulating agents (ESA) APPRISE Oncology Program to prescribe or dispense; ESAs increase the risk of serious cardiovascular events, myocardial infraction, stroke, venous thromboembolism, vascular access thrombosis, and mortality when administered to target hemoglobin levels greater than 11 g/dL
Generic Name Eltrombopag **Brand Name** Promacta ■ ■ (PD)	Aplastic anemia Chronic hepatitis C associated thrombocytopenia Chronic immune thrombocytopenia	Dose varies by indication and patient's clinical response **Illustrative oral dose for chronic immune thrombocytopenia:** 50 mg daily (maximum daily dose: 75 mg)	• May cause rash, headache, fatigue, insomnia, nausea, diarrhea, anemia, decreased appetite, hyperbilirubinemia cough, and fever • Reduce initial dose for patients of Eastern Asian descent • Monitor platelet count • Use the minimum dose to maintain platelet count of at least 50,000/mm^3 • Dose adjustments are required based on platelet count; refer to package insert • Take on an empty stomach at least 1 hour before or 2 hours after a meal • Do not crush or chew tablets Associated with: • Severe hepatic impairment and hepatotoxicity; use with caution in any patient with preexisting hepatic disease • Risk of hepatic decompensation may be increased in patients with chronic hepatitis C with cirrhosis
Generic Name Epoetin alfa **Brand Name** Epogen Procrit ■ (PD)	Anemia Anemia due to chemotherapy Surgery patients	Doses vary with indication for use and patient's clinical response **Illustrative dosing for anemia:** Initial IV/SQ: 50 to 100 units/kg 3 times per week May require higher doses for different indications	• Initiate therapy when hemoglobin (Hgb) is less than 10 mg/dL • May cause hypertension, fever, headache, pruritus, and rash • Monitor transferrin saturation and serum ferritin prior to and during treatment • Monitor Hgb weekly after initiation; do not increase dose more than once every 4 weeks • Start therapy 10 days prior to procedure • Specific recommendations for patients undergoing dialysis Associated with: • Shortened survival and increased tumor progression in some patients with certain neoplastic disease • Increased the risk of death, myocardial infarction or stroke, congestive heart failure, and thromboembolic events in the higher target groups • Greater risk of death and adverse outcomes for patients with hemoglobin concentration greater than 11 g/dL

Drug Name	FDA-Approved Indications	Adult Dosage Range	Precautions and Clinical Pearls
Generic Name Filgrastim **Brand Name** Neupogen Zarxio Granix (PD)	Myelosuppressive chemotherapy recipients with nonmyeloid malignancies (MCNM) Acute myeloid leukemia (AML) following induction or consolidation chemotherapy Bone marrow transplantation Acute hematopoietic radiation injury syndrome Peripheral blood progenitor cell collection and therapy	Doses are based on indication for use, formulation selected, and patient's clinical response **Illustrative parenteral doses for MCNM:** IV/SQ: 5 mcg/kg per day; may increase by 5 mcg/kg for each cycle of chemotherapy (Neupogen or Zarxio can be increased only)	• Acute respiratory distress syndrome (ARDS) has been reported; evaluate patient if symptoms develop (dyspnea and fever, etc.) • May cause chest pain, fatigue, dizziness, pain, skin rash, nausea, and thrombocytopenia • Dose escalation is based on product-specific guidelines; refer to PI • Administer as IV infusion over 15 to 30 minutes • Do not administer more than 24 hours before or after cytotoxic chemotherapy • Discontinue when absolute neutrophil count (ANC) is greater than 10,000/mm^3 • Monitor CBC and platelets
Generic Name Oprelvekin **Brand Name** Neumega ▲ ■	Thrombocytopenia	**Usual parenteral dose:** SQ: 50 mcg/kg per day	• May cause tachycardia, arrhythmias, edema, fever, hemolytic anemia, insomnia, rash, conjunctival redness • Discontinue therapy when post-nadir platelet count is at least 50,000/mm^3 • Monitor electrolytes and fluid balance (pericardial effusion and ascites have been reported) • Avoid in patients predisposed to arrhythmias • Monitor CBC and platelet count • Administer after chemotherapy; treatment course of greater than 21 days is not recommended Associated with: • Severe acute hypersensitivity reactions have been reported (angioedema, bronchospasm, dyspnea)
Generic Name Pegfilgrastim **Brand Name** Neulasta Neulasta Onpro Kit (PD)	Prevention of chemotherapy-induced neutropenia (CIN) Hematopoietic radiation injury syndrome	Doses are based on indication for use and patient's clinical response **Illustrative parenteral dosing for prevention of CIN:** SQ: 6 mg once per chemotherapy cycle	• Glomerulonephritis has been reported; monitor for hematuria and proteinuria • Splenomegaly and spleen rupture have been reported • Administer to outer upper arms, abdomen, front middle thigh, or upper outer buttocks • Monitor CBC and platelet count • ARDS has been reported; evaluate patient if symptoms develop (dyspnea and fever, etc.) • Do not administer in the period between 14 days before and 24 hours after chemotherapy • Commonly causes bone pain

Generic Name Plerixafor **Brand Name** Mozobil ▲	Hematopoietic stem cell mobilization	Doses are based on weight **Illustrative parenteral dosing for patients weighing 83 kg or more with normal renal function:** SQ: 0.24 mg/kg actual body weight (maximum dose, 40 mg); daily for up to 4 consecutive days	• Dose is based on actual body weight • Administer approximately 11 hours prior to apheresis • Monitor CBC, platelets, and signs and symptoms of splenomegaly • Use hazardous precautions for handling and disposal of this agent • Monitor renal function, and adjust dose accordingly; refer to PI • May cause fatigue, headache, dizziness, nausea, diarrhea injection-site reaction, and arthralgia • Serious and life-threatening hypersensitivity reactions, including anaphylactic reactions, hypotension, and shock have been reported with use
Generic Name Romiplostim **Brand Name** Nplate	Chronic immune thrombocytopenia	**Usual parenteral dose:** SQ: 1 mcg/kg once weekly; adjust dose to achieve platelet count of at least 50,000/mm^3 (max dose: 10 mcg/kg per week)	• Initial dose is based on actual body weight • Dose adjustments based on platelet count; refer to PI for guidance • Use caution due to small volumes (gradations of 0.01 mL) • May increase the risk of hematologic malignancies; use caution in patients with neoplastic disease • May cause hemolytic anemia, dizziness, insomnia, abdominal pain, arthralgia, myalgia, and limb pain
Generic Name Sargramostim **Brand Name** Leukine (PD)	Treatment of neutropenia Acute myeloid leukemia Bone marrow transplant failure or engraftment delay Myeloid reconstitution after allogeneic or autologous bone marrow transplantation Peripheral stem cell transplantation mobilization (autologous) or peripheral stem cell transplantation (autologous) post transplant	Infusion rate (over a specific number of hours) and schedule of administration (specific days) vary based on indication for use and patient's clinical status **Usual parenteral dose for treatment of neutropenia:** IV/SQ: 250 mcg/m^2 per day	• Monitor CBC with differential, renal and liver function, lung function, vital signs, hydration status, and weight (severe fluid retention and pulmonary toxicity has been reported) • Begin 2 to 4 hours following infusion of bone marrow and not less than 24 hours after the last dose of chemotherapy or radiotherapy • Stop treatment or reduce dose 50% if WBC is greater than 50,000/mm^3 and/or ANC is greater than 20,000/mm^3 • Arrhythmias have been reported; use caution in patients who may be predisposed • Hepatic and renal impairment have been reported • Do not administer with an in-line filter • May be administered either IV or SQ (administer SQ in undiluted form) • Rotate injection sites • First-dose effect (respiratory distress, hypoxia, flushing) and anaphylaxis has been reported with use Contraindications: • Concurrent use with myelosuppressive chemotherapy or radiation therapy

Hemorrheologic Agents

Drug Name	FDA-Approved Indications	Adult Dosage Range	Precautions and Clinical Pearls
Generic Name Pentoxifylline **Brand Name** Trental ▲	Intermittent claudication	**Usual oral dose:** 400 mg 3 times daily	• Monitor renal function • Give with meals; may cause nausea and vomiting • Monitor hemoglobin and hematocrit in patients with risk factors for hemorrhage Contraindications: • Recent cerebral or retinal hemorrhage
Dextran 40	Refer to the Electrolytic, Caloric, and Water Balance Agents chapter.		

Antihemorrhagic Agents

Antiheparin Agents

Drug Name	FDA-Approved Indications	Adult Dosage Range	Precautions and Clinical Pearls
Generic Name Protamine sulfate ■	Heparin neutralization	Dose varies based on clinical need of patient: 1 mg of protamine neutralizes approximately 100 units of heparin (maximum: 100 mg IV within 2 hours)	• Coagulation test; aPTT or ACT • Cardiac monitor and blood pressure monitor are required during administration Associated with: • Severe hypotension, cardiovascular collapse, pulmonary edema, and pulmonary hypertension; carefully consider use in patients who may be predisposed to these effects

Hemostatic Agents

Drug Name	FDA-Approved Indications	Adult Dosage Range	Precautions and Clinical Pearls
Generic Name Aminocaproic acid **Brand Name** Amicar	Acute bleeding	**Illustrative dose:** Loading dose: Oral/IV: 4 to 5 grams during the first hour, followed by 1 gram per hour for 8 hours (up to 1.25 gram for oral dose) per hour or until bleeding is controlled up to a MDD of 30 g	• May be diluted in D5W or NS • Evidence of an active intravascular clotting process • May cause bradycardia, hypotension, myopathy, rash, rhabdomyolysis, renal failure, and thrombosis Associated with: • Contraindicated in patients with disseminated intravascular coagulation ([DIC] without heparin)

Generic Name Antihemophilic factor (human) **Brand Name** Hemofil M Koate-DVI Monoclate-P	Hemophilia	Dose is based on weight **Illustrative parenteral dose of Koate-DVI:** IV: 10 international units/kg per dose. May repeat dose if there is evidence of continued bleeding.	• Dosing is based on desired factor VIII increase (to achieve a peak post-infusion FVIII activity concentration of 20% of normal is administered) • Administer by slow IV • Acute hemolytic anemia has been reported • Thrombosis and thromboembolism have been reported in patients predisposed to this risk • May cause life-threatening hypersensitivity reactions
Generic Name Antihemophilic factor (porcine) **Brand Name** Obizur	Acquired hemophilia A	**Usual parenteral dose:** 200 units/kg initially; may redose every 4 to 12 hours	• Administer at a rate of 1 to 2 mL per minute • Use isolated tubing only (not with other medications) • Factor VIII levels should not exceed 200% of normal or 200 units/dL • May cause antibody development and severe hypersensitivity reactions have been reported
Generic Name Antihemophilic factor (recombinant) **Brand Name** Eloctate (PD)	Hemophilia A	Dose is based on weight **Illustrative parenteral dose:** IV: (Dose in International Units) = Body Weight (kg) × Desired factor VIII Rise (International Units/dL or % of normal) × 0.5 (International Units/kg per International Units/dL)	• Administration of factor VIII 1 unit/kg will increase circulating factor VIII levels by approximately 2 units/dL • Use the administration sets provider by the manufacturer • May cause rash, headache, injection-site reactions, arthralgia, cough and fever • Infusion rates are product specific
Generic Name Anti-inhibitor coagulant complex **Brand Name** FEIBA (PD) ■	Control and prevention of bleeding episodes	**Usual parenteral dose:** 50 to 100 units/kg per dose **Maximum:** 100 units/kg for single dose 200 units/kg per day	• Frequency of dosing is based on indication for use • For IV injection or infusion only, at a maximum rate of 2 units/kg per minute • Monitor for control of bleeding • Monitor for DIC if dosage recommendations are exceeded Associated with: • Contraindication in patients with DIC or acute thrombosis or embolism (including myocardial infarction)

Drug Name	FDA-Approved Indications	Adult Dosage Range	Precautions and Clinical Pearls
Generic Name Factor VIIa (recombinant) **Brand Name** NovoSeven RT ■	Congenital hemophilia A or B with inhibitors Congenital factor VII deficiency Acquired hemophilia Glanzmann's thrombasthenia	Dose is based on indication for use and patient's clinical response **Illustrative parenteral dose for congenital factor VII deficiency:** IV: 15 to 30 mcg/kg per dose every 4 to 6 hours	• Discuss the risks and explain the signs and symptoms of thrombotic and thromboembolic events to patients who will receive this agent • Monitor patients for signs and symptoms of activation of the coagulation system and for thrombosis • Administer IV bolus over 2 to 5 minutes • Use NS to flush the line before and after use • Discontinue dosing when hemostasis achieved • Monitor for evidence of hemostasis and thrombosis Associated with: • Serious arterial and venous thrombotic events especially in patients predisposed
Generic Name Factor IX (human); factor IX complex (human) **Brand Name** AlphaNine SD Mononine	Control or prevention of bleeding in patients with factor IX deficiency (hemophilia B or Christmas disease)	Dose is based on weight Rate of administration is based on formulation selected	• Infuse slowly over several minutes; rate is specific to the product formulation selected; refer to the specific PI for guidance • Monitor factor IX levels: measure 15 minutes after infusion to verify calculated doses • Refer to PI for equation to determine the number of units of factor IX required • May cause flushing, thrombosis, burning sensation, chills, photosensitivity, nausea, vomiting, and diarrhea
Generic Name Factor IX (recombinant) **Brand Name** Alprolix BeneFIX Ixinity Rixubis	Control or prevention of bleeding in patients with factor IX deficiency (hemophilia B or Christmas disease)	Dose is based on weight Rate of administration is based on formulation selected	• Some formulations are to be administered by bolus infusion, while others are to be infused slowly over several minutes • Monitor factor IX levels, blood pressure, heart rate, aPTT, and signs and symptoms of DIC and thrombosis • Refer to the PI for the equation to determine the number of factor IX units required Contraindications: • Life-threatening, immediate hypersensitivity reactions (including anaphylaxis) • DIC • Signs of fibrinolysis • May cause injection-site reactions, nausea, and headache

Generic Name Factor XIII (human) **Brand Name** Corifact	Congenital factor XIII deficiency	**Usual parenteral dose:** IV: Initial: 40 units/kg	• Maintenance doses (including increased, decreased, or no-change maintenance doses) are established based on "trough" levels; refer to the PI for guidance • Administer by IV infusion at a rate not to exceed 4 mL per minute • May cause rash, fever, headache, and arthralgia • Monitor the patient's trough factor XIII activity level during treatment Contraindications: • History of anaphylaxis or severe systemic reactions to human plasma-derived products
Generic Name Fibrinogen concentrate (human) **Brand Name** RiaSTAP	Congenital fibrinogen deficiency	Dose is based on weight and baseline fibrinogen levels **Illustrative parenteral dose if fibrinogen level is unknown:** IV: 70 mg/kg	• Infuse at a rate not to exceed 5 mL per minute • Do not administer with other products • Monitor fibrinogen level: target level is 100 mg/dL; maintain this level until hemostasis is obtained • A single dose of 70 mg/kg is expected to increase the fibrinogen plasma concentration by approximately 120 mg/dL • May cause fever and headache
Generic Name Prothrombin complex concentrate (PCC, human) **Brand Name** Kcentra ■	Vitamin K antagonist reversal in patients with acute major bleeding or need for an urgent surgery/invasive procedure	Dose is based on INR and patient's clinical response **Illustrative parenteral dose for patients with pretreatment INR 2 to less than 4:** 25 units/kg (max: 2500 units)	• Contains factors II, VII, IX, and X; protein C; and protein S • Administer vitamin K concurrently to maintain vitamin K-dependent clotting factor concentrations once the effects of prothrombin complex concentrate have diminished • Administer at room temperature at a rate of 0.12 mL/kg per minute • Monitor INR at baseline and 30 minutes post dose • May cause hypotension, tachycardia, headache, intracranial hemorrhage, hypokalemia, nausea, vomiting, arthralgia, and pleural effusion • Use should be weighed against the risk of a thromboembolic event Associated with: • Increased risk of thromboembolic complications • Contraindicated in patients with DIC
Generic Name Thrombin alfa **Brand Name** Recothrom ■	Hemorrhage	**Usual topical dose:** Apply directly to the bleeding site or in conjunction with a gelatin sponge	• Do not inject directly into the circulatory system Contraindications: • Treatment of massive or brisk arterial bleeding Associated with: • Severe thrombosis and bleeding even with topical administration

Drug Name	FDA-Approved Indications	Adult Dosage Range	Precautions and Clinical Pearls
Generic Name Thrombin (bovine) **Brand Name** Thrombin-JMI ■	Hemorrhage	**Usual topical dose for severe bleeding:** Solution: apply 1000 to 2000 units/mL to area of profuse bleeding **Powder:** apply directly to site on oozing surfaces	• Do not inject directly into the circulatory system • Sponge the application surface (do not wipe) prior to use • Hold in place for 10 to 15 seconds Associated with: • Severe thrombosis and bleeding even with topical administration
Generic Name Thrombin (human) **Brand Name** Evithrom ■	Hemorrhage	**Usual topical dose:** Directly apply by flooding the treatment area	• Do not inject directly into the circulatory system • Thrombin (human) is supplied as a frozen solution that must be thawed prior to administration • The volume of thrombin (human) required to achieve hemostasis varies depending on the size of the bleeding area and the method of application Associated with: • Contraindication for use in treatment of massive or brisk arterial bleeding
Desmopressin	Refer to the Hormones and Synthetic Substitutes chapter.		

Chapter 6

Cardiovascular Agents

Author: **Carolyn Hempel, PharmD, BCPS**

Editor: **Gina Prescott, PharmD, BCPS**

Learning Objectives

- Identify current pharmacologic agents that are appropriate for each condition/diagnosis.
- Recommend optimal pharmacologic interventions based on patient-specific characteristics.
- Provide appropriate patient-specific counseling points and optimal overall medication management.

Key Terms: antiarrhythmic agents, cardiotonic agents, antilipemic agents, hypotensive agents, vasodilating agents, adrenergic agents, calcium-channel agents, renin-angiotensin-aldosterone system inhibitors

Overview of Cardiovascular Agents

Understanding the pharmacology of cardiovascular drugs requires a basic knowledge of cardiac anatomy, physiology, and pathophysiology. Such a knowledge base leads to a greater understanding of how to use the drugs based on their mechanism of action. Disease management of cardiologic conditions is based on evidence-based medicine (EBM), with the medication recommendations for most conditions being the outcomes of multiple large, randomized, controlled trials. This chapter provides an introduction to the primary cardiac disease states and the drug classes and drugs used to treat these conditions.

Cardiovascular disease—specifically, coronary artery disease (CAD)—is the number one cause of death in the United States for men and women. Both CAD and ischemic heart disease results from a buildup of plaque in the coronary arteries, known as atherosclerosis. A number of factors, both modifiable and nonmodifiable, put patients at risk for atherosclerosis and CAD. Some of these modifiable risk factors have also represented opportunities for drug therapy interventions such as antihypertensives and antilipemic agents. The nonmodifiable risk factors include advanced age (older than 65 years), sex (male), and family history of cardiovascular disease. Modifiable risk factors include tobacco use, hypertension, dyslipidemia, diabetes, and lack of physical activity or obesity. It is important to recognize a patient's risk factors for cardiovascular disease so as to appropriately counsel and treat patients. Depending on the patient's individual circumstance, counseling points may include smoking cessation, exercising and dietary modifications, and identifying and treating hypertension, dyslipidemia, and diabetes.

Dyslipidemia is primarily classified as increased low-density lipoprotein (LDL) levels and decreased high-density lipoprotein (HDL) levels, and has been associated with increased incidence of atherosclerosis and cardiovascular disease. Current recommendations for lipid-lowering therapies involve assessing a patient's atherosclerotic risk and calculating an atherosclerotic cardiovascular disease (ASCVD) risk score. This risk score incorporates modifiable and nonmodifiable risk factors as well as lipid levels.

HMG-CoA reductase inhibitors, better known as statins, have emerged as the primary class of lipid-lowering therapies used to treat and prevent cardiovascular disease and death. Statins inhibit the enzyme responsible for cholesterol biosynthesis and are the most effective therapies for decreasing LDL levels. Statins also increase HDL levels through an unknown mechanism and have other pleiotropic effects.

Although many other classes of agents may lower or raise certain lipid levels, their use is limited due to the lack of evidence supporting their prevention of cardiovascular events. Agents such as niacin, which directly increases HDL levels, were once thought to be beneficial; however, in a large randomized controlled trial, the use of niacin did not result in improved outcomes. The best way to increase HDL levels is by increasing physical activity. Other classes of agents such as fibric acid derivatives, bile acid sequestrants, and cholesterol intestinal absorption inhibitors are usually reserved for selected patients or patients who do not tolerate statin therapy.

Hypertension, or high blood pressure, should also be accurately assessed and treated to prevent the progression of cardiovascular disease. Treatment for hypertension should begin with lifestyle modifications, but often requires pharmacologic interventions. Lifestyle modifications include limiting sodium intake to less than 2 g per day, weight reduction, smoking cessation, and limiting alcohol intake.

Multiple classes of agents and more than 100 oral drugs are available, as well as additional intravenous therapies, to treat elevated systolic or diastolic blood pressure. These agents can be classified based on their mechanism of action to understand how they affect blood pressure. Hypertensive medications work by two main mechanisms: by targeting cardiac output (heart rate and stroke volume) or by targeting peripheral resistance. According to the most recent JNC 8 guidelines, patients should initially be started on one of four classes of agents: angiotensin-converting enzyme (ACE) inhibitors, angiotensin-receptor blockers (ARBs), thiazide-type diuretics, or calcium-channel blockers. Preference should be given to calcium-channel blockers and thiazide-type diuretics in African American patients.

Coronary Artery Disease and Acute Coronary Syndromes

Coronary artery disease is a disease of atherosclerosis in the coronary arteries that causes an imbalance between myocardial oxygen supply and demand, which then leads to chest pain, also known as angina pectoris. Typical cardiac chest pain is described as diffuse substernal pressure-like pain that may radiate to the back, neck, and jaw, and usually to the left side. It may be accompanied with diaphoresis, nausea, and tachycardia.

Stable angina may be present in patients with a history of CAD and increasing myocardial demand, such as exercise. Angina that occurs at rest, does not resolve after a few minutes, or becomes progressively more severe may be indicative of a more serious condition, known as acute coronary syndrome (ACS). Patients with ACS should seek emergency medical attention to prevent the complications of myocardial necrosis. ACS is diagnosed when a patient presents with chest pain, abnormal ECG findings, and detection of cardiac-specific biomarkers.

Although CAD and ACS are disorders along a continuum, it is important to identify the specific type of chest pain a patient is having, as patients with different disorders will be treated in a different manner. In the acute setting, ACS is treated very differently; however, long-term treatment of these disease states is nearly identical.

The long-term goals when treating patients with CAD or ACS are to decrease angina and to prevent future myocardial infarction (MI). In both cases, treatment should include risk factor modification, as discussed previously. In patients with a history of CAD and ACS, long-term aspirin and statin therapy is indicated to prevent future or recurrent MI. Statin doses vary based on a patient's condition: High-intensity therapy is prescribed for ACS versus moderate- to high-intensity therapy for CAD. P2Y12 inhibitors are also used in the acute management of ACS; they are discussed elsewhere in this text. Other agents that should be used following an MI include beta blockers and ACE inhibitors for those patients with a reduced ejection fraction (EF).

Beta blockers are used in both stable angina and treatment of ACS to decrease myocardial oxygen demand by decreasing the force of ventricular contraction and heart rate. These agents have also been shown to decrease the rates of recurrent MI and mortality after an MI, and are usually continued indefinitely after an ACS.

Calcium-channel blockers (CCBs) may also be used to treat angina and stable CAD. CCBs are classified into two groups: dihydropyridines (DHPs; e.g., nifedipine and amlodipine) and nondihydropyridines (NDHPs; e.g., diltiazem and verapamil). DHPs are potent vasodilators that help release the pressure and resistance on the ventricle, thereby decreasing oxygen demand and causing coronary vasodilation. NDHP CCBs also act as vasodilators, but mainly exert their antianginal effects by reducing contractility and heart rate. NDHPs should not be used in patients with a reduced EF.

Nitrates, which include nitroglycerin and isosorbide dinitrate or mononitrate, may also be used to treat angina. They work by decreasing myocardial oxygen demand and increasing myocardial oxygen supply.

Heart Failure

The most severe complication of CAD is heart failure (HF). Heart failure is classified according to its two main causes: impaired relaxation resulting in diastolic dysfunction, also known as heart failure with preserved ejection fraction (HFpEF), or decreased contractility resulting in systolic dysfunction, also known as heart failure with reduced ejection fraction (HFrEF). Both types of HF cause a similar manifestation of symptoms and volume overload; however, EBM treatments have been shown to decrease morbidity, mortality, and hospital admission only for patients with HFrEF. Therapies that have been shown to reduce mortality include ACE inhibitors and ARBs, beta blockers (specifically carvedilol, metoprolol succinate, and bisoprolol), and aldosterone antagonists (e.g., spironolactone, eplerenone). In African Americans, a combination of hydralazine and nitrates, in addition to the treatments mentioned earlier, have been shown to reduce mortality. Guideline-directed medical therapy (GDMT) is the goal for all patients with chronic HF. Loop diuretics are used in conjunction with GDMT in both types of HF for symptomatic management and treatment of volume overload, but do not have any improved morbidity or mortality benefit.

To compensate for the decreased cardiac output state in HF, there is an increase in sympathetic activity and the activity of the renin-angiotensin-aldosterone system. This results in increased heart rate and volume overload. The agents that have been shown to decrease morbidity and mortality directly block these compensatory mechanisms, which prevent ventricular remodeling. ACE inhibitors, ARBs, and aldosterone antagonists work in HF by blocking the negative effects of angiotensin II and aldosterone, such as volume overload, vasoconstriction, and fibrosis. Aldosterone antagonists should be used in conjunction with ACE inhibitors and have been shown to improve survival in patients on recommended treatment with HFrEF. Caution should be observed, however, as the major adverse effect of these agents includes hyperkalemia. Aldosterone antagonists should not be used in patients with a history of hyperkalemia, and their doses should be carefully titrated, especially when they are used in conjunction with ACE inhibitors or ARBs. These medications are renally eliminated, so the patient's serum creatinine (SCr) should be monitored to determine the appropriateness of therapy.

As mentioned earlier, a notable compensatory effect of HF is activation of the sympathetic nervous system. Certain beta blockers work by inhibiting these negative effects, such as increased heart rate, augmentation of ventricular contractility, and possible stimulation of vasoconstriction through the alpha-receptors. It is important that beta blockers are used cautiously in the acute setting due to their negative inotropic effects. These agents are used for their long-term beneficial effects on morbidity and mortality in HF.

In patients with HF with volume overload, both preload and afterload are increased. Preload is the pressure or volume of blood in the left ventricle at the end of diastole; afterload is the pressure that your heart needs to pump against, such as that caused by hypertension and vasoconstriction of the systemic arteries. In patients with HF, decreasing preload and afterload will improve the contractility and forward pumping function of the heart. Loop diuretics are the mainstay of treatment for symptomatic HF. They work by promoting sodium and water excretion in the ascending limb of the loop of Henle in the kidney, thereby resulting in decreased preload. Loop diuretics, which are the most potent diuretics, include furosemide, torsemide, and bumetanide.

Other therapies for HF include vasodilator medications, which work by dilating the veins, arterioles, or both. Nitrates are mainly venous vasodilators, which help decrease preload in patients with HF. Hydralazine is an arterial vasodilator; it reduces systemic vascular resistance and, therefore, decreases afterload. Hydralazine and nitrates should be used together for optimal effect in those patients who have symptomatic HF and who are African American. ACE inhibitors and ARBs also have vasodilatory effects and decrease both preload and afterload.

Digoxin is no longer recommended as first-line therapy for patients with HFrEF. In HF, digoxin works by inhibiting the sodium-potassium (Na-K) ATPase pump, which in turn promotes calcium influx into the cells and leads to increased contractility. EBM has not shown that digoxin decreases morbidity or mortality in HF, and it may actually increase mortality when used inappropriately. Use of digoxin in HFrEF is restricted to patients who remain symptomatic despite being on optimal therapies and to patients with concomitant atrial fibrillation.

In acute decompensated heart failure (ADHF), patients present with either volume overload or decreased cardiac output. The mainstay of treatment for ADHF includes treating volume overload with loop diuretics and supplementing cardiac output with inotropes so as to maintain perfusion to the vital organs. Dobutamine and dopamine are beta$_1$-adrenergic agonists that are used in acutely ill, hospitalized patients who are in need of hemodynamic support. Milrinone, a phosphodiesterase (PDE) inhibitor, also works in the acutely decompensated patient with HF by promoting vasodilation to improve cardiac output. Once a patient has stabilized, the goal is to get patients on GDMT (i.e., ACE inhibitors, beta blockers, and aldosterone antagonists).

In the setting of HF, it is important to avoid agents that can decrease a patient's cardiac output or increase sodium or water retention. Specifically, NDHP CCBs should be avoided when a patient's ejection fraction is reduced (EF < 40%). Amlodipine is the only CCB that has been shown to be safe in the treatment of patients with HF, but does not add symptomatic, morbidity, or mortality benefits. Other agents that should be used carefully or avoided in patients with HF include nonsteroidal anti-inflammatory agents (NSAIDs), thiazolidinediones, and Class I antiarrhythmics.

Arrhythmias

Disorders that arise from alterations in impulse formation and conduction result in bradyarrhythmias and tachyarrhythmias. Careful analysis of the ECG is required to determine the appropriate therapy that should be administered. Bradyarrhythmias are rhythms in which the heart rate is less than 60 beats per minute and arise from disorders of the sinoatrial (SA)/atrioventricular (AV) node or impaired conduction. Beta blockers and certain calcium-channel blockers may suppress SA nodal activity and cause sinus bradycardia. Disorders of the AV node may also cause conduction impairments that result in AV blocks. Such a disorder may be caused by a number of factors, including use of drug therapies such as beta blockers, calcium-channel blockers, digoxin, and certain antiarrhythmic agents. Usually asymptomatic bradycardia bradyarrhythmias are not treated with drug therapies, but drug therapies that may potentially cause bradyarrhythmias should be assessed and discontinued. Isoproterenol is a $beta_1/beta_2$ agonist that may be used in certain bradyarrhythmias to increase pacing of the heart.

There are two main types of tachyarrhythmias: supraventricular arrhythmias and ventricular arrhythmias, which are defined as a heart rate greater than 100 beats per minute. Supraventricular arrhythmias include atrial fibrillation and atrial flutter. Treatment of atrial fibrillation includes measures directed toward rate control or rhythm control. EBM shows no difference in outcomes when comparing rate versus rhythm control. Nevertheless, rate control is generally preferred as first-line therapy due to the toxicities associated with rhythm-controlled medications. First-line drug therapy for rate control includes the use of beta blockers or nondihydropyridine calcium-channel blockers. Digoxin may also be used along with beta blockers and NDHP CCBs as part of rate control strategies, but is usually reserved for those patients who cannot tolerate an increase in medications but still need additional rate control.

Rhythm control strategies are reserved for patients who are not adequately rate controlled or who are symptomatic. Agents used to treat atrial fibrillation include Class III antiarrhythmics, which are administered to convert patients into normal sinus rhythm or maintain normal sinus rhythm. Amiodarone is the agent in this class that is most widely used in the inpatient setting; however, due to its adverse effects, it is not an optimal long-term medication. Other Class III agents must be carefully monitored. Generally, Class IC antiarrhythmics are avoided because of their proarrhythmic and adverse effects.

Treatment of cardiovascular disease is based on the evidence, so it may change as new evidence becomes available. Careful understanding of pathophysiology and concomitant disorders in patients with cardiovascular disease needs to be applied to select the appropriate medications to maximize the morbidity and mortality benefits of therapy and to minimize the potential adverse effects.

6.1 Cardiac Agents

Antiarrhythmic Agents

Class I antiarrhythmics are designated as IA, IB, or IC based on slight variations in their mechanism of action, but are all considered sodium-blocking agents. Class IA agents, which include quinidine and procainamide, work by blocking sodium and also have potassium-blocking properties. This dual effect results in an increased action potential duration and increased effective refractory period. Although these agents are primarily prescribed to treat ventricular arrhythmias and atrial fibrillation, their use is uncommon today due to their many drug interactions and adverse effects. The most common adverse effects of quinidine include nausea, abdominal pain, diarrhea, and central nervous system (CNS) adverse effects known as cinchonism (i.e., tinnitus, delirium, and hearing and visual impairment). Quinidine is metabolized through the liver, so it has multiple drug interactions. Procainamide is primarily eliminated by the kidney and requires dose adjustments in patients with renal impairment. Agranulocytosis and a lupus-like syndrome that includes arthralgias, myalgias, and rash can also occur with this drug. The major side effects of disopyramide (another Class IA agent) include urinary retention, constipation, and dry mouth. This medication is also metabolized by the liver, so drug interactions are also possible. Polymorphic ventricular tachycardia and torsades de pointes are the most serious side effects associated with this antiarrhythmic class as a whole.

The Class IB agents, which include lidocaine and mexiletine, are strictly used for the management of ventricular tachyarrhythmias. These agents reduce the action potential's duration, but also decrease the effective refractory period. Lidocaine is primarily metabolized by the liver, so dose adjustments are required for patients with liver impairment given the potential for lidocaine accumulation and toxicity. Although lidocaine is administered intravenously for antiarrhythmic indications, topical formulations are available for indications requiring its anesthetic action. Adverse effects are primarily limited to the CNS and include paresthesia, confusion, and seizures. Mexiletine is an oral formulation that is primarily metabolized by regions in the liver where opioids also interact. This Class IB agent also has CNS side effects (e.g., tremors and confusion) as well as gastrointestinal effects (e.g., nausea and vomiting).

The Class IC agents, which include flecainide and propafenone, are used to treat ventricular and supraventricular tachyarrhythmias (i.e., atrial fibrillation, Wolff-Parkinson-White syndrome). They are considered strong sodium-channel blockers and increase the duration of the action potential. These medications are contraindicated in patients with structural heart disease (i.e., post MI or heart failure) due to their potential for precipitating life-threatening arrhythmias. They can depress systolic function and lead to heart failure. Other adverse effects include dizziness, headache, and blurred vision. Propafenone can cause an altered taste as well as nausea and vomiting. Class IC agents are mostly metabolized by the liver.

The Class III agents are the most widely used class of antiarrhythmics and exert most of their effects by blocking potassium channels, which delays the repolarization of phase 3 and increase the action potential's duration and the effective refractory period. The most significant side effect associated with this class of medications is QTc prolongation—a condition that poses an increased risk of ventricular tachycardias such as torsades de pointes. Class III agents (e.g., dofetilide and sotalol) require frequent EKG monitoring to ensure proper dose adjustments for patients.

Amiodarone is the most unique member of the Class III antiarrhythmics, as it also exhibits effects as a sodium-channel blocker, alpha and beta blocker, and calcium-channel blocker. As a result, the possibility of ventricular tachycardias is decreased with use of amiodarone compared to the other agents. In addition, this agent has some vasodilatory effects. It is used in patients with atrial fibrillation and recurrent ventricular arrhythmias. It is given orally or intravenously, and has an extremely long half-life of 40 to 50 days. Loading doses are commonly administered when patients are newly started on this agent. Amiodarone is associated with an extensive list of toxicities—for example, hypothyroidism and hyperthyroidism, optic neuritis, and pulmonary fibrosis—that require frequent monitoring.

Antiarrhythmic Agents

Class IA Antiarrhythmic Agents

Disopyramide
- Procainamide
- Quinidine

Class IB Antiarrhythmic Agents

Lidocaine
Mexiletine

Class IC Antiarrhythmic Agents

Flecainide
Propafenone

Class III Antiarrhythmic Agents

Amiodarone
Dofetilide
Dronedarone
Ibutilide
Sotalol *(see also the Adrenergic Agents section)*

Class IV Antiarrhythmic Agents

Adenosine
Diltiazem *(see also the Calcium-Channel Blocking Agents section)*
Verapamil *(see also the Calcium-Channel Blocking Agents section)*

Miscellaneous Antiarrhythmic Agents

Digoxin *(see also the Cardiotonic Agents section)*
Magnesium sulfate *(see also the Anticonvulsant Agents section in the Central Nervous System Agents chapter)*

Cardiotonic Agents

Cardiotonic agents work to increase ventricular contraction and were once thought to increase myocardial systolic function. The cardiac glycosides are called "digitalis" because they are based on extracts of the foxglove plant, *Digitalis purpurea*. The most commonly used member of this class is digoxin. Digoxin blocks the Na-K ATPase pump, which in turn increases intracellular calcium levels, subsequently causing the heart to be subjected to a greater force of contraction. Digoxin also slows down the heart rate by working directly on the AV node and prolonging the refractory period.

In the past, digoxin was predominantly used for augmenting cardiac output and increasing the force of contraction in HF, but it is no longer used as frequently now that more effective therapies have been developed. EBM studies have not shown a decrease in mortality and morbidity with the use of this agent in patients with HF. As a consequence, digoxin is now largely relegated to the HFrEF indication, in patients who remain symptomatic despite optimal therapies or those with concomitant atrial fibrillation. This drug is excreted unchanged by the kidney and requires a series of loading doses to achieve a therapeutic drug concentration. Maintenance doses are based on renal function.

Because digoxin has a narrow therapeutic index, it is important to maintain a serum concentration in the range of 0.5 to 0.9 ng/mL. Digoxin toxicity—evidenced by CNS changes, gastrointestinal symptoms, and visual changes (including color distortions/yellow halos), among other effects—can result in a life-threatening arrhythmia. Abnormalities with serum creatinine, hypokalemia or hyperkalemia, and hypomagnesemia may result in higher concentrations of digoxin or development of arrhythmias. This risk is of particular concern in patients using loop diuretics, ACE inhibitors, ARBs, or aldosterone antagonists. It is important to ensure that potassium levels are within normal limits. Concurrent administration of digoxin with amiodarone may raise the serum digoxin concentrations. Digoxin is considered a Beers list medication and should be used with caution in elderly patients.

Milrinone and dobutamine are inotropic agents that are used in the setting of acute decompensated heart failure. Although the indications for these agents are similar, their mechanisms of action are different. Dobutamine primarily exerts its effects on $beta_1$ and $beta_2$ receptors, but has minimal effects on $alpha_1$ receptors. Patients with HF often demonstrate blunted responses to the beta-adrenergic receptor responses; milrinone can be useful by working through the phosphodiesterase 3 system to increase cAMP levels, which leads to increased myocardial contractility and vasodilation. Dopamine is a vasopressor agent and inotrope that is useful in the treatment of cardiogenic shock.

Cardiotonic Agents

Digoxin
Milrinone
Dobutamine *(see also the Autonomic-Sympathomimetic Adrenergic Agents section in the Autonomic Agents chapter)*
Dopamine *(see also the Autonomic-Sympathomimetic Adrenergic Agents section in the Autonomic Agents chapter)*

Miscellaneous Cardiac Agents

Ranolazine

Case Studies and Conclusions

TG is a 68-year-old female who has been admitted to the hospital for symptomatic atrial fibrillation. Her past medical history includes hypertension, heart failure, and atrial fibrillation. TG states that she becomes dizzy and short of breath when she goes into atrial fibrillation, and her heart rate is between 130 and 160 beats per minute. TG's blood pressure is normal and the physician does not want to add on any medication that may decrease her blood pressure. TG has been controlled on metoprolol XL 200 mg oral daily, and her physician would like to add an additional rate-controlling agent.

1. Which of the following agents would you recommend?

   a. Dofetilide
   b. Digoxin
   c. Dopamine
   d. Dronedarone

Answer B is correct. Digoxin is a rate-controlling agent that should be added on when a patient is already optimized on a beta blocker or calcium-channel blocker. It is also appropriate for use in a patient with heart failure. When digoxin is prescribed, the healthcare provider will need to monitor renal function and potassium levels, and make sure the medication is dosed appropriately.

A rate-controlling agent was not sufficient to control TG's symptoms, and the physician would like to begin a rhythm-controlling agent to keep TG in normal sinus rhythm.

2. Which of the following agents would be an appropriate choice?

   a. Amiodarone
   b. Propafanone
   c. Lidocaine
   d. Flecainide

Answer A is correct. Amiodarone is the only acceptable answer in this case. Propafanone is a rhythm-controlling agent, lidocaine should be used only for ventricular arrhythmias, and flecainide should not be used in someone who has structural heart disease. Amiodarone and dofetilide are the only two antiarrhythmics that should be used in a patient with HF.

3. Which of the following is a common and significant adverse effect of Class III antiarrhythmic agents?

   a. Agranulocytosis
   b. Parasthesias
   c. QTc prolongation
   d. Myalgias

Answer C is correct. Class III agents work by blocking potassium channels, which results in an increased action potential duration and effective refractory period. The other side effects are not typical of the Class III agents as a whole.

Patient DR is a 55-year-old male who was admitted for ventricular tachycardia and firing of his automatic implantable cardioverter-defibrillator (AICD). DR has a past medical history that is significant for CAD, HF with EF less than 40%, and gastroesophageal reflux disease (GERD). DR was sitting in his living room watching television when he was shocked suddenly. His wife called an ambulance, and he was shocked two more times on the way to the hospital.

1. When DR arrives in the emergency department, which of the following agents would be an appropriate treatment for this patient's ventricular tachycardia and AICD firing?

   a. Dofetilide
   b. Digoxin
   c. Lidocaine
   d. Mexiletine

Answer C is correct. Lidocaine or amiodarone infusion would be the most appropriate answer. Dofetilide and digoxin are primarily used for treatment of atrial fibrillation. Mexiletine is not appropriate because it is only available in an oral formulation, and it is important to first treat this patient acutely with IV therapies.

2. Which of the following is a common adverse effect of Class IB agents?
    a. QTc prolongation
    b. CNS-related effects
    c. Agranulocytosis
    d. Pulmonary fibrosis

Answer B is correct. CNS-related adverse effects are the most commonly seen side effects with the Class IB agents.

6.2 Antilipemic Agents

HMG-CoA reductase inhibitors, also known as statin medications, are the standard therapy for primary and secondary prevention of cardiovascular disease and the most commonly used antilipemic agents. They work through inhibition of HMG-CoA reductase, which prevents the production of cholesterol. Statins are generally well tolerated, but can cause myalgias or, in more severe cases, rhabdomyolysis. If a patient develops symptoms, many can tolerate a retrial with a water-soluble statin such as rosuvastatin or pravastatin. Liver function tests should be performed at baseline, as there have been rare reports of liver failure with statin use. Patients should not drink grapefruit juice with simvastatin, lovastatin, or atorvastatin, as this beverage can inhibit the metabolism of these agents and increase the risk of adverse events. There are also many drug interactions with statins and other agents, most notably with simvastatin. It is important to check for drug interactions, especially with other cardiovascular drugs such as diltiazem and other substrates or inhibitors of the CYP3A4 system.

Bile acid sequestrants exhibit their effects by binding bile acids in the intestinal lumen to promote the elimination of bile acids through the feces. Decreasing bile acids will result in lowering LDL levels; however, use of these medications is limited due their GI side effects, which include constipation, nausea, bloating, and flatulence. Because of their mechanism of action, bile acid sequestrants may prevent absorption of other medications and fat-soluble vitamins (A, D, E, and K), levothyroxine, hydrochlorothiazide, iron, and warfarin. Due to these limitations, bile acid sequestrants are not used frequently, and a large percentage of patients discontinue them within the first year of use.

Ezetimibe lowers cholesterol levels by inhibiting absorption of cholesterol via the sterol transporter in the small intestine. This effect decreases the absorption of cholesterol from the gut, depletes stores from the liver, and increases cholesterol clearance from the blood. Although ezetimibe can be added to statin therapy for additional LDL lowering, little evidence exists that demonstrates this therapy benefits patients with cardiovascular disease. This agent is generally well tolerated, but can cause additive side effects when combined with statins.

Niacin reduces hepatic synthesis of very low-density lipoprotein (VLDL), which decreases production of LDL. Major adverse events associated with niacin use include significant flushing and itching in patients, which limits adherance with this medication and hence its utility. The risk of flushing/itching can be mitigated by pretreatment with aspirin 325 mg. Niacin also increases HDL levels, although in large randomized controlled trials this effect did not translate into better cardiovascular outcomes.

Fibrates promote the elimination of triglycerides and can decrease VLDL levels and increase HDL levels. They are more commonly used for their triglyceride-lowering action and to treat genetic-origin hyperlipidemias. Again, only a limited cardiovascular benefit has been shown with fibrate use. Gemfibrozil is contraindicated with concomitant simvastatin use due to the increased risk of myopathy and rhabdomyolysis associated with this combination.

PCSK9 inhibitors are a new drug class that lower LDL cholesterol in patients who are already taking the maximum doses of statins and following dietary recommendations; they are also approved for use in genetic-origin hyperlipidemias. These monoclonal antibodies target the PCSK9 enzyme, which inhibits the breakdown of the LDL-R receptor and allows for further clearing of LDL from the body. To date, the most common side effects observed with PCSK9 inhibitors are diarrhea and an increased risk of influenza. The cardiovascular disease prevention effects of these medications have not been established. PCSK9 inhibitors are subcutaneous injectable formulations and are costly, which may limit their use in patients.

Antilipemic Agents

Bile Acid Sequestrants

Cholestyramine
Colesevelam
Colestipol

Cholesterol Absorption Inhibitors

Ezetimibe

Fibric Acid Derivatives

- Fenofibrate
Gemfibrozil

HMG-CoA Reductase Inhibitors

Atorvastatin
Fluvastatin
Lovastatin
Pitavastatin
Pravastatin
Rosuvastatin
Simvastatin

PCSK9 Inhibitors

Alirocumab
Evolocumab

Miscellaneous Antilipemic Agents

Icosapent ethyl
Lomitapide
Mipomersen
Niacin
Omega-3-acid ethyl esters

Case Studies and Conclusions

VT is a 55-year-old white male with a history of hypertension. He is currently taking hydrochlorothiazide 25 mg daily and amlodipine 5 mg daily. The current lipid panel shows that this patient's total cholesterol is 200 mg/dL and his HDL is 40 mg/dL. VT does not drink alcohol and smokes 2 packs of cigarettes per day.

1. What is VT's 10-year ASCVD risk?

   a. 6%
   b. 13%
   c. 15%
   d. 25%

Answer C is correct. ASCVD risk calculators may be found on the Internet at http://tools.acc.org. All of the information provided in the scenario is needed to calculate a patient's 10-year ASCVD risk.

2. Which cholesterol therapy would you recommend at this time?

   a. Atorvastatin 20 mg oral daily
   b. Pravastatin 20 mg oral daily
   c. Niacin 500 mg oral daily
   d. Ezetimibe 10 mg oral daily

Answer A is correct. Based on this patient's 10-year ASCVD risk, which is greater than or equal to 7.5%, it is recommended that this patient be initiated on moderate- to high-intensity statins. Pravastatin 20 mg is considered a low-intensity statin. Other non-statin therapies are not recommended; therefore, therapy with atorvastatin 20 mg oral daily, a moderate-intensity statin, is indicated.

3. Which side effects should you monitor while a patient is on statin therapy?
    a. Baseline LFTs
    b. Baseline LFTs and then every 3 months
    c. Baseline creatinine kinase (CK)
    d. Baseline CK and then every 3 months

Answer A is correct. Baseline LFTs should be drawn prior to initiation of statin therapy in every patient, but these tests do not need to be monitored thereafter unless concerns for hepatotoxicity arise. CK monitoring is not indicated unless the patient has myalgias or there is concern for rhabdomyolysis.

4. What is VT's goal LDL level?
    a. Less than 70 mg/dL
    b. Less than 100 mg/dL
    c. Less than 130 mg/dL
    d. No recommendation

Answer D is correct. The new cholesterol guidelines (2013 ACC/AHA Guideline on the Treatment of Blood Cholesterol to Reduce Cardiovascular Atherosclerotic Risk) no longer recommend targeting a specific LDL level, but instead identify specific doses of statin therapies to treat a patient's risk.

6.3 Hypotensive Agents

Alpha$_2$ receptor agonists' mechanism of action in hypertension involves their binding to receptors in the CNS, which inhibits sympathetic outflow from the brain. Binding to peripheral alpha$_2$ receptors on smooth muscle cells results in vasoconstriction. All centrally acting agents are on the Beers list.

Use of clonidine, a central alpha$_2$ agonist, may result in hypotension and bradycardia. Adverse effects associated with this medication include dry mouth and sedation, as clonidine also stimulates parasympathetic outflow. These effects diminish with continued use, but may also be mitigated with transdermal administration. It is important that patients not abruptly discontinue this agent, as they can experience rebound hypertension and withdrawal that can be severe. This medication should be tapered over 2 to 4 days, and patients who are taking a beta blocker should discontinue the use of the beta blocker several days before clonidine withdrawal begins.

Guanfacine is a more selective alpha$_2$ receptor agonist than clonidine. It is as effective as clonidine for blood pressure control, and patients may experience milder side effects than with clonidine. Extended-release guanfacine is also used in children aged 6 to 17 years who have attention-deficit/hyperactivity disorder (ADHD).

Guanabenz and methyldopa are centrally acting alpha$_2$ agonists and have a similar mechanism of action as clonidine. These agents are not frequently used in clinical practice, but methyldopa is still considered the drug of choice for treating hypertension in pregnancy due to its long-term use and the safety data available for its use in this population.

Diuretics are agents that promote water loss through excretion in urine. Commonly termed "water pills," these medication agents also reduce blood pressure as the total fluid volume decreases. These medications have varying degrees of effects on electrolyte panels, often promoting hyponatremia and hypokalemia. Named for their protective effects, potassium-sparing agents can be used when limited loss of potassium is desired, but are not generally considered to be as potent in terms of their diuresis effects.

Hypotensive Agents

Central Alpha Agonists

Clonidine
Guanabenz
Guanfacine
Methyldopa

Direct Vasodilators

Fenoldopam
Hydralazine
Minoxidil

Sodium nitroprusside
Diazoxide *(see also the Antidiabetic and Antihypoglycemic Agents section in the Hormones and Synthetic Substitutes chapter)*

Diuretic Agents

Carbonic Anhydrase Inhibitors

Acetazolamide *(see also the the Antiglaucoma Agents section in the Eye, Ear, Nose, and Throat Preparations chapter)*

Loop Diuretics

Bumetanide *(see also the Diuretic Agents section in the Electrolytic, Caloric, and Water Balance Agents chapter)*
Ethacrynic acid *(see also the Diuretic Agents section in the Electrolytic, Caloric, and Water Balance Agents chapter)*
Furosemide *(see also the Diuretic Agents section in the Electrolytic, Caloric, and Water Balance Agents chapter)*
Torsemide *(see also the Diuretic Agents section in the Electrolytic, Caloric, and Water Balance Agents chapter)*

Osmotic Diuretics

Mannitol *(see also the Diuretic Agents section in the Electrolytic, Caloric, and Water Balance Agents chapter)*
Urea *(see also the Diuretic Agents section in the Electrolytic, Caloric, and Water Balance Agents chapter)*

Potassium-Sparing Diuretics

Amiloride *(see also the Diuretic Agents section in the Electrolytic, Caloric, and Water Balance Agents chapter)*
Eplerenone *(see also the Renin–Angiotensin–Aldosterone System Inhibitors section)*
Spironolactone *(see also the Renin–Angiotensin–Aldosterone System Inhibitors section)*
Triamterene *(see also the Diuretic Agents section in the Electrolytic, Caloric, and Water Balance Agents chapter)*

Thiazide Diuretics

Bendroflumethiazide *(see also the Diuretic Agents section in the Electrolytic, Caloric, and Water Balance Agents chapter)*
Chlorothiazide *(see also the Diuretic Agents section in the Electrolytic, Caloric, and Water Balance Agents chapter)*
Hydrochlorothiazide *(see also the Diuretic Agents section in the Electrolytic, Caloric, and Water Balance Agents chapter)*
Methyclothiazide *(see also the Diuretic Agents section in the Electrolytic, Caloric, and Water Balance Agents chapter)*

Thiazide-like Diuretics

Chlorthalidone *(see also the Diuretic Agents section in the Electrolytic, Caloric, and Water Balance Agents chapter)*
Indapamide *(see also the Diuretic Agents section in the Electrolytic, Caloric, and Water Balance Agents chapter)*
Metolazone *(see also the Diuretic Agents section in the Electrolytic, Caloric, and Water Balance Agents chapter)*

Miscellaneous Hypotensive Agents

Phenoxybenzamine *(see also the Autonomic-Sympatholytic [Adrenergic Blocking] Agents section in the Autonomic Agents chapter)*
Phentolamine *(see also the Autonomic-Sympatholytic [Adrenergic Blocking] Agents section in the Autonomic Agents chapter)*

Case Studies and Conclusions

MJ is a 61-year-old African American male with a history of hypertension, HFrEF, and hyperlipidemia. He is currently on lisinopril 10 mg daily, spironolactone 25 mg daily, furosemide 40mg daily, metoprolol tartrate 100 mg twice daily, and amlodipine 10 mg daily. His blood pressure is still uncontrolled at 160/90 mm Hg, and his physician decides to start clonidine.

1. Which adverse effect is this patient at risk for with the use of clonidine?
   a. Acute renal failure
   b. Atrial fibrillation
   c. Bradycardia
   d. Hyperkalemia

Answer C is correct. Since it is a centrally acting agent (alpha agonist), clonidine will cause bradycardia. There are no concerns for development of acute renal failure or hyperkalemia. Clonidine can also cause sedation and dry mouth.

The patient is admitted to the hospital a few weeks later. His blood pressure is a little low (108/72 mm Hg), but he is hemodynamically stable. The medical team decides to stop his clonidine.

2. Which recommendation would you make?
   a. Stop the clonidine immediately.
   b. Taper the clonidine off first over 2 to 4 days.
   c. Stop the beta blocker first, then taper the clonidine.
   d. Change the patient's clonidine formulation to a transdermal patch.

Answer C is correct. Rapid discontinuation of clonidine can result in a withdrawal syndrome with rebound hypertension; it is important to taper the medication over 2 to 4 days. In patients taking concomitant beta blockers, the beta blocker should be discontinued first and then tapering of clonidine should occur.

6.4 Vasodilating Agents

Nitrates promote the release of nitric oxide from the endothelium, resulting in arterial and venous vasodilation. Venous dilation lowers preload and oxygen demand, whereas arterial dilation lowers blood pressure and oxygen demand. Arterial dilation also reduces vasospasm, which improves myocardial blood flow and oxygenation. Common side effects of nitrates include headache (dose limiting), flushing, tachycardia, and hypotension.

Nitrates have failed to show mortality benefits in clinical trials as treatment for acute MI, but they are widely used for symptomatic treatment of angina. Nitroglycerin tablets are often used sublingually every 5 minutes up to 3 doses upon onset of angina symptoms in patients with persistent ischemia, heart failure, or uncontrolled high blood pressure. Nitroglycerin should not be used within 24 hours of taking phosphodiesterase type 5 (PDE-5) inhibitors such as sildenafil and vardenafil, or within 48 hours of taking tadalafil, due to the risk of profound decrease in blood pressure.

Isosorbide dinitrate can be used in combination with hydralazine in African American patients with HFrEF to decrease cardiovascular events. This medication is also administered in combination with ACE inhibitors, beta blockers, and diuretics.

The PDE-5 inhibitors sildenafil and tadalafil are approved for erectile dysfunction (ED) as well as for pulmonary arterial hypertension (PAH). Sildenafil increases the intracellular concentration of cyclic guanosine monophosphate (cGMP), leading to vasorelaxation and antiproliferative effects on vascular smooth muscle cells. This reduces mean pulmonary arterial pressure (mPAP) and improves the patient's functional PAH classification. Potential side effects include changes in vision (blue-tinted vision or sudden vision loss), dyspepsia, and diarrhea, all of which may be more common with higher doses.

Nitrates and Nitrites

Amyl nitrite
Isosorbide dinitrate/mononitrate
Nitroglycerin

Phosphodiesterase Type 5 Inhibitors

Sildenafil
Tadalafil
Vardenafil
Cilostazol *(see also the Antithrombotic Agents section in the Blood Formation, Coagulation, and Thrombosis Agents chapter)*

Miscellaneous Vasodilating Agents

Alprostadil
Dipyridamole
Isoxsuprine
Nesiritide
Papaverine

Ambrisentan *(see also the Phosphodiesterase Type 4 Inhibitors and Miscellaneous Respiratory Agents section in the Respiratory Tract Agents chapter)*
Amlodipine *(see also the Calcium-Channel Blocking Agents section)*
Bosentan *(see also the Phosphodiesterase Type 4 Inhibitors and Miscellaneous Respiratory Agents section in the Respiratory Tract Agents chapter)*
Diltiazem *(see also the Calcium-Channel Blocking Agents section)*
Epoprostenol *(see also the Phosphodiesterase Type 4 Inhibitors and Miscellaneous Respiratory Agents section in the Respiratory Tract Agents chapter)*
Iloprost *(see also the Phosphodiesterase Type 4 Inhibitors and Miscellaneous Respiratory Agents section in the Respiratory Tract Agents chapter)*
Macitentan *(see also the Phosphodiesterase Type 4 Inhibitors and Miscellaneous Respiratory Agents section in the Respiratory Tract Agents chapter)*
Nicardipine *(see also the Calcium-Channel Blocking Agents section)*
Nifedipine *(see also the Calcium-Channel Blocking Agents section)*
Nimodipine *(see also the Calcium-Channel Blocking Agents section)*
Riociguat *(see also the Phosphodiesterase Type 4 Inhibitors and Miscellaneous Respiratory Agents section in the Respiratory Tract Agents chapter)*
Treprostinil *(see also the Phosphodiesterase Type 4 Inhibitors and Miscellaneous Respiratory Agents section in the Respiratory Tract Agents chapter)*
Verapamil *(see also the Calcium-Channel Blocking Agents section)*

Case Studies and Conclusions

CB is a 68-year-old Caucasian male who has a medical history of hypertension, HFpEF, diabetes mellitus type 2, hypothyroidism, and acute myocardial infarction (AMI) 2 years ago status post stenting. He arrives to the hospital complaining of chest pain and on the following medications for AMI: ASA 81 mg oral daily, metoprolol 25 mg oral twice daily, clopidogrel 75 mg oral daily, atorvastatin 80 mg oral daily, morphine 5 mg IV every 4 hours as needed for pain, and nitroglycerin ointment ½ inch. The next morning he complains of a headache and his chest pain seems to be responding to the medications.

1. How should you treat the headache?
   a. Give the patient a dose of acetaminophen.
   b. Give the patient a dose of ibuprofen.
   c. Increase the patient's morphine dose to 10 mg.
   d. Change the patient's nitroglycerin ointment to "as needed" (PRN) dosing.

Answer D is correct. While you could give the patient a dose of acetaminophen, his headache is likely due to the continuous use of nitroglycerin ointment. Thus, the dosing of the nitroglycerin ointment should be changed to "as needed," or the patient should be placed on sublingual nitroglycerin "as needed." Ibuprofen is contraindicated in AMI and should not be used in this patient. Increasing his morphine dose would not be appropriate, as his headache is a drug-induced effect that can be handled by removing/lessening the offending agent.

The patient is discharged and continues all the medications except for the morphine; he is placed on sublingual nitroglycerin for emergency use. He visits his endocrinologist and describes his diabetes-associated ED, for which he is placed on sildenafil.

2. What could occur if his endocrinologist is not aware that this patient is taking sublingual nitroglycerin tablets?
   a. GI bleed
   b. Hypotension
   c. Itching
   d. Tinnitus

Answer B is correct. Due to dilation of the coronary artery and nitrates' mechanism of action, profound hypotension has occurred in patients who took both of these medications within a 24-hour period. Sildenafil is contraindicated in patients who are taking nitroglycerin.

6.5 Adrenergic Agents

Adrenergic agents work on many receptors, including $alpha_1$, $alpha_2$, $beta_1$, and $beta_2$ receptors. It is important to understand the location and role of these receptors to appreciate how these therapies work.

$Alpha_1$ receptors are located on arterial and venous vessels as well as on visceral smooth muscle; they cause vasoconstriction when activated. Blocking $alpha_1$ receptors will cause vasodilation and reduce peripheral vascular resistance, resulting in a decrease in blood pressure. The $alpha_1$ blockers prazosin, terazosin, and doxazosin have been used to treat hypertension, but are not first-line therapies in this indication. These agents are also used to treat benign prostatic hypertrophy (BPH). $Alpha_{1a}$ receptors are found in the prostate, and blocking these receptors will decrease the resistance to outflow of urine.

Adverse effects of this class of medications include severe orthostatic hypotension and syncope—a combination known as the "first-dose effect" that can be seen as soon as 30 minutes after the initial dose. $Alpha_1$ blockers should be titrated slowly, and concomitant antihypertensive therapy should be used cautiously when initiating therapy. Standing and recumbent blood pressure should be monitored. Other potential adverse effects with these medications include headache and dizziness.

Beta-receptor antagonists can be classified as having either $beta_1$ or $beta_2$ activity. $Beta_1$ receptors are found in the heart; they control heart rate and contractility. $Beta_2$ receptors are found in smooth muscle cells of both vascular and nonvascular tissues. Beta-receptor antagonists have many indications, including hypertension, secondary prevention for MI, arrhythmias, angina, and heart failure.

$Beta_1$ blockade primarily affects the heart, slowing heart rate and decreasing myocardial contractility. $Beta_1$ antagonists are particularly effective at blocking the body's sympathetic response during exercise or exertion. Metoprolol is an example of a $beta_1$-selective blocker with no intrinsic sympathomimetic activity. Two formulations of this medication are available: metoprolol tartrate (Lopressor), which is an immediate-release formulation, and metoprolol succinate (Toprol XL), which is an extended-release formulation. Metoprolol succinate is also a preferred agent for patients with congestive heart failure. Atenolol is similar to metoprolol but has a longer half-life. It exhibits fewer CNS side effects than the other beta blockers. Esmolol is an ultra-short-acting beta antagonist that is available only intravenously. It is indicated for hypertensive emergencies. Bisoprolol is highly selective for $beta_1$ receptors and is also approved for the treatment of HF.

Nonspecific beta blockers have activity at both $beta_1$ and $beta_2$ receptors.

Propranolol, for example, has equal affinity for $beta_1$ and $beta_2$ receptors. This medication is metabolized extensively in the liver, but with high interpatient variability. Nadolol is also a nonspecific beta blocker but has a longer half-life than propranolol.

Third-generation beta blockers, which include carvedilol and labetolol, produce additional vasodilatory effects through a variety of mechanisms, particularly $alpha_1$ blockade. As a consequence, these agents can both lower heart rate and reduce cardiac preload and blood pressure. In acute hypertensive crisis secondary to cocaine overdose, they are the preferred therapies to reduce the risk of rebound vasoconstriction and further elevations of blood pressure. Labetalol is indicated for hypertensive emergencies due to its fast onset of action. Carvedilol is similar to labetalol but is available only as an oral formulation; it is a preferred agent for patients with congestive heart failure. Whenever starting a beta blocker in patient with HF, it is recommended to start with the lowest dose and titrate the dose up slowly due to potential negative inotropic effects.

Beta blockers can mask symptoms of hypoglycemia (e.g., tremors, tachycardia, nervousness) in patients with diabetes by blocking the sympathetic response to glycogenolysis that occurs when hypoglycemia is present. Nonspecific beta blockers can cause bronchospasm and life-threatening bronchoconstriction in patients with chronic obstructive pulmonary disease (COPD) or asthma because of their effects on bronchial smooth muscle. $Beta_1$-selective agents (such as bisoprolol) are preferred in these patients. Adverse effects commonly observed with all beta blockers include dizziness, bradycardia, headache, and orthostatic hypotension. Caution should be used when using beta blockers in ADHF.

Alpha-Adrenergic Blocking Agents

Doxazosin
Prazosin
Terazosin
Carvedilol *(see also the Beta-Adrenergic Blocking Agents section)*
Labetalol *(see also the Beta-Adrenergic Blocking Agents section)*

Beta-Adrenergic Blocking Agents

Acebutolol
Atenolol
Betaxolol
Bisoprolol
Carvedilol
Esmolol
Labetalol
Metoprolol
Nadolol
Nebivolol
Pindolol
Propranolol
Sotalol
Timolol

Case Studies and Conclusions

TO is a 56-year-old male with a past medical history of ischemic cardiomyopathy (EF = 35%) and diabetes. He is currently stable and his cardiac symptoms are under control with use of furosemide 40 mg daily. TO is on lisinopril 20 mg daily and spironolactone 25 mg oral daily.

1. Which of the following beta blockers is appropriate to use in this patient?
   a. Metoprolol tartrate
   b. Metoprolol succinate
   c. Nadolol
   d. Propranolol

Answer B is correct. The three beta blockers that are approved for HFrEF are bisoprolol, metoprolol succinate, and carvedilol.

2. Given that the physician decides to begin carvedilol therapy for this patient, which of the following would be an appropriate dose for this patient?
   a. Carvedilol 3.125 mg oral twice daily
   b. Carvedilol 6.25 mg oral twice daily
   c. Carvedilol 12.5 mg oral twice daily
   d. Carvedilol 25 mg oral twice daily

Answer A is correct. Whenever starting a beta blocker in patient with HF, it is recommended to start with the lowest dose and titrate the dose up slowly due to its negative inotropic effects. Carvedilol should be started at 3.125 mg oral twice daily and then titrated up to a maximum tolerated dose of 25 mg oral twice daily.

3. Which of the following statements is true regarding carvedilol?
   a. Carvedilol is less likely to cause bronchospasm than metoprolol.
   b. Carvedilol also has antihypertensive effects due to its alpha blockade.
   c. Carvedilol does not mask hypoglycemia symptoms.
   d. Carvedilol is not approved for HF.

Answer B is correct. Carvedilol is a third-generation beta blocker that has nonselective beta-blocking properties and $alpha_1$-blocking properties, which causes it to deliver better blood pressure control than other beta blockers. The other statements are not true.

JT is a 53-year-old male with a history of asthma, hypertension, and CAD. He is currently using an albuterol inhaler and is taking hydrochlorothiazide 25 mg daily, aspirin 81 mg daily, atorvastatin 20 mg daily, and amlodipine 5 mg daily. This patient now reports increasing angina symptoms.

1. Which of the following medications would you recommend that would carry the least risk of bronchospasm?
    a. Propranolol
    b. Labetolol
    c. Bisoprolol
    d. Nebivolol

Answer C is correct. Bisoprolol is a highly selective $beta_1$ antagonist. Nonspecific beta blockers that block $beta_2$ receptors in the bronchial smooth muscles have a higher risk of causing bronchospasm.

6.6 Calcium-Channel Blocking Agents

Calcium-channel antagonists, also known as calcium-channel blockers (CCBs), work by selectively blocking calcium channels in cardiac and vascular smooth muscle cells. An increased concentration of intracellular calcium leads to augmented contractility in the myocardium and vascular smooth muscle. By blocking the buildup of intracellular calcium, CCBs have a net effect of vasodilation in the smooth muscle and negative inotropic effects in the myocardium.

CCBs are classified into two types: nondihydropyridines (NDHP), which are selective for cardiac myocytes, and dihydropyridines (DHP), which are selective for vascular calcium channels. These medications have many uses. They are considered first-line agents according to the JNC 8 guidelines and are preferred agents in African American patients. They are also used to treat stable angina, coronary artery vasospasm, and certain supraventricular arrhythmias.

Verapamil and diltiazem are classified as NDHP CCBs. These drugs are primarily utilized for rate control in patients with arrhythmias, including atrial fibrillation and atrial flutter, due to their negative inotropic and chronotropic effects. Nevertheless, they are associated with an increased likelihood of bradycardia, heart failure exacerbation, and AV block owing to this mechanism, so their use is contraindicated in certain patients. Verapamil and diltiazem both strongly inhibit the same liver metabolism enzyme and should not be used concomitantly with many other drugs, including azole antifungals, simvastatin, cyclosporine, and digoxin, as serum concentrations of the latter agents will be increased.

Amlodipine and nifedipine are examples of agents classified as DHP CCBs. They primarily act on the calcium channels in the large vessels to produce vasodilation and subsequent reduction in blood pressure. Nifedipine is selective for arterial vessels and produces prominent vasodilation. Amlodipine produces less reflex tachycardia than nifedipine due to its prolonged half-life. Amlodipine is preferred in patients with HF who need additional blood pressure control when they are already on optimal therapy. Felodipine is highly selective for vascular tissue and does not produce any inotropic effects. Nicardipine is more selective for cerebral and coronary vessels than other drugs in this class, though it is not recommended that nifedipine be used as an immediate-release formulation. Clevidipine is an intravenous drug used for hypertensive emergencies due to its rapid onset of action and short half-life.

Adverse effects of CCBs include headache, postural hypotension, and bradycardia (specifically for NDHP CCBs). Peripheral edema is more commonly associated with DHP CCBs due to the vasodilation and "pooling" of blood in the lower extremities caused by these agents. A rash can develop more commonly with verapamil and diltiazem, and can sometimes be as severe as Steven-Johnson syndrome. Heart block is also more common with the NDHP CCBs, and these agents should be used with extreme caution in patients with heart failure.

Several case studies have identified calcium supplementation as a significant interaction risk when these supplements are used concomitantly with CCBs. Increasing serum calcium can theoretically decrease the hypotensive effects of calcium-channel antagonists; however, this relationship has not been confirmed in clinical trials. Although not clinically relevant in a majority of patients, this interaction should be evaluated if patients are unsuccessful in achieving the desired outcome while taking calcium-channel blockers.

Dihydropyridine Calcium-Channel Blockers

Amlodipine
Clevidipine

Felodipine
Isradapine
Nicardipine
Nifedipine
Nimodipine
Nisoldipine

Miscellaneous Calcium-Channel Blocking Agents

Diltiazem
Verapamil

Case Studies and Conclusions

EB is a 75-year-old male with atrial fibrillation who is being started on rate-controlling therapy. He has a normal ejection fraction.

1. Which of the following calcium-channel blockers would be preferred in this patient?
   a. Diltiazem
   b. Nifedipine IR
   c. Nifedipine XL
   d. Clevidipine
   e. Nicardipine

Answer A is correct. NDHP CCBs reduce heart rate and, therefore, are good choices for rate control in patients with atrial fibrillation.

2. Which of the following adverse effects is more commonly seen with NDHP CCBs than with DHP CCBs?
   a. Hypotension
   b. Bradycardia
   c. Peripheral edema
   d. Rash

Answer B is correct. Bradycardia is commonly seen with NDHP CCBs but not DHP CCBs. Both types of CCBs will produce hypotension. Rash occurs at similar rates for both drug classes, but peripheral edema is more commonly associated with DHP CCBs.

A patient has a diagnosis of HF and is already optimized on all HF therapies.

1. Which of the following drugs would you recommend to add on for additional blood pressure control?
   a. Nifedipine IR
   b. Nifedipine XL
   c. Amlodipine
   d. Diltiazem
   e. Verapamil

Answer C is correct. Amlodipine is the only CCB that has been studied in patients with HF. It was found to have neutral effects in these patients—that is, neither negative nor positive.

6.7 Renin–Angiotensin–Aldosterone System Inhibitors

ACE inhibitors work in the renin-angiotensin-aldosterone system (RAAS) by blocking the conversion of angiotensin I to angiotensin II. Angiotensin II leads to vasoconstriction and sodium and water retention.

By blocking the effects of angiotensin II, ACE inhibitors reduce peripheral vascular resistance, which in turn lowers blood pressure. They are considered a first-line therapy according to JNC 8 guidelines for hypertension, and are preferred agents in patients with diabetes mellitus or chronic kidney disease due to their renal-protective effects—that is, they decrease glomerular efferent arteriolar resistance. ACE inhibitors are also class A recommendations for patients with HFrEF and post MI. Side effects of these agents include severe hypotension, acute kidney failure (especially in patients with renal artery stenosis), hyperkalemia, dry cough, and angioedema. ACE inhibitors are contraindicated in pregnancy. They should be used cautiously with potassium supplements due to the risk of hyperkalemia; likewise, they should not be used with NSAIDs.

Angiotensin-converting enzyme also inactivates the natural vasodilator bradykinin, which causes the cough adverse effect associated with ACE inhibitors. Since ARBs block the angiotensin II receptor with no effect on bradykinin receptors, they are used in patients who develop an ACE-induced cough. The adverse-effect profile for ARBs is otherwise similar to that for ACE inhibitors. There is also less incidence of angioedema with ARBs, but their use in patients who experience ACE inhibitor–induced angioedema is generally not recommended.

Potassium-sparing diuretics block the aldosterone receptors in the collecting ducts of the kidney, which increases both sodium excretion and potassium absorption. This effect is particularly useful in HFrEF, as it reduces hypertension, ventricular hypertrophy, and myocardial fibrosis. Spironolactone can cause gynecomastia in patients, which can be avoided by administering eplerenone, but at a higher cost. Eplerenone is contraindicated with use of strong CYP3A4 inhibitors such as clarithromycin and azole antifungals, verapamil, and diltiazem. Potassium-sparing diuretics are renally eliminated and can cause hyperkalemia, so patients' SCr and potassium should be monitored closely.

Aliskiren, a renin inhibitor, interrupts the generation of angiotensin II by inhibiting renin within the RAAS cascade and stopping the production of both angiotensin I and II. Aliskiren should not be combined with ACE inhibitors or ARBs, especially in those patients with diabetes or a CrCl less than 60 mL per minute. Potential adverse effects of aliskiren are similar to those noted with ACE inhibitors and ARBs and include hyperkalemia and acute renal failure. Aliskiren should not be used in pregnancy.

Angiotensin-Converting Enzyme Inhibitors

Benazepril
Captopril
Enalaprilat/enalapril
Fosinopril
Lisinopril
Moexipril
Perindopril
Quinapril
Ramipril
Trandolapril

Angiotensin II Receptor Antagonists

Azilsartan
Candesartan
Eprosartan
Irbesartan
Losartan
Olmesartan
Telmisartan
Valsartan

Mineralocorticoid (Aldosterone) Receptor Antagonists

Eplerenone
Spironolactone

Renin Inhibitors

Aliskiren

Case Studies and Conclusions

BB is a new patient of yours. He is currently taking quinapril but is interested in taking valsartan instead. He would like to know which of the following adverse effects is more commonly seen with ACE inhibitors than with ARBs.

1. What do you tell him?
   a. Acute renal failure
   b. Bradycardia
   c. Cough
   d. Hypotension

Answer C is correct. Although acute renal failure can occur in patients on ACE inhibitors or ARBs, it is not common in patients unless they are taking concomitant nephrotoxins or other agents that affect the renin–angiotensin system (RAS). Bradycardia is not an adverse effect of either of these medications because they are arterial vasodilators. The risk of hypotension is not different for the two medications, although this adverse effect can occur. Bradykinin (which leads to the cough) is produced by the ACE inhibitors but not by the ARBs.

2. If BB needed to start an aldosterone antagonist, which baseline lab values should you obtain before you initiate that medication?
   a. Na and SCr
   b. Na and K
   c. K and SCr
   d. SCr and LFTs

Answer C is correct. Aldosterone antagonists are renally eliminated and can cause hyperkalemia as a side effect; this electrolyte imbalance is a dose/use-limiting effect. Although it is important to know the patient's sodium level, it would not necessarily change much with use of an aldosterone antagonist. LFTs are not monitored when aldosterone antagonists are prescribed.

JC is a 52-year-old male patient with a past medical history of hypertension, type 2 diabetes mellitus, stage 3 chronic kidney disease, COPD, and HFrEF.

1. Which of the following is NOT an indication for an ACE inhibitor in this patient?
   a. Type 2 diabetes mellitus
   b. Stage 3 CKD
   c. COPD
   d. HFrEF

Answer C is correct. ACE inhibitors are preferred agents in patients with hypertension, type 2 diabetes mellitus, or stage 3 CKD. They also carry a Grade A recommendation for use in patients with HFrEF. There is no preferred agent in regard to COPD.

2. JC is later placed on spironolactone for treatment of his HFrEF. Which of the following is an adverse effect that you need to be concerned with in this patient?
   a. Hypokalemia
   b. Gynecomastia
   c. Suicidal ideation
   d. Visual changes

Answer B is correct. Spironolactone (compared to eplerenone) has been shown to cause gynecomastia. This agent causes hyperkalemia, not hypokalemia. Suicidal ideation and visual changes have not been associated with this medication.

Tips from the Field

1. The use of cardiovascular agents, as with most other medications, is based on expert consensus and guidelines.
2. Cardiovascular interventions, including cholesterol and lipid treatment, are based on risk calculations and focused on the intensity rankings of statin therapy.
3. Some of the older medications are no longer considered first line, so be familiar with guidelines and which combinations are acceptable in addition to which combinations would be suboptimal or therapeutically "duplicative."
4. Remember the importance of non-pharmaceutical interventions and be supportive when motivating your patient to increase exercise, improve diet, and consider smoking cessation.
5. ACE inhibitors are frequently the culprit when patients present with dry, non-productive cough. Consider changing your patient to an ARB if there appears to be no other reasonable cause of cough.
6. ACEs/ARBs have been associated with angioedema, which can be fatal. Be sure you evaluate and intervene appropriately.
7. Remind patients to separate their bile acid sequestrant products, such as cholestyramine or colestipol, from other medications. It is generally best to take critical oral medications at least 1 hour prior to the sequestrant product.
8. Not all diuretics are equally strong, and some, such as furosemide, are reserved for more extreme diuresis. Educate patients to take diuretics first thing in the morning so sleep is not interrupted with frequent nighttime urination.
9. Speak openly about the risk (and definition) of priapism with your patients using ED products. Priapism can result in serious, permanent disfigurement and dysfunction if immediate medical attention is not received.
10. Patients who use nitroglycerin patches require a nitrate-free interval for the nitrate to work most effectively. This is generally best accomplished with removal prior to bedtime and reapplication upon awakening.
11. Topical patch application should be rotated, never applied to broken or irritated skin, and preferably applied to a hairless area.
12. If your patient is scheduled for an MRI, be sure they discuss their topical patch use (for cardiovascular or other conditions) and alternatives for medication during that test and evaluation period.

Tammie Lee and Jacque

Bibliography

American Geriatrics Society. 2015 updated Beers criteria for potentially inappropriate medication use in older adults. *J Am Geriatr Soc.* 2015;63:2227-2246.

DiPiro JT, Talbert RL, Yee GC, Matzke GR, Wells BG, Posey LM. *Pharmacotherapy: A Pathophysiologic Approach.* 9th ed. New York, NY: McGraw-Hill Medical; 2014.

Brunton LL, Chabner BA, Knollmann BC, eds. *Goodman & Gilman's The Pharmacological Basis of Therapeutics.* 12th ed. New York, NY: McGraw-Hill Medical; 2011.

Katzung BG, Trevor AJ, Teton Data Systems. *Basic and Clinical Pharmacology.* 13th ed. New York, NY: McGraw-Hill Education; 2015.

McEvoy GK, ed. *AHFS: Drug Information.* Bethesda, MD: American Society of Health-System Pharmacists; 2016.

Symbols

Symbol	Meaning	Symbol	Meaning
▲	Renal impairment: Dose adjustment is recommended.	(BL)	Beers list criteria (avoid in elderly).
□	Hepatic impairment: Dose adjustment is recommended.	(PD)	FDA-approved pediatric doses are available.
■	Black box warning exists for this drug.	(GD)	FDA-approved geriatric doses are available.
(QT)	QTc prolongation effects have been reported.		See primary body system.

Cardiovascular Agents

Universal prescribing alerts:

- Known serious hypersensitivity to the specific drug or any other component of the product/formulation selected warrants a contraindication for its use.
- Adverse reactions associated with the use of some **cardiovascular agents** include dizziness, drowsiness, vertigo, and fatigue; these agents may also impair the ability to perform tasks requiring mental alertness. Caution should always be recommended when using any new drug for the first time, when there is a dose change, and for continued use of known offending agents.
- Many medications increase the risk of QT prolongation. The risk of QT prolongation is increased in susceptible individuals including patients with cardiac disease or other conditions that may increase the risk of QT prolongation including cardiac arrhythmias, congenital long QT syndrome, heart failure, bradycardia, MI, hypertension, CAD, hypomagnesemia, hypokalemia, hypocalcemia, or in patients receiving medications known to prolong the QT interval or cause electrolyte imbalances. Females, geriatric patients, patients with diabetes, thyroid disease, malnutrition, alcoholism, or hepatic dysfunction may also be at increased risk for QT prolongation. Patients receiving these medications who have cardiac disease or arrhythmias should be monitored closely, ECGs should be administered during and after therapy, or in some cases clinical decision should be made to avoid the agent entirely if the risk is too great.
- Doses expressed are for usual adult dosage ranges only. "Geriatric doses" are assumed to be the same as adult doses unless otherwise noted with a symbol. Where pediatric dosing is available, a symbol will guide the reader to additional prescribing references. Refer to real-time prescribing references for these age-specific doses.
- Use of cardiovascular agents in pregnancy is based on weighing clinical risk versus benefit, and safety concerns are not represented in this grid. Refer to the package insert (PI) for more information. Clinicians should continue to provide education about the reproductive risks of any medication and offer risk-reduction strategies (which may include contraceptive use) to women of childbearing age and understand that these reproductive risks may also extend to males. Other medications may decrease the effectiveness of oral contraceptives. Where necessary, an alternative means of birth control should be explored.
- Brand names are provided for those agents still available on the market. Due to ever-changing product availability, refer to Food and Drug Administration (FDA) resources to confirm the actual brands available. This drug summary is intended for educational purposes only. Prescribing decisions should be based on real-time comprehensive drug databases that are updated on a regular basis.

Cardiac Agents

Antiarrhythmic Agents

Class IA Antiarrhythmic Agents

Drug Name	FDA-Approved Indications	Adult Dosage Range	Precautions and Clinical Pearls
Generic Name Disopyramide **Brand Name** Norpace Norpace CR QT BL PD	Ventricular arrhythmias	**Usual oral dose for patients weighing 50 kg or more:** Immediate release (IR): Initial loading dose (LD): 300 mg for rapid onset, then 150 mg every 6 hours (up to 200 mg every 6 hours) Alternatively may give: controlled release (CR): 300 mg every 12 hours	• Monitor hypotension during initial therapy • Should be initiated in the hospital with cardiac monitoring • Avoid in patients with structural heart disease • Subject to all the universal prescribing alerts for anticholinergic agents Contraindications: • Cardiogenic shock • Preexisting second- or third-degree heart block • Congenital long QT syndrome • Sick sinus syndrome Associated with: • Increased mortality
Generic Name Procainamide **Brand Name** Apo-Procainamide Procainamide Hydrochloride injection Procan SR QT	Life-threatening ventricular arrhythmias	**Illustrative parenteral dose:** IV: LD: 100 mg per dose every 5 minutes as needed to a maximum LD of 15 mg/kg and maximum infusion rate of 500 mg in 30 minutes. Maintenance: IV: 1 to 4 mg per minute continuous infusion	• *N*-Acetylprocainamide is the active metabolite that is renally cleared • Specific dose recommendations for patients undergoing dialysis; refer to PI • Avoid use in patients with structural heart disease or HF • May be administered IM with specific dosing recommendations. Adjust dosage based on renal function, clinical goals, and serum drug level monitoring. Contraindications: • Complete heart block • Second-degree atrioventricular (AV) block or venous types of hemiblock • Systemic lupus erythematosus (SLE) • Torsades de pointes Associated with: • Blood dyscrasias • Drug-induced lupus erythematosus-like syndrome • Increased mortality

Drug Name	FDA-Approved Indications	Adult Dosage Range	Precautions and Clinical Pearls
Generic Name Quinidine **Brand Name** Apo-Quinidine BioQuin Durules Novo-Quinidin Quinate ■ QT	Atrial fibrillation/flutter Maintenance of sinus rhythm in paroxysmal atrial fibrillation/flutter or life-threatening ventricular arrhythmias Severe malaria treatment	Dose varies with indication for use, formulation selected, and patient's clinical response **Illustrative oral dose for arrhythmias:** **Quinidine sulfate:** Immediate release (IR) Initial: 200 mg every 6 hours Extended release (ER) Initial: 300 mg every 8 to 12 hours **Quinidine gluconate:** Initial: 324 mg every 8 to 12 hours	• Correct any electrolyte disturbances, especially hypokalemia or hypomagnesemia • Use with caution in renal impairment and hepatic impairment • Avoid use in patients with structural heart disease Contraindications: • Thrombocytopenia • Myasthenia gravis • Heart block greater than first degree • Idioventricular conduction delays • Concurrent use medications that prolong QT interval Associated with: • Increased mortality
Class IB Antiarrhythmic Agents			
Drug Name	FDA-Approved Indications	Adult Dosage Range	Precautions and Clinical Pearls
Generic Name Lidocaine **Brand Name** Xylocaine ■ ■ PD	Common indications for use: Antiarrhythmic Anesthesia, local injectable	Dose varies with indication for use, formulation selected, and patient's clinical response **Illustrative parenteral dose:** Ventricular fibrillation (VF) or pulseless ventricular tachycardia (VT) or stable monomorphic VT: IV: Initial: 1 to 1.5 mg/kg; repeat with 0.5 to 0.75 mg/kg every 5 to 10 minutes as needed (maximum cumulative dose: 3 mg/kg) Follow with continuous infusion of 1 to 4 mg per minute	• Constant ECG monitoring during IV administration • Part of ACLS algorithm for VF or pulseless VT Contraindications: • Adam-Stokes syndrome • Wolff-Parkinson-White syndrome • Severe degrees of sinoatrial (SA), AV, or intraventricular heart block • Requires experienced clinician who is knowledgeable in the use of this agent and specialized care setting Associated with: • Increased risk of serious adverse effects when viscous formulation is used in special populations; refer to PI • Epidural, local, nerve block and spinal administration: specific contraindicated populations, including patients with sepsis and those with impaired bleeding times; refer to PI

Generic Name Mexiletine ▲ □ ■ (PD)	Life-threatening ventricular arrhythmias Conversion	**Usual oral dose:** Initial: 200 mg every 8 hours (maximum: 1.2 g per day)	• Switching strategy from oral antiarrhythmics is available in the package insert; initiate dose after the last dose of the former agent • Hematologic abnormalities have been reported • Switching from IV lidocaine: initiate dose when lidocaine infusion is stopped • Seizure and tremor have been reported; may exacerbate Parkinson's disease • Smoking cessation may result in significantly reduced clearance despite nicotine replacement • Gastrointestinal (GI) distress and nausea/vomiting are very common adverse effects • Acute liver injury has been reported (though rare) Contraindications: • Cardiogenic shock • Second- or third-degree AV block Associated with: • Increased mortality • Proarrhythmic effects

Class IC Antiarrhythmic Agents

Drug Name	FDA-Approved Indications	Adult Dosage Range	Precautions and Clinical Pearls
Generic Name Flecainide ▲ ■ (QT) (BL) (PD)	Ventricular arrhythmias (prevention) Paroxysmal atrial fibrillation/flutter and paroxysmal supraventricular tachycardia (PSVT) (prevention)	Dose varies with indication for use, formulation selected, and patient's clinical response **Illustrative oral dose:** Initial: 50 mg every 12 hours; increase by 50 mg twice daily at interval of 4 days (maximum: 300 mg per day)	• Conversion from another antiarrhythmic agent: allow for 2 to 4 half-lives of the other agents after discontinuation to pass before initiating flecainide • Drug interactions may require dosage adjustment or avoidance of certain drug combinations Contraindications: • Cardiogenic shock • Preexisting second- or third-degree AV block or with right bundle branch block when associated with a left hemiblock Associated with: • Ventricular proarrhythmic effects in patients with atrial fibrillation/flutter • Increased mortality

Drug Name	FDA-Approved Indications	Adult Dosage Range	Precautions and Clinical Pearls
Generic Name Propafenone **Brand Name** Rythmol Rythmol SR ■ QT	Atrial fibrillation (prevention of recurrence) PSVT (prevention of recurrence) Ventricular arrhythmias	**Illustrative oral dose:** Immediate release (IR) Initial: 150 mg every 8 hours; may increase to 225 mg every 8 hours at interval of 3 to 4 days (further increase to 300 mg every 8 hours) Extended release (ER) Initial: 225 mg every 12 hours; may increase to 325 mg every 12 hours at interval of 3 to 4 days (may further increase to 425 mg every 12 hours)	• May cause dizziness, fatigue, and blurred vision • Agranulocytosis has been reported; white blood cell resolution occurs upon discontinuation of therapy Contraindications: • Brugada syndrome • Sinus bradycardia • Cardiogenic shock • Uncompensated cardiac failure • Marked hypotension • Bronchospastic disorder or severe obstructive pulmonary disease • Uncorrected electrolyte abnormalities Associated with: • Increased risk of QT prolongation
Class III Antiarrhythmic Agents			
Drug Name	**FDA-Approved Indications**	**Adult Dosage Range**	**Precautions and Clinical Pearls**
Generic Name Amiodarone **Brand Name** Cardarone Nexterone Pacerone ■ QT BL	Ventricular arrhythmias Atrial fibrillation	**Illustrative parenteral dose:** LD: 150 mg over 10 minutes, 1 mg per minute for 6 hours, 0.5 mg per minute for 18 hours then consider conversion to oral dose **Alternative oral dose:** LD: 800 mg to 1600 mg per day in 1 or 2 divided doses for 1 to 3 weeks, decrease to lowest effective maintenance dose (usual maintenance dose is 400 mg per day single or divided dose)	• Infusion-related bradycardia and hypotension • Drug interactions may require dose adjustment • Long half-life requires large loading dose • Conversion from IV to oral therapy should be done as soon as clinically possible; refer to PI for dosing strategies and schedules • Visual disturbances have been reported; regular eye exams recommended for all patients • Use caution in thyroid disease and goiter • May cause sun sensitivity; avoid exposure • Requires experienced clinician who is knowledgeable in the use of this agent Contraindications: • Severe sinus-node dysfunction causing marked sinus bradycardia • Second- and third-degree heart block • Bradycardia causing syncope • Cardiogenic shock Associated with: • Liver toxicity • Proarrhythmic effects • Pneumonitis

Generic Name Dofetilide **Brand Name** Tikosyn ▲ ■ QT	Atrial fibrillation/flutter	**Usual oral dose:** Initial: 500 mcg twice daily	• Obtain baseline QT or QTc prior to first dose • Dose adjustments based on QTc interval and renal impairment • Monitor patient in a facility for a minimum of 3 days • Use caution in patients with hepatic impairment Contraindications: • Congenital or acquired long QT syndrome • Baseline QT interval or QTc is greater than 440 ms • Severe renal impairment Associated with: • Life-threatening arrhythmias • Requires experienced clinician who is knowledgeable in the use of this agent and specialized care setting
Generic Name Dronedarone **Brand Name** Multaq ■ QT BL	Paroxysmal or persistent atrial fibrillation (AF)	**Usual oral dose:** 400 mg twice daily	• Administer with morning and evening meals • Drug interactions may require dose adjustment; avoid use of grapefruit or grapefruit juice • Available through Risk Evaluation and Mitigation Strategy (REMS) program Contraindications: • Symptomatic heart failure (HF) • Liver or lung toxicity related to previous amiodarone use • Bradycardia less than 50 beats per minute • Severe hepatic impairment Associated with: • Contraindication in permanent atrial fibrillation • Increased risk of death, stroke, and HF
Generic Name Ibutilide **Brand Name** Corvert ■ QT	Atrial fibrillation/flutter	**Usual parenteral dose:** For patients weighing 60 kg or more: IV: 1 mg over 10 minutes	• Discontinue infusion if arrhythmia terminates, if ventricular tachycardia occurs, or if marked prolongation of QT/QTc occurs • Additional dosing recommendations for patients weighing less than 60 kg; refer to PI Associated with: • Arrhythmias • Potential torsades de pointes (QT prolongation) • Not for patients with chronic atrial fibrillation or in any patient QTc interval greater than 440 ms • Requires experienced clinician who is knowledgeable in the use of this agent
Sotalol	Refer to the Adrenergic Agents section.		

Class IV Antiarrhythmic Agents			
Drug Name	FDA-Approved Indications	Adult Dosage Range	Precautions and Clinical Pearls
Generic Name Adenosine **Brand Name** Adenocard Adenoscan (PD)	PSVT (Adenocard) Pharmacologic stress testing (Adenoscan)	Dose varies with indication for use, formulation selected, and patient's clinical response **Illustrative parenteral dose for PSVT:** IV: Initial: 6 mg; may repeat 12 mg bolus if needed (maximum single dose: 12 mg)	• Use caution in those with history of seizure • Cerebrovascular accidents have been reported; use caution in any patient who may be predisposed (i.e., hypovolemia, valvular heart disease, etc.) Contraindications: • Sick sinus syndrome • Symptomatic bradycardia • Bronchoconstrictive or bronchospastic lung disease • Asthma
Diltiazem	Refer to the Calcium-Channel Blocking Agents section.		
Verapamil	Refer to the Calcium-Channel Blocking Agents section.		
Miscellaneous Antiarrhythmic Agents			
Digoxin	Refer to the Cardiotonic Agents section.		
Magnesium sulfate	Refer to the Central Nervous System Agents chapter.		
Cardiotonic Agents			
Drug Name	FDA-Approved Indications	Adult Dosage Range	Precautions and Clinical Pearls
Generic Name Digoxin **Brand Name** Digitek Digox Lanoxin (BL) (PD) (GD)	Heart failure Supraventricular tachyarrhythmias (rate control)	**Illustrative dose:** IV/IM digitalizing loading dose: 8 to 12 **mcg**/kg total* Alternatively Oral digitalizing loading dose: 0.75 mg (750 **mcg**) to 1.5 mg (1500 **mcg**) total* *Total loading dose divided into 3 doses, with the first dose equaling one-half the total with the remaining half in 2 equally divided doses at 6 to 8 hour intervals **Usual oral maintenance for heart failure:** 0.125 mg (125 **mcg**) to 0.5 mg (500 **mcg**) once daily	• Extravasation from IV; vesicant • IM injections associated with considerable pain • Avoid in patients who may experience undesirable increases in myocardial oxygen demand (i.e., those with pulmonary disease) • Usual daily maintenance dose requirements for the treatment of congestive heart failure are based on corrected CrCl and lean body weight (LBW). • Careful assessment of clinical response must be ensured before each additional dose • Monitor electrolytes; correct imbalances • High-alert medication; use caution with doses being written in "mg" or "mcg" Contraindications: • Ventricular fibrillation

Generic Name Milrinone	Inotropic support in heart failure	**Usual parenteral dose:** IV loading dose: 50 mcg/kg over 10 minutes Maintenance: 0.375 to 0.75 mcg/kg per minute	• Renally eliminated; use lower doses based on renal function; avoid loading doses • Monitor blood pressure • Correct any electrolyte imbalance, especially hypokalemia and hypomagnesemia • Dosing with loading dose is optional but not recommended by American College of Cardiology Foundation and the and the American Heart Association HF guidelines
Dobutamine	Refer to the Autonomic Agents chapter.		
Dopamine	Refer to the Autonomic Agents chapter.		

Miscellaneous Cardiac Agents

Drug Name	FDA-Approved Indications	Adult Dosage Range	Precautions and Clinical Pearls
Generic Name Ranolazine **Brand Name** Ranexa QT	Chronic angina	**Usual oral dose:** Initial: 500 mg twice daily (maximum: 1000 mg twice daily)	• Do not crush, break, or chew • Drug interactions may require dose adjustments or avoidance of certain drug combinations (also grapefruit juice) Contraindications: • Hepatic cirrhosis • Renal failure or significant impairment

Antilipemic Agents

Bile Acid Sequestrants

Universal prescribing alerts:

- These agents have the potential to bind to other drugs and may prevent absorption of other medications (i.e., thyroid supplementation, digoxin, etc.). Take other drugs at least 1 hour before or at least 4 to 6 hours after dose of bile acid sequestrant.
- Patients with constipation are at increased risk of developing fecal impaction, GI obstruction and hemorrhoid exacerbation. Bile acid sequestrants should also be used with caution (or avoided) in patients with dysphagia, swallowing disorders, severe gastrointestinal motility disorders (e.g., ileus), or major gastrointestinal tract surgery.

Drug Name	FDA-Approved Indications	Adult Dosage Range	Precautions and Clinical Pearls
Generic Name Cholestyramine **Brand Name** Prevalite Questran Questran Light PD	Hypercholesterolemia (especially with elevated LDL) Pruritis associated with biliary stasis	**Usual oral dose:** Initial: 4 g daily to twice daily Maintenance: 4 to 16 g per day divided in 2 doses (maximum: 24 g per day)	• Avoid with baseline fasting triglyceride levels of 300 mg/dL or greater • Take before meals; do not administer as dry powder (must be reconstituted); refer to PI • Binds to other drugs and may prevent absorption of other medications (i.e., thyroid supplementation); take other drugs at least 1 hour before or at least 4 to 6 hours after dose • May increase risk of bleeding by blocking absorption of vitamin K Contraindications: • Complete biliary obstruction

Drug Name	FDA-Approved Indications	Adult Dosage Range	Precautions and Clinical Pearls
Generic Name Colesevelam **Brand Name** Welchol (PD)	Hyperlipidemia Diabetes mellitus type 2	**Usual oral dose:** 3.75 g (suspension or 6 tablets) once daily Alternatively 1.875 g (3 tablets) twice per day	• Avoid in patients with gastroparesis, cholelithiasis, or complete biliary obstruction • Administer with liquid (4 to 8 ounces of water, fruit juice, etc.) and a meal • Separate administration from other medications Contraindications: • History of bowel obstruction • Serum triglycerides (TG) concentration of more than 500 mg/dL • History of hypertriglyceridemia-induced pancreatitis
Generic Name Colestipol **Brand Name** Colestid Colestid Flavored Micronized Colestipol HCl	Primary hypercholesterolemia	**Usual oral dose:** Granules: Initial: 5 g daily or twice daily Maintenance: 5 to 30 g daily or in divided doses Tablets: Initial: 2 g daily or twice daily Maintenance: 2 to 16 g daily or in divided doses	• Avoid in patients with gastroparesis, cholelithiasis, or complete biliary obstruction • Use with caution in patients susceptible to fat-soluble vitamin deficiencies • Dose increases should be considered no sooner than at 1 to 2 month intervals • Separate administration from other medications • Fecal impaction may occur
Cholesterol Absorption Inhibitors			
Drug Name	FDA-Approved Indications	Adult Dosage Range	Precautions and Clinical Pearls
Generic Name Ezetimibe **Brand Name** Zetia	Homozygous familial hypercholesterolemia Primary hyperlipidemia Homozygous sitosterolemia	**Usual oral dose:** 10 mg per day	• Not recommended for patients with moderate to severe hepatic impairment • Myopathy and rhabdomyolosis have been reported with use Contraindications: • Drug interactions may require dose adjustments or avoidance of certain drug combinations
Fibric Acid Derivatives			
Drug Name	FDA-Approved Indications	Adult Dosage Range	Precautions and Clinical Pearls
Generic Name Fenofibrate	Hypertriglyceridemia	**Usual oral dose:** Lipofen brand: 50 to 150 mg per day with meals (maximum daily: 150 mg)	• Multiple different brand names with unique product dosing; refer to PI before prescribing (some administered without regard to food) • Monitor closely for myositis, myopathy, or rhabdomyolysis; patients with hypothyroidism may be at higher risk

Brand Name Antara Fenoglide Fibricor Lipofen Lofibra Tricor Triglide Trilipix ▲	Hypercholesterolemia or mixed hyperlipidemia		• Drug interactions may require dose adjustment or avoidance of certain drug combinations • Improvement in cardiovascular disease mortality has not been demonstrated • Thrombosis has been reported with use Contraindications: • Active liver disease and hepatic impairment • Severe renal dysfunction or end-stage renal disease (ESRD) and dialysis • Preexisting gallbladder disease
Generic Name Gemfibrozil **Brand Name** Lopid	Hyperlipidemia/ hypertriglyceridemia	**Usual oral dose:** 600 mg twice daily 30 minutes before breakfast and dinner	• Discontinue if response is inadequate after 3 months of therapy Contraindications: • Hepatic or severe renal dysfunction • Primary biliary cirrhosis • Preexisting gallbladder disease • Drug interactions may require dose adjustment or avoidance of certain drug combinations (including, but not limited to, concurrent use of statins)

HMG-CoA Reductase Inhibitors

Universal prescribing alerts:

- Contraindicated in patients with active liver disease and with unexplained persistent elevations of serum transaminases.
- Monitor closely for myopathy/rhabdomyolysis. Patients should be advised to promptly report unexplained myalgias, muscle tenderness or weakness, and general malaise. HMG-CoA reductase inhibitors should be discontinued immediately if marked elevations in creatine phosphokinase (CPK) or rhabdomyolysis are evident or if myopathy is diagnosed or suspected. Females, patients with renal impairment, and those with uncontrolled hypothyroidism appear to be predisposed to developing myopathy. The risk of developing myopathy also appears to be increased when HMG-CoA reductase inhibitors are used in combination with selected drugs (e.g., fibrates and others), so drug interactions should always be confirmed before concomitant administration.
- Rhabdomyolysis may result in subsequent renal failure in any patient, however individuals with hypotension, sepsis or severe acute infection, severe uncontrolled endocrine disorders, electrolyte imbalances, seizure disorder, major surgery, and trauma are at higher risk.
- Drug interactions may require dose adjustments or avoidance of certain drug combinations.

Drug Name	FDA-Approved Indications	Adult Dosage Range	Precautions and Clinical Pearls
Generic Name Atorvastatin **Brand Name** Lipitor (PD)	Prevention of hypercholesterolemia and mixed hyperlipidemia Prevention of cardiovascular disease	**Usual oral dose:** Initial: 10 to 20 mg per day Range: 10 to 80 mg per day	• Give without regard to meals • May be used as a high-intensity statin • Monitor closely for myopathy/rhabdomyolysis Contraindications: • Hepatic disease and impairment
Generic Name Fluvastatin **Brand Name** Lescol XL (PD)	Hypercholesterolemia Mixed dyslipidemia Prevention of cardiovascular disease	**Usual oral dose:** IR: 40 mg per day in the evening or 40 mg twice daily ER: 80 mg per day	• Monitor closely for myopathy/rhabdomyolysis Contraindications: • Hepatic disease and impairment
Generic Name Lovastatin **Brand Name** Altoprev Mevacor ▲	Dyslipidemia and primary prevention of CAD Prevention of cardiovascular disease	**Usual oral dose:** IR: Initial: 20 mg per day with evening meal (maximum: 80 mg per day) ER: Initial: 20, 40, or 60 mg daily at bedtime (maximum: 60 mg per day)	• Drug interactions may require dose adjustments • Monitor closely for myopathy/rhabdomyolysis • Food reduces absorption of ER formulation Contraindications: • Hepatic disease and impairment
Generic Name Pitavastatin **Brand Name** Livalo ▲	Primary hyperlipidemia and mixed dyslipidemia Prevention of cardiovascular disease	**Usual oral dose:** Initial: 2 mg per day (maximum: 4 mg per day)	• Monitor closely for myopathy/rhabdomyolysis Contraindications: • Active liver disease, including unexplained persistent elevations of hepatic transaminases • Drug interactions may require dose adjustments or avoidance of certain drug combinations
Generic Name Pravastatin **Brand Name** Pravachol ▲ (PD)	Hyperlipidemias Primary prevention of coronary events Secondary prevention of cardiovascular events	**Usual oral dose:** Initial: 40 mg per day Usual range: 10 to 80 mg per day (maximum: 80 mg per day)	• Monitor closely for myopathy and rhabdomyolysis Contraindications: • Active liver disease and hepatic impairment • Unexplained persistent elevations of serum transaminases

Drug Name	FDA-Approved Indications	Adult Dosage Range	Precautions and Clinical Pearls
Generic Name Rosuvastatin **Brand Name** Crestor ▲	Hyperlipidemia Mixed dyslipidemia Hypertriglyceridemia Primary dysbetalipoproteinemia Slowing progression of atherosclerosis Primary prevention of cardiovascular disease	**Usual oral dose:** Initial: 10 to 20 mg per day Dose range: 5 to 40 mg per day (maximum: 40 mg per day)	• Consider higher starting dose for patients with LDL cholesterol greater than 190 mg/dL • Consider lower starting dose for Asian patients • Drug interactions may require dose adjustments or avoidance of certain drug combinations • Monitor closely for myopathy and rhabdomyolysis • May be used as a high-intensity statin Contraindications: • Active liver disease or unexplained persistent elevations of serum transaminases
Generic Name Simvastatin **Brand Name** Zocor	Homozygous familial hypercholesterolemia Prevention of cardiovascular disease	**Usual oral dose:** Initial: 10 to 20 mg once daily in the evening (usual range is 5 to 40 mg once daily)	• Increasing to dose of 80 mg is not recommended Contraindications: • Active liver disease and hepatic impairment • Unexplained persistent elevations of serum transaminases • Drug interactions may require dose adjustment or avoidance of certain drug combinations
PCSK9 Inhibitors			
Drug Name	**FDA-Approved Indications**	**Adult Dosage Range**	**Precautions and Clinical Pearls**
Generic Name Alirocumab **Brand Name** Praluent	Adjunct to diet and maximally tolerated statin therapy for the treatment of heterozygous familial hypercholesterolemia or clinical atherosclerotic disease in patients who require additional lowering of LDL-C	**Usual parenteral dose:** SQ: 75 mg once every 2 weeks	• Increase dose to 150 mg every 2 weeks if LDL lowering is inadequate • Evaluate LDL concentrations 4 to 8 weeks following initiation or with dose changes • If a dose is missed, give dose within 7 days from missed dose and then resume original schedule, however if the missed dose is not administered within 7 days, wait until the next scheduled dose • Specific administration and storage recommendations; refer to PI
Generic Name Evolocumab **Brand Name** Repatha	Adjunct to diet and maximally tolerated statin therapy (or other LDL lowering therapies) for the treatment of heterozygous familial hypercholesterolemia or primary hyperlipidemia with established clinical atherosclerosis in patients who require additional lowering of LDL-C	**Usual parenteral dose:** SQ: 140 mg every 2 weeks or 420 mg once monthly	• Administer a missed dose as soon as possible if there are more than 7 days until the next scheduled dose, or omit the missed dose and administer the next dose according to the original schedule • Specific administration and storage recommendations; refer to PI

Miscellaneous Antilipemic Agents			
Drug Name	FDA-Approved Indications	Adult Dosage Range	Precautions and Clinical Pearls
Generic Name Icosapent ethyl **Brand Name** Vascepa	Hypertriglyceridemia	**Usual oral dose:** 2 g (2 capsules) twice daily (4 g total daily)	• Periodically monitor hepatic transaminases in patients with hepatic impairment and LDL levels • Inhibits platelet aggregation and may prolong bleeding time in predisposed individuals • Not interchangeable with Lovaza brand capsules which are omega-3-acid ethyl esters eicosapentaenoic acid (EPA) and docosahexaenoic acid (DHA); Vascepa is exclusively eicosapentaenoic acid (EPA)
Generic Name Lomitapide **Brand Name** Juxtapid ▲ ■	Homozygous familial hypercholesterolemia (HoFH)	**Usual oral dose:** 5 mg per day; may increase up to 10 mg as tolerated after 2 weeks Further dose increases should be considered no sooner than every 4 weeks but may increase to 20 mg daily, then 40 mg daily, up to a maximum of 60 mg daily	• Take at least 2 hours after evening meal with full glass of water; do no open, crush, or chew • Monitor hepatic function prior to treatment and regularly during treatment • Drug interactions may require dose adjustment • Specific recommendations for patients undergoing dialysis Contraindications: • Moderate to severe hepatic impairment Associated with: • Hepatotoxicity (REMS program) • Requires experienced clinician who is knowledgeable in the use of this agent
Generic Name Mipomersen **Brand Name** Kynamro	Homozygous familial hypercholesterolemia (HoFH)	**Usual parenteral dose:** 200 mg subcutaneously every week	• Maximal LDL cholesterol reduction seen after approximately 6 months • Available through REMS program • Not recommended for patients with renal impairment Contraindications: • Moderate or severe hepatic impairment • Active liver disease • Unexplained persistent elevations of hepatic transaminases Associated with: • Steatohepatitis • Cirrhosis

Generic Name Niacin **Brand Name** Niacor Niaspan	**Common indications for use:** Dietary supplement Hyperlipidemia	**Usual oral dose:** Immediate release initial: 250 mg per day, with evening meal (maximum: 6 g per day in 3 divided doses)	• Avoid alcohol, hot drinks, and spicy foods around the time of the niacin dose • May cause facial flushing; non-enteric coated aspirin 30 minutes prior to dose may mitigate • ER and IR are not equally interchangeable • Also known as vitamin B3 • Nicotinic acid is active as a hypolipidemic agent but nicotinamide (niacinamide) is not • May cause vasodilation; avoid in patients where this may complicate medical condition • Rhabdomyolosis has been reported (see universal prescribing alerts) Contraindications: • Active hepatic disease or significant or unexplained persistent elevations in hepatic transaminases • Active peptic ulcer • Arterial hemorrhage
Generic Name Omega-3-acid ethyl ester **Brand Name** Lovaza	Hypertriglyceridemia	**Usual oral dose:** 4 capsules per day as a single dose or as 2 capsules twice daily	• Periodically monitor hepatic transaminases in patients with hepatic impairment and high LDL cholesterol levels • Inhibits platelet aggregation and may prolong bleeding time in predisposed individuals

Hypotensive Agents

Central Alpha Agonists

Universal prescribing alerts:

- Centrally active alpha-adrenergic agonists are well known for their potential to cause dizziness, drowsiness, and sedation. Use care and recognize these agents have the potential to impair the ability to perform tasks requiring mental alertness. Caution should always be recommended when using any new drug for the first time, when there is a dose change, and for continued use of known offending agents.
- Recommendation to change doses gradually (increase or decrease). Carefully monitor blood pressure during initial titration, subsequent upward adjustment, or discontinuation.

Drug Name	FDA-Approved Indications	Adult Dosage Range	Precautions and Clinical Pearls
Generic Name Clonidine **Brand Name** Catapres Duraclon Kapvay (BL) (PD)	Hypertension ADHD Pain management	**Usual oral dose for hypertension:** IR: Initial: 0.1 mg twice daily Usual dose: 0.1 to 0.3 mg twice daily (maximum: 2.4 mg per day) **Transdermal:** Initial: 0.1 mg per 24 hour patch once every 7 days Usual dose: 0.1 to 0.3 mg per 24 hour once every 7 days (maximum 2 × 0.3 mg [0.6 mg total] patches applied once weekly)	• Use with caution in patients with severe coronary insufficiency, cerebrovascular disease, and chronic renal impairment (may decrease perfusion) • Do not discontinue clonidine abruptly; if discontinuation is needed, gradually reduce the dose over 2 to 4 days to avoid rebound hypertension • The adhesive overlay is intended for application over the patch that contains active drug Contraindications • Specific to epidural injections; refer to PI
Generic Name Guanabenz (BL) (PD)	Hypertension	**Usual oral dose:** 2 to 4 mg twice daily Maintenance: 4 to 16 mg twice daily (maximum: 32 mg twice daily)	• Potential sedative effect that may impair driving or operating machinery • Use caution in hepatic impairment • Carefully monitor blood pressure during initial titration, subsequent upward adjustment, or discontinuation
Generic Name Guanfacine **Brand Name** Intuniv Tenex (BL)	Hypertension ADHD	**Usual oral dose for hypertension:** IR: 1 mg per day at bedtime	• Use caution when performing tasks that require mental alertness • Abrupt discontinuation can result in nervousness, anxiety, depression, and, rarely, rebound hypertension • ER formulation is indicated for ADHD

Generic Name Methyldopa ▲ BL PD	Hypertension	**Usual oral dose:** Initial: 250 mg 2 to 3 times per day Usual dose: 250 to 500 mg twice daily (maximum: 3 g per day) **Usual parenteral dose:** IV: 250 to 1000 mg every 6 to 8 hours (maximum: 4 g per day)	• Administer new dosage increases in the evening to minimize sedation • Drug interactions may require dose adjustment • Specific recommendations for patients undergoing dialysis • Use caution in patients with preexisting mental health disorders; depression has been reported • Parkinson's symptoms may be worsened • Caution in patients with cardiac insufficiency • Hemolytic anemia has been reported Contraindications: • Active hepatic disease • Liver disorders previously associated with use of methyldopa
Direct Vasodilators			
Drug Name	FDA-Approved Indications	Adult Dosage Range	Precautions and Clinical Pearls
Generic Name Fenoldopam **Brand Name** Corlopam BL PD	Hypertension	**Usual parenteral dose for severe hypertension:** IV initial: 0.03 to 0.1 mcg/kg per minute (maximum: 1.6 mcg/kg per minute)	• Use with caution in patients with angina, open-angle glaucoma, and increased intracranial pressure • May cause dose-dependent sinus tachycardia • Monitor potassium concentration
Generic Name Hydralazine ▲ BL	**Common indication for use:** Hypertension Hypertensive emergency	**Usual oral dose:** Initial: 10 mg 4 times per day (maximum: 300 mg per day, in divided doses)	• Needs dose adjustment in patients with renal impairment • Systemic lupus erythematosus has been reported and risk appears to be greater in patients receiving higher doses • May cause reflex tachycardia and increases myocardial oxygen demand; avoid in conditions that may be worsened (i.e., CAD, angina, MI, etc.) Contraindications: • Mitral valve rheumatic heart disease

Drug Name	FDA-Approved Indications	Adult Dosage Range	Precautions and Clinical Pearls
Generic Name Minoxidil ▲ ■ (PD)	Hypertension Alopecia	**Usual oral dose for hypertension:** Initial: 5 mg per day Usual dose: 10 to 40 mg per day	• May experience hair growth or nausea • Avoid in severe renal impairment • Should be given with a diuretic and a beta blocker to prevent tachycardia and serious fluid accumulation • Topical formulations indicated for hair growth Contraindications: • Pheochromocytoma; hypotensive effects can stimulate catecholamine release Associated with: • Pericarditis, pericardial effusion (and cardiac tamponade) • Exacerbation of angina pectoris and other cardiac disease
Generic Name Sodium nitroprusside **Brand Name** Nitropress ▲ ■ (BL)	Acute hypertension Acute decompensated heart failure	Dose varies with indication for use and patient's clinical response **Usual parenteral dose:** IV initial: 0.3 to 0.5 mcg/kg per minute (maximum: 10 mcg/kg per minute)	• Elderly patients may have an increased sensitivity to nitroprusside • Avoid in patients with thyroid disorders • Avoid in severe renal impairment • For patients undergoing anesthesia; use caution in states of hypovolemia and/or anemia • May increase intracranial pressure • Dilute according to PI Contraindications: • Treatment of compensatory hypertension • Congenital optic atrophy • High output acute heart failure (such as that seen in patients with endotoxic sepsis) or other acute congestive heart failure associated with reduced peripheral vascular resistance Associated with: • Excessive hypotension resulting in compromised perfusion of vital organs • Cyanide toxicity
Diazoxide	Refer to the Hormones and Synthetic Substitutes chapter.		
Diuretic Agents			
Carbonic Anhydrase Inhibitors			
Acetazolamide	Refer to the Eye, Ear, Nose, and Throat Preparations chapter.		

Loop Diuretics	
Bumetanide	Refer to the Electrolytic, Caloric, and Water Balance Agents chapter.
Ethacrynic acid	Refer to the Electrolytic, Caloric, and Water Balance Agents chapter.
Furosemide	Refer to the Electrolytic, Caloric, and Water Balance Agents chapter.
Torsemide	Refer to the Electrolytic, Caloric, and Water Balance Agents chapter.
Osmotic Diuretics	
Mannitol	Refer to the Electrolytic, Caloric, and Water Balance Agents chapter.
Urea	Refer to the Electrolytic, Caloric, and Water Balance Agents chapter.
Potassium-Sparing Diuretics	
Amiloride	Refer to the Electrolytic, Caloric, and Water Balance Agents chapter.
Eplerenone acid	Refer to the Renin–Angiotensin–Aldosterone System Inhibitors section.
Spironolactone	Refer to the Renin–Angiotensin–Aldosterone System Inhibitors section.
Triamterene	Refer to the Electrolytic, Caloric, and Water Balance Agents chapter.
Thiazide Diuretics	
Bendroflumethiazide	Refer to the Electrolytic, Caloric, and Water Balance Agents chapter.
Chlorothiazide	Refer to the Electrolytic, Caloric, and Water Balance Agents chapter.
Hydrochlorothiazide	Refer to the Electrolytic, Caloric, and Water Balance Agents chapter.
Methyclothiazide	Refer to the Electrolytic, Caloric, and Water Balance Agents chapter.

Drug Name	FDA-Approved Indications	Adult Dosage Range	Precautions and Clinical Pearls
Thiazide-like Diuretics			
Chlorthalidone	Refer to the Electrolytic, Caloric, and Water Balance Agents chapter.		
Indapamide	Refer to the Electrolytic, Caloric, and Water Balance Agents chapter.		
Metolazone	Refer to the Electrolytic, Caloric, and Water Balance Agents chapter.		
Miscellaneous Hypotensive Agents			
Phenoxybenzamine	Refer to the Autonomic Agents chapter.		
Phentolamine	Refer to the Autonomic Agents chapter.		
Vasodilating Agents			
Nitrates and Nitrites			
Generic Name Amyl nitrite	Angina	**Usual dose:** 2 to 6 nasal inhalations from 1 broken ampule; may repeat in 3 to 5 minutes	• Diminished oxygen-carrying capacity may cause methemoglobinemia and severe hypotension; avoid in severe anemia • May cause increased intracranial pressure • Use caution in any patient with conditions worsened by hypotension (cardiac disease, sensitive to reflex tachycardia, etc.) Contraindications: • Glaucoma • Recent head trauma or cerebral hemorrhage
Generic Name Isosorbide **Brand Name** Isordil (isosorbide dinitrate) Imdur (isosorbide mononitrate)	Angina	**Usual oral dose isosorbide dinitrate:** Initial: 5 to 20 mg 3 times per day Maximum: 40 mg of 3 times per day **Usual oral dose isosorbide mononitrate ER (Imdur):** 30 to 60 mg once daily	• Isosorbide mononitrate is the once-daily formulation of isosorbide dinitrate Contraindications: • Drug interactions may require dose adjustments or avoidance of certain drug combinations (i.e., selective PDE inhibitors) • Glaucoma; may cause increased intraocular pressure • Shock or markedly low blood pressure • Diminished oxygen-carrying capacity may cause methemoglobinemia and severe hypotension; avoid in severe anemia

Generic Name Nitroglycerin **Brand Name** Minitran Nitrolingual NitroMist Rectiv	**Common indications for use:** Angina CAD Chronic anal fissure	**Illustrative dose for angina using sublingual tablets:** SL: 0.3 to 0.6 mg every 5 minutes, up to a maximum of 3 tablets in 15 minutes	• Avoid use of long-acting agents in patients with acute myocardial infarction (AMI) or acute HF • Multiple dosage forms available including: oral, parenteral, topical patch, ointment, and lingual spray • The maximum dosage is dependent on route of administration and indication for therapy Contraindications: • Drug interactions may require dose adjustments or avoidance of certain drug combinations (i.e., selective PDE inhibitors) • IV: constrictive pericarditis • SL: early MI; increased intracranial pressure; severe anemia • Any condition that would be exacerbated by reduced venous return, decreased preload, and cardiac output

Phosphodiesterase Type 5 Inhibitors

Universal prescribing alerts:

- Contraindications: Drug interactions require dose adjustments or avoidance of certain drug combinations (including but not limited to concurrent use of organic nitrates in any form).
- Flushing and headache are common side effects.
- Watch for signs and symptoms of impairment of color discrimination or hearing loss.
- Drug interactions may require dose reduction or avoidance of certain drug combinations.
- Prolonged erections greater than 4 hours and priapism (painful erections greater than 6 hours in duration) have been associated with PDE5 inhibitor administration, which if not treated promptly, can result in irreversible damage to the erectile tissue. Patients who have an erection lasting greater than 4 hours, whether painful or not, should seek emergency medical attention. Use of these agents for the treatment of ED should be used with caution in patients with penile structural abnormality or in patients who have conditions which may predispose them to priapism (i.e., leukemia, multiple myeloma, or history of priapism etc.).

Drug Name	FDA-Approved Indications	Adult Dosage Range	Precautions and Clinical Pearls
Generic Name Sildenafil **Brand Name** Revatio Viagra ▲ ■	Erectile dysfunction (Viagra) Pulmonary arterial hypertension (Revatio)	**Usual oral dose:** Viagra: 50 mg per day 1 hour before sexual activity as needed Revatio: **Usual parenteral dose:** IV: 2.5 or 10 mg 3 times per day Oral: 5 or 20 mg 3 times per day, 4 to 6 hours apart	• Sudden hearing loss or vision loss may occur; if it does, consult with the physician and discontinue therapy • Prescribers must evaluate the cardiovascular status of their patients and avoid use in those who would be adversely affected by vasodilatory events Contraindications: • Drug interactions may require dose adjustments or avoidance of certain drug combinations (i.e., nitrate therapy)

Drug Name	FDA-Approved Indications	Adult Dosage Range	Precautions and Clinical Pearls
Generic Name Tadalafil **Brand Name** Adcirca Cialis ▲ ■	Pulmonary arterial hypertension (Adcirca) BPH (Cialis) ED (Cialis)	Dose varies with indication for use and patient's clinical response **Illustrative oral dose for ED:** 10 or 20 mg per day at least 30 minutes prior to sexual activity	• Sudden hearing loss or vision loss may occur; if it does, consult with the physician and discontinue therapy • Prescribers must evaluate the cardiovascular status of their patients and avoid use in those who would be adversely affected by vasodilatory events • May worsen GERD Contraindications: • Drug interactions may require dose adjustments or avoidance of certain drug combinations (i.e., nitrate therapy)
Generic Name Vardenafil **Brand Name** Levitra Staxyn ■ QT	ED	**Usual oral dose:** Levitra: 5 to 20 mg per day 1 hour prior to sexual activity Staxyn: 10 mg per day 1 hour prior to sexual activity	• Sudden hearing loss or vision loss may occur; if it does, consult with the physician and discontinue therapy • Prescribers must evaluate the cardiovascular status of their patients and avoid use in those who would be adversely affected by vasodilatory events Contraindications: • Drug interactions may require dose adjustments or avoidance of certain drug combinations (i.e., nitrate therapy)
Cilostazol	Refer to Blood Formation, Coagulation, and Thrombosis Agents chapter.		

Miscellaneous Vasodilating Agents

Drug Name	FDA-Approved Indications	Adult Dosage Range	Precautions and Clinical Pearls
Generic Name Alprostadil **Brand Name** Caverject Edex Muse Prostin VR ■	**Common indications for use:** ED	**Usual dose for ED Caverject:** Initiate dosage titration at 2.5 mcg Doses greater than 60 mcg (Caverject, Caverject Impulse) are not recommended	• When used in ED, priapism and syncope may occur • Do not administer more than 3 times per week and no less than 24 hours between doses • Multiple dosage forms available • Risk of priapism Contraindications: • Conditions predisposing patients to priapism • Patients with anatomic deformation or fibrotic conditions of the penis • Penile implants
Generic Name Dipyridamole **Brand Name** Persantine BL	Adjunctive therapy for prophylaxis of thromboembolism with cardiac valve replacement Evaluation of CAD	**Usual oral dose thromboembolism prophylaxis:** 75 to 100 mg 4 times per day in combination with warfarin **Usual parenteral dose for evaluation:** IV: 0.14 mg/kg per minute for 4 minutes (maximum: 60 mg)	• Use with caution in patients with hypotension, unstable angina, or recent MI • Severe adverse reactions have occurred (rarely) with IV administration • Combinations with aspirin are also available

Generic Name Isoxsuprine BL	Peripheral vascular disease or symptoms of cerebrovascular insufficiency	**Usual oral dose:** 10 to 20 mg 3 to 4 times per day	• Possible side effects are dizziness, nausea, vomiting, and rash • May precipitate arrhythmias, avoid in patients who may be predisposed Contraindications: • Presence of arterial bleeding
Generic Name Nesiritide **Brand Name** Natrecor	Acute decompensated heart failure	**Usual parenteral dose:** IV initial: 2 mcg/kg (bolus optional), followed by continuous infusion at 0.01 mcg/kg per minute	• Serious anaphylactic or hypersensitivity reactions may occur Contraindications: • Cardiogenic shock • Hypotension (persistent systolic blood pressure less than 100 mm Hg) prior to therapy
Generic Name Papaverine QT	Arterial spasm	**Usual parenteral dose:** IM/ IV: 30 to 120 mg; may repeat dose every 3 hours Inject slowly over 1 to 2 minutes	• Discontinue use if GI symptoms, jaundice, eosinophilia, or abnormal LFTs occur Contraindications: • Complete AV block
Ambrisentan	Refer to the Respiratory Tract Agents chapter.		
Amlodipine	Refer to the Calcium-Channel Blocking Agents section.		
Bosentan	Refer to the Respiratory Tract Agents chapter.		
Diltiazem	Refer to the Calcium-Channel Blocking Agents section.		
Epoprostenol	Refer to the Respiratory Tract Agents chapter.		
Iloprost	Refer to the Respiratory Tract Agents chapter.		
Macitentan	Refer to the Respiratory Tract Agents chapter.		
Nicardipine	Refer to the Calcium-Channel Blocking Agents section.		
Nifedipine	Refer to the Calcium-Channel Blocking Agents section.		
Nimodipine	Refer to the Calcium-Channel Blocking Agents section.		
Riociguat	Refer to the Respiratory Tract Agents chapter.		
Treprostinil	Refer to the Respiratory Tract Agents chapter.		
Verapamil	Refer to the Calcium-Channel Blocking Agents section.		

Adrenergic Agents

Alpha-Adrenergic Blocking Agents

Universal prescribing alerts:

- Patients should use caution when performing tasks that require mental alertness.
- Can cause significant orthostatic hypotension and syncope, especially with first dose.

Drug Name	FDA-Approved Indications	Adult Dosage Range	Precautions and Clinical Pearls
Generic Name Doxazosin **Brand Name** Cardura (BL)	BPH Hypertension	Dose varies with indication for use and patient's clinical response **Illustrative oral dose for BPH:** IR initial: 1 mg at bedtime dose may be increased up to 8 mg per day ER initial: 4 mg with breakfast, up to 8 mg per day	• Avoid in patients with hepatic disease or compromise • Intraoperative floppy iris syndrome during ocular surgery has been reported • Can cause significant orthostatic hypotension and syncope, especially with first dose • Rare side effect: priapism • Avoid in geriatric females with urinary incontinence, regardless of cause or type, because aggravation of incontinence may occur
Generic Name Prazosin **Brand Name** Minipress (BL) (PD)	Hypertension	**Usual oral dose:** Initial: 1 mg 2 to 3 times per day Usual maintenance: 6 to 15 mg per day in divided doses	• May cause significant orthostatic hypotension and syncope with sudden loss of consciousness, especially within 30 to 90 minutes of the first dose • Priapism has been reported • Avoid in patients with hepatic disease or compromise • Intraoperative floppy iris syndrome during ocular surgery has been reported • Avoid in geriatric females with urinary incontinence, regardless of cause or type, because aggravation of incontinence may occur
Generic Name Terazosin **Brand Name** (BL)	BPH Hypertension	Dose varies with indication for use and patient's clinical response **Illustrative oral dose for BPH:** Initial: 1 mg daily at bedtime up to 10 mg per day	• Patients should use caution when performing tasks that require mental alertness • Can cause significant orthostatic hypotension and syncope, especially with first dose • May require dose adjustment in hepatic impairment, although there are no specific recommendations are available • Priapism and floppy iris syndrome have been reported • Avoid in geriatric females with urinary incontinence, regardless of cause or type, because aggravation of incontinence may occur
Carvedilol	Refer to Beta-Adrenergic Blocking Agents section.		
Labetalol	Refer to Beta-Adrenergic Blocking Agents section.		

Beta-Adrenergic Blocking Agents

Universal prescribing alerts:

- May potentiate hypoglycemia.
- Beta blockers should be used with caution in patients with hyperthyroidism or thyrotoxicosis because beta-blockade can mask tachycardia. Abrupt withdrawal of beta blockers in a patient with hyperthyroidism can precipitate thyroid storm. Abrupt withdrawal should be avoided with beta blocker therapy.
- Although beta$_1$-adrenergic selective beta blockers are preferred over nonselective agents in patients with asthma or other pulmonary disease where there is increased risk of acute bronchospasm, all beta blockers should be used with caution in these patients (especially when high doses are used).
- Beta blockers should be used with caution in patients with cerebrovascular insufficiency, cerebrovascular disease or stroke. Alternative drug therapy should be considered if there are signs or symptoms associated with reduced blood flow to the brain during use.

Drug Name	FDA-Approved Indications	Adult Dosage Range	Precautions and Clinical Pearls
Generic Name Acebutolol **Brand Name** Sectral ▲ GD	Angina Ventricular arrhythmia Hypertension	Dose varies with indication for use and patient's clinical response **Illustrative oral dose for hypertension:** 400 mg per day in either 1 dose or 2 divided doses Usual maintenance: 400 to 800 mg per day in divided doses	• Use caution in patients with hepatic disease Contraindications: • Overt cardiac failure • Cardiogenic shock • Persistently severe bradycardia • Second- and third-degree heart block
Generic Name Atenolol **Brand Name** Tenormin ▲ ■ GD	Hypertension Angina pectoris Post MI	Dose varies with indication for use and patient's clinical response **Illustrative oral dose:** 100 mg per day or 50 mg twice daily for 6 to 9 days post MI	Contraindications: • Sinus bradycardia • Greater than first-degree heart block • Cardiogenic shock • Uncompensated cardiac failure • Pulmonary edema Associated with: • Need to not abruptly discontinue
Generic Name Betaxolol **Brand Name** Kerlone ▲	Hypertension Glaucoma	**Usual oral dose:** 10 mg per day; may increase to 20 mg per day	• Psoriasis exacerbation has been reported • Visual changes in patients with myasthenia gravis Contraindications: • Sinus bradycardia • Greater than first-degree heart block • Cardiogenic shock • Uncompensated cardiac failure

Drug Name	FDA-Approved Indications	Adult Dosage Range	Precautions and Clinical Pearls
Generic Name Bisoprolol **Brand Name** Zebeta ▲ ■	Hypertension	**Usual oral dose:** 2.5 to 5 mg per day; may increase to 20 mg per day	Contraindications: • Cardiogenic shock • Overt cardiac failure • Marked sinus bradycardia • Greater than first-degree heart block
Generic Name Carvedilol **Brand Name** Coreg	Hypertension Heart failure Left ventricular dysfunction following MI	Dose varies with indication for use and patient's clinical response **Illustrative oral dose:** IR initial: 6.25 mg twice daily up to 25 mg twice daily ER initial: 20 mg per day up to maximum 80 mg per day	• Can cause significant orthostatic hypotension and syncope, especially with first dose Contraindications: • Decompensated cardiac failure requiring intravenous inotropic therapy • Bronchial asthma or related bronchospastic conditions • Second- or third-degree AV block • Sick sinus syndrome • Severe bradycardia • Cardiogenic shock • Severe hepatic impairment
Generic Name Esmolol **Brand Name** Brevibloc	Intraoperative and postoperative tachycardia and/or hypertension Supraventricular tachycardia (SVT) or noncompensatory sinus tachycardia	**Usual parenteral dose:** Immediate control: Initial bolus: 1 mg/kg over 30 seconds, followed by 150 mcg/kg per minute infusion **Alternatively may use:** Gradual control loading dose (optional): 0.5 mg/kg over 1 minute; followed with a 50 mcg/kg per minute infusion for 4 minutes	• Monitor hyperkalemia and hypotension • May potentiate hypoglycemia • Abrupt withdrawal should be avoided with beta blocker therapy Contraindications: • Severe sinus bradycardia • Greater than first-degree heart block • Sick sinus syndrome • Cardiogenic shock • Decompensated heart failure • Drug interactions may require dose adjustment or avoidance of certain drug combinations • Pulmonary hypertension and edema

Generic Name Labetalol **Brand Name** Trandate ■	Hypertension Acute hypertension (hypertensive emergency/ urgency)	**Usual oral dose:** Initial: 100 mg twice daily (maximum: 2400 mg per day) **Usual parenteral doses:** IV bolus: Initial: 20 mg over 2 minutes, up to 300 mg total cumulative dose IV infusion: Initial: 2 mg per minute, up to 300 mg total cumulative dose	• Periodically monitor LFTs with prolonged use • Can cause significant orthostatic hypotension and syncope, especially with first dose Contraindications: • Severe bradycardia • Greater than first-degree heart block • Cardiogenic shock • Bronchial asthma • Uncompensated cardiac failure • Conditions associated with severe and prolonged hypotension Associated with: • Need to not abruptly discontinue
Generic Name Metoprolol tartrate Metoprolol succinate **Brand Name** Lopressor Toprol XL ■ (PD)	Angina Heart failure Hypertension Ventricular rate control MI	Dose varies with indication for use, formulation selected, and patient's clinical response **Illustrative oral dose for hypertension** **IR tartrate:** 100 mg in single or divided doses (maximum: 450 mg per day) **XL succinate:** 25 to 100 mg once daily up to 400 mg per day **Illustrative parenteral dose:** IV: 5 mg every 5 minutes as tolerated, for up to 3 doses	• Use caution in hepatic impairment • Psoriasis exacerbation has been reported • Visual changes in patients with myasthenia gravis • Metoprolol succinate (Toprol XL) should be used in patients with heart failure with reduced ejection fraction Contraindications for use in hypertension and angina: • Sinus bradycardia • Second- and third-degree heart block • Cardiogenic shock • Overt heart failure • Sick sinus syndrome • Severe peripheral arterial disease • Pheochromocytoma Contraindications in use for MI: • Severe sinus bradycardia • Significant first-degree heart block • Second- and third-degree heart block • Systolic blood pressure less than 100 mm Hg • Moderate to severe cardiac failure Associated with: • Exacerbation of ischemic heart disease following abrupt withdrawal

Drug Name	FDA-Approved Indications	Adult Dosage Range	Precautions and Clinical Pearls
Generic Name Nadolol **Brand Name** Corgard ▲ ■	Angina Hypertension	Dose varies with indication for use and patient's clinical response **Usual oral dose:** 40 to 80 mg per day	Contraindications: • Bronchial asthma • Sinus bradycardia • Sinus node dysfunction • Greater than first-degree heart block • Cardiogenic shock • Uncompensated cardiac failure Associated with: • Exacerbation of ischemic heart disease following abrupt withdrawal
Generic Name Nebivolol **Brand Name** Bystolic ▲ ■	Hypertension	**Usual oral dose:** 5 to 10 mg per day (maximum: 40 mg per day)	• Has not been shown to reduce morbidity or mortality in the general HF population Contraindications: • Severe bradycardia • Greater than first-degree heart block • Cardiogenic shock • Decompensated heart failure • Sick sinus syndrome • Severe hepatic impairment
Generic Name Pindolol	Hypertension	**Usual oral dose:** Initial: 5 mg twice daily (maximum: 60 mg)	• May potentiate hypoglycemia • Use caution in renal and hepatic impairment Contraindications: • Bronchial asthma • Cardiogenic shock • Heart block • Overt cardiac failure • Severe bradycardia Associated with: • Need to not abruptly discontinue

Generic Name Propranolol **Brand Name** Hemangeol Inderal InnoPran XL ■ (PD)	Essential tremor Hypertension Migraine headache prophylaxis Obstructive hypertrophic cardiomyopathy Pheochromocytoma Post-MI mortality reduction Stable angina Tachyarrhythmias	Dose varies with indication for use, formulation selected, and patient's clinical response **Illustrative oral dose for hypertension:** 40 mg twice per day May give up to 640 mg per day maximum in divided doses	• Prescriptions for Hemangeol may be obtained via the Hemangeol Patient Access program Contraindications: • Uncompensated congestive heart failure • Cardiogenic shock • Severe sinus bradycardia • Sick sinus syndrome • Greater than first-degree heart block • Bronchial asthma
Generic Name Sotalol **Brand Name** Betapace Betapace AF Sorine Sotylize ▲ ■ (QT)	Atrial fibrillation/flutter (symptomatic) Ventricular arrhythmias (Betapace, Sorine, Sotylize)	Dose varies with indication for use, formulation selected, and patient's clinical response **Illustrative parenteral dose:** IV Initial: 75 mg infused over 5 hours twice daily Usual dose: most patient achieve response at 150 mg twice daily **Illustrative oral dose:** Initial: 80 mg twice daily Usual dose: most patient achieve response at 120 mg twice daily	• Also has a beta blocking component • Before initiating therapy (and throughout therapy) evaluate CrCl, HR, and QTc, correct electrolyte imbalances, allow at least 36 hours between dose adjustments (base adjustments on clinical response, QTc interval and other clinical factors) Contraindications: • Bronchial spasm (and asthma) • Sinus bradycardia (less than 50 beats per minute) • Congenital or acquired long QT syndromes • Cardiogenic shock • Uncontrolled HF Betapace AF, Sotylize, Sotalol injection: • Baseline QTc interval greater than 450 ms • Creatinine clearance (CrCl) less than 40 mL per minute • Serum potassium less than 4 mEq/L • Sick sinus syndrome Associated with: • Potential torsades de pointes (QT prolongation) • Renal impairment • Betapace should not be substituted for Betapace AF • Requires experienced clinician who is knowledgeable in the use of this agent and specialized care setting

Drug Name	FDA-Approved Indications	Adult Dosage Range	Precautions and Clinical Pearls
Generic Name Timolol **Brand Name** Apo-Timol Nu-Timolol Teva-Timolol	Hypertension Prevention of MI Migraine prophylaxis Glaucoma	Dose varies with indication for use, formulation selected, and patient's clinical response **Illustrative oral dose for hypertension:** 10 to 30 mg per day	• Use caution in patients with renal or hepatic impairment Contraindications: • Sinus bradycardia • Sinus node dysfunction • Greater than first-degree heart block • Cardiogenic shock • Uncompensated cardiac failure • Bronchospastic disease Associated with: • Exacerbation of ischemic heart disease following abrupt withdrawal

Calcium-Channel Blocking Agents

Dihydropyridine Calcium-Channel Blockers

Universal prescribing alerts:

- Calcium channel blockers should be used cautiously in patients with gastroesophageal reflux disease (GERD) or hiatal hernia associated with reflux esophagitis. These drugs may relax the lower esophageal sphincter.

Drug Name	FDA-Approved Indications	Adult Dosage Range	Precautions and Clinical Pearls
Generic Name Amlodipine **Brand Name** Norvasc ■ (PD)	**Common indications for use:** CAD Hypertension	**Usual oral dose:** 5 to 10 mg per day	• Use with caution in elderly patients • Increased angina and MI have occurred with initiation or dosage titration
Generic Name Clevidipine	**Common indications for use:** Hypertensive urgency Perioperative hypertension	**Usual parenteral dose:** IV: Initially, 1 to 2 mg per hour continuously Maximum 32 mg per hour	• No more than 1000 mL should be infused in 24 hours (an average of 21 mg per hour) due to lipid load restrictions • Use caution; may produce negative inotrope effects and exacerbate heart failure Contraindications: • Advanced aortic stenosis due to decreased myocardial oxygen delivery • Hyperlipidemia and acute pancreatitis

Generic Name Felodipine **Brand Name** Plendil ■	**Common indications for use:** Hypertension	**Usual oral dose:** Initial: 5 mg once daily Usual range: 2.5 to 10 mg once daily Maximum: 10 mg per day	• Dosage should be adjusted according to patient response, and any increase made at intervals of at least 2 weeks. • May worsen GERD • Use cautiously in patients who may have condition worsened with potential negative inotropic effects of the drug
Generic Name Isradipine	Hypertension	**Usual oral dose:** 5 mg once daily Maximum: 20 mg daily	• Use caution; may produce negative inotrope effects and exacerbate heart failure • Use caution in renal and hepatic impairment
Generic name Nicardipine **Brand Name** Cardene IV ■	Angina Hypertension Acute hypertension	**Usual oral dose for hypertension:** IR: 20 to 40 mg 3 times daily ER: 30 to 60 mg twice daily **Usual parenteral dose:** IV: Initial: 5 mg per hour up to a maximum of 15 mg per hour	• Close monitoring for heart rate is required • Use caution in renal impairment • May cause significant hypotension; use caution in intracranial bleeding or with acute stroke Contraindications: • Advanced aortic stenosis due to decreased myocardial oxygen delivery
Generic Name Nifedipine **Brand Name** Adalat CC Afeditab CR Nifediac CC Nifedical XL Procardia (BL) (PD)	Chronic stable or vasospastic angina Hypertension	Dose varies with indication for use and patient's clinical response **Illustrative oral dose:** IR: Usual: 10 to 20 mg 3 times per day ER: Initial: 30 to 60 mg per day Maximum: 120 mg per day	• Drug interactions may require dose adjustment or avoidance of certain drug combinations • Rare reports of symptoms of GI obstruction with extended formulations; use caution in patients at risk for obstruction • Use caution in hepatic impairment Contraindications: • Cardiogenic shock • The use of immediate-release nifedipine (sublingually or orally) in hypertensive emergencies and urgencies is neither safe nor effective
Generic Name Nimodipine	Subarachnoid hemorrhage	**Usual oral dose:** 60 mg every 4 hours for 21 consecutive days	• Peripheral edema occurs within 2 to 3 weeks of therapy • Use cautiously in patients who may have condition worsened with potential negative inotropic effects of the drug • Drug interactions may require a dose adjustment • For oral use only

Drug Name	FDA-Approved Indications	Adult Dosage Range	Precautions and Clinical Pearls
Brand Name Nymalize ■			Associated with: • Deaths and serious, life-threatening adverse events have occurred when the contents of nimodipine capsules have been injected parenterally.
Generic Name Nisoldipine **Brand Name** Sular ■	Hypertension	**Usual oral dose:** Initial: 17 mg daily Usual range: 17 to 34 mg once daily.	• Administer on an empty stomach • Avoid grapefruit juice • Extended release formulation only; do not crush or chew (swallow whole) • Use cautiously in patients who may have condition worsened with potential negative inotropic effects of the drug
Miscellaneous Calcium-Channel Blocking Agents			
Drug Name	**FDA-Approved Indications**	**Adult Dosage Range**	**Precautions and Clinical Pearls**
Generic Name Diltiazem **Brand Name** Cardizem Cartia XT Matzim LA Taztia XT Tiazac (BL)	**Common indications for use:** Angina Hypertension Atrial fibrillation/flutter PSVT	**Usual oral dose for hypertension:** ER: Initial 120 to 240 mg once daily. Usual range: 240 to 360 mg per day	• Dosage formulations are specific to FDA indications (i.e., regular release tablets are not FDA approved for hypertension) • The most common side effect is peripheral edema. • May worsen GERD • Use caution in hepatic impairment • Avoid in aortic stenosis Contraindications: • Acute MI or other cardiac conditions that can be worsened with cardiac conduction changes and/or bradycardia and severe hypotension (i.e.: cardiogenic shock)
Generic Name Verapamil **Brand Name** Isoptin SR Calan SR ■ (BL)	**Common indications for use:** Angina PSVT prophylaxis Hypertension Atrial fibrillation (rate control)	**Usual oral dose for hypertension:** **IR:** 80 to 160 mg 3 times per day **SR:** 180 once daily in the morning (may increase to 240 mg twice daily) **ER:** 240 mg once daily in the morning (may increase to 480 mg daily) **Illustrative parenteral dose for atrial fibrillation:** IV Initially: 5 to 10 mg (0.075 to 0.15 mg/kg) over at least 2 minutes.	• Use caution in renal impairment. Additional ECG monitoring in patients with renal insufficiency • May worsen GERD • Frequently causes constipation; use caution or avoid in patients with GI obstruction, etc. • Decreased neuromuscular transmission has been reported (may worsen symptoms of myasthenia gravis) • Parenteral dose may be repeated based on response and clinical needs; refer to PI Contraindications: • Acute MI or other cardiac conditions that can be worsened with cardiac conduction changes and/or bradycardia and severe hypotension (i.e., cardiogenic shock)

Renin–Angiotensin–Aldosterone System Inhibitors

Angiotensin-Converting Enzyme Inhibitors

Universal prescribing alerts:

- Monitor potassium levels for hyperkalemia.
- Dry cough is common side effect (results from the accumulation of kinins in the respiratory tract, sometimes causing a persistent, nonproductive cough)
- The incidence of ACE-inhibitor induced angioedema is higher in Black patients than non-Black patients. ACE inhibitors are less effective in lowering blood pressure in Black patients, including the African-American population.

Contraindications:

- History of angioedema (with an ACE inhibitor).
- Relative contraindication in patients who exhibit hypotension that can occur with hypovolemia or hyponatremia.
- Should be used cautiously in patients with congestive heart failure (initial doses should be lower than in the treatment of hypertension) because of a greater risk of developing hypotension which can exacerbate ischemia in patients with CAD or cerebrovascular disease, and which may precipitate an MI or cerebrovascular accident (caution also in those with cardiac structural defects, stenosis, hypertrophy, and/or cardiomyopathy).
- See each specific agent for recommendations for use in patients undergoing dialysis.

Associated with:

- Contraindication for specific age population and developmental stages; refer to PI.

Drug Name	FDA-Approved Indications	Adult Dosage Range	Precautions and Clinical Pearls
Generic Name Benazepril **Brand Name** Lotensin ▲ ■ (PD)	Hypertension	**Usual oral dose:** 20 to 80 mg per day as a single dose or 2 divided doses	• This is a prodrug that must be converted to active form via hepatic metabolism; patients with hepatic impairment may not see full benefit of drug • Potentially life-threatening angioedema has been reported even in patients that are not allergic
Generic Name Captopril **Brand Name** Apo-Capto Dom-Captopril Mylan-Captopril PMS-Captopril ▲ ■ (PD)	Acute hypertension (urgency/ emergency) Heart failure with reduced ejection fraction Hypertension Left ventricular (LV) dysfunction following MI Diabetic nephropathy	Dose varies with indication for use, formulation selected, and patient's clinical response **Illustrative oral dose:** Initial 12.5 to 25 mg then increase up to 50 mg 3 times per day if needed	• Short-acting ACE inhibitor requires 3 times per day dosing • May cause neutropenia or agranulocytosis • Patients with renal disease and/or immunosuppression may be more likely to experience adverse effects • Potentially life-threatening angioedema has been reported even in patients that are not allergic

Drug Name	FDA-Approved Indications	Adult Dosage Range	Precautions and Clinical Pearls
Generic Name Enalaprilat/ enalapril **Brand Name** Epaned Vasotec ▲ ■ (PD)	Asymptomatic LV dysfunction Heart failure with reduced ejection fraction Hypertension	Dose varies with indication for use, formulation selected, and patient's clinical response **Illustrative oral dose:** 10 to 20 mg twice daily	• Enalaprilat is IV formulation • May precipitate severe ventricular arrhythmias in patients with specific underlying conditions • Potentially life-threatening angioedema has been reported even in patients that are not allergic
Generic Name Fosinopril **Brand Name** Monopril ■ (PD)	Heart failure Hypertension	Dose varies with indication for use and patient's clinical response **Illustrative oral dose:** 10 to 40 mg per day	• As with other ACE inhibitors, may increase the risk of anaphylactoid reactions in patients undergoing hymenoptera venom (insect sting) allergy desensitization. • Neutropenia has been reported
Generic Name Lisinopril **Brand Name** Prinivil Zestril ▲ ■ (PD)	AMI within 24 hours in hemodynamically stable patients) Heart failure Hypertension	Dose varies with indication for use and patient's clinical response **Illustrative oral dose:** 5 to 40 mg per day	• Potentially life-threatening angioedema has been reported even in patients that are not allergic
Generic Name Moexipril **Brand Name** Univasc [DSC] ▲ ■ (QT)	Hypertension	**Usual oral dose:** 7.5 to 30 mg per day in 1 to 2 divided doses 1 hour before meals	• Use caution in patients with underlying cardiac conditions (i.e., aortic stenosis or hypertrophic cardiomyopathy) • Drug interactions may require dose adjustment or avoidance of certain drug combinations • This is a prodrug that must be converted to active form via hepatic metabolism; patients with hepatic impairment may not see full benefit of drug
Generic Name Perindopril **Brand Name** Aceon ▲ ■	Hypertension Stable CAD	**Usual oral dose:** 4 to 8 mg per day	• Potentially life-threatening angioedema has been reported even in patients that are not allergic

Generic Name Quinapril **Brand Name** Accupril ▲ ■	Heart failure Hypertension	**Usual oral dose:** Initial: 10 to 20 mg per day Usual range: 20 to 80 mg per day	• Potentially life-threatening angioedema has been reported even in patients that are not allergic • Use caution in patients with bone marrow suppression
Generic Name Ramipril **Brand Name** Altace ▲ ■	Heart failure post MI Hypertension Reduction in risk of MI, stroke, and death from cardiovascular causes	Dose varies with indication for use and patient's clinical response **Illustrative oral dose for hypertension:** 2.5 to 20 mg per day in 1 to 2 divided doses	• Potentially life-threatening angioedema has been reported even in patients that are not allergic
Generic Name Trandolapril **Brand Name** Mavik ▲ ■ ■	Hypertension Post-MI heart failure or LV dysfunction	Dose varies with indication for use and patient's clinical response (and whether patient is already on diuretics) **Illustrative oral dose for hypertension:** 2 to 8 mg per day	• To reduce the possibility of developing symptomatic hypotension, the diuretic should, if possible, be discontinued 2 to 3 days prior to starting therapy • Diuretic may be resumed if blood pressure is not adequately controlled • Neutropenia has been reported

Angiotensin II Receptor Antagonists

Universal prescribing alerts:

- Monitor potassium levels for hyperkalemia.
- Anaphylactic reactions and angioedema have been reported with angiotensin II receptor antagonists (although it may be less likely than with ACE inhibitors); use caution when using in patients with a history of angioedema related to ACE inhibitor therapy. Angiotensin II receptor antagonists (ARBs) have still been recommended as alternatives to ACE inhibitors in patients who experienced angioedema with ACE-inhibitor (although safety in these patients has not been definitively established).
- Use caution in patients who exhibit hypotension that can occur with hypovolemia or hyponatremia.
- Black patients are a low-renin population and therefore there is generally a smaller antihypertensive response compared to other ethnic populations. For these patients, recommendations advise to consider combining with a diuretic to increase the antihypertensive response.

Associated with:

- Contraindication for specific age population and developmental stages; refer to PI.

Drug Name	FDA-Approved Indications	Adult Dosage Range	Precautions and Clinical Pearls
Generic Name Azilsartan **Brand Name** Edarbi ■	Hypertension	**Usual oral dose:** 80 mg per day	• Consider lower starting doses for patients on high dose diuretic therapy
Generic Name Candesartan **Brand Name** Atacand ▲ ■ (PD)	Hypertension Heart failure	Dose varies with indication for use and patient's clinical response **Usual oral dose for hypertension:** 8 to 32 mg per day in 1 to 2 divided doses	• Consider lower starting doses for patients on high dose diuretic therapy
Generic Name Eprosartan **Brand Name** Teveten ▲ ■	Hypertension	**Usual oral dose:** 400 to 800 mg day in 1 to 2 divided doses	• Consider lower starting doses for patients on high dose diuretic therapy
Generic Name Irbesartan **Brand Name** Avapro ■	Hypertension Nephropathy in patients with type 2 diabetes and hypertension	**Usual oral dose:** 150 to 300 mg per day	• Consider lower starting dose in volume depleted patients • Use caution in hepatic disease
Generic Name Losartan **Brand Name** Cozaar ■ ■ (PD)	Hypertension Diabetic nephropathy Hypertension with left ventricular hypertrophy	Dose varies with indication for use and patient's clinical response **Usual oral dose for hypertension:** 25 to 100 mg per day in 1 to 2 divided doses	• Not recommended in severe renal impairment • Consider lower starting dose in volume depleted patients

Generic Name Olmesartan **Brand Name** Benicar ■ (PD)	Hypertension	**Usual oral dose:** 20 to 40 mg per day	• Consider lower starting dose in volume depleted patients
Generic Name Telmisartan **Brand Name** Micardis ■ ■	**Common indications for use:** Hypertension Cardiovascular risk reduction	Dose varies with indication for use and patient's clinical response **Illustrative oral dose for hypertension:** 20 to 80 mg per day	• Consider lower starting dose in volume depleted patients
Generic Name Valsartan **Brand Name** Diovan ■ (QT)	Hypertension Heart failure Left ventricular dysfunction after MI	Dose varies with indication for use and patient's clinical response **Illustrative oral dose for hypertension:** 80 to 320 mg per day	• Not recommended for severe renal impairment

Mineralocorticoid (Aldosterone) Receptor Antagonists

Universal prescribing alerts:

- Monitor potassium levels for hyperkalemia.

Drug Name	FDA-Approved Indications	Adult Dosage Range	Precautions and Clinical Pearls
Generic Name Eplerenone **Brand Name** Inspra ▲	Hypertension Heart failure	Dose varies with indication for use and patient's clinical response **Illustrative oral dose for hypertension:** 50 mg once or twice per day	• Drug interactions may require dose adjustments or avoidance of certain drug combinations Contraindications: • Serum creatinine greater than 2.0 mg/dL in males or greater than 1.8 mg/dL in females • Serum potassium greater than 5.5 mEq/L at initiation • CrCl less than 50 mL per minute for hypertension • CrCl less than or equal to 30 mL per minute for heart failure requires dose adjustment

Drug Name	FDA-Approved Indications	Adult Dosage Range	Precautions and Clinical Pearls
Generic Name Spironolactone **Brand Name** Aldactone ▲ ■	Edema Hypokalemia Hypertension Diagnosis of primary aldosteronism Heart failure	Dose varies with indication for use and patient's clinical response **Illustrative oral dose for hypertension:** 50 to 200 mg per day in 1 to 2 divided doses	• Monitor for dehydration and electrolyte disturbances, especially potassium • Drug interactions may require dose adjustments or avoidance of certain drug combinations Contraindications: • Anuria • Acute renal insufficiency • Significant impairment of renal excretory function • Hyperkalemia • Addison's disease Associated with: • Classified as a tumorigen in chronic toxicity animal studies; avoid unnecessary use

Renin Inhibitors			
Drug Name	FDA-Approved Indications	Adult Dosage Range	Precautions and Clinical Pearls
Generic Name Aliskiren **Brand Name** Tekturna ■	Hypertension	**Usual oral dose:** 150 to 300 mg per day	• Monitor for hyperkalemia • Use caution in renal impairment • Refer to universal prescribing alerts for ACE and ARBs

Chapter 7

Central Nervous System Agents

Authors: **Tammie Lee Demler, PharmD, BS Pharm, MBA, RPh, BCPP; Kimberly Mulcahy, PharmD, BCPS; and Rebecca Waite, PharmD, BCPP**

Editor: **Christopher Thomas, PharmD, BCPP, BCPS, CGP**

Learning Objectives

- Identify current pharmacologic agents that are appropriate for each condition/diagnosis.
- Recommend optimal pharmacologic interventions based on patient-specific characteristics.
- Provide appropriate patient-specific counseling points and optimal overall medication management.

Key Terms: adamantanes, amphetamines and derivatives, analgesics and antipyretics, anorexigenic agents and stimulants, anticholinergic agents, anticonvulsants (benzodiazepines, hydantoins, barbiturates, succinimides, miscellaneous), antidepressants, antimanic agents, antipsychotics, anxiolytics, sedatives, and hypnotics, barbiturates (anxiolytics, sedatives, and hypnotics), COMT inhibitors, COX-2 inhibitors, dopamine precursors, ergot-derivative dopamine receptor agonists, fibromyalgia agents, general anesthetics (barbiturates, miscellaneous), MAOB inhibitors, MAOI-antidepressants, non-ergot-derivative dopamine receptor agonists, nonsteroidal anti-inflammatory agents, opiate agonists, opiate antagonists, opiate partial agonists, respiratory and CNS stimulants, salicylates, selective serotonin agonists, serotonin modulators, serotonin–norepinephrine reuptake inhibitors (SNRI), selective serotonin reuptake inhibitors (SSRI), tricyclic antidepressants (TCA)

Overview of Central Nervous System Agents

Whether considering opiate analgesics, antipsychotics, or antiepileptic agents, drugs that influence the central nervous system (CNS) do so through a variety of mechanisms, including through direct, indirect, or a combination of actions on receptors and neurotransmitters, as well as by altering ion channels and facilitating neuronal communication through second messengers. To understand this complex system, a basic understanding of the organization of the bodily processes and structures is needed.

The autonomic nervous system (ANS) controls the most basic functions of the body, such as blood pressure, body temperature, and gastrointestinal motility. Rapid and intense sweating to cool our overheated bodies within seconds and shivering to warm our cold bodies are just some examples of these functions that happen without our conscious knowledge. The ANS is controlled by "activity centers" in the brain, spinal cord, and hypothalamus; in addition, it is influenced by the cerebral cortex.

The ANS has two major divisions: the sympathetic and parasympathetic systems. Both systems secrete mainly acetylcholine (cholinergic) or norepinephrine (adrenergic), which are synaptic transmitter substances. Preganglionic neurons are cholinergic factors in both systems, whereas the majority of postganglionic sympathetic neurons are adrenergic factors, with a few exceptions (e.g., sweat glands are linked to cholinergic activity). Acetylcholine (AChE) is one of the many neurotransmitters in the ANS. Acetylcholine has documented action in both the peripheral nervous system (PNS) and the CNS; it stimulates both muscarinic and nicotinic receptors. Adrenergic receptors can be both excitatory and inhibitory. They include the alpha and beta types, which are further divided into alpha 1 and 2 subunits and beta 1, 2, and 3 subunits, respectively. Norepinephrine activates mainly alpha receptors, and beta receptors to a lesser extent, whereas epinephrine activates both types of receptors equally. While the alpha and beta receptors offset and complement each other's actions, bodily tissues and organs are generally under the primary influence of one or the other adrenergic systems.

Fibers in the sympathetic nervous system originate in the spinal cord and innervate organs and tissues that are stimulated by sympathetic activity. For bodily action to take place, acetylcholine, norepinephrine, and/or epinephrine must bind to specific receptors. This binding results in conformational changes to receptor proteins, thereby stimulating or inhibiting ion channels or affiliated enzymes. In the case of second messenger systems, receptors can activate or inactivate chemicals inside a cell. An example is the extracellular action of the norepinephrine receptor on the intracellular adenyl cyclase enzyme, which subsequently forms cyclic adenosine monophosphate (cAMP).

When framing a general summary of how the CNS operates, the best representation is essentially a milieu of neurochemicals, the most common of which are described in this chapter. Chemicals that induce actions within the brain must be able to pass into the brain, via the fat-loving (lipophilic) blood-brain barrier.

Blood–Brain Barrier

The blood-brain barrier is a highly impermeable, lipophilic, thick basement membrane with connected tight junctions between the endothelial cells, which lines the cerebral microvessels and separates blood from the brain's extracellular fluid (BECF). The blood-brain barrier is an essential part of the CNS and prevents the passive diffusion of solutes from the blood into the CNS, thereby maintaining a highly regulated microenvironment. Moreover, this barrier acts to protect the CNS from infection.

For drug targeting purposes, tremendous challenges must be overcome to get therapeutic agents across the blood-brain barrier to active sites in the brain. Potential mechanisms for drug targeting include going through (using drugs that are small, lipophilic molecules) or behind (intracerebral implantation) the blood-brain barrier, as well as using endogenous transport systems such as carrier-mediated transporters or injecting therapeutic agents directly into the cerebrospinal fluid.

Neurotransmitters

Dopamine

Dopamine is the neurotransmitter released by the dopaminergic neurons. It is synthesized from the amino acid tyrosine in the extracellular space and bloodstream. A tyrosine pump moves tyrosine into the neuron, where it is converted into dopamine first by tyrosine hydroxylase and, subsequently, by DOPA decarboxylase. Dopamine "uptake" is further accomplished by the synaptic vesicles, where it is stored to be used during neurotransmission.

Dopamine is broken down and eliminated by a presynaptic reuptake transporter called dopamine active transport (DAT). DAT is responsible for terminating synaptic action during neurotransmission by decreasing the amount of dopamine in the synapse. This termination is accomplished by moving dopamine back into the presynaptic nerve terminal, where it is stored in the synaptic vesicles. Inactivating mechanisms work to prevent the buildup of excess dopamine in the synapses. Dopamine can also be destroyed by the monoamine oxidase (MAO-A or MAO-B) enzymes or catechol-*O*-methyl-transferase (COMT).

At least five pharmacologic subtypes of dopamine receptors exist, with D_2 being the most studied and best understood. D_2 receptors are a target in Parkinson's disease, where treatments seek to stimulate these receptors, and in schizophrenia, where treatments seek to block the receptors.

The dopamine hypothesis of schizophrenia proposes possible involvement of the mesolimbic dopamine pathway in the development of this mental disorder. The mesolimbic dopamine pathway, in theory, plays an important role in emotional behaviors such as positive symptoms, which include the delusions and hallucinations experienced by patients with schizophrenia. Mesolimbic dopamine hyperactivity also plays a role in the aggressive and hostile symptoms of related illnesses. Current theories also propose that dysfunction in prefrontal cortex and hippocampal glutamate activity causes downstream consequences, which may also contribute to the schizophrenia diagnosis.

For more than four decades, it has been observed that drugs that increase dopamine release promote and produce positive psychotic symptoms, whereas drugs that decrease dopamine mitigate these symptoms. Therefore, all known antipsychotic medications that treat positive symptoms work by blocking D_2 receptors.

The cause of the negative and cognitive symptoms of schizophrenia, however, remains an open question. Many researchers believe that deficits of dopamine activity in the mesocortical projections, the dorsolateral prefrontal cortex, or the ventromedial prefrontal cortex are responsible for the negative symptoms.

Dopamine plays an important role in the reward and euphoria systems of the human brain. The highest density of dopamine receptors is found in the ventral tegmental area (VTA) which also contains two of the largest projection pathways—namely, the mesolimbic and mesocortical pathways. Moreover, the VTA output pathways, along with VTA electrical stimulation, which itself leads to dopamine release, can act as a potent reward feedback mechanism.

Euphoria and reward, then, can be enhanced and prolonged by certain drugs. Many drugs with potent pharmacologic effects including euphoria ("highs") are mediated by monoamine reuptake inhibition. For example, cocaine is a dopamine reuptake inhibitor that causes a sustained increase in dopamine level and leads to euphoria and reward-motivated behavior.

Serotonin

Serotonin is another monoamine neurotransmitter derived from tryptophan. Most of the serotonin found in the body is located in the enterochromaffin cells of the gastrointestinal tract; the rest resides in the CNS, where it regulates mood, sleep, and appetite.

Serotonergic abnormalities are well known to be involved in major depressive disorders and other mental health conditions. Depletion of the serotonin concentration in the cerebrospinal fluid has been found to influence mood and may contribute to decreased psychiatric stability, thereby increasing the risk of serious suicidal behavior. The monoamine hypothesis of depression proposes that depletion of monoamines such as serotonin contributes to symptoms of depression.

The pharmacologic action of most antidepressants is based on inhibition of one or more serotonin reuptake transporters, which prevents the metabolism of serotonin and, in turn, results in increased serotonin concentrations in the synapse. However, the hypothesis that increased monoamine concentrations are the underlying explanation for antidepressants' effects clearly does not tell the whole story. Reuptake inhibition results in increased monoamine concentrations over the course of hours and days; however, the antidepressant effects of these agents take weeks and months to appear. Scientific theory now supports the contention that the rapid increase in monoamine concentrations leads to adaptive downregulation and desensitization of receptors.

Both the dopaminergic and serotonergic systems are believed to play important roles in mood and emotion regulation. Evidence suggests that a variety of serotonin receptors influence dopamine through either enhancement or inhibition effects.

Norepinephrine

Norepinephrine is another monoamine neurotransmitter in the catecholamine family. Metabolically modified from dopamine, it serves as both a neurotransmitter and a hormone. The sympathetic nervous system, which becomes activated during stressful events, employs norepinephrine as the neurotransmitter primarily responsible for the "fight or flight" response. The sympathetic system is involved in regulation of heart rate and blood pressure, and is influenced by changes in the serum norepinephrine concentration. Norepinephrine is used as a medication intervention to increase vascular tone through the activation of alpha-adrenergic receptors.

Similar to the effects posited in the theory of depression, the level of monoamines influences manic symptoms. Unlike in patients with depression, however, the amount of monoamine in patients with mania is excessive (rather than deficient). In terms of their antimanic effects, all antipsychotic agents—both first generation (FGA) and second generation (SGA)—are effective for psychotic mania, with SGAs having the greater efficacy. Dopamine (D_2) antagonists in combination with serotonin antagonists are effective in managing nonpsychotic mania.

Glutamate

Glutamate is a neurotransmitter that is also an amino acid. This excitatory neurotransmitter can stimulate all the CNS neurons—a capability that is unique to glutamate and explains why it is commonly known as the "master switch." Glutamate plays an important role in disorders such as schizophrenia and depression. It is synthesized in the glia cells from glutamine. Excitatory amino acid transporters (EAAT) take up glutamate once it has been released from the neurons by neighboring glia cells. During this reuptake process, the cells can either reuse the glutamate or synthesize it back to glutamine for storage for future use, rather than using glutamate for protein synthesis.

Many different types of glutamate receptors exist, though they are classified into just two main categories: metabotropic and ionotropic. Ionotropic receptors are further divided into three main types of receptors: AMPA, harmac, and NMDA. The NMDA receptor requires glutamate to have a co-transmitter before it can bind to this receptor; the co-transmitter can be either the amino acid glycine or D-serine. Drugs can target these receptors to reduce glutamate release. Among the types of drugs that do so are anticonvulsants, mood stabilizers, and *N*-methyl-D-aspartate (NMDA) receptor antagonists (such as memantine). It is thought that a core element for the emergence of schizophrenia is suboptimal NMDA function.

Gamma-Aminobutyric Acid

Gamma-aminobutyric acid (GABA) is a powerful inhibitory neurotransmitter in the CNS. Glutamate and GABA, together, work in coordination with voltage-gated ion channels and G protein–coupled receptors (GPCRs) in the CNS, which assist in the regulation of the neurotransmitters.

GABA is synthesized from glutamate by glutamate decarboxylase (GAD). GABA is stored in synaptic vesicles by the vesicular inhibitory amino acid transporter (VGAT). GABA-A receptors are found throughout the CNS and is the primary effector of the GABA-mediated inhibitory postsynaptic potential (IPSP). GABA-B receptors are responsible for the metabotropic effects of GABA and for the inhibition of voltage-gated calcium channels and the opening of potassium channels. GABA-B receptors are also responsible for the release of glutamate and monoamines. Four transporters of GABA are numbered as GAT-1 through GAT-4. GAT-1 and GAT-2 are primarily found in the CNS and help regulate GABA neurotransmission.

Two main neurotransmitters regulate the sleep/wake switch: histamine (an excitatory neurotransmitter) and GABA (an inhibitory neurotransmitter). The sleep promoter is located within the ventrolateral pre-optic nucleus (VLPO), which releases GABA. The wake promoter is located within the tuberomammillary nucleus (TMN) of the hypothalamus, which releases histamine. The main class of medications for insomnia consists of the benzodiazepine receptor agonists, more commonly known as "Z drugs" or "Z-hypnotics." These drugs are positive allosteric modulators of GABA-A receptors; they enhance GABA release, which in turn inhibits wake promotion. Antihistamines also inhibit the wake promotion effect, leading to drowsiness. Traditional benzodiazepines bind to GABA receptors and enhance the effects of GABA, but have broader effects on the GABA system, resulting in anxiolysis, muscle relaxation, and reduced seizure activity. They differ in the way they bind to the GABA-A receptors, in that their effects are shorter than those associated with the Z drugs, and they increase the chances of tolerance and dependence.

Acetylcholine

Acetylcholine is another important neurotransmitter produced in the brain. It is a product of choline and acetyl coenzyme A (AcCoA). AcCoA is derived in the mitochondria from glucose, whereas choline comes from dietary and intraneuronal sources. Compared to its protein-based counterparts, the composition, action, and pathway of deactivation for acetylcholine are unique. It is terminated by two types of enzymes, acetylcholinesterase (AchE) and butyrylcholinesterase (BuChE), which convert acetylcholine back into choline and AcCoA. AchE, which more commonly deactivates acetylcholine, is found throughout the brain. Choline is then transported back into the cell, where it can be synthesized into acetylcholine again. One class of drugs used for Alzheimer's disease blocks the actions of AchE, leading to higher levels of acetylcholine and improved cognition and memory.

Acetylcholine has many different receptors, of which the two main subgroups are nicotinic and muscarinic cholinergic receptors. Muscarinic receptors can be inhibitory or excitatory and are often targeted by the class of medications called "anticholinergics." These receptors are divided further into M_1, M_2, M_3, M_4, and M_5 subgroups. The M_1 receptors are mainly responsible for the memory functions of acetylcholine, whereas the M_2 receptors are responsible for preventing the excessive release of acetylcholine. The M_3 subgroup is found outside the brain, and these receptors are associated with some of the common side effects caused by some anticholinergics.

Nicotinic receptors are excitatory types. The two main subgroups of nicotinic receptors are the subtypes with all α_7 subunits and the subtypes with both α_4 and β_2 subunits. Presynaptic α_7-nicotinic receptors help regulate dopamine and glutamate release when acetylcholine is released. The $\alpha_4\beta_2$ subtype is the primary target of the nicotine found in cigarettes.

Other

The CNS is also influenced by prostaglandins. Fever is often triggered by infectious stimuli that cause an elevation in the core body temperature. The relationship between the increase in prostaglandin E_2 (PGE_2) and fever results in alteration of thermoregulation in the hypothalamus. Most antipyretic medications work by inhibiting the enzyme cyclooxygenase (COX) and reducing PGE_2 levels. Other theorized mechanisms of action suggest that antipyretic medications have the ability to promote anti-inflammatory signals and reduce pro-inflammatory mediators.

The main neurons that are involved in nociceptive pain are the dorsal horn neurons. Many neurotransmitters involved in the pain pathway are present at the dorsal horn, so drugs tend to target these neurons. These neurotransmitters include norepinephrine, serotonin, GABA, and glutamate. Common drug classes that target these neurotransmitters to help alleviate nociceptive pain are opioids, serotonin-norepinephrine reuptake inhibitors (SNRIs), and alpha-2 ligands, which are discussed in detail in this chapter.

7.1 Analgesic and Antipyretic Agents

All pain is not the same and, therefore, different treatments are required based on patient presentation. Every patient has a different and unique pain threshold, report, and description, so therapy must be carefully individualized, implemented, and monitored, including the choice of medication, strength, and duration. Pain is perceived by nociceptors, which are the ends of afferent fibers; these nociceptors may be stimulated by heat, acids, or pressure.

Pain is organized into two categories: acute or chronic. Acute pain, or nociception, is a sharp, quick pain; common examples would be touching a hot stove, a needle prick, or an incision. Tissue injury, or inflammation, can be categorized as either acute or chronic pain, or it may last longer than acute nociception but not long enough to be considered chronic. Inflammation is described as throbbing, burning, or even aching and is characterized by warmth, pain, redness, and swelling at the site of injury. Inflammatory mediators are released during tissue injury; they enhance the sensitivity of the nociceptors and increase pain perception. The pain associated with tissue injury stems from the release of prostaglandins and other inflammatory mediators at the site of injury. Causes of tissue injury may include burns, abrasions, joint inflammation, incisions or surgeries, or musculoskeletal injury. Inflammation can also be a response to other injurious stimuli, such as infections and antibodies.

Chronic pain is pain that lasts longer than the time the injury needs to heal, typically having at least 3 months' duration. Chronic pain can be further classified as neuropathic, nociceptive, mixed, or visceral pain.

Neuropathic pain is due to injury to the peripheral nerves that causes shooting or burning pain. Sometimes, even a light touch to the area can evoke a painful sensation. Nerve injury can be caused by diabetes (diabetic neuropathy), shingles, nerve trauma, or nerve compression, and it may be a side effect of some medications, such as chemotherapy. While opiates are effective in relieving nociceptive pain, the treatment of neuropathic pain utilizes atypical medications, such as certain antidepressants and anticonvulsants.

Chronic nociceptive pain has characteristics similar to those linked to acute pain, but the duration is significantly longer. Arthritis, cancer pain, and back pain are some examples of chronic pain.

Visceral pain is pain originating from thoracic, pelvic, or abdominal areas. Sensations are typically dull, aching, or cramping. Examples of causes of visceral pain include organ inflammation, tumors pressing on other internal structures, and obstructions.

Nonsteroidal anti-inflammatory drugs (NSAIDs) are most beneficial for symptomatic relief of pain and inflammation due to musculoskeletal disorders of low to moderate intensity. Migraines, menstrual pain, and gout pain can also be treated first-line with NSAIDs. Opioids are more efficacious in situations involving moderate to severe pain, but have the potential to produce unwanted CNS effects, addiction and dependence, and potentially fatal respiratory depression. Co-administration of NSAIDs and opiates may result in a lower dose of opiates being required to obtain analgesia, and in turn reduce opiate-related side effects. Multiple combination opiate/NSAID or opiate/acetaminophen products are available through prescription.

Nonsteroidal Anti-inflammatory Agents

Cyclooxygenase-2 Inhibitors

NSAIDs exert their therapeutic effects by inhibiting prostaglandin production. The first enzyme involved in prostaglandin synthesis is cyclooxygenase (COX). COX-1 and COX-2 are the two forms of COX, but COX-2 is the primary enzyme responsible for prostaglandin synthesis in response to inflammation. COX-1 is predominantly found on gastric epithelial cells and creates protective prostaglandins; thus, its inhibition can cause unwanted gastric effects, ranging from stomach upset to gastric ulceration.

Most available NSAIDs inhibit both COX-1 and COX-2 enzymes. COX-2 inhibitors were formulated to provide analgesic and inflammation relief with less of a side-effect burden for patients. Placebo-controlled trials found that COX-2 inhibitors have an increased risk of cardiovascular side effects, specifically myocardial infarction, stroke, and thrombosis. In patients with cardiovascular disease, it is recommended to reserve the use of COX-2 inhibitors for instances where there is a high risk of complications and use of other NSAIDs is contraindicated. The combination of aspirin and a COX-2 inhibitor does not reduce the potential for cardiovascular side effects, but instead increases the risk of GI upset and ulceration.

Cyclooxygenase-2 Inhibitors

Celecoxib

Salicylates

Aspirin and other salicylates irreversibly bind to, and inhibit, the COX-1 and COX-2 enzymes. Unlike with the other NSAIDs, aspirin's duration of action depends on the rate of production of COX enzymes in the tissues and not on the drug disposition. This relationship presents a challenge for patients: because COX enzymes on platelets have a turnover rate of 8–12 days, use of salicylates may put patients at an increased and irreversible risk of bleeding if they undergo surgery before the enzymes have sufficient time to recover. The average person can have prolonged bleeding time for 4–7 days after a 325 mg dose of aspirin, and an unplanned surgery or serious injury can cause possible hemostatic instability in complex cases.

Aspirin is frequently used for cardioprotection in patients at high risk of myocardial infarction and can reduce serious vascular events by 20% to 25%. Low-dose aspirin (81 mg, frequently referred to as "baby aspirin") carries a lower risk of GI adverse effects. Nevertheless, patients who take this formulation can still be at risk for GI bleed, including individuals on other antiplatelet or anticoagulant therapies, the elderly, individuals who consume more than 3 alcoholic beverages per day, and individuals with a history of GI bleeding.

When aspirin is dosed for pain management (approximately 3–4 g per day) and used chronically, it is no longer cardioprotective, but rather may compromise cardiac function and cause cardiac failure and pulmonary edema. Chronic use of higher doses of salicylates can also cause a reduction in renal function, gastric ulceration, hepatic injury, and tinnitus. Taking salicylates with food can help minimize GI upset.

Salicylate toxicity occurs when high doses (10–30 g sodium salicylate or aspirin in adults, and much less in children) are consumed and can be life threatening. Signs and symptoms include hyperpyrexia, convulsions, and, in serious cases, coma or cardiovascular collapse. Salicylism results from salicylate toxicity, with its symptoms including headache, dizziness, tinnitus and difficulty hearing, vision changes, confusion, drowsiness, sweating, hyperventilation, nausea, vomiting, and diarrhea.

Combination of aspirin and NSAIDs does not reduce the potential for cardiovascular side effects, but instead increases the risk of GI upset and ulceration.

Salicylates should be avoided in children and young adults (younger than 20 years) with fevers associated with viral illness due to the increased risk of Reye's syndrome. Reye's syndrome is a potentially fatal disease characterized by acute-onset encephalopathy and liver dysfunction.

Salicylates

- Aspirin
  Choline salicylate

Magnesium salicylate
Salsalate
Trolamine salicylate

Other Nonsteroidal Anti-inflammatory Agents

NSAIDs are used to treat inflammation, pain, and fever by inhibiting the prostaglandin synthase enzymes known as cyclooxygenases. Inhibiting COX-2 causes the anti-inflammatory, antipyretic, and analgesic effects associated with NSAID use, and inhibition of COX-1 causes the GI adverse effects, such as stomach upset or GI ulceration.

Gastrointestinal side effects occur in 15% to 30% of regular users of NSAIDs, and can range from mild stomach upset to full-thickness ulceration of the GI mucosa. Ulceration can cause blood loss and ultimately anemia, which may become life threatening. Patients using multiple NSAIDs are at an increased risk of GI bleeds, as are those who are older (older than 70 years), are taking concurrent anticoagulation or antiplatelet therapies (including selective serotonin reuptake inhibitors [SSRIs]), and/or have a past history of ulcers. Patients who generally consume more than 3 alcoholic beverages per day are at increased risk of GI events. Co-administration with proton-pump inhibitors or misoprostol can prevent duodenal and gastric ulceration in patients where the benefit of NSAID use outweighs the risk. Patients may be advised to take these medications with food to reduce stomach upset.

Cardiovascular side effects are associated with NSAIDs having a higher selectivity for COX-2 receptors, such as diclofenac, meloxicam, and nimesulide. These side effects include an increased risk for myocardial infarction, stroke, and other thrombotic events.

Patients with chronic kidney failure, congestive heart failure, and hepatic cirrhosis should use NSAIDs with caution. The prostaglandin activity and COX-2 receptors in the kidney cause these patients to be at increased risk of water retention, which can also complicate other disease states. Chronic use of high doses of NSAIDs or use of NSAIDs in combination with other renally cleared medications (such as angiotensin-converting enzyme [ACE] inhibitors and lithium) can increase a patient's risk for acute kidney injury.

Combination of aspirin and NSAIDs does not reduce the potential for cardiovascular side effects, but instead increases the risk of GI upset and ulceration. Also, ibuprofen, when taken in close proximity to aspirin, eliminates the cardioprotective qualities of aspirin altogether.

Allergies to NSAIDs have been reported and in serious cases can result in anaphylaxis. If a patient exhibits an NSAID allergy, cross-reactivity is possible and future NSAID use should be undertaken with extreme caution.

FDA Black Box Warnings

NSAIDs may cause an increased risk of number of serious medical complications. Some examples of these potentially fatal events include myocardial infarction, stroke, and other cardiovascular thrombotic events. Although the absolute risk of any of these events, as well as the timeline within which they are most likely to occur, is difficult to determine, this risk is often associated with a longer duration of use. Older adult patients are at greater risk of these serious cardiovascular side effects as well as potential GI events.

FDA Special Alert

Non-aspirin NSAIDs increase the risk of a heart attack or stroke. The risk of heart attack or stroke can occur as early as the first 2 weeks of NSAID use. This risk may increase with longer use of the NSAID, and it appears to be greater at higher doses. Insufficient data are available to determine whether the risk of any particular NSAID is definitely higher or lower than that of any other particular NSAID.

In addition to an increased risk of heart failure, NSAIDs have also been associated with an increased risk of heart attack and stroke. This increased risk applies not only to individuals with heart disease, but also those without risk factors or evidence of cardiovascular disease.

Other Nonsteroidal Anti-inflammatory Agents

Diclofenac
Diflunisal

Etodolac
Fenoprofen
Flurbiprofen
Ibuprofen
Indomethacin
Ketoprofen
Ketorolac
Meclofenamate
Mefenamic acid
Meloxicam
Nabumetone
Naproxen
Oxaprozin
Piroxicam
Sulindac
Tolmetin

Opiate Agonists

Opiate agents have been subject to scrutiny lately given their potential for overuse. Because of this potential, they have been included in the FDA risk evaluation and mitigation strategies (REMS) program to ensure additional safety measures in prescribing. Because these agents are subject to misuse and abuse (i.e., tolerance, dependence, and addiction), their place in the therapeutic algorithm for pain is controversial and complicated. In addition to their analgesic actions, opioid agonists induce the pharmacologic actions of anxiolysis, miosis, and cough suppression.

Patients who require prolonged opiate interventions often require dose conversions from short- to long-acting products or to agents with higher potency. Prescribers may find these conversions challenging, as the different products and formulations often do not share the same degree of potency or pharmacodynamics behaviors. Long-term use of opioids can be problematic due to the rapid development of profound tolerance to the analgesic effects, coupled with the slow development of tolerance to many of the untoward effects of these agents. It is the inability to tolerate these undesirable side effects that eventually limits dose escalations and analgesic efficacy. A similar tolerance to a new opiate after use of another opiate (cross-tolerance) is often incomplete, leaving the patient subject to unexpected and unpredictable therapeutic and adverse effects, some of which can result in inadvertent overdose and fatality. For this reason, opiate conversions often are based on morphine equivalents, with recommendations to decrease the final opiate calculated dose by at least 25%.

As a class, opiate agonists are well known to cause serious CNS depressant effects, including respiratory depression and extreme somnolence, in addition to the more seemingly benign side effects of nausea and constipation. Some class effects, however, are less widely recognized, including the adverse effects on the endocrine system through the inhibited secretion of adrenocorticotropic hormone (ACTH), cortisol, and luteinizing hormone (LH), and by stimulating secretion of prolactin, growth hormone (GH), insulin, and glucagon. A decrease in production of LH, and a corresponding decrease in testosterone, may result in a decrease in libido and, in some cases, hypoglycemia.

Evidence of histamine release—such as urticaria, wheals, and local tissue irritation—can trigger complaints of pruritus. This phenomenon may lead to an incorrect diagnosis of opiate allergy, when in fact all patients are susceptible to opiate-induced release of histamines. The symptoms that result from histamine release can be mitigated by giving a lower dose of the agent or by adding a supplemental antihistamine to the opiate regimen. In contrast, histamine-induced bronchoconstriction can restrict the use of morphine in patients with a diagnosis of asthma.

Opiate agents also may influence serotonin and have been implicated in serotonin syndrome when included in a regimen that includes concomitant serotonergic agents. Signs of opioid overdose include pinpoint pupils, shallow and infrequent breaths, cool or clammy skin, and difficulty in arousal or being nonresponsive to stimuli. Overdose agents are available and will be discussed in conjunction with opiate antagonists.

Opiate products are classified as natural, synthetic, or semisynthetic agents. The three major mammalian types of opioid receptors (OR) are designated as μ, δ, and κ. The mu (μ)-opioid receptor (MOR), delta (δ)-opioid receptor (DOR), and kappa (κ)-opioid receptor (KOR) all play roles in the action and adverse effects of opiate agents.

Opiate Agonists

Codeine
Fentanyl citrate
Hydrocodone
Hydromorphone
Levorphanol
Meperidine
Methadone
• Morphine
Oxycodone
Oxymorphone
Remifentanil
Sufentanil citrate
Tapentadol
Tramadol

Opiate Partial Agonists

Opiate partial agonists and mixed antagonists/agonists were developed in an effort to reduce or eliminate the respiratory depression and lower the abuse potential associated with the opiate agonists. These agents still have undesirable side effects, and they exert weaker analgesic effects than opiate agonists. Some oral formulations are combined with naloxone, an opiate antagonist, to further reduce the abuse potential. When naloxone is taken orally, it is rapidly metabolized by the liver and does not have any pharmacologic action. If used intravenously, however, it blocks the opiate receptors from binding with the opiate.

Opiate Partial Agonists

Buprenorphine
Butorphanol
Nalbuphine
Pentazocine

Miscellaneous Analgesic and Antipyretic Agents

Acetaminophen has antipyretic and analgesic properties, but does not have anti-inflammatory activity. It is typically recommended as a first-line treatment for pain and is effective in conditions such as osteoarthritis (OA), but is less effective in inflammatory conditions such as rheumatoid arthritis (RA). Because it does not carry the risk of triggering Reye's syndrome, acetaminophen is the drug of choice to treat fevers in children and young adults.

Acetaminophen is available in a variety of combination products, including fixed-dose preparations with opiates, barbiturates, caffeine, sleep aids, antihistamines, antitussives, decongestants, expectorants, and cold and flu preparations. Although this medication does not possess GI effects, hepatic damage is a serious side effect and can occur with chronic high-dose use.

Dosing limits of no more than 4 g per day (or more than 2 g per day in patients with alcohol use disorder) are recommended due to the potential for hepatic injury. Acetaminophen toxicity or overdose typically occurs after ingestion of more than 7.5 g (or lower doses in patients with hepatic insufficiency or with heavy alcohol consumption) or with consistent supratherapeutic doses. Acetaminophen overdose is a medical emergency, and early diagnosis and treatment is required for a positive patient outcome. Initially activated charcoal may be given if taken within 4 hours of ingestion; otherwise, *N*-acetylcysteine is the antidote for hepatic protection.

Salicylamide is an analgesic and antipyretic with similar properties to aspirin, but is metabolized differently and, therefore, is not considered a true salicylate. It is commonly found in combination over-the-counter (OTC) pain relievers with acetaminophen, aspirin, and caffeine. In clinical trials, salicylamide alone was not reported to have significant analgesic effects compared to placebo, and both acetaminophen and aspirin have been found to be more effective for the treatment of pain and fever in adults and children. Currently, there are insufficient data to report on the safety of salicylamide at the reported doses required to obtain analgesia (6–24 g per day). The most common adverse effects with this agent are similar to those associated with the salicylates, including GI disturbances, dizziness, and headaches. Most of these adverse effects are dose related.

Ziconotide is an intrathecal analgesic indicated for chronic pain. In the United States, its label carries a black box warning for severe psychiatric and neurologic impairment, including hallucinations, mood changes, and changes in consciousness. Cognitive effects from ziconotide are typically reversible up to 2 weeks after discontinuation.

Miscellaneous Analgesic and Antipyretic Agents

Acetaminophen
Salicylamide
Ziconotide
Antimigraine agents (*see also the Antimigraine Agents section*)
Gabapentin (*see also the Anticonvulsant Agents section*)

Fibromyalgia Agents

Milnacipran
Duloxetine (*see also the Psychotherapeutic Agents section)*
Pregabalin (*see also the Anticonvulsant Agents section*)

Anti-gout Agents

Allopurinol
Colchicine
Febuxostat

Case Studies and Conclusions

Robert is a 73-year-old man with RA. He presents to his doctor for medication management, but the physician is hesitant to initiate therapy with an NSAID because of the potential for GI risk.

1. Which of the following is not a risk factor for serious gastrointestinal effects?
    a. Age greater than 70 years
    b. Male gender
    c. Previous stomach ulcer
    d. Concurrent antiplatelet use

Answer B is correct. Age, history of GI ulcers, and concurrent anticoagulants, antiplatelets, or NSAID use increase the risk of a serious GI adverse effect. Female patients are at a greater risk than male patients.

2. Which medication would be the best option for pain management of Robert's RA?
    a. Ketorolac
    b. Diclofenac
    c. Celecoxib
    d. Meloxicam

Answer C is correct. Celecoxib has the lowest potential for GI effects due to its selectivity for the COX-2 enzyme. Ketorolac is not recommended for long-term use (more than 5 days).

Robert states that he was previously told to take a "baby aspirin" (81 mg aspirin) daily for cardioprotection.

3. Which of the following statements is true in regard to aspirin use?
   a. Due to the cardioprotective properties of aspirin, patients can take it simultaneously with an NSAID, such as ibuprofen, and there is no longer a concern for MI, stroke, or thromboembolic events.
   b. High-dose aspirin (3 g per day) can adequately manage pain and maintain cardioprotective properties.
   c. Patients taking baby aspirin are not at risk of a GI bleed.
   d. Aspirin irreversibly binds to COX on platelets and can cause increased risk of bleeding up to 7 days after its administration.

Answer D is correct. When aspirin is used concurrently with NSAIDs, it loses its cardioprotective properties and the patient can experience increased risk of GI bleeding. High-dose aspirin at 3–4 g per day is effective in analgesia, but at higher doses aspirin loses its cardioprotective properties. Although the risk is small, patients can still experience GI bleeds with low-dose aspirin, especially patients older than 70 years, with a history of GI bleed/ulcer, or of female gender, and those concurrently taking anticoagulants, antiplatelets, or NSAIDs. Aspirin irreversibly binds to COX receptors on platelets, so the efficacy of the medication lasts until new platelets are formed, which leads to an increased risk of bleeding that lasts 4–7 days after the last dose.

Mary is a 48-year-old woman with complaints of chronic back pain. She has a past medical history that includes gastroesophageal reflux disease (GERD), obesity, hypertension, and chronic obstructive pulmonary disease (COPD).

1. Which medication is the best first-line option to treat Mary's low back pain?
   a. Ibuprofen
   b. Aspirin
   c. Acetaminophen
   d. Salicylamide

Answer C is correct. Ibuprofen could be an appropriate choice in many patients, but Mary has a diagnosis of GERD and would be at an increased risk of GI bleed, as would aspirin. Hydrocodone/acetaminophen combination tablets could be acceptable as a second- or third-line agent. Salicylamide does not have sufficient evidence to support its use as monotherapy for analgesia. Acetaminophen is generally the first-line agent for pain management in patients.

Two months pass, and Mary returns to the office stating that despite taking the recommended medication, stretching, and physical therapy, she still experiences pain throughout the day.

2. Which of the following options could be the next step up in her pain management?
   a. Methadone
   b. Hydrocodone/acetaminophen
   c. Fentanyl
   d. Buprenorphine/naloxone

Answer B is correct. Methadone is reserved for severe chronic pain or opiate detoxification. Fentanyl is also reserved for severe, chronic pain, and in most cases (other than with transdermal administration) it is reserved for patients with severe cancer pain or in palliative care practices. Buprenorphine/naloxone is also utilized for opiate withdrawal/dependence or severe pain and would not be the best option for this patient.

3. Given Mary's multiple comorbidities and new medication regimen, which of the following counseling points is/are FALSE?
   a. Use of opiates can cause respiratory depression, and Mary should use the medication only as directed because she is at increased risk for this adverse effect owing to of her COPD and obesity.
   b. Constipation is a common side effect of opiates, but it will subside after 1 week of medication use.
   c. Taking an opiate with acetaminophen or an NSAID can reduce the dose required of the opiate to attain analgesia.
   d. All of the statements are FALSE.

Answer B is correct. Constipation occurs in 40% to 95% of patients who use opioids, but patients do not become tolerant to this side effect. Patients should be advised to take a stool softener and a stimulant laxative if constipation becomes a concern.

Opiates do cause respiratory depression: Patients with COPD, asthma, or sleep apnea; older patients; and patients who are obese are at an increased risk for experiencing this adverse effect. Use of both acetaminophen and NSAIDs can reduce the dose of the opioid that is required to attain analgesic effects. Combination therapy also reduces the risk and severity of the side effects associated with opioids.

7.2 Opiate Antagonists

Opiate antagonists are used to treat opioid dependence and can be administered to treat or prevent opioid intoxication in an overdose situation. Opiate antagonists have a higher affinity for the opiate receptors in the brain; thus, when used concurrently with an opiate, the antagonist will block the effects of the opiate. When these medications are administered to patients who have opioids in their system, the antagonists can induce immediate withdrawal symptoms. If these medications are prescribed to help manage opioid abstinence or prevent a relapse, it is important that the patient is opiate free when therapy is initiated. The washout period for opiates is 3–6 days after the last use of a short-acting opioid or 7–10 days after the last use of a long-acting opioid. Opiate antagonists exert pharmacologic effects only in the presence of opiate agents.

Naloxone is used to prevent or reverse the effects of opiates on opioid receptors in case of an overdose. When naloxone is administered intravenously, intranasally, or intramuscularly, it exerts its effects for only a few minutes, and due to its short duration of action may require readministration. Oftentimes, especially if naloxone is administered to a patient with chronic opiate use or abuse, the patient may experience immediate withdrawal signs and symptoms. The severity of withdrawal symptoms experienced by the patient depends on the type and degree of dependence on opioids of the patient. Furthermore, naloxone exerts no pharmacologic activity when administered orally.

Naltrexone is used to help maintain opiate and alcohol abstinence in patients with a history of opiate or alcohol abuse or dependence. Oral naltrexone must be administered daily to be effective and requires a highly motivated patient. Intramuscular naltrexone is administered every 4 weeks and may be a better alternative for patients with a high risk of relapse or who have a history of poor therapy adherence.

Naloxone and naltrexone have been used in combination with opiates to reduce the abuse potential of medications. Naloxone, in particular, has no oral bioavailability, so if the combination medication product is taken orally as intended, the patient will experience analgesia from the opiate. However, if the patient tries to adulterate the medication and inject it, naloxone will block the opiate and the patient will not experience the euphoric effects he or she is trying to achieve.

Opiate Antagonists

- Naloxone
  Naltrexone

Case Study and Conclusions

John is brought to the emergency department by emergency medical services (EMS) responders. He has pinpoint pupils and shallow breathing, and is unresponsive to noxious stimuli (including a sternal rub). The paramedics state that they found an empty prescription bottle of oxycodone at the scene in his room after John's parents called 911. The emergency room attending physician believes that this is an opiate overdose situation.

1. Which medication should be used to immediately reverse the effects of opiate intoxication?
   a. Naltrexone IM
   b. Naltrexone PO
   c. Naloxone IV
   d. Naloxone PO

Answer C is correct. While naltrexone competes for opiate receptors, the onset of the medication is not fast enough to reverse opiate effects in an emergency situation. Naloxone PO has negligible oral bioavailability and would be largely ineffective. Naloxone given by the IV, IM, subcutaneous, or intranasal route of administration would be appropriate in case of opiate toxicity or overdose.

After a brief hospitalization, John decides that he would like to abstain from opiates altogether. His past medical history shows previous admissions to recovery programs, but he admits to relapsing after every treatment program. Today, he would like to start pharmacologic treatment to aid in his sobriety.

2. Which medication would be most appropriate to aid in John's sobriety from opiates?
   a. Naltrexone IM
   b. Naltrexone PO
   c. Naloxone IV
   d. Naloxone PO

Answer A is correct. Naltrexone IM is administered every 4 weeks, so it would remain in the patient's system and have a longer duration of action compared to the PO formulation. Oral naltrexone requires a patient to be highly motivated to want to remain abstinent due to its daily dosing schedule. Naloxone is indicated in emergency situations for opiate reversal, and oral naloxone has no pharmacologic action.

3. Which of the following statements is FALSE in regard to naltrexone use?
   a. Injection-site reactions are a common side effect with intramuscular administration of naltrexone.
   b. Acute kidney injury can occur with use of naltrexone, but reverses after medication discontinuation.
   c. Patients who receive naltrexone should report signs of depression or suicidality to healthcare providers right away.
   d. Administration of naltrexone should be delayed until opiates are no longer in the patient's system (i.e., 7–10 days after the last use of a long-acting opiate).

Answer B is correct. Hepatocellular injury is a rare but serious side effect that can occur with naltrexone use. This injury will be reversed after medication discontinuation.

7.3 Anticonvulsant Agents

A seizure occurs because of disordered firing of brain neurons, which causes an excess of excitatory neurotransmitters, enhancement of excitatory synaptic activity, and reduction of inhibitory synaptic activity and, ultimately, increased stimulation of receptors. Epilepsy is a disorder characterized by episodic and erratic seizures. Gamma-aminobutyric acid is the primary inhibitory neurotransmitter and glutamate is the primary excitatory neurotransmitter in such seizures. Pharmacologic medications can enhance GABA synaptic inhibitory action or antagonize excitatory action of glutamate. Voltage-gated ion channels such as potassium, sodium, and calcium channels have also been identified as important factors leading to disrupted synaptic function and, potentially, epileptiform activity.

Multiple types of seizures are possible, and therapy is based on the patient's specific diagnosis. Partial seizures involve a specific focal site from which the seizure originates. During a simple partial seizure, which typically lasts 20-60 seconds, the patient maintains consciousness and the symptoms depend on the area of cortex affected. During a complex partial seizure, which lasts from 30 seconds to 2 minutes, the patient will lose or have impaired consciousness and may experience purposeless movements such as lip smacking or hand wringing. Treatment options for simple or complex partial seizures include carbamazepine, phenytoin, or valproate.

Sometimes patients may have a partial seizure that develops into a tonic-clonic seizure, which involves a loss of consciousness with sustained contractions (tonic) of the muscles and periods of muscle contraction and relaxation (clonic) lasting around 1-2 minutes. Medication options for partial with tonic-clonic seizures include carbamazepine, phenobarbital, phenytoin, primidone, and valproate. Simple partial, complex partial, and partial with tonic-clonic seizures can also be treated with gabapentin, lacosamide, lamotrigine, levetiracetam, rufinamide, tiagabine, topiramate, or zonisamide.

Generalized seizures, unlike partial seizures, involve both hemispheres of the brain. They are classified as absence, myoclonic, or generalized tonic-clonic seizures. During an absence seizure, which typically lasts less than 30 seconds, the patient experiences changes in consciousness, a disruption in activity, and staring. Absence seizures typically occur in children and resolve before adulthood. Therapeutic options include lamotrigine, ethosuximide, valproate, and clonazepam. A myoclonic seizure is a brief (several seconds), shock-like contraction of muscles that either could involve one extremity or be generalized to the whole body. Medications prescribed for myoclonic seizures include valproate, clonazepam, and levetiracetam. Generalized tonic-clonic seizures have the same presentation as partial tonic-clonic seizures, except that they do not follow a partial seizure. Treatment options include carbamazepine, phenobarbital, phenytoin, primidone, valproate, lamotrigine, levetiracetam, and topiramate.

Currently, there are no anti-epileptogenic agents available in the United States; that is, the medications now available provide only symptomatic relief. The exact mechanism of action of anticonvulsants is unknown, although theories about the proposed mechanisms are widely accepted. Many medications are also thought to induce their antiepileptic effect through a variety of mechanisms.

Sodium-channel modulators can enhance fast inactivation of the neuron (phenytoin, carbamazepine, lamotrigine, felbamate, oxcarbazepine, topiramate, and valproic acid) or can enhance slow inactivation (lacosamide). This effect blocks the action potential's transmission through the neuron and stabilizes the neuronal membranes, decreasing neurotransmitter release and the seizure spread. Calcium-channel blockers (valproic acid, lamotrigine) decrease slow depolarization and neuron discharges.

Alpha ($\alpha_{2\delta}$)-ligands include gabapentin and pregabalin, which modulate neurotransmitter release and increase membrane hyperpolarization and the seizure threshold. GABA receptor allosteric modulators (benzodiazepines, phenobarbital, felbamate, topiramate, carbamazepine, oxcarbazepine) decrease focal firing, and increase GABA levels and membrane hyperpolarization. GABA uptake inhibitors and GABA-transaminase inhibitors (tiagabine, vigabatrin) decrease focal firing and decrease slow excitatory neurotransmission. NMDA receptor antagonists (felbamate) decrease excitatory amino acid neurotoxicity and delay epileptogenesis. AMPA/kinase receptor antagonists (phenobarbital and topiramate) decrease fast excitatory neurotransmission and buffer large hyperpolarizing and depolarizing inputs.

Enhancers of hyperpolarization-activated cyclic nucleotide–gated (HCN) channel activity (lamotrigine) suppress the action potential initiation from dendritic inputs. Synaptic vesicle protein (SV2A) protein ligand (levetiracetam) is hypothesized to decrease neurotransmitter release and increase HCN-mediated currents. Inhibitors of brain carbonic anhydrase (topiramate and zonisamide) decrease NMDA-mediated currents and increase GABA mediated inhibition.

Complete control of seizures is achieved in only approximately 50% of patients, though another 25% of patients may experience significant improvement. Efficacy of medications is largely dependent on seizure type, severity, and cause of seizures. Patients are also at risk of experiencing a myriad of side effects, including CNS impairment, Stevens-Johnson syndrome (SJS), hepatic failure, and death. The Food and Drug Administration (FDA) requires that the labels of all antiseizure medications include a warning about the increased risk of suicidal thoughts or actions.

Monotherapy is the preferred regimen when treating seizures to limit the potential for side effects and drug interactions from the medications. However, polypharmacy is often indicated, including in cases where a patient may have two or more types of seizures.

Plasma levels of several medications can be measured to ensure the medication is present at a therapeutic level and to avoid medication toxicity. Recommended serum concentrations are intended as guidelines for therapy, however, all medication regimens should be individualized based on efficacy and tolerability.

Important drug interactions to note include the ability of carbamazepine, oxcarbazepine, phenobarbital, phenytoin, and primidone to induce specific hepatic enzymes (CYP3A4) and to increase the metabolism of other antiepileptic medications as well as oral contraceptives. The latter effect can cause unplanned pregnancies, which are particularly dangerous due to the teratogenicity of these products.

Antiepileptic therapy may be tapered and discontinued after two years of seizure-free therapy if this is considered appropriate for the patient. Most reoccurrences of seizures will happen within 4 months of medication discontinuation.

Status epilepticus is a medical emergency in which a patient experiences continual seizures without return of consciousness between them. It requires immediate treatment due to the potential for permanent brain injury. Medications should be given intravenously only for cases of status epilepticus.

Barbiturates

Phenobarbital is the most frequently used barbiturate for seizure treatment and is effective for generalized tonic-clonic and partial seizures. It works by causing synaptic inhibition of the GABA receptors, which in turn increases the GABA receptor–mediated current.

The serum concentration of phenobarbital for seizure control is recommended to be 10–35 μg/mL. Nevertheless, the exact relationship between efficacy and plasma level is not precisely known.

Phenobarbital induces specific hepatic enzymes (CYP2C and CYP3A4), so it can reduce the efficacy of oral contraceptives and some antiepileptic medications. Sedation is a common side effect with this medication, but tolerance typically develops with continued use. Irritability and hyperactivity can occur in children, and agitation and confusion can occur in elderly patients.

Barbiturates

Mephobarbital
Phenobarbital
Primidone
Methohexital (*see also the Anxiolytic, Sedative, and Hypnotic Agents section*)

Benzodiazepines

Many benzodiazepines have antiseizure properties, with clonazepam and clorazepate being FDA approved for long-term treatment of seizures. Clonazepam is effective in absence and myoclonic seizures in children, but tolerance to its anticonvulsant properties can develop after 1–6 months of use. Clorazepate is effective when used in combination with other anticonvulsant medications for the treatment of partial seizures. Midazolam can be used for intermittent treatment in patients with refractory seizures while on a stable anticonvulsant therapy, and diazepam and lorazepam are effective in the management of status epilepticus. Benzodiazepines enhance GABA-mediated synaptic inhibition; at high doses, they can reduce high-frequency firing of neurons.

Benzodiazepines cause drowsiness and lethargy, but tolerance develops with prolonged chronic use of these agents. Administering the medication in divided doses throughout the day can reduce the severity of the side effects. Aggression, hyperactivity, irritability, difficulty concentrating, and other behavioral changes can occur in children who take benzodiazepines. If benzodiazepines are discontinued abruptly in patients after chronic use, seizures can occur so dose tapering is recommended.

Benzodiazepines

Clobazam
Clonazepam
Clorazepate (*see also the Anxiolytic, Sedative, and Hypnotic Agents section*)
Diazepam (*see also the Anxiolytic, Sedative, and Hypnotic Agents section*)
Lorazepam (*see also the Anxiolytic, Sedative, and Hypnotic Agents section*)

Hydantoins

Phenytoin is effective for relief of all partial and tonic–clonic seizures, but is ineffective for absence seizures. Phenytoin reduces the action potential of neurons by slowing the recovery rate of voltage-activated sodium channels. Fosphenytoin, the prodrug to phenytoin, was developed for intramuscular or intravenous administration in patients with seizures.

The free (or unbound) concentration of serum phenytoin is often monitored both for efficacy and to avoid toxicity. Seizure control is seen with a free phenytoin level of 0.75–1.25 μg/mL. The serum concentrations may change if a patient is switched between the immediate-release and extended-release formulations.

Phenytoin is extensively bound to serum proteins—predominantly albumin. Consequently, patients with hypoalbuminemia or uremia can demonstrate dramatic variations in the amount of free (or active) phenytoin. Some medications can compete with phenytoin for protein binding and specific hepatic metabolism enzymes, leading to adverse effects of either phenytoin or the other medication. In particular, phenytoin inhibits warfarin's metabolism, which can lead to increased risk of bleeding in patients. The metabolism of oral contraceptives is increased by phenytoin hepatic enzyme induction, which can lead to unplanned pregnancy. This risk is particularly dangerous due to the teratogenicity of phenytoin.

Carbamazepine can increase the metabolism of phenytoin, causing a decrease in phenytoin concentration. Conversely, phenytoin can decrease the concentration of carbamazepine.

Adverse effects of chronic phenytoin use may include behavioral changes, GI symptoms, gingival hyperplasia, osteomalacia, megaloblastic anemia, and hirsutism. Serious adverse reactions may include Stevens-Johnson syndrome, toxic epidermal necrolysis, systemic lupus erythematosus, neutropenia, leukopenia, and potentially fatal hepatic necrosis. Unlike many other anticonvulsant medications, phenytoin does not cause general CNS depression.

Hydantoins

Ethotoin
Fosphenytoin
Phenytoin

Succinimides

Ethosuximide is used exclusively for the treatment of absence seizures. Methsuximide is active against electroshock seizures and is no longer commonly used. Ethosuximide reduces low-threshold calcium currents in the neurons of the thalamus. A target plasma concentration of 40–100 μg/mL will provide control over the majority of absence seizures. GI upset (nausea, vomiting, anorexia) and CNS effects (drowsiness, euphoria, dizziness, headache) are the most common side effects, and tolerance typically develops with chronic use.

Succinimides

Ethosuximide
Methsuximide

Miscellaneous Anticonvulsant Agents

Carbamazepine is the primary drug used to treat partial and tonic-clonic seizures. It works by slowing the rate of recovery of voltage-activated sodium channels from inactivation and limits repetitive firing. Carbamazepine induces a number of hepatic enzymes responsible for drug metabolism, so its use decreases the efficacy of oral contraceptives, valproate, lamotrigine, tiagabine, and topiramate. Phenobarbital, phenytoin, and valproate can increase the metabolism of carbamazepine. Carbamazepine also has the potential to auto-induce its own metabolism, so dose increases are often required shortly after the initiation of therapy or after dose adjustments.

Adverse effects of carbamazepine may include nausea, vomiting, blood dyscrasias, hypersensitivity reactions, and water retention, which can be dangerous in individuals with cardiovascular disease. This agent's label carries has an FDA black box warning due to its potential to induce serious dermatologic reactions. In addition, genetic testing is often done for the HLA-B*1502 allele, which is linked to aplastic anemia and agranulocytosis risk, specifically in patients of Asian descent. Renal and hepatic function should be monitored when patients take carbamazepine.

Oxcarbazepine is an analog of carbamazepine that can be used for partial seizures. It is a less potent enzyme inducer than carbamazepine. If the patient is switched from carbamazepine to oxcarbazepine, the latter medication can cause an increase in the effects of concomitant phenytoin and valproic acid if the patient is on polypharmacy for seizure control. Despite the reduction in enzyme induction, oxcarbazepine can reduce the efficacy of oral contraceptives. Both carbamazepine and oxcarbazepine have been noted to cause hyponatremia by inducing the syndrome of inappropriate antidiuretic hormone (SIADH) secretion. If not treated, SIADH can lead to serious complications; unfortunately, most patients remain asymptomatic so early diagnosis may be missed.

Felbamate inhibits NMDA responses and potentiates GABA responses; it is effective in patients with partial and generalized seizures. Because felbamate is associated with liver failure, this medication is no longer widely used and is reserved for cases of extreme refractory seizures.

Gabapentin and pregabalin are centrally active GABA agonists that can be effective in treating partial seizures when used in combination with other antiepileptic medications. The most common adverse effects associated with these agents include somnolence, dizziness, and fatigue, and tolerability to the side effects develops with continued therapy.

Lacosamide limits repetitive firing of neurons and slows the inactivation of sodium channels. It is effective as adjunctive therapy for partial-onset seizures.

Lamotrigine's mechanism of action is not completely understood, but it is thought to delay the recovery from inactivation of sodium channels and inhibit the synaptic release of glutamate. This agent is effective for partial and generalized seizures. Carbamazepine, phenytoin and phenobarbital all increase the metabolism and reduce the plasma concentration of lamotrigine. Use of lamotrigine with valproate increases the concentration of lamotrigine and reduces the concentration of valproate. Lamotrigine can also increase the formation of metabolites of carbamazepine and may cause toxicity in some patients. Lamotrigine is available in blister packs available in specific dosing regimens for patients who are concurrently taking enzyme-inducing antiepileptic drugs (such as carbamazepine, phenytoin, phenobarbital, or primidone), for patients who are concurrently taking valproic acid, and for those who are taking lamotrigine as monotherapy. The serious and rare side effect of Stevens-Johnson syndrome warrants specific titration, and it is important for patients to remain adherent to medication therapy. Other side effects of lamotrigine may include dizziness, nausea, vomiting, and rash.

Levetiracetam is effective as adjunct therapy for myoclonic, partial-onset, and generalized tonic-clonic seizures. Its exact mechanism of action is unknown. This agent has minimal drug interactions, including no known interactions with other anticonvulsant medications or oral contraceptives. The most common adverse effects include somnolence and dizziness.

Rufinamide slows the inactivation of sodium channels and reduces the repetitive firing of neurons. It is effective in partial seizures.

Tiagabine inhibits the GABA transporter and reduces GABA reuptake into the neurons. It is effective as adjunct therapy for partial seizures. This agent is metabolized by the liver, and its metabolism is increased when it is used with phenobarbital, phenytoin, carbamazepine, and other enzyme-inducing medications. The primary adverse effects associated with tigabine are dizziness, somnolence, and tremor. Tolerance to the side effects tends to develop with chronic use.

Topiramate reduces voltage-gated sodium currents, enhances post-synaptic GABA-receptors, and limits activation of glutamate receptors. It is effective as monotherapy and adjunctive therapy for partial-onset or primary generalized tonic-clonic seizures. Topiramate is associated with reduced estradiol concentrations, so higher doses of oral contraceptives may be warranted when used concurrently with this medication. Potential adverse effects include confusion, drowsiness, weight loss, and nervousness.

e Valproic acid and derivatives are effective for partial, tonic-clonic, myoclonic, and absence seizures; they work by limiting the repetitive firing of neurons and inhibiting the enzymes that degrade GABA. The most common adverse effects associated with these medications include GI symptoms such as nausea, vomiting, and anorexia. Dividing daily doses greater than 250 mg can reduce the severity of these side effects. Chronic treatment with valproic acid and similar drugs can cause appetite stimulation and weight gain, rash, and alopecia. Increases in liver enzymes are frequently noted and asymptomatic; on rare occasions, valproic acid can cause hepatitis, which may be fatal. Pancreatitis and hyperammonemia are also rare, but are potentially serious side effects. Plasma concentrations of valproic acid necessary to achieve anticonvulsant effects are 50–100 μg/mL. Valproate inhibits specific hepatic enzymes and can affect serum concentrations of phenytoin and phenobarbital. If lamotrigine and lorazepam are used concurrently with this medication, their metabolism will be inhibited due to valproate's inhibition of uridine diphosphate glucuronosyltransferase (UGT). Phenytoin metabolism is further altered due to valproate's protein binding.

Vigabatrin irreversibly inhibits the enzyme that degrades GABA, causing an increase the amount of GABA available at the neuron. This agent is effective as adjunctive therapy for refractory partial complex seizures. Because vigabatrin causes progressive and permanent bilateral vision loss, its use is restricted to patients who have failed to respond to multiple therapies. This medication must be dispensed in accordance with the SHARE distribution program.

Zonisamide inhibits repetitive firing of spinal cord neurons and is effective as an adjunct therapy for partial seizures. Phenobarbital, phenytoin, and carbamazepine decrease the plasma concentration of zonisamide, whereas lamotrigine increases the plasma concentration of this drug. Zonisamide, however, has minimal effect on the plasma concentrations of other antiepileptic medications. Common adverse effects associated with its use include somnolence, anorexia, nervousness, and fatigue. Patients with renal disease, severe respiratory disorders, diarrhea, surgery, or ketogenic diet are at an increased risk of metabolic acidosis when taking zonisamide, and serum bicarbonate monitoring is recommended in such patients.

Miscellaneous Anticonvulsant Agents

Carbamazepine
Eslicarbazepine
Ezogabine
Felbamate
Gabapentin
Lacosamide
Lamotrigine
Levetiracetam
Magnesium sulfate
Oxcarbazepine

Perampanel
Pregabalin
Rufinamide
Tiagabine
Topiramate
Valproate/divalproex
Vigabatrin
Zonisamide
Acetazolamide *(see also the Antiglaucoma Agents section in the Eye, Ear, Nose, and Throat Preparations chapter)*

Case Studies and Conclusions

Charlie is a 21-year-old male who experiences absence seizures.

1. Which of the following medications is indicated for monotherapy for absence seizures?
   a. Clonazepam
   b. Phenobarbital
   c. Phenytoin
   d. Valproic acid

Answer D is correct. Clonazepam is effective in absence and myoclonic seizures in children. Phenobarbital is used for generalized tonic–clonic and partial seizures. Phenytoin is ineffective for absence seizures. Valproic acid is effective for partial, tonic–clonic, myoclonic, and absence seizures.

Serum monitoring is indicated with the use of many anticonvulsant medications to improve the medication's efficacy and reduce toxicity.

2. What is the ideal plasma concentration to ensure valproic acid's anticonvulsant effects are achieved?
   a. 0.75–1.25 μg/mL
   b. 10–35 μg/mL
   c. 50–100 μg/mL
   d. 40–100 μg/mL

Answer C is correct. The ideal therapeutic range for phenytoin is 0.75–1.25 μg/mL, the ideal range for phenobarbital is 10–35 μg/mL, the ideal level for valproic acid is 50–100 μg/mL, and the ideal range for ethosuximide to ensure anticonvulsant effects is 40–100 μg/mL.

Use of valproic acid requires monitoring for many adverse effects.

3. Which of the following is NOT something that should be monitored in patients receiving valproic acid?
   a. Ammonia levels
   b. Liver enzymes
   c. Changes in mood/behavior
   d. Renal function

Answer D is correct. Ammonia levels may increase in patients on chronic valproic acid therapy. Liver enzymes may become elevated with valproic acid use, and this medication may cause dose-related hepatotoxicity. Changes in mood, behavior, suicidality, and psychiatric symptoms may develop or worsen with use of valproic acid. Renal function is not compromised with valproic acid use.

Charlotte is a 32-year-old female who has been prescribed lamotrigine for seizure control. Recently, she has been experiencing additional seizures despite being at an adequate dose level of lamotrigine.

1. Which of the following statements is INCORRECT about polypharmacy of anticonvulsants?
   a. Carbamazepine decreases the plasma concentration of lamotrigine.
   b. Phenobarbital increases the plasma concentration of lamotrigine.
   c. Phenytoin decreases the plasma concentration of lamotrigine.
   d. Valproic acid increases the plasma concentration of lamotrigine.

Answer B is correct. Carbamazepine, phenytoin, and phenobarbital increase the metabolism and reduce the plasma concentration of lamotrigine. Use of lamotrigine with valproate increases the concentration of lamotrigine and reduces the concentration of valproate. Lamotrigine can increase formation of the metabolites of carbamazepine and may cause toxicity in some patients.

Prior to selecting an additional agent, it is noted that Charlotte is currently prescribed oral contraceptives.

2. Which of the following medication options will NOT interact with the efficacy of this patient's oral contraceptive?
   a. Carbamazepine
   b. Oxcarbazepine
   c. Phenobarbital
   d. Levetiracetam

Answer D is correct. Levetiracetam has not been found to interact with oral contraceptives or other antiepileptic medications. Carbamazepine, oxcarbazepine, phenobarbital, phenytoin, primidone, and topiramate can decrease the efficacy of oral contraceptives, and patients should be warned about this effect.

After the addition of the second anticonvulsant to her medication regimen, Charlotte has not experienced a seizure in the past 4 months and is wondering when or if she can ever discontinue taking her medications.

3. When can anticonvulsant therapy be reduced or discontinued?
   a. After the patient has been seizure free for 6 months
   b. After the patient has been seizure free for 12 months
   c. After the patient has been seizure free for 24 months
   d. Anticonvulsant therapy is always lifelong.

Answer C is correct. After a patient has been seizure free for 24 months, titration of the dose or discontinuation of the medication may be considered. A seizure recurrence, if it occurs, is likely to happen within 4 months of therapy discontinuation.

7.4 Psychotherapeutic Agents

Antidepressant Agents

Numerous hypotheses have been proposed regarding the role of antidepressants in the treatment of depression. Antidepressants, upon the first few doses, cause changes in the action of certain neurochemicals, but the overall optimal effects are not seen for weeks in depression and even longer in other mental health conditions. One of the actions that accounts for the majority of antidepressants' influence is the neurochemical's inhibition or reuptake into the synaptic vesicle once initially released. This reuptake inhibition allows for a longer neurochemical influence in the synapse and likely an extended action of the neurotransmitter. In contrast, the older antidepressants established their activity by inhibiting the monoamine oxidase (MAO) enzyme, which was responsible for "breaking down" or metabolizing the active neurotransmitter; thus, they extended the neurotransmitter's physiologic action.

Antidepressant agents are primarily selected based on patient-specific factors, including their side-effect profiles, the patient's comorbid disease states (these medications can work additively or may need to be avoided in certain populations), and cost. Universal precautions apply when using any CNS agents: Specifically, patients should be warned that they may experience drowsiness or dizziness, and advised to use caution while driving or operating machinery until the effects of the drug are known. Also, for most antidepressants, gradual dose increases with therapy initiation and slow tapers when discontinuing the medication are recommended. Oftentimes, if antidepressants are abruptly discontinued, patients may experience withdrawal symptoms, which is also known as antidepressant discontinuation syndrome. Patients may experience symptoms such as anxiety, headaches, insomnia, drowsiness, flu-like symptoms, electric shock-like sensations, and a return of the depression symptoms. The duration and severity of the discontinuation syndrome vary based on which agent was discontinued, but some patients may experience symptoms for a few weeks. Regardless of the agent prescribed, patients should be encouraged to talk to their healthcare provider prior to stopping antidepressant therapy. Clinicians who prescribe antidepressants should ensure that the dose and the duration of therapy are optimized before considering the possibility of a treatment failure. Dose escalations and assessments of response should be considered in light of the delayed effects of antidepressants after their initiation.

The class side effects range from the potential to cause anticholinergic side effects, to sexual side effects (including decreased libido), to QTc prolongation, to serotonin syndrome. Serotonin syndrome, though relatively rare, may result in death if not recognized and treated properly. This syndrome is more likely to be experienced by patients who are taking multiple concomitant agents with serotonergic influence and may initially resemble GI upset or flu-like symptoms. Antidepressants may also lead to pupillary dilation, exacerbating closed-angle glaucoma; if left unaddressed, this effect could cause blindness. Seizures have been reported in some antidepressant trials, so a universal precaution is warranted regarding these agents' use in patients with history of seizure.

Critical to success with the overall use of antidepressants is the clinical team's willingness to use the optimal dose and duration of these agents before changing regimens (including, but not limited to, augmentation or alternative agents) or before declaring a treatment failure. If antidepressants are prescribed for extended periods, the patient should be periodically reevaluated for drug effectiveness and safety. Some patients, depending on their severity of depression, may require antidepressant therapy on a lifelong basis.

Age-associated reduced medication clearance (elimination) may be addressed with decreased doses or even every-other-day dosing of antidepressant agents, especially in patients sensitive to drugs with a longer half-life and duration of action. When the drug is being used to stabilize mood, manage behavior, or treat psychiatric disorders, an attempt must be made to periodically taper the medication or provide documentation of medical necessity in accordance with OBRA guidelines. All antidepressant agents carry a black box warning about increased risk of suicidality, although this risk is linked to a specific age for those 24 years or younger.

Monoamine Oxidase Inhibitors

Monoamine oxidase inhibitors (MAOIs) inhibit monoamine oxidase, which is responsible for metabolizing monoamines (norepinephrine, serotonin, dopamine). In addition to the side effects shared by most antidepressants, such as serotonin syndrome, MAOIs have a unique class requirement of avoidance of tyramine-rich foods, medications that raise blood pressure (i.e., sympathomimetics), and medications that possess MAOI-like activity. Failure to avoid these combinations can lead to hypertensive crisis or serotonin syndrome. A "washout period" is required when changing to an MAOI from another antidepressant medication. Establishing an optimal antidepressant regimen is challenging and may require a trial of different antidepressant agents. Generally MAOIs are reserved for later use after initial trials of newer agents have failed. When transitioning to MAOIs from other antidepressants, a washout waiting period of no less than 14 days is required for most agents and even longer for other agents such as fluoxetine and vortioxetine. Patients who are diagnosed with pheochromocytoma—a tumor associated with secretion of vasopressor substances (i.e., norepinephrine)—can experience hypertensive crisis if also on a MAOI due to the inhibited metabolism of catecholamine monoamines.

Monoamine Oxidase Inhibitors

Phenelzine
Tranylcypromine
Rasagiline *(see also the Antiparkinsonian Agents section)*
Selegiline *(see also the Antiparkinsonian Agents section)*

Serotonin and Norepinephrine Reuptake Inhibitors

Gastrointestinal side effects are among the most commonly reported side effects of newly initiated serotonin-modulating antidepressant therapy, but are generally transient (i.e., they decrease after 1–2 weeks of usage). If a patient suddenly develops GI symptoms after a successful, prolonged period of use of an antidepressant, the clinician should rule out potential serotonin syndrome or other drug-induced causes or a new medical condition. Complaints of sexual dysfunction are also common with serotonin-modulating antidepressants, but are not considered transient;

therefore, a shared decision should be made about whether changing to another class of antidepressants that have less negative sexual effects may improve the patient's overall quality of life (i.e., bupropion). This medication class may also cause hyponatremia, resulting from inappropriate antidiuretic hormone secretion (SIADH). Consequently, electrolytes should be evaluated as clinically appropriate. Due to their noradrenergic effects, SNRIs can cause elevations in blood pressure. Caution should be used in patients with uncontrolled hypertension.

Clinicians who initiate serotonin-modulating antidepressants (i.e., SNRIs and SSRIs) must monitor patients for signs and symptoms of bleeding. Impaired platelet aggregation may result from drug-induced platelet serotonin depletion, possibly increasing the risk of a bleeding complication (i.e., GI bleed). The risk of bleeding is further worsened if the patient is on concurrent anticoagulant therapy, thrombolytic therapy, or other medications that increase the potential of bleeding.

Some data suggest an association between exposure to serotonin reuptake inhibitors and reduced bone density. Thus, patients who may be at increased risk for osteoporosis should have more frequent bone density monitoring.

Selective Serotonin–Norepinephrine Reuptake Inhibitors

Desvenlafaxine
Duloxetine
Levomilnacipran
Venlafaxine
Milnacipran *(see also the Analgesic and Antipyretic Agents section)*

Selective Serotonin Reuptake Inhibitors

Citalopram
Escitalopram
Fluoxetine
Fluvoxamine
Paroxetine
Sertraline

Serotonin Modulators

Nefazodone
Trazodone
Vilazodone
Vortioxetine

Tricyclic Antidepressants and Other Norepinephrine-Reuptake Inhibitors

Tricyclic antidepressants (TCAs) should be used with caution in patients with any cardiac disease (e.g., heart failure, coronary artery disease), with these patients undergoing careful monitoring of ECGs and clinical exams. Cardiovascular adverse events, including potentially fatal arrhythmias, are a significant risk after acute overdose, whether intentional or unintentional. These agents should be avoided in patients at risk of overdose secondary to suicidal ideation.

Due to their potential anticholinergic side effects (e.g., dry eyes, constipation, worsening of benign prostatic hyperplasia, glaucoma, and reduced sweating and temperature regulation), standard anticholinergic precautions should be respected in patients on concomitant medications with anticholinergic properties or with conditions that can be worsened by these side effects (including higher risk of falls). Notably, anticholinergic effects may alter symptoms of Parkinson's disease and can even cause—though rarely—extrapyramidal symptoms (involuntary movements) that resemble tardive dyskinesia. In addition to patients vulnerable to TCAs' anticholinergic effects, patients with respiratory depression or disease should be treated cautiously with these agents because of the CNS-depressant effects of TCAs. Blood dyscrasias have been reported as well, so TCAs should be used cautiously in patients who are predisposed to or who have current hematologic disease. Use caution in patients with hepatic disease, because liver failure and death have occurred when TCAs were continued in patients who developed hepatitis. Liver function tests should be performed and drug discontinuation considered if persistent elevation of liver enzymes is noted. Patients may experience greater sun sensitivity when taking TCAs and should be counseled on taking photosensitivity precautions during treatment. All antidepressants have common class side effects;

however, some agents have unique adverse effects that clinicians should be aware of prior to selection and use. Refer to the companion drug grid for additional detail on drug-specific facts.

Tricyclic Antidepressants and Other Norepinephrine-Reuptake Inhibitors

Amitriptyline
Amoxapine
Clomipramine
Desipramine
Doxepin
Imipramine
Maprotiline
Nortriptyline
Protriptyline
Trimipramine

Miscellaneous Antidepressant Agents

Bupropion
Mirtazapine

Antipsychotic Agents

Antipsychotic medications are central to the overall management of many mental health conditions, including, but not limited to, schizophrenia. Advances since the 1950s, when the first antipsychotic agent was used therapeutically, have included the introduction of newer second-generation agents. Both first-generation (FGA) and second-generation (SGA) antipsychotic agents are considered first-line agents for initial treatment of schizophrenia because they share similar efficacy and a common mechanism of action—namely, the ability to block the dopamine D_2 receptor. The SGAs have additional receptor actions that give them a unique pharmacologic profile and properties. These properties include antagonism at various receptors, primarily dopamine and serotonin receptors, along with histamine, alpha 1 and 2, and cholinergic receptors.

Extrapyramidal side effects (EPS), including Parkinsonism and akathisia, which are seen more commonly with the use of the FGAs, fueled interest in the development of newer agents that would have less potential to cause these movement disorders. Thus, the SGAs have been progressively displacing the FGAs in overall practice despite their lack of established superior efficacy. With the exception of clozapine, which has documented superiority, the selection of antipsychotic agents should be based on patient preference and side-effect profile. The SGAs have been associated with less EPS, but they are associated with more non-dose-related weight gain and metabolic abnormalities such as dyslipidemia, cardiac irregularities, and abnormal blood glucose.

The FDA labels of all antipsychotics carry a black box warning for use in patients with dementia-related psychosis. Some antipsychotic agents are approved for use as augmentation for depression and thus are associated with the additional warnings relative to antidepressant agents increasing the risk compared with placebo of suicidal thinking and behavior (suicidality). These agents should be used with caution in patients who are taking other benzodiazepines, sleep medications, and medications that can lower the seizure threshold.

Antipsychotic Agents

Second-Generation (Atypical) Agents

Aripiprazole
Asenapine
Brexpiprazole
Cariprazine
Clozapine
Iloperidone
Lurasidone
Olanzapine

Paliperidone
Quetiapine
Risperidone
Ziprasidone

First-Generation (Conventional/Typical) Agents: Butyrophenones

Haloperidol

First-Generation (Conventional/Typical) Agents: Phenothiazines

Chlorpromazine
Fluphenazine
Perphenazine
Prochlorperazine
Thioridazine
Trifluoperazine

First-Generation (Conventional/Typical) Agents: Thioxanthenes

Thiothixene

Miscellaneous Antipsychotic Agents

Loxapine
Molindone
Pimozide

Case Studies and Conclusions

SD is a 35-year-old male currently in week 10 of treatment for his first episode of major depressive disorder. Although he reports some improvement in mood, he describes "not feeling as good" when compared to how he felt before the depression began. He also mentions that he saw a TV commercial for quetiapine (Seroquel) to use as an "add-on" to his antidepressant and is now interested in using it along with his current prescription for fluoxetine 10 mg (the dose on which he started).

1. What would you recommend for this patient?
   a. Add quetiapine 50 mg and continue fluoxetine 10 mg
   b. Increase to fluoxetine 20 mg and add quetiapine 50 mg
   c. Add quetiapine 50 mg and discontinue fluoxetine 10 mg
   d. Increase to fluoxetine 2 0mg and do not add quetiapine 50 mg

Answer D is correct. The addition of an antipsychotic augmentation agent should be considered only after optimization of the initial agent's dose and duration. The assessment of the patient should also include verification of adherence in a patient who has had a dose and duration that appears otherwise clinically appropriate. Unnecessary addition of antipsychotic drugs poses a risk of increased side effects (including metabolic long-term effects) and drug interactions.

SD reports his insurance will no longer cover his fluoxetine, so he would like to consider another SSRI option.

2. Which information would you provide to SD about the SSRI class?
   a. SSRIs commonly cause sexual side effects.
   b. SSRIs commonly cause cardiac toxicity.
   c. SSRIs commonly cause dangerous increases in blood pressure.
   d. SSRIs commonly cause renal dysfunction.

Answer A is correct. Although other antidepressants have sexual side effects, the SSRI class of agents have a higher rate of reported side effects when compared to the others. Bupropion and other antidepressants that may influence dopamine may represent alternatives with significantly less frequent reports of sexual side effects.

SD reports that he is experiencing ongoing insomnia with his current SSRI regimen. He was told by a friend to consider amitriptyline because it worked well for her.

3. Which information would you provide SD about the TCA class?
   a. TCAs are known to cause renal dysfunction.
   b. TCAs are known to cause dangerous increases in blood pressure.
   c. TCAs are known to cause cardiotoxic effects.
   d. TCAs are known to cause acne.

Answer C is correct. Many antidepressant agents can affect the cardiovascular system, but TCAs are more likely to cause cardiac toxicity because they are prone to complications associated with impaired cardiac conduction. By comparison, the SSRIs/SNRIs are more likely to cause prolongation of the QTc interval. TCAs are notably more associated with lethality in overdose due to this cardiac side effect.

FF is a 40-year-old male who arrives to the emergency room (ER) with a diagnosis of serotonin syndrome. He is currently on sertraline 200 mg daily and reports some recent activities that he believes may have contributed to the cause for his ER visit, which including increased use of sumatriptan for migraine.

1. Which of the following additional activities would be most likely to cause FF's serotonin syndrome?
   a. Consumed cheese pizza with alcoholic beverages
   b. Took dextromethorphan for cough
   c. Skipped the morning dose of sertraline
   d. Took diphenhydramine for allergy relief

Answer B is correct. Dextromethorphan-containing products are known to contribute to serotonin syndrome when administered with other agents with a serotonin "influence." Because dextromethorphan is an OTC medication, prescribers may confuse this interaction with that associated with guaifenesin-containing cough syrups, which is not the case here. Aged cheeses, dairy products, and processed meats are on the MAOI avoidance list, but are not contraindicated with the other antidepressant agents; these products should be avoided to prevent hypertensive crisis owing to the overabundance of tyramine, the precursor of the monamines such as norepinephrine.

While FF is being treated in the ER, he reports that his depression is not improving. The psychiatrist considers changing FF to phenelzine.

2. What is the shortest allowable duration of time that is recommended for this conversion?
   a. Discontinue full-dose sertraline on day 1, start full-dose phenelzine on day 2
   b. Discontinue sertraline 2 weeks prior to starting phenelzine
   c. Discontinue sertraline 3 weeks after to starting phenelzine
   d. Discontinue sertraline 5 weeks prior to starting phenelzine

Answer B is correct. A 2-week washout is required for most SSRI/SNRI agents with some exceptions. One of those exceptions is fluoxetine, for which the washout period is 5 weeks due to this agent's extensive half-life. This washout period reduces the chance of hypertensive crisis and serotonin syndrome.

7.5 Anorexigenic Agents and Respiratory and CNS Stimulants

Stimulants are used for a variety of indications, including attention-deficit/hyperactivity disorder (ADD/ADHD), daytime sleepiness in narcolepsy, as an adjunct to diet and exercise for weight loss, headache treatment, and respiratory apnea in neonates. Amphetamines are controlled substances, meaning there is a potential for their abuse, and restrictions are enforced on their prescribing.

ADHD is a chronic condition, whose onset typically occurs in childhood. The patient experiences symptoms of hyperactivity, impulsivity, and/or inattention that occur in multiple settings (e.g., home, work, school, social events) and affect the patient's functioning academically, socially, and emotionally. Stimulants may not treat all behavioral symptoms of ADHD, and they are used adjunctively with behavioral therapy, since both forms of treatment used together are more efficacious than either used alone. Typically, if a patient fails a trial with one stimulant (due to either efficacy or adverse effects), a different stimulant should be tried, because failure of one agent does not mean failure of all. If left untreated, ADHD can have serious consequences, including increased risk of substance use disorders, oppositional defiant disorder, conduct disorder, motor vehicle accidents, incarcerations, interpersonal and relationship difficulties, and unemployment.

Narcolepsy is a disorder involving a disruption of sleep/wake control. All patients with narcolepsy suffer from chronic sleepiness despite obtaining adequate nighttime sleep, with sleepiness sometimes occurring without warning. Patients may become incredibly sleepy and fall asleep at inappropriate times. Other symptoms include cataplexy (transient muscle weakness triggered by strong emotions, such as laughing or excitement), hypnagogic hallucinations (vivid visual, tactile, or auditory hallucinations that occur when a patient is falling asleep), and sleep paralysis (inability to move for 1-2 minutes after waking or before falling asleep). Amphetamines are the mainstay of treatment for narcolepsy, with the medication being selected based on side effects or patient preference. If amphetamines are not effective, the patient's diagnosis of narcolepsy should be reconsidered. Long-term use of high-dose amphetamines may result in tolerance, so it is important to continue to monitor the patient and the efficacy of medications.

Short-term use of stimulants can be used in addition to a calorie-restricted diet, exercise, and behavioral therapy in the treatment of obesity in patients. Long-term use of these medications has not been studied for the indication of obesity and is not recommended.

Although the exact mechanism of action of stimulants is unknown, these agents are thought to increase the levels of neurotransmitters (norepinephrine and dopamine) in the synapse between neurons by inhibiting their reuptake. The increased levels of norepinephrine, dopamine, and other catecholamines in the brain result in increased wakefulness, alertness, initiative, ability to concentrate, and motor activities. Although the speed of work may be increased, amphetamines may nevertheless increase the risk of errors.

Amphetamines

Amphetamines are available as extended-release and immediate-release products. Immediate-release formulations are approved for use in children 3 years and older, whereas extended-release products are approved in children 6 years and older. Although the extended-release products are dosed on a once-daily basis, occasionally patients may experience breakthrough symptoms and require an afternoon dose of an immediate-release formulation.

The products called "mixed amphetamine salts" are composed of amphetamine (amphetamine aspartate and amphetamine sulfate) and dextroamphetamine (dextroamphetamine saccharate and dextroamphetamine sulfate). Amphetamines are stimulating medications, so they have the potential to cause insomnia. It is recommended that the doses be taken immediately upon waking in the morning; late-afternoon/evening doses should be avoided if possible to prevent sleep disturbance. Amphetamine products can also cause nervousness, anxiety, jitteriness, aggression, and manic symptoms.

Amphetamines can alter an individual's ability to perform hazardous tasks, such as driving a motor vehicle or operating heavy machinery. Patients should be aware of the medication's effects on their attention and focus prior to engaging in any potentially hazardous activities.

Weight loss is a common adverse effect of amphetamines, although the mechanism of action behind this effect is unknown. Children and adolescents should be encouraged to eat a balanced diet. If weight loss and appetite reduction are significant, snacks throughout the day should be strongly encouraged and large or high-caloric meals should be consumed prior to dose administrations (i.e., breakfast or an afternoon snack if the individual receives a second dose) or when the medication effects are wearing off. Children may experience growth suppression (less than 1 cm decrease over 1-3 years), and drug holidays may be implemented if this is a concern.

Cardiovascular abnormalities have been reported with amphetamine use, including echocardiogram changes, abnormal heart valve functioning, high blood pressure, tachycardia, chest pain, and murmurs. At large doses, these agents can induce cardiac arrhythmias. Consequently, the U.S. labels of amphetamines carry a black box warning for risk of these cardiac abnormalities and sudden cardiac death. Patients with structural cardiac abnormalities or structural heart defects should not use amphetamines due to this increased risk.

Some evidence indicates that stimulant use is associated with an increased risk of seizures, lowering of the seizure threshold, or electroencephalogram changes. If a patient experiences a seizure, stimulant therapy should be discontinued.

The FDA labels of amphetamines also carry a black box warning about their high abuse potential, and these medications are classified as controlled substances due to this risk. Sometimes amphetamines are abused by individuals due to their CNS excitation effects, but more commonly they are abused by individuals in positions requiring endurance, such as students, athletes, and drivers of motor vehicles. Many people do not consider utilizing an amphetamine product to assist with "studying" or "focus" to constitute abuse. However, if a medication is not prescribed for the individual consuming the product, it is, in fact, medication misuse. Furthermore, research does not support the contention that use of amphetamines in individuals without ADHD helps improve grades or quality of work.

Long-term use of high doses of amphetamines can result in development of tolerance and can put individuals at risk for dependence and addiction. Although drug abuse is possible, having a history of a substance use disorder is not an absolute contraindication to amphetamine use in patients with ADHD. Chronic amphetamine abusers (average consumption 1–2 g per day) can experience teeth grinding or chewing and tongue rubbing along the backside of the teeth. This can result in tooth loss and ulceration of the tongue and gums. Prolonged abuse can result in symptoms similar to schizophrenia, including hallucinations and paranoia.

Amphetamines

Amphetamine
Benzphetamine
Dextroamphetamine
Lisdexamfetamine
Methamphetamine

Anorexigenic Agents

Amphetamine Derivatives

Amphetamine derivatives are used in the treatment of obesity because they may reduce patient food intake by causing early satiety; their use in this indication should be combined with a low-calorie diet and exercise. These medications are approved only for short-term use (up to 12 weeks) for obesity treatment. Although efficacious, they are not recommended for general weight loss due to their side-effect profiles and potential for abuse. The obesity indication specifies that these medications should be used only in patients with a body mass index (BMI) greater than 30 kg/m^2, or greater than 27 kg/m^2 with additional risk factors (i.e., diabetes, hyperlipidemia, controlled hypertension).

Use of amphetamine derivatives in patients with coronary heart disease, hypertension, or hyperthyroidism is contraindicated. Side effects of these sympathomimetic drugs include increased heart rate and blood pressure, insomnia, nervousness, dry mouth, and constipation. In the past, some medications in this class were removed from the market due to safety concerns, including increased risk of nonfatal MI, nonfatal stroke, and hemorrhagic stroke.

Amphetamine Derivatives

Diethylpropion
Phendimetrazine
Phentermine

Selective Serotonin Receptor Agonists

Lorcaserin is approved for weight loss in conjunction with a low-calorie diet and exercise, and is indicated for use only in patients with a BMI greater than 30 kg/m^2, or greater than 27 kg/m^2 with risk factors (i.e., diabetes, hyperlipidemia, controlled hypertension). Lorcaserin activates serotonin receptors, which decreases food consumption and increases satiety. Its exact mechanism of action, however, is unknown.

Most adverse effects of lorcaserin are mild, including headache, dizziness, and nausea. Patients with a diagnosis of diabetes who experience episodes of hypoglycemia during trials may require a reduction in the doses of their diabetes medications.

There is an increased risk of serotonin syndrome when lorcaserin is used in combination with other serotonergic agents (e.g., antidepressants, triptans) due to its potentiating effects on serotonin receptors.

Selective Serotonin Receptor Agonists

Lorcaserin

Respiratory and Other Central Nervous System Stimulants

Although the exact mechanism of action of stimulants is unknown, these agents are thought to increase the levels of neurotransmitters (norepinephrine and dopamine) in the synapse between neurons by inhibiting their reuptake. The increased levels of norepinephrine, dopamine, and other catecholamines in the brain result in increased wakefulness, alertness, initiative, and ability to concentrate and perform motor activities. It is important to note that although the speed of work may be increased, stimulants may also increase the risk of errors.

Stimulants are available as extended-release and immediate-release products. Although the extended-release products are dosed on a once-daily basis, occasionally patients may experience breakthrough symptoms and require an afternoon dose of an immediate-release formulation.

Methylphenidate and dexmethylphenidate are stimulating medications, so they have the potential to cause insomnia. It is recommended that the doses be taken immediately upon waking in the morning; late-afternoon/evening doses should be avoided if possible. If a patch formulation is used, it should be removed at least 3 hours prior to anticipated sleep. Stimulant products can also cause nervousness, anxiety, jitteriness, aggression, and manic symptoms. They can alter the user's ability to perform hazardous tasks, such as driving a motor vehicle or operating heavy machinery. Patients should be aware of the medication's effects on their attention and focus prior to engaging in any potentially hazardous activities.

Weight loss is a common adverse effect of dexmethylphenidate and methylphenidate, although the mechanism of action behind this effect is unknown. Children and adolescents should be encouraged to eat a balanced diet. If weight loss and appetite loss are significant, snacks throughout the day should be strongly encouraged, and large or high-caloric meals should be consumed prior to dose administrations (i.e., breakfast or afternoon snack if the patient receives a second dose) or when the medication effects are wearing off. Children may experience growth suppression (less than 1 cm decrease over 1- 3 years), and drug holidays may be implemented if this is a concern.

Cardiovascular abnormalities have been reported with stimulant use, including echocardiogram changes, abnormal heart valve functioning, high blood pressure, tachycardia, chest pain, and murmurs. At large doses, these agents can induce cardiac arrhythmias. Some evidence indicates that stimulant use is associated with an increased risk of seizures, lowering of the seizure threshold, or electroencephalogram changes. If a patient experiences a seizure, stimulant therapy should be discontinued.

Dexmethylphenidate and methylphenidate are classified as controlled substances due to the possible risk of abuse. Sometimes they are abused by individuals due to their CNS excitation effects, but more commonly they are abused by individuals in positions requiring endurance, such as students, athletes, and drivers of motor vehicles. Many people do not consider utilizing a stimulant product to assist with "studying" or "focus" to constitute abuse. However, if a medication is not prescribed for the individual consuming the product, it is, in fact, medication misuse. Furthermore, research does not support the contention that use of stimulants in individuals without ADHD helps improve grades or quality of work.

Long-term use of dexmethylphenidate and methylphenidate can result in development of tolerance, as well as risk for dependence and addiction. Chronic stimulant abusers can experience teeth grinding or chewing and tongue rubbing along the backside of the teeth. This can result in tooth loss and ulceration of the tongue and gums. Prolonged abuse can result in symptoms similar to schizophrenia, including hallucinations and paranoia. Although drug abuse is possible, having a history of a substance use disorder is not an absolute contraindication to stimulant use in patients with ADHD.

Respiratory and Other Central Nervous System Stimulants

Ammonia spirit
Caffeine/caffeine and sodium benzoate
Dexmethylphenidate
Doxapram
Methylphenidate
Theophylline *(see also the Respiratory Smooth Muscle Relaxants section in the Smooth Muscle Relaxants chapter)*

Wakefulness-Promoting Agents

Patients with narcolepsy exhibit signs and symptoms of daytime sleepiness. Although napping may provide some relief, oftentimes this is not an option—so pharmacotherapy is utilized to diminish the sleepiness. Modafinil and armodafinil promote wakefulness and maximize daytime alertness (as much as 70% to 80% of normal).

Modafinil is a non-amphetamine wakefulness agent that is believed to exert its effects by increasing dopaminergic signaling. It should be taken first thing in the morning, and its effects typically wear off in the early evening, so it does not disrupt nighttime sleeping. Armodafinil is an enantiomer of modafinil and, therefore, has very similar effects to modafinil. Once therapy is initiated and optimized, patients should be routinely monitored with the Epworth Sleepiness Score or the Maintenance of Wakefulness Test.

There is a lower abuse potential with modafinil and armodafinil compared to other stimulants because they are non-amphetamine products. They are also considered to be safer in older patients due to their mild side-effect profiles. Adverse effects of these medications are uncommon, but include headache, dry mouth, anorexia, nausea, and diarrhea. Modafinil may increase blood pressure and should be used with caution in patients with arrhythmias or heart disease. Stevens-Johnson syndrome has been reported on rare occasions with modafinil use.

Oral contraceptive efficacy may be reduced by many medications, including modafinil. Women of childbearing potential who are taking oral contraceptives should use an alternative and/or backup method of contraception when taking modafinil.

Wakefulness-Promoting Agents

Armodafinil
Modafinil

Miscellaneous Central Nervous System Stimulants

Several medications are currently categorized as "central nervous system, miscellaneous" agents by the American Hospital Formulary Service. Refer to the current drug grid for specific drug information, including indications, dose, and other important therapeutic information.

Miscellaneous Central Nervous System Stimulants

Acamprosate
Atomoxetine
Dextromethorphan and quinidine
Flumazenil
Memantine
Riluzole
Sodium oxybate
Tetrabenzine
Guanfacine *(see also the Hypotensive Agents section in the Cardiovascular Agents chapter)*

Case Studies and Conclusions

Thomas is an 18-year-old who was recently diagnosed with ADHD. His parents have exhausted all nonpharmacologic interventions without significant reduction in their son's symptoms.

1. It is decided to initiate pharmacotherapy at this time. Which medication should be recommended?
    a. Mixed amphetamine salts, extended-release formulation
    b. Mixed amphetamine salts, immediate-release formulation
    c. Lisdexamfetamine
    d. Methamphetamine

Answer A is correct. Extended- and modified-release products are approved in patients older than 6 years.

Thomas's parents state that his cousin in high school often visits him. They heard on the news that young adults and teenagers often abuse stimulants.

2. Which of the following statement is FALSE in regard to abuse of ADHD stimulant medications?
    a. Amphetamines are controlled substances.
    b. The use of stimulants does not improve learning capacity.
    c. Use at normal doses of stimulants can lead to tolerance and dependence.
    d. History of substance use disorder is not a contraindication to therapy with stimulants.

Answer C is correct. Amphetamines are DEA-controlled substances (C-II). Many states limit the quantity allowed to be dispensed, and no refills can be authorized—a new prescription is required for each fill. Although frequently abused by teenagers/young adults to help with academic performance, stimulants do not increase learning capacity or intelligence; they are effective only in reducing ADHD symptoms such as lack of concentration. Use at higher than therapeutic doses for ADHD can lead to tolerance and dependence, and chronic use at doses more than 1 g per day can lead to serious side effects. History of substance use disorder is not a contraindication to therapy with stimulants for treatment of ADHD, although a healthcare provider may decide to use a non-controlled medication for treatment instead.

Sara is a 27-year-old female who is recently diagnosed with ADHD. She was diagnosed with depression when she was 17 years old and has been on antidepressant therapy since then. She feels that, despite her treatment for depression, her ADHD symptoms still interrupt her daily functioning. Sara would like to begin therapy with an amphetamine product.

1. Sara is currently taking tranylcypromine 20 mg twice a day, but is willing to switch to a different antidepressant. How long does she have to wait between the last dose of her MAOI before starting an amphetamine product?
   a. 7 days
   b. 14 days
   c. 21 days
   d. The amphetamine product can be started immediately.

Answer B is correct. MAOIs require a 14-day washout period prior to starting amphetamine products.

Sara is hoping to have to take her medication only once a day.

2. Which of the following medications is not available as a long-acting or extended-release formulation?
   a. Amphetamine
   b. Dextroamphetamine
   c. Lisdexamfetamine
   d. Methamphetamine

Answer D is correct. All of these medications are available as extended-release formulations except for methamphetamine.

Sara read online that amphetamines can cause sudden cardiac death, and she is concerned because some of her family members have high blood pressure.

3. Which of the following is NOT an appropriate counseling point for Sara?
   a. Patients with an underlying structural heart defect are at risk of sudden cardiac death when they take amphetamines.
   b. Arrhythmias are common with use of amphetamines, even at low doses.
   c. Amphetamines can increase blood pressure in patients.
   d. Your doctor may want to obtain a baseline electroencephalogram when prescribing an amphetamine.

Answer B is correct. Patients with underlying structural heart defects should not use amphetamine products due to the risk of sudden cardiac death. Arrhythmias may occur at high doses of these medications. Amphetamines increase both systolic and diastolic blood pressure. If a healthcare provider is concerned about cardiac changes, oftentimes an electroencephalogram (EEG) is ordered, especially in children or other at-risk patients.

Jared is an obese 42-year-old African American male who is interested in losing weight. He has tried diet and exercise, including seeing a personal trainer and dietician regularly, but he cannot seem to lose the excess weight. After researching this topic online, he found that there are prescription options for weight loss available.

1. Which of the following disease states would cause the most concern during drug therapy for weight loss?
   a. Dyslipidemia
   b. Diabetes
   c. GERD
   d. Hypertension

Answer D is correct. Severe or uncontrolled hypertension can lead to increased risk of cardiovascular adverse effects with weight loss medications.

Jared currently takes medications to manage his diabetes and dyslipidemia at bedtime, and he is wondering if he can do the same with his new amphetamine derivative.

2. Which of the following statements is true in regard to dosing time?
   a. Phendimetrazine should be taken prior to the morning meal.
   b. Phentermine should be taken prior to the morning meal.
   c. Diethylpropion should be taken at bedtime.
   d. Timing of the amphetamine derivative medication dose is not important, as long as the patient takes the dose at the same time every day.

Answer A is correct. Phendimetrazine should be taken 30–60 minutes prior to the morning meal. Diethylpropion should also be taken prior to the morning meal, and should not be given at bedtime. Phentermine should be taken 1 hour after the morning meal.

Eric is a 19-year-old male who has been diagnosed with ADHD. His parents say they have exhausted all nonpharmacologic measures, and Eric is beginning to struggle in college classes. It is decided to start medication therapy. Eric expresses concerns about starting stimulant therapy.

1. Which of the following statements is an appropriate recommendation to make to his parents?
   a. Stimulants can stunt the growth of young adults, so he should increase calcium intake to ensure bone growth.
   b. Drug holidays can be used to reduce the risk of growth inhibition and weight loss in children; however, young adults do not need to worry about this possible side effect.
   c. The patient should eat large meals in the middle of the day, when the drug effects peak.
   d. If the patient is losing weight, supplement treatment with an appetite stimulant.

Answer B is correct. Stimulants may reduce the growth of children, but only by 1–3 cm per year. This does not apply to young adults. Drug holidays can help prevent growth suppression. If a patient is losing weight or has reduced appetite, consuming larger or higher-calorie meals prior to taking the medication or when the medication is wearing off can help the patient maintain weight. Also, eating small meals throughout the day can reduce weight loss.

Eric is experiencing success with the product selected for his ADHD; however, he states that he has always had a hard time swallowing tablets.

2. Which of the following statements is FALSE in regard to ADHD medication delivery forms?
   a. Extended-release capsules can be opened and sprinkled on food (e.g., applesauce).
   b. The methylphenidate patch can cause skin depigmentation changes.
   c. Extended-release tablets can be crushed and put on food (e.g., applesauce).
   d. Extended-release suspensions must be shaken for at least 10 seconds prior to taking them.

Answer C is correct. Extended-release tablets must be taken whole; they cannot be crushed or divided. These formulations require the integrity of the tablet to have biphasic release times. In contrast, extended-release capsules can be opened and their contents sprinkled on food (though the patient must not chew them); the sprinkles within the capsule determine the drug's extended delivery system. The methylphenidate patch (Daytrana) has been associated with depigmentation of the skin in areas where the patch has been applied, and its label now contains a black box warning to that effect. Extended-release suspensions must be shaken for at least 10 seconds to ensure the contents have not settled.

Eric requests to be changed to the methylphenidate patch.

3. Which of the following statements is NOT an important counseling point in regard to the new medication?
   a. The patch must be removed prior to swimming/bathing and reapplied immediately thereafter.
   b. Skin depigmentation can occur at areas of patch application.
   c. The patch should be removed at least 3 hours prior to the desired bedtime.
   d. All of these statements are true.

Answer A is correct. The patch can remain in place during activities such as bathing, swimming, and exercising. Skin depigmentation is an undesirable adverse effect and is now identified as a risk in a black box warning on the product. Methylphenidate distribution occurs with patch application and the medication effects last up to 3 hours after removal; thus, to reduce the risk of insomnia, the patch should be removed approximately 3 hours prior to the desired bedtime.

Grace is a 23-year-old female who complains of excessive daytime sleepiness despite getting a full night's sleep. She also states that she experiences sleep paralysis upon wakening and falls asleep in the middle of the day without warning. After obtaining further information from this patient, the doctor makes a diagnosis of narcolepsy. Due to the severe disruption in her work and social life, Grace would like to start pharmacotherapy immediately.

1. Which of the following statements should Grace be told prior to medication initiation?
   a. Side effects are common and can include severe nausea and vomiting.
   b. Modafinil interacts with oral contraceptives, so Grace should use a backup method to prevent contraception if she is sexually active.
   c. Armodafinil and modafinil are controlled substances and subject to abuse like amphetamines.
   d. The medication should be taken right before bedtime so it will be working as soon as she wakes up in the morning.

Answer B is correct. Although nausea and vomiting are possible side effects of the medications prescribed for narcolepsy, the actual incidence of these side effects is low. Modafinil does interact with oral contraceptives, so female patients of childbearing potential should be forewarned about this interaction. Armodafinil and modafinil do not have the same abuse potential as the amphetamine products. Both of these medications should be taken first thing in the morning.

As you look further into the patient's chart, you notice that Grace's past medical history includes a psychiatric hospitalization for major depressive disorder.

2. Which of the following statements is INCORRECT in regard to comorbid conditions and armodafinil or modafinil use?
   a. These medications should not be used in patients with structural heart defects.
   b. Armodafinil and modafinil may exacerbate psychiatric symptoms.
   c. Dosage reduction is required for patients with renal impairment.
   d. Use caution when prescribing armodafinil and modafinil in patients with hepatic impairment.

Answer C is correct. Armodafinil and modafinil should not be used in patients with left ventricular hypertrophy, mitral valve prolapse, or history of myocardial infarction or angina. These medications may exacerbate psychiatric symptoms, in which case therapy may be required to be discontinued. Armodafinil and modafinil are not dependent on renal function, but should be used in caution in patients with hepatic impairment; specifically, dose reductions are recommended in patients with severe hepatic impairment.

7.6 Anxiolytic, Sedative, and Hypnotic Agents

Medications in the anxiolytic, sedative, and hypnotic category have a variety of FDA-approved indications. The primary uses for these agents are to treat and manage the symptoms of anxiety and/or sleep disorders. Some agents can also be used for managing ethanol withdrawal, status epilepticus and seizure disorders (see also the discussion of anticonvulsants), general anesthesia, sedation of patients in the intensive care unit (ICU), and anticipatory anxiety prior to surgical operations or procedures.

Due to the sedating nature of the agents in this category, they must be used with caution in older patients and individuals at higher risk for cognitive impairment and falls. Most are included on the Beers list for this reason. While these medications most commonly produce sedation in adults, children and older adults may experience a paradoxical hyperactivity or irritability.

Many of these agents are scheduled as controlled substances (C-II to C-IV) due to their abuse potential. They can also produce rebound anxiety and/or jitteriness if rapidly discontinued.

Barbiturates

Barbiturates are believed to exhibit their sedative-hypnotic properties through the enhancement of GABA activity. GABA is an inhibitory neurotransmitter that reduces neuronal excitation and firing. Enhancing GABA activity leads to a reduced propensity for seizures as well as CNS depression.

The sedating properties of barbiturates are well recognized, and sedation can be a therapeutic indication for these agents when used on a short-term or as-needed basis. However, tolerance typically develops with continued use.

Several barbiturates induce the actions of enzymes in the liver, leading to a high risk of drug interactions with other agents. Phenobarbital induces specific hepatic enzymes and can, therefore, reduce the efficacy of oral contraceptives and some antiepileptic medications. Pentobarbital, phenobarbital, secobarbital, and amobarbital are strong hepatic inducers that can reduce the effectiveness of valproic acid.

Barbiturates

Amobarbital
Butabarbital
Mephobarbital
Pentobarbital
Phenobarbital
Secobarbital

Benzodiazepines

Benzodiazepines are believed to exhibit their anxiolytic and sedative effects through their binding to benzodiazepine (BZ) receptors. BZ receptors influence adjacent GABA receptors. When benzodiazepines bind to BZ receptors, GABAergic effects are enhanced and chloride channels are opened. This influx of chloride ions lowers the potential for neuronal activity and firing.

The potency of these agents varies, but all benzodiazepines provide the same degree of anxiolytic properties with equipotent dosing. Drug selection is based primarily on the specific medication's pharmacokinetic profile, with onset and duration of action varying between agents. Patients with hepatic impairment should be prescribed only lorazepam, oxazepam, or temazepam (LOT): These agents do not undergo extensive metabolism in the liver, so they are less likely to accumulate to toxic levels.

The sedative effects of benzodiazepines, in case of either therapeutic use or overdose, can be reversed by intravenous administration of flumazenil when necessary.

Abrupt discontinuation of benzodiazepines can lead to withdrawal symptoms and seizures, especially following chronic use at higher doses. When discontinuing therapy, dosing should be tapered over several months.

Benzodiazepines

Alprazolam
Chlordiazepoxide
Clorazepate
Diazepam
Estazolam
Flurazepam
Lorazepam
Midazolam
Oxazepam
Quazepam
Temazepam
Triazolam
Clonazepam *(see also the Anticonvulsant Agents section)*

Miscellaneous Anxiolytic, Sedative, and Hypnotic Agents

Buspirone is a partial agonist at $5HT_{1A}$ serotonin receptors. It also reduces presynaptic serotonin firing, producing an anxiolytic effect. This agent takes several weeks to begin producing this anxiolytic effect and is not a good option for immediate relief of panic symptoms. Buspirone is not a controlled substance and, due to its lack of abuse potential, may serve as an alternative anxiolytic agent to benzodiazepines in patients with a history of substance abuse. However, buspirone may be less effective in patients who have previously been treated with benzodiazepines.

Zolpidem, zaleplon, and eszopiclone are nonbenzodiazepine hypnotics used in the treatment of insomnias. They share a similar mechanism of action with benzodiazepines through binding of benzodiazepine receptors, but are unique in their molecular structures. These agents should be given at the lowest possible dose to minimize the risk of daytime sedation. Zolpidem, in particular, can remain in the body longer and has a longer duration of effect in women and obese patients because it is stored in fatty areas, which slows the drug's clearance. Complex sleep behaviors such as sleep eating and sleep driving have been reported with nonbenzodiazepine hypnotics, and patients should be counseled about this possibility.

Used in the management of insomnia, ramelteon and tasimelteon produce hypnotic effects through their agonism of melatonin receptors. These agents mimic the normal actions of endogenous melatonin, a hormone that influences circadian rhythms.

Miscellaneous Anxiolytic, Sedative, and Hypnotic Agents

Buspirone
Dexmedetomidine
Droperidol
Eszopiclone
Hydroxyzine
Meprobamate
Promethazine
Ramelteon
Suvorexant
Tasimelteon
Zaleplon
Zolpidem
Diphenhydramine *(see also the First-Generation Antihistamine Agents section in the Antihistamine Agents chapter)*
Doxylamine *(see also the First-Generation Antihistamine Agents section in the Antihistamine Agents chapter)*
Fospropofol *(see also the Miscellaneous General Anesthetic Agents section)*
Propofol *(see also the Miscellaneous General Anesthetic Agents section)*

General Anesthetic Agents

General anesthetics are used during surgeries and procedures to produce unconsciousness, amnesia, analgesia, inhibition of autonomic reflexes, and relaxation of skeletal muscles. Medications are typically used in combination to produce all of these effects.

General Anesthetic Agents

Barbiturates

Methohexital

Miscellaneous General Anesthetic Agents

Etomidate
Fospropofol
Propofol

Case Studies and Conclusions

MP is a 22-year-old female who has been experiencing panic attacks several times a week for the past 3 months. She has been initiated on SSRI therapy but is aware that it may take several weeks to see a therapeutic response. MP would like a medication that she can use on an "as needed" basis to relieve her panic symptoms until they have responded to the SSRI.

1. Which of the following medications would be the best choice for short-term, as-needed management of MP's panic attacks?
    a. Alprazolam
    b. Buspirone
    c. Secobarbital
    d. Zolpidem

Answer A is correct. A benzodiazepine with a rapid onset and short duration would be appropriate in the short term for managing this patient's panic attacks on an as-needed basis. Buspirone takes weeks to begin to work and would not be helpful for immediate relief of symptoms. Secobarbital is a barbiturate with a high abuse potential and is not used to manage panic attacks. Zolpidem is a nonbenzodiazepine sedative/hypnotic with a longer onset of action and is used for insomnia, not anxiety disorders.

When her laboratory bloodwork is received, it is discovered that MP has impaired hepatic function. The physician would like to select a benzodiazepine to manage her more severe panic attacks.

2. Which of the following agents is the best choice for MP, considering her hepatic dysfunction?
    a. Alprazolam
    b. Chlordiazepoxide
    c. Lorazepam
    d. Midazolam

Answer C is correct. Lorazepam does not undergo hepatic metabolism and has a rapid-enough onset to relieve panic attack symptoms. Alprazolam and chlordiazepoxide are metabolized in the liver and could accumulate in patients with hepatic impairment. Midazolam is not typically given as an oral dose and is not approved for use in anxiety disorders.

CC is a 46-year-old male who has been treated with diazepam 5 mg twice daily for his anxiety disorder for approximately 20 years. The prescriber would like to switch CC's medication to an SSRI, but is concerned about discontinuing the diazepam.

1. What is the primary concern with abrupt discontinuation of this benzodiazepine?
    a. Somnolence
    b. Urticaria
    c. Flu-like symptoms
    d. Withdrawal seizures

Answer D is correct. Withdrawal seizures, although considered a rare event, are potentially dangerous and must always be considered in benzodiazepine discontinuation. Tapering to discontinue this medication is a safer strategy and prevents the patient from experiencing other uncomfortable adverse effects such as rebound anxiety.

2. How long can CC anticipate the taper of his diazepam to take?
    a. 3–5 days
    b. 1–2 weeks
    c. 2–4 months
    d. 1–2 years

Answer C is correct. The dose of diazepam is usually decreased by 5% to 10% weekly, and tapering to discontinue this medication takes several months to complete. Dose tapering over a few days to weeks is too rapid and can result in withdrawal symptoms and possibly seizures. It is usually not necessary to perform an extremely slow taper over a year or more, and doing so prolongs the patient's exposure to the medication and its potential adverse effects.

7.7 Antimanic Agents

A mood stabilizer is a psychiatric pharmaceutical product used to treat mood disorders that are characterized by intense and sustained mood shifts, typically bipolar disorder type I or type II or schizophrenia. Historically, the definition of a mood stabilizer has been topic of intense debate. The contested definitions are based on the drugs' antimanic, antidepressant, and prophylactic properties to varying degrees, and two of these three effects are usually required to warrant inclusion of a drug in this class.

Not long ago, only lithium was categorized as a "mood stabilizer"; it is used to treat patients who experience "mania" and/or depressive symptoms in bipolar disorder. Eventually, clinical experience led practitioners to use anticonvulsant medications—the first of which was carbamazepine—to control impulsivity and extreme shifts of mood. Valproate soon became widely available for this purpose and was considered a novel and effective mood stabilizer. Since then, it seems that every new anticonvulsant has been evaluated for its mood-stabilizing properties. Based on research, not all anticonvulsants are effective mood-stabilizing antiepileptic drugs (AEDs). For those AEDs that have shown efficacy in this indication, only some of these agents can be used as monotherapy; others are indicated for "augmentation or adjunctive" therapy only.

More recently, the second-generation (atypical) antipsychotic agents have demonstrated beneficial effects in stabilizing mood. The use of mood stabilizers or "antimanic" agents is based on current clinical guidelines, which are continually under review and are updated when new drugs or information becomes available within the psychiatric community. Note that some of these agents are more effective during acute mania episodes and may not be as effective for long-term maintenance treatment.

Antimanic Agents

Lithium salts
Aripiprazole *(see also the Psychotherapeutic Agents section)*
Asenapine *(see also the Psychotherapeutic Agents section)*
Carbamazepine *(see also the Anticonvulsant Agents section)*
Cariprazine *(see also to the Psychotherapeutic Agents section)*
Lamotrigine *(see also the Anticonvulsant Agents section)*
Lurasidone *(see also to the Psychotherapeutic Agents section)*
Olanzapine *(see also the Psychotherapeutic Agents section)*
Quetiapine *(see also the Psychotherapeutic Agents section)*
Risperidone *(see also the Psychotherapeutic Agents section)*
Valproate/divalproex *(see also the Anticonvulsant Agents section)*
Ziprasidone *(see also the Psychotherapeutic Agents section)*

Case Studies and Conclusions

TS is a 34-year-old white female patient who arrives at the clinic today (accompanied by her mother) with symptoms of nausea, vomiting, loss of balance, and tremors. The patient's mother reports that TS has been vigorously exercising to lose weight and decrease her blood pressure, but stopped this physical activity when the stomach "bug" hit and the vomiting started. The mother states that TS's mood has been really good lately since she started taking lithium last year.

TS's current medication list upon admission (duration 12 months, no changes in drug therapy) is as follows:

- Lithium carbonate 300 mg in the morning and 300 mg at bedtime for bipolar disorder (she took only the morning dose today)
- Olanzapine/fluoxetine 12 mg/50 mg daily in the morning for bipolar disorder
- Lorazepam 0.5 mg at bedtime as needed for insomnia

Denies use of any other prescription or OTC medications or illicit agents
Does not drink alcohol; does not smoke
STAT vital signs:

- Blood pressure: 150/90 mm Hg (high)
- Blood glucose (fingerstick): 140 mg/dL (within normal limits)

STAT labs:

- Lithium: 1.8 mEq/L (high); prior month lab: 1.3 mEq/L

TS's mother wonders what the best explanation for her elevated lithium today is, since her last "level" was therapeutic according to her psychiatrist last month.

1. What do you tell her?
   a. Hypertension
   b. Dehydration
   c. Drug interaction
   d. Missed lithium dose

Answer B is correct. The patient had a normal concentration last month with no dose changes in lithium. Her symptoms could otherwise be attributed to another medical illness if the serum lithium were not in a toxic range. The likely culprit is dehydration due to overexertion, resulting in lithium toxicity.

TS has had a significant improvement in her bipolar symptoms since starting her current medication regimen. According to her medical record, she recently reported easy bruising and bleeding.

2. How should you respond when the ER physician asks you to identify the medication MOST commonly associated with this effect?
   a. Olanzapine
   b. Lithium
   c. Lorazepam
   d. Fluoxetine

Answer D is correct. Lithium does not cause increased bleeding potential, whereas SSRIs such as fluoxetine do increase that risk.

TS has had a significant improvement in her bipolar symptoms since starting her current medication regimen. She now reports increased urination frequency and thirst.

3. Which medication is MOST commonly associated with this effect?
   a. Divalproex
   b. Olanzapine/fluoxetine
   c. Lithium
   d. Lorazepam

Answer C is correct. Lithium's effect on renal function is the likely culprit here. Although olanzapine may cause elevated blood glucose, the patient's fingerstick measurement was within normal limits. Excessive lithium serum concentration also supports this adverse effect.

TS's mother is worried about her continued use of lithium.

4. Which of the following statements about lithium therapy is TRUE?
   a. Lithium is highly metabolized by the liver prior to excretion.
   b. Lithium is excreted unchanged in the urine.
   c. Lithium should be used only as monotherapy.
   d. Patients taking lithium should be placed on a sodium-restricted diet.

Answer B is correct. Chronic lithium administration is known to have long-term adverse consequences on the kidneys. There is no liver metabolism with this agent, it is often used in combination with other medications, and sodium restriction is not advised during treatment.

5. Which of TS's organ systems will be most likely to be adversely affected by chronic lithium use?
   a. Liver
   b. Thyroid
   c. Gallbladder
   d. Ovaries

Answer B is correct. Chronic lithium administration is known to have long-term adverse consequences on the thyroid. Lithium is not associated with liver or gallbladder disease, nor is it linked to ovarian complications.

7.8 Antimigraine Agents

Migraines are severe headaches that are often accompanied by nausea, light sensitivity, and sound sensitivity. Migraines develop in four phases: prodrome, aura, headache, and postdrome. The prodrome, which may occur 24 to 48 hours prior to the actual headache, includes symptoms such as irritability and other mood changes, food cravings, stiff neck, and increased yawning.

Most migraines are classified as migraine without aura; however, patients who do have an aura experience neurologic symptoms that may precede the headache or sometimes occur at the same time as the headache. These neurologic symptoms may include visual disturbances of shapes, bright lights, or objects; auditory effects; tactile sensations of burning, pain, or paresthesias; and motor disturbances such as jerking or other movements. Sometimes an aura may be the loss of a sensation, with patients experiencing difficulties with vision, hearing, or feeling. Typically, auras are mostly visual. Patients who experience an aura are able to use this aspect of the migraine to their advantage, since they are aware that the headache will soon happen; this "heads up" can alert the patient to take abortive migraine therapy as soon as possible.

The next phase is the actual headache. Patients experience a throbbing or pulsing unilateral pain with increasing intensity as the migraine persists. Nausea and vomiting are common during the headache as well. An untreated migraine headache can last from 4 hours to several days. After the headache, during the postdrome phase, the patient may still experience pain with sudden head movements, as well as fatigue.

Many triggers for a migraine attack have been identified. Oftentimes, patients are able to either avoid their specific trigger or prepare themselves for the migraine if they cannot avoid it. Emotional stress is one of the most frequent causes of migraines, as well as hormonal changes in women, fasting or not eating, weather changes and pressure changes, sleep disturbances, alcohol, certain foods, and lights.

In mild to moderate migraines, patients may experience adequate symptom relief by taking OTC analgesics, such as acetaminophen or NSAIDs. Serotonergic agents—the "triptans"—are frequently prescribed as abortive therapy to be taken in the prodromal or aura phase in patients with more severe migraines. They may be taken during the headache, but are more efficacious when taken as soon as possible. For patients who experience frequent migraines (more than 4 episodes per month), a daily prophylactic treatment may be prescribed. Propranolol, some antidepressants, and some antiepileptic medications are commonly prescribed for prophylaxis.

Selective Serotonin Agonists

The "triptans" are serotonin 1B and serotonin 1D agonists. Their exact mechanism of action is unknown, but the predominant hypotheses include releasing vasoactive peptides, promoting vasoconstriction, and blocking pain pathways in the brain stem. Of note, triptans will treat a migraine, but they are not to be used for migraine prophylaxis. Triptans are unique in the treatment of migraine, in that they decrease symptoms of nausea and vomiting.

Choosing a triptan should be individualized for the patient. If a patient does not respond to one triptan, he or she may respond to another agent. Other considerations include available dosage forms. For instance, if a patient experiences severe nausea or vomiting with migraines, a medication with an intranasal or injectable formulation may be a better choice than oral formulations. Patients may repeat their dose if they do not experience adequate relief 2 hours after the first dose, but they should not exceed the maximum daily dose.

Triptan use is contraindicated in patients with a history of coronary artery disease, cerebrovascular or peripheral vascular disease, other significant cardiovascular diseases, uncontrolled hypertension, or ischemic bowel disease. Triptans should not be used for hemiplegic or basilar migraines. Use of these agents within 14 days of an MAOI and near-term prior exposure to ergot alkaloids is also contraindicated. Chronic use of triptans (i.e., for 10 or more days during the month) may result in worsening of headaches.

Selective Serotonin Agonists

Almotriptan
Eletriptan
Frovatriptan
Naratriptan
Rizatriptan
Sumatriptan
Zolmitriptan

Miscellaneous Antimigraine Agents

Some patients who experience migraines may find relief with use of NSAIDs and acetaminophen. Other patients may require opiate agonists or combination opiate products. In addition, some patients may require preventive migraine treatment. Such prophylaxis is indicated when the headaches are frequent (more than 4 migraines per month) or long-lasting (more than 12 hours), when they diminish the quality of life of the patient, when abortive therapy is contraindicated or does not work, and in patients who experience menstrual migraines. Medications approved for prophylactic therapy include some beta blockers, antidepressants, and antiepileptics. Therapy should be individualized to the patient, taking the side effects, comorbid conditions, possible medication interactions, and dosing regimen into consideration. Preventive medications should be initiated at a low dose and slowly titrated up until there is a therapeutic effect.

Miscellaneous Antimigraine Agents

Acetaminophen *(see also the Analgesic and Antipyretic Agents section)*
Butorphanol *(see also the Analgesic and Antipyretic Agents section)*
Caffeine/caffeine and sodium benzoate *(see also the Anorexigenic Agents and Respiratory and CNS Stimulants section)*
Dihydroergotamine *(see also the Autonomic-Sympatholytic [Adrenergic Blocking] Agents section in the Autonomic Agents chapter)*
Ergotamine *(see also the Autonomic-Sympatholytic [Adrenergic Blocking] Agents section in the Autonomic Agents chapter)*
Ketoprofen *(see also the Analgesic and Antipyretic Agents section)*
Opiate agonists *(see also the Analgesic and Antipyretic Agents section)*
Propranolol *(see also the Adrenergic Agents in the Cardiovascular Agents chapter)*
Salicylates *(see also the Analgesic and Antipyretic Agents section)*
Timolol *(see also the Adrenergic Agents in the Cardiovascular Agents chapter)*
Topiramate *(see also the Anticonvulsant Agents section)*
Valproate/divalproex *(see also the Anticonvulsant Agents section)*

Case Studies and Conclusions

Miriam is a 35-year-old female who was recently diagnosed with migraines. She experiences severe nausea and vomiting, and taking products does not alleviate her pain.

1. Which of the following medications would be a good option for Miriam to use?
   a. Almotriptan
   b. Eletriptan
   c. Naratriptan
   d. Sumatriptan

Answer D is correct. Sumatriptan is available in an oral tablet and as intranasally, subcutaneously, and transdermally administered formulations. If a patient has substantial nausea and vomiting, a route of administration other than oral could be more beneficial.

A few months have passed, and Miriam states she did not experience relief with the sumatriptan products.

2. What is an appropriate option following this treatment failure?
   a. Rizatriptan
   b. Zolmitriptan
   c. If the patient fails one triptan therapy, the whole class is most likely ineffective.
   d. If the patient fails triptan therapy, she should receive prophylaxis.

Answer B is correct. Rizatriptan is available only in an oral formulation. Zolmitriptan has a nasal formulation that the patient could use due to her severe nausea and vomiting. If a patient fails one triptan therapy, it does not mean treatment failure for the whole class. Prophylaxis is reserved for patients who experience frequent and severe migraines. Other indications for prophylaxis include contraindications, intolerance, and multiple treatment failures with triptans.

Miriam returns to the office for another check-up. At this appointment, she says that she needs to use her triptan prescription 6 times each month. She would like to pursue prophylactic therapy.

3. Which of the following medications is NOT appropriate for migraine prophylaxis?
   a. Valproic acid
   b. Ketoprofen
   c. Topiramate
   d. Propranolol

Answer B is correct. Some antiepileptics (such as valproic acid and topiramate), antidepressants, and antihypertensives (such as propranolol) can be used for migraine prophylaxis. Ketoprofen is an NSAID that can be used as an abortive therapy. Chronic use of OTC analgesics, triptans, and other abortive therapies can result in rebound and worse headaches.

7.9 Antiparkinsonian Agents

Antiparkinsonian agents are used to manage the triad of hallmark symptoms in Parkinson's disease: tremor, muscle rigidity, and slowed or lack of voluntary movement (bradykinesia). The goal of currently available medication therapy is to manage the symptoms of the disease. At this time, there are no treatments that can reverse the disease or prevent its further progression.

Parkinson's disease presents when there is a dysfunction of dopamine activity in the basal ganglia of the brain. Dopamine activity in the basal ganglia is responsible for sustaining smooth movements and posture. Deficits in dopamine or dopamine binding lead to involuntary movements, such as tremor. Antiparkinsonian agents aim to restore or mimic binding of dopamine to the dopamine receptors in the basal ganglia.

The challenge with treatment selection and dosing is to increase dopamine activity sufficiently without exceeding the amount needed for therapeutic effect. Increasing dopamine activity excessively can lead to dyskinetic movements. Patients who experience these choreiform dyskinesias exhibit persistent writhing movements that can be more bothersome to them than the Parkinsonian symptoms being treated.

Dopamine replacement therapy with levodopa/carbidopa is the gold standard of care for Parkinson's disease. Initiation of this therapy is delayed as long as possible, however, because it becomes less effective over time; that is, it provides the greatest symptom reduction in the first few years of treatment. Symptoms are managed with other agents during the earlier stages of the disease, and dopamine replacement is reserved for later use when symptoms progress.

Adamantanes

Adamantanes promote dopamine release by blocking glutamate transmission at the NMDA receptors. This effect can be transient and may diminish after several months of treatment, resulting in a rebound of Parkinsonian symptoms. Patients may benefit from a drug holiday when this occurs. Adamantanes are effective in treating symptoms of tremor, rigidity, and slowed movements.

The adamantane, amantadine, has been associated with compulsive behaviors and a reduction in impulse control. Concerns have also arisen about significant CNS depression and impairment, suicidal ideation, edema, and melanoma. Some patients have experienced livedo reticularis (purple mottling of the skin, especially in lower extremities) while taking this agent.

Adamantanes

Amantadine

Anticholinergic Agents

Anticholinergic agents block acetylcholine, thereby increasing the relative ratio of dopamine to acetylcholine in the body. These drugs improve only symptoms of tremor in Parkinson's disease; they do not have any effect on muscle rigidity or slowed movement. Nevertheless, they can assist in the management of drooling, a common symptom in patients with Parkinson's disease who suffer from swallowing difficulties. In addition to their role in Parkinson's disease, these agents can be useful for treating acute dystonic reactions and preventing the pseudoparkinsonian side effects of antipsychotic medications.

Anticholinergic medications should be used with caution, especially in adults older than 65 years, due to the risks of cognitive impairment and falls. Common side effects of medications with anticholinergic properties are dry mouth, constipation, urinary retention, dry eyes, and memory impairment. These side effects can be additive with the effects caused by other drugs possessing anticholinergic properties.

Anticholinergic Agents

Benztropine
Trihexyphenidyl
Diphenhydramine *(see also the First-Generation Antihistamine Agents section in the Antihistamine Agents chapter)*
Orphenadrine *(see also the Skeletal Muscle Relaxants and Miscellaneous Autonomic Agents section in the Autonomic Agents chapter)*

Catechol-*O*-Methyltransferase Inhibitors

Catechol-O-methyltransferase (COMT) inhibitors block the destruction of levodopa by the COMT enzyme, thereby maximizing the availability and benefits of this dopamine precursor in the CNS. COMT inhibitors are used only with levodopa/carbidopa as adjunctive therapy; they are not effective as monotherapy agents. Because they increase the dopaminergic impact of levodopa, patients using these drugs may experience dyskinesias or hallucinations that require a decrease in their dose of levodopa.

Patients taking COMT inhibitors may experience gastrointestinal side effects such as nausea and anorexia. Tolcapone is associated with a higher incidence of delayed-onset diarrhea and hepatotoxicity. Strict liver function monitoring is recommended.

Catechol-*O*-Methyltransferase Inhibitors

Entacapone
Tolcapone

Dopamine Precursors

Dopamine precursors are used to replace missing dopamine in the brain. Levodopa—the active ingredient in such medications—is converted to dopamine after it crosses the blood-brain barrier. Carbidopa is always given with levodopa to protect levodopa from peripheral metabolism prior to reaching the CNS. If levodopa is metabolized to dopamine peripherally, it cannot cross the blood-brain barrier and exert its intended mechanism of action.

The benefits of levodopa/carbidopa therapy are the greatest in the first few years after therapy initiation, when the brain can still supplement its effects with endogenous dopamine. As Parkinson's disease progresses, the brain loses this ability, and the drug benefits diminish. Dosing regimens may also need to be adjusted more frequently as the drug effects wear off more quickly. Other motor complications include episodes of sudden motor freezing, delayed or lack of response to levodopa, and dystonias prior to the next dose. More-frequent dosing or addition of an adjunctive therapy (e.g., COMT inhibitor, MAO-B inhibitor, dopamine agonist) may be warranted to manage these symptoms.

Patients sometimes elect to take breaks during their daily dopamine precursor regimen to provide relief from the dyskinesias that can appear following doses of levodopa/carbidopa. These dyskinesias correspond with peak dopamine activity in the striatum. The addition of amantadine is sometimes helpful in controlling these movements.

Absorption of levodopa/carbidopa can be influenced by several factors, so patients need to be educated on the impact of these factors on absorption and subsequent drug effect. Levodopa/carbidopa is absorbed in the small intestine, so absorption can be reduced when taken with food (especially protein), in the presence of excess stomach acid, or with concurrent use of anticholinergic medications that can slow gastric emptying. Certain antacids can improve the absorption of levodopa/carbidopa when taken concurrently.

Dopamine Precursors

Levodopa/carbidopa

Dopamine Receptor Agonists

Dopamine receptor agonists are structurally similar to dopamine and mimic the actions of dopamine when directly bound to dopamine receptors in the brain. Non-ergot-derived dopamine agonists are safer and more effective than ergot-derived agents. These medications can be used as adjunctive therapy with levodopa/carbidopa to enhance and increase the duration of levodopa's therapeutic effect.

Because each agent has a slightly different dopamine receptor binding pattern, if one agent is ineffective, another one can be tried.

Dopamine receptor agonists are better tolerated in younger patients due to their potential side effects: sedation, postural hypotension, confusion, hallucinations, and pedal edema.

Apomorphine is available as a subcutaneous injection. It is used only as needed as a rescue medication when patients have an inadequate response to a dose of levodopa/carbidopa. Temporary relief lasts for approximately 60 minutes.

Dopamine Receptor Agonists

Ergot-Derived Dopamine Receptor Agonists

Bromocriptine
Cabergoline

Non-Ergot-Derived Dopamine Receptor Agonists

Apomorphine
Pramipexole
Ropinirole
Rotigitine

Monoamine Oxidase B Inhibitors

Monoamine oxidase B (MAO-B) inhibitors irreversibly block the enzyme that metabolizes dopamine in the brain, thereby extending dopamine's half-life. These agents can be used alone or as adjunctive therapy with levodopa/carbidopa to increase the duration of levodopa's therapeutic effect.

Overall, rasagiline has a better tolerability profile than selegiline. Unlike rasagiline, selegiline is associated with insomnia and jitteriness because it is metabolized to an amphetamine. Selegiline is more likely than rasagiline to worsen psychiatric symptoms, such as hallucinations. Either agent may be a good choice in a patient with Parkinson's disease who also experiences depressive symptoms, as long as the patient is not taking another antidepressant agent. MAO-B inhibitors should not be used with other serotonergic agents, and they require a washout period of at least 2 weeks if switching to/from another antidepressant due to the potential risk of developing serotonin syndrome.

Monoamine Oxidase B Inhibitors

Rasagiline
Selegiline

Case Studies and Conclusions

FM is a 55-year-old male who presents with Parkinsonian tremor in his left hand. He does not experience muscle rigidity or slowed movement at this time. FM works as a carpenter and would like to start a medication to control his tremor. He has no other medical complaints.

1. Which of the following medications would be a good choice given FM's tremor-only presentation?
   a. Apomorphine
   b. Bromocriptine
   c. Entacapone
   d. Benztropine

Answer D is correct. Anticholinergic agents are only useful for Parkinsonian tremor (not rigidity or slowed movements). FM is young enough that he should be able to tolerate this agent safely. Its initiation will reserve other categories of agents for later use as the disease progresses. Apomorphine is a rescue agent and is not used in early treatment. Bromocriptine is rarely used due to tolerability issues. Entacapone is a COMT inhibitor that is used only as an adjunct to levodopa/carbidopa, which the patient is not taking at this time.

Fifteen months later, FM reports a worsening of symptoms. His tremor is now accompanied by muscle rigidity and slowed muscle movement. He is having trouble sleeping at night because he cannot roll over, and his mood is depressed. He is on no other medications at this time.

2. Which of the following medications would be the best choice for FM's current symptom presentation?
   a. Amantadine
   b. Rasagiline
   c. Tolcapone
   d. Trihexyphenidyl

Answer B is correct. Rasagiline is an MAO-B inhibitor that can be used to treat tremor, muscle rigidity, and bradykinesia. It can also be effective in managing depressive symptoms and is safe because the patient is not on any interacting serotonergic medications (e.g., SSRIs). Amantadine could make psychiatric symptoms (depression) worse. Tolcapone is a COMT inhibitor that is used only as an adjunct to levodopa/carbidopa, which the patient is not taking at this time. Trihexyphenidyl is an anticholinergic agent that is effective in treating tremor, but not muscle rigidity or bradykinesia.

TS is a 74-year-old woman with a 7-year history of Parkinson's disease. Her symptoms of bradykinesia, muscle rigidity, and tremor have been treated with ropinirole, but this drug is now insufficient for managing her disease. The physician is considering initiating levodopa/carbidopa therapy for TS.

1. Which of the following counseling points would be the most important in maximizing this patient's benefit from her dose of levodopa/carbidopa?
   a. Levodopa/carbidopa must be taken with at least 8 oz of water.
   b. Antacids should not be taken with levodopa/carbidopa because they bind to levodopa and prevent its absorption in the stomach.
   c. Taking levodopa/carbidopa with protein-rich meals may reduce the absorption and effect of the product.
   d. Levodopa/carbidopa should be taken at bedtime because it is best absorbed overnight.

Answer C is correct. Proteins can compete with levodopa for transporters in the lining of the small intestine, creating the possibility of reduced absorption. A full glass of water is not necessary for the absorption of levodopa, especially early in its use. Antacids can enhance—not prevent—the absorption of levodopa; this absorption occurs in the small intestine, not the stomach. Levodopa is not best absorbed at any particular time of day.

TS has now been taking levodopa/carbidopa for 3 years. Her dose of levodopa/carbidopa was increased 2 months ago due to disease progression and complaints that the dose wore off too soon. At her current visit, TS reports that she is experiencing involuntary twitching and jerking movements of her neck, arms, and legs. This happens about an hour after each dose of levodopa/carbidopa, and lasts about an hour.

2. Which of the following is the best option for managing the adverse effects TS is experiencing?
   a. Add tolcapone to TS's medication regimen
   b. Add benztropine to TS's medication regimen
   c. Increase TS's dose of levodopa/carbidopa
   d. Decrease TS's dose of levodopa/carbidopa

Answer D is correct. The dose of levodopa is too high, resulting in dyskinetic choreiform movements. A decrease in dose should resolve this adverse effect. Tolcapone is a COMT inhibitor with poor tolerability that will worsen the problem through augmented dopaminergic activity. Benztropine does not have an effect on dyskinetic movements. Increasing the dose of levodopa/carbidopa will exacerbate the dyskinesia, instead of making it better.

Tips from the Field

NSAID Pain Relievers

1. The FDA has issued warnings that as little as 400 mg of ibuprofen can interfere with the antiplatelet effects of low dose aspirin (81 mg per day). A number of drug interactions and clinical consequences resulting from the coadministration of aspirin and NSAIDs must be addressed if no alternative exists to concomitant use. For patients taking cardioprotective 81 mg aspirin, it is recommended that the NSAID be taken either 8 hours before the ASA or 30 minutes after non-enteric coated ASA.

2. Combinations of NSAID with ASA can increase the risk of bleeding. Review guidelines on aspirin use for primary and secondary prevention before recommending it. Not everyone should be getting a "once a day aspirin" anymore. Risk calculations must be considered.

3. FDA black box warnings: NSAIDs may cause an increased risk of serious cardiovascular thrombotic events, myocardial infarction, and stroke, which can be fatal. This risk may increase with duration of use; however, it can also occur as early as the first 2 weeks of use. Because there is insufficient data on whether the risk of any one particular agents is definitely higher or lower—consider all these agents at equal risk and educate your patient. Patients with cardiovascular disease or risk factors of cardiovascular disease may be at greater risk. NSAIDs are contraindicated for the treatment of perioperative pain in the setting of CABG surgery. Your older adult patient will be also at higher risk of serious GI side effects.

4. Salicylates are drugs that are divided into two groups, acetylated and nonacetylated. Aspirin (acetylsalicylic acid [ASA]) is acetylated, while others such as Disalcid (salsalate) and (Trilisate) choline magnesium trisalicylate are nonacetylated. Nonacetylated salicylates may be preferred in patients who are at higher risk of bleeding but may be in need of salicylate therapy due to the lack (or lesser) effect on platelets.

Opiates

1. At all points of opiate treatment, providers should assess patients for risks of addiction, abuse, or misuse before drug initiation, and monitor patients who receive opioids routinely for development of these behaviors. Focused pain management that includes intensive monitoring and counseling is appropriate even if there is a potential risk of abuse.

2. Physical tolerance and dependence are common, especially when opiate interventions are implemented; however, abuse and addiction are different. Patients who exhibit symptoms of tolerance and dependence often do not exhibit symptoms of addiction and abuse.

3. To discourage misuse and abuse, only the smallest quantity of opiates should be dispensed, and proper disposal instructions for unused drug should be given to patients which may include DEA drop off events.

Tammie Lee and Jacque

Bibliography

American Geriatrics Society. 2015 updated Beers criteria for potentially inappropriate medication use in older adults. *J Am Geriatr Soc.* 2015;63:2227-2246.

Anton RF. Naltrexone for the management of alcohol dependence. *N Engl J Med.* 2008;359:715-721.

Becker WJ. Acute migraine treatment in adults. *Headache.* 2015;55:778-793.

Catella-Lawson F, Reilly MP, Kapoor SC, et al. Cyclooxygenase inhibitors and the antiplatelet effects of aspirin. *N Engl J Med.* 2001;345:1809-1817.

Doyon S, Aks SE, Schaeffer S. Expanding access to naloxone in the United States. *J Med Toxicol.* 2014;10:431-434.

Dumas EO, Pollack GM. Opioid tolerance development: a pharmacokinetic/pharmacodynamic perspective. *AAPS J.* 2008;10(4):537-551.

Fernández-López JA, Remesar X, Foz M, Alemany M. Pharmacological approaches for the treatment of obesity. *Drugs.* 2002;62:915-944.

FitzGerald GA, Patrono C. The coxibs, selective inhibitors of cyclooxygenase-2. *N Engl J Med.* 2001;345:433-442.

Fleckenstein A. New insights into the mechanism of actions of amphetamines. *Annu Rev Pharmacol.* 2007;47:691-698.

French JA, Kanner AM, Bautista J, et al. Efficacy and tolerability of the new antiepileptic drugs. I. Treatment of new-onset epilepsy: Report of the TTA and QSS subcommittees of the American Academy of Neurology and American Epilepsy Society. *Neurology.* 2004;62:1252-1260.

French JA, Pedley TA. Initial management of epilepsy. *N Engl J Med.* 2008;359:166-176.

García Rodríguez LA, Varas-Lorenzo C, Maguire A, González-Pérez A. Nonsteroidal antiinflammatory drugs and the risk of myocardial infarction in the general population. *Circulation.* 2004;109:3000-3006.

Haile CN, Kosten TA, Kosten TR. Pharmacogenetic treatments for drug addiction: alcohol and opiates. *Am J Drug Alcohol Abuse.* 2008;34:355-381.

Kelley NE, Tepper DE. Rescue therapy for acute migraine, part 1: triptans, dihydroergotamine, and magnesium. *Headache.* 2012;52:114-128.

Lowenstein DH, Alldredge BK. Status epilepticus. *N Engl J Med.* 1998;338:970-976.

McEvoy GK, ed. *AHFS: Drug Information.* Bethesda, MD: American Society of Health-System Pharmacists; 2016.

McNamara JO. Pharmacotherapy of the epilepsies. In: Brunton LL, Chabner BA, Knollmann BC, eds. *Goodman & Gilman's The Pharmacological Basis of Therapeutics.* 12 ed. New York, NY: McGraw-Hill; 2011: 583-608.

Mészáros A, Czobor P, Bálint S, Komlósi S, Simon V, Bitter I. Pharmacotherapy of adult attention deficit hyperactivity disorder (ADHD): a meta-analysis. *Int J Neuropsychopharmacol.* 2009;12:1137-1147.

PDR. Desvenlafaxine: drug summary. http://www.pdr.net/drug-summary/?druglabelid=625. Accessed January 20, 2017.

PDR. Fluoxetine hydrochloride: drug summary. http://www.pdr.net/drug-summary/Fluoxetine-Tablets-fluoxetine-hydrochloride-1416.5847. Accessed January 20, 2017.

PDR. Ibuprofen: drug summary. http://www.pdr.net/drug-summary/Ibuprofen-Tablets-ibuprofen-2618. Accessed January 20, 2017.

PDR. Oxycodone hydrochloride: drug summary. http://www.pdr.net/drug-summary/OxyContin-oxycodone-hydrochloride-492. Accessed January 20, 2017.

Online Pharmacy. Melocam strong analgesic, antirheumatic, and anti-inflammatory. March 30, 2015. https://www.medicinep.com/melocam-strong-analgesic-antirheumatic-and-anti-inflammatory-2620.html. Accessed January 20, 2017.

Rizzoli PB. Acute and preventive treatment of migraine. *Continuum (Minneap Minn).* 2012;18:764-782.

Rogawski MA, Löscher W. The neurobiology of antiepileptic drugs. *Nat Rev Neurosci.* 2004;5:553-564.

Santosh PJ, Sattar S, Canagaratnam M. Efficacy and tolerability of pharmacotherapies for attention-deficit hyperactivity disorder in adults. *CNS Drugs.* 2011;25:737-763.

Sasich L. US FDA strenghtens warning about risk of heart attack or stroke with NSAIDs. August 30, 2015. http://www.patientdrugnews.com/us-fda-strengthens-warning-about-risk-of-heart-attack-or-stroke-with-nsaids/. Accessed January 20, 2015.

Silberstein SD. Treatment recommendations for migraine. *Nat Clin Pract Neurol.* 2008;4:482-489.

Swanson JM, Volkow ND. Serum and brain concentrations of methylphenidate: implications for use and abuse. *Neurosci Biobehav Rev.* 2003;27:615-621.

U.S. Food and Drug Administration. *COX-2 Selective (includes Bextra, Celebrex, and Vioxx) and Non-Selective Non-Steroidal Anti-Inflammatory Drugs (NSAIDs).* Updated January 9, 2015. http://www.fda.gov/Drugs/DrugSafety/PostmarketDrugSafetyInformationforPatientsandProviders/ucm429364.htm. Accessed December 19, 2016.

Wilens TE, Morrison NR, Prince J. An update on the pharmacotherapy of attention-deficit/hyperactivity disorder in adults. *Expert Rev* Neurother. 2011;11:1443-1465.

Symbols

- ▲ Renal impairment: Dose adjustment is recommended.
- ■ Hepatic impairment: Dose adjustment is recommended.
- ■ Black box warning exists for this drug.
- (QT) QTc prolongation effects have been reported.
- (BL) Beers list criteria (avoid in elderly patients).
- (PD) FDA-approved pediatric doses are available.
- (GD) FDA-approved geriatric doses are available.
-  See primary body system.

Central Nervous System Agents

Universal prescribing alerts:

- Known serious hypersensitivity to the specific drug or any other component of product/formulation selected warrants a contraindication for its use.
- Adverse reactions associated with the use of some **central nervous system agents** include dizziness, drowsiness, vertigo, and fatigue; these agents may also impair the ability to perform tasks requiring mental alertness. Caution should always be recommended when using any new drug for the first time, when there is a dose change, and for continued use of known offending agents.
- Doses expressed are for usual adult dosage ranges only. "Geriatric doses" are assumed to be the same as adult doses unless otherwise noted with a symbol. Where FDA-approved, pediatric dosing is available, a symbol will guide the reader to additional prescribing references. Refer to real-time prescribing references for these age-specific doses.
- Use of CNS agents in pregnancy is based on weighing clinical risk versus benefit and safety concerns are not represented in this grid. Refer to the package insert (PI) for more information. Clinicians should continue to provide education about the reproductive risks of any medication and offer risk-reduction strategies (which may include contraceptive use) to women of childbearing age and understand that these reproductive risks may also extend to males. Other medications may decrease the effectiveness of oral contraceptives. Where necessary, an alternative means of birth control should be explored.
- Brand names are provided for those products still available on the market. Due to the ever-changing product availability, refer to the Food and Drug Administration (FDA) resources to confirm the actual brands available. This drug summary is intended for educational purposes only. Prescribing decisions should be based on real-time comprehensive drug databases that are updated on a regular basis.

Analgesic and Antipyretic Agents

Nonsteroidal Anti-inflammatory Agents

Universal prescribing alerts:

- Serious GI tract bleeding and ulceration have been reported without symptoms or warning. Use nonsteroidal anti-inflammatory agents (NSAIDs) with extreme caution in patients at higher risk of this adverse event including those with a prior history of GI bleeding, GI perforation, or ulcerative GI disease, the elderly, those in poor general health, heavy smokers and/or drinkers or debilitated patients and in those taking other high-risk medications such as concurrent oral corticosteroid therapy or anticoagulant therapy. For high-risk patients, alternate therapies that do not involve NSAIDs should be considered. These agents are stomach irritants; take with food.
- NSAIDs may interfere in the compensatory role that renal prostaglandins play in the maintenance of renal perfusion, thus causing potential renal toxicity. The administration of an NSAID may cause a dose-dependent reduction in prostaglandin formation and, secondarily, in renal blood flow, which may precipitate overt renal decompensation. Patients who are at highest risk of this toxicity are those with renal and/or hepatic impairment, renal failure, heart failure, hypovolemia (dehydration), those taking diuretics and ACE inhibitors, angiotensin II receptor antagonists (ARBs), or older patients. Monitor renal function and ensure proper hydration before using (and throughout use) of NSAIDs. Discontinuation of NSAID therapy is usually followed by renal recovery.
- Consider the cardiovascular risk and the potential treatment benefit prior to NSAID therapy initiation. All NSAIDs may exacerbate hypertension and congestive heart failure and may cause an increased risk of serious cardiovascular thrombotic events, myocardial infarction or stroke, which can be fatal.

NSAIDs may mask the signs of infection such as fever or pain in patients with bone marrow suppression.

FDA special alerts:

- Patients with heart disease or risk factors for heart disease have a greater likelihood of heart attack or stroke following NSAID use than patients without these risk factors.
- Patients treated with NSAIDs following a first heart attack were more likely to die in the first year after the heart attack compared with patients who were not treated with NSAIDs after their first heart attack. There is an increased risk of heart failure with NSAID use.
- These products require a special FDA "medguide" to be distributed when dispensing.

Cyclooxygenase-2 Inhibitors

Drug Name	FDA-Approved Indications	Adult Dosage Range	Precautions and Clinical Pearls
Generic Name Celecoxib **Brand Name** Celebrex ■ ■ (BL) (PD) (GD)	**Common indications for use:** Acute pain Ankylosing spondylitis Osteoarthritis (OA) Primary dysmenorrhea Rheumatoid arthritis (RA)	**Usual oral dose for RA:** 100 to 200 mg twice daily	• Use the lowest effective dose for the shortest duration • Black patients may experience higher drug concentrations than white patients, use caution • May cause serious skin reactions, including exfoliative dermatitis, Stevens-Johnson syndrome, and toxic epidermal necrolysis; discontinue at the first sign of a rash • Bronchospasm and severe, potentially fatal anaphylactoid reactions have been reported; patients with asthma may be at higher risk; this reaction may warrant contraindication for further use of NSAIDs • Drug interactions may require dose adjustment or avoidance of certain drug combinations Associated with: • Increased risk of MI and stroke in certain conditions and thus contraindicated to be given within 14 days of coronary artery bypass graft surgery (CABG) • GI bleeding and perforation • Serious cardiovascular events include MI and stroke

Salicylates

Universal prescribing alerts:

- Patients are at an increased risk of bleeding for up to 4–7 days after taking the last salicylate dose.
- Due to the increased risk of bleeding, salicylates should be avoided in patients with hypoprothrombinemia, vitamin K deficiency, coagulopathy, thrombotic thrombocytopenic purpura (TTP), in patients receiving anticoagulant therapy or thrombolytic therapy, or in patients with severe hepatic impairment. Because salicylates may cause or aggravate hemolysis in patients with pyruvate kinase deficiency or rare variants of G6PD deficiency, these drugs should be avoided in these patients.
- Chronic use of high doses can compromise cardiac function and cause cardiac failure, pulmonary edema, reduced renal function, gastric ulceration, hepatic injury, and tinnitus.
- Avoid use in certain age-specific populations who have viral illness (may cause Reyes syndrome); refer to PI.

- May increase serum uric acid levels, resulting in hyperuricemia and reducing the efficacy of uricosuric agents in patients with gout.
- Renal toxicity has also been reported and is due to the compensatory role renal prostaglandins play in the maintenance of renal perfusion. The use of an NSAID may cause a dose-dependent reduction in prostaglandin formation and subsequent decrease in renal blood flow, precipitating renal decompensation. Patients who are predisposed to this renal risk are older patients, those with renal impairment/failure, heart failure, hepatic impairment, hypovolemia (dehydration), and those taking ACE inhibitors and/or diuretics.
- Take salicylates with food to reduce GI upset.

Drug Name	FDA-Approved Indications	Adult Dosage Range	Precautions and Clinical Pearls
Generic Name Aspirin **Brand Name** Aspercin Aspirtab Buffasal Bufferin Buffinol Ecotrin Halfprin ▲ (BL) (PD)	**Common indications for use:** Analgesic Antipyretic Revascularization procedures Rheumatoid disease Vascular indications	Dose varies depending on combination product selected **Usual oral dose for pain:** 325 to 650 mg as needed every 4 hours as needed (maximum daily dose [MDD]: 4 g) **Usual rectal dose:** 300 to 600 mg every 4 hours	• Enteric formulations are not intended for initial use (or rapid onset of effects) due to delayed absorption and action • GI adverse effects are common; enteric-coated formulations are available and may minimize these effects • Guidelines are available for use in primary and secondary prevention of cardiovascular events; these prescribing decisions are based on risk stratification and assurance that risks do not exceed benefits of therapy • Avoid in severe renal or hepatic impairment; specific guidelines for dosing in primary and secondary prevention scenarios, as well as for patients undergoing dialysis; refer to PI • Avoid in patients with asthma with a history of aspirin-induced acute bronchospasm • May mask signs and symptoms of infection; may increase risk of bleeding • Acid-base imbalances have been reported with use • Drug interactions may require dose adjustment or avoidance of certain drug combinations • Available in multiple combination products; see the individual product for indications, dosing, and brand name
Generic Name Choline salicylate **Brand Name** Arthropan (PD)	Mild to moderate pain OA RA Fever	**Usual oral dose for pain:** 435 to 870 mg every 4 hours as needed (MDD: 5352 mg per day)	• Most common side effects are nausea, vomiting, dyspepsia, heartburn, diarrhea, constipation, and abdominal pain • May contribute to additional imbalances in patients with acid–base disorders • GI ulceration and bleeding have been reported • Hepatotoxicity has been reported • All salicylates may increase risk of bleeding, however non acetylated agents such as choline salicylate may have lower risk • May mask signs and symptoms of infection

Drug Name	FDA-Approved Indications	Adult Dosage Range	Precautions and Clinical Pearls
Generic Name Magnesium salicylate **Brand Name** Doan's Regular Caplets Doan's Extra Strength Caplets Momentum Caplets Mobidin Keygesic-10 (PD)	Mild to moderate pain OA RA Fever	**Usual oral dose:** 600 mg every 4 hours or 1160 mg 3 times per day as needed (MDD: 4.8 g per day)	• Do not use in patients with severe chronic renal impairment due to risk of hypermagnesemia • Serum magnesium levels should be monitored with high dosages • Side effects include nausea, vomiting, dyspepsia, heartburn, diarrhea, constipation, and abdominal pain • GI bleeding has been reported; use caution (or avoid) in patients at high risk of this adverse effect
Generic Name Salsalate **Brand Name** Disalcid ■	Rheumatic disorders OA	**Usual oral dose:** 3 g daily in 2 to 3 divided doses	• May cause acid–base imbalances • May cause hypertension • Decreased hepatic function has been reported Associated with: • GI bleeding and perforation • Increased risk of cardiovascular thrombotic events • A contraindication for use in the treatment of pain from coronary artery bypass graft • Reye's syndrome in certain age-specific populations infected with viral illness
Generic Name Trolamine salicylate **Brand Name** Myoflex Others	Muscle or joint pain	**Usual topical dose:** Apply to affected area 2 to 4 times per day	• If pain does not improve in 7 days, the patient should discontinue therapy and notify a physician • May wrap the affected area loosely with a 2- to 3-inch elastic bandage • Avoid applying heat to the area where cream has been applied (especially in patients with diabetes)

Other Nonsteroidal Anti-inflammatory Agents			
Drug Name	**FDA-Approved Indications**	**Adult Dosage Range**	**Precautions and Clinical Pearls**
Generic Name Diclofenac **Brand Name** Cambia Dyloject Voltaren Zipsor Zorvolex ■ (BL)	**Common indications for use:** Acute pain OA	**Usual oral dose for OA (Voltaren delayed release tabs):** 50 mg 3 times per day **Usual parenteral dose:** IV: 37.5 mg every 6 hours as needed (MDD: 150 mg per day) **Usual topical dose for OA:** 1% gel: apply 2 to 4 g of gel to affected area 4 times per day **Patch for acute pain:** Apply 1 patch to affected area twice daily	• Do not cover topical products with occlusive dressings, heat, sunscreens, cosmetics, or other topical medications • Avoid showering at least 1 hour after application • Different formulations of diclofenac are not bioequivalent even if of equivalent milligram strength; solution is also available • Products and formulations are associated with specific indications for use; refer to PI prior to selecting and administering • Hepatic adverse effects have been reported Contraindications: • Do not apply topical products to open skin, wounds, eyes, or mucous membranes • Do not use for the treatment of perioperative pain in the setting of CABG • For use in moderate to severe renal impairment Associated with: • Increased risk of MI and stroke • GI perforation and bleeding
Generic Name Diflunisal **Brand Name** Dolobid ▲ ■ (BL) (GD)	Mild to moderate pain OA RA	**Usual oral dose for OA:** 500 mg to 1 g daily divided into 2 doses	• Hepatic adverse effects have been reported Contraindications: • Do not use for the treatment of perioperative pain in the setting of CABG Associated with: • Increased risk of MI and stroke • GI perforation and bleeding
Generic Name Etodolac **Brand Name** Lodine ■ (BL) (PD)	**Common indications for use:** Acute pain RA OA	**Usual oral dose for pain:** 200 to 400 mg every 6 to 8 hours as needed	Contraindications: • Do not use for the treatment of perioperative pain in the setting of CABG Associated with: • Increased risk of MI and stroke • GI perforation and bleeding

Drug Name	FDA-Approved Indications	Adult Dosage Range	Precautions and Clinical Pearls
Generic Name Fenoprofen **Brand Name** Nalfon ■ (BL)	Mild to moderate pain RA	**Usual oral dose:** 400 to 600 mg 3 to 4 times per day (MDD: 3.2 g per day)	Contraindications: • Do not use for the treatment of perioperative pain in the setting of CABG Associated with: • Increased risk of MI and stroke • GI perforation and bleeding
Generic Name Flurbiprofen **Brand Name** Ansaid ▲ ■ (BL)	**Common indications for use:** RA OA	**Usual oral dose for pain:** 50 mg 4 times per day or 100 mg twice daily	• Visual disturbances have been reported Contraindications: • Do not use for the treatment of perioperative pain in the setting of CABG Associated with: • Increased risk of MI and stroke • GI perforation and bleeding
Generic Name Ibuprofen **Brand Name** Caldolor Motrin ▲ ■ (BL) (PD)	Analgesia/pain Antipyretic OA RA Dysmenorrhea	Dose varies depending on combination product selected **Illustrative oral dose:** 400 mg every 4 to 6 hours as needed **Usual parenteral dose:** IV: 400 to 800 mg every 6 hours as needed (MDD 3.2 g per day)	• Available in multiple combination products; see the individual product for indications, dosing, and brand name Contraindications: • Do not use for the treatment of perioperative pain in the setting of CABG Associated with: • Increased risk of MI and stroke • GI perforation and bleeding

Generic Name Indomethacin **Brand Name** Indocin Tivorbex ■ (BL) (PD)	**Common indications for use:** Mild to moderate acute pain Inflammatory/rheumatoid disorders Bursitis/tendonitis Acute gouty arthritis	**Usual oral dose:** 20 mg 3 times per day **Illustrative rectal dose:** 50 mg 3 times per day	• Retain suppository for no less than 60 minutes • Age-specific warnings/alerts for parenteral administration; refer to PI for details • Visual disturbances have been reported • Tivorbex is indicated for acute pain only; it is not indicated for long-term use Contraindications: • Do not use for the treatment of perioperative pain in the setting of CABG Associated with: • Increased risk of MI and stroke • GI perforation and bleeding
Generic Name Ketoprofen **Brand Name** Orudis ▲ □ ■ (BL)	**Common indications for use:** Mild to moderate pain OA RA Dysmenorrhea	**Usual oral dose for OA:** IR: 50 mg 4 times per day or 75 mg 3 times per day (MDD: 300 mg per day) Alternatively may give: ER: 200 mg per day	Contraindications: • Do not use for the treatment of perioperative pain in the setting of CABG • Monitor renal and hepatic function; dose reduction may be warranted in cases of impairment Associated with: • Increased risk of MI and stroke • GI perforation and bleeding
Generic Name Ketorolac **Brand Name** Toradol ▲ ■ (BL) (GD)	**Common indications for use:** Moderate acute pain Ocular pain	**Usual oral dose:** 20 mg, then 10 mg every 4 to 6 hours as needed (MDD: 40 mg per day) **Usual parenteral dose:** IM/IV: 30 mg every 6 hours (MDD: 120 mg per day)	• Maximum duration of combined treatment is 5 days • Use caution in hepatic impairment • Many dose formulations are available, including nasal spray and eye drops Contraindications: • Risk of cerebrovascular bleeding, hemorrhage, diathesis, incomplete hemostasis, and high risk of bleeding • Use as prophylactic analgesia prior to surgery Associated with: • Epidural administration or intrathecal administration • GI perforation and bleeding • Contraindicated for use in renal failure or severe impairment • Need for limited duration of use (maximum of 5 days)

Drug Name	FDA-Approved Indications	Adult Dosage Range	Precautions and Clinical Pearls
Generic Name Meclofenamate **Brand Name** Meclomen ■ (BL)	Mild to moderate pain OA RA Primary dysmenorrhea	**Usual oral dose:** 50 to 100 mg every 4 to 6 hours (MDD: 400 mg per day)	• May require dose adjustment for renal and hepatic impairment; no specific recommendations are available • May cause dizziness, rash, and abdominal pain Contraindications: • Do not use for the treatment of perioperative pain in the setting of CABG Associated with: • Increased risk of MI and stroke • GI perforation and bleeding
Generic Name Mefenamic acid **Brand Name** Ponstel ■ (BL)	Mild to moderate pain Primary dysmenorrhea	**Usual oral dose:** 500 mg, then 250 mg every 6 hours as needed	• Duration of therapy should not exceed 1 week • Side effects include headache, nervousness, itching, rash, abdominal cramps, tinnitus, and increased liver function tests (LFTs) • May require dose adjustment for renal and hepatic impairment; no specific recommendations are available Contraindications: • Do not use for the treatment of perioperative pain in the setting of CABG Associated with: • Increased risk of MI and stroke • GI perforation and bleeding
Generic Name Meloxicam **Brand Name** Mobic ■ (BL) (PD)	OA RA	**Usual oral dose:** Tablets: 7.5 mg per day (MDD: 15 mg per day)	• Not recommended for use in severe hepatic or renal impairment • Capsules are not interchangeable with other formulations of meloxicam • Side effects include edema, pain, rash, pruritus, upper respiratory tract infections, urinary tract infection, and abdominal pain Contraindications: • Do not use for the treatment of perioperative pain in the setting of CABG Associated with: • Increased risk of MI and stroke • GI perforation and bleeding
Generic Name Nabumetone **Brand Name** Relafen ▲ ■ (BL)	Arthritis	**Usual oral dose:** 1000 mg once per day or 500 mg twice per day (MDD: 2000 mg per day)	• Side effects include abdominal pain, edema, dizziness, headache, pruritus, and rash Contraindications: • Do not use for the treatment of perioperative pain in the setting of CABG Associated with: • Increased risk of MI and stroke • GI perforation and bleeding

Generic Name Naproxen **Brand Name** Naprosyn Alleve ▲ ■ ■ (BL)	**Common indications for use:** Mild to moderate pain Ankylosing spondylitis OA RA Gout Dysmenorrhea	Dose varies depending on combination product selected **Illustrative oral dose for OA:** 500 mg every 12 hours (MDD: 1000 mg per day)	• Enteric formulations are not intended for initial use due to delayed absorption and effects • Naproxen sodium doses are different than other formulations; verify product and dose prior to use • Adverse effects include edema, dizziness, drowsiness, headache, pruritus, rash, abdominal pain, and increased liver enzymes • Available in multiple combination products; see the individual product for indications, dosing, and brand name Contraindications: • Do not use for the treatment of perioperative pain in the setting of CABG Associated with: • Increased risk of MI and stroke • GI perforation and bleeding
Generic Name Oxaprozin **Brand Name** Daypro ▲ ■ (BL) (PD)	OA RA	**Usual oral dose:** 1200 mg per day (MDD: patients weighing more than 50 kg: 1800 mg)	• Side effects include edema, confusion, dizziness, pruritus, rash, abdominal distress, and increased liver enzymes • Specific recommendations for patients undergoing dialysis; refer to PI for details Contraindications: • Do not use for the treatment of perioperative pain in the setting of CABG Associated with: • Increased risk of MI and stroke • GI perforation and bleeding
Generic Name Piroxicam **Brand Name** Feldene ■ (BL)	OA RA	**Usual oral dose:** 20 mg per day	• Hepatic adverse effects have been reported • Side effects include edema, dizziness, headache, pruritus, rash, abdominal pain, anorexia, constipation, diarrhea, and increased liver enzymes Contraindications: • Do not use for the treatment of perioperative pain in the setting of CABG Associated with: • Increased risk of MI and stroke • GI perforation and bleeding
Generic Name Sulindac **Brand Name** Clinoril ■ (BL) (PD)	OA RA Acute gout	**Usual oral dose:** 150 mg twice daily	• Side effects include dizziness and headache Contraindications: • Do not use for the treatment of perioperative pain in the setting of CABG Associated with: • Increased risk of MI and stroke • GI perforation and bleeding

Drug Name	FDA-Approved Indications	Adult Dosage Range	Precautions and Clinical Pearls
Generic Name Tolmetin **Brand Name** Tolectin ■ (BL) (PD)	OA RA	**Usual oral dose:** 400 mg 3 times per day (MDD: 1800 mg per day)	• Side effects include edema, hypertension, dizziness, headache, and weight changes Contraindications: • Do not use for the treatment of perioperative pain in the setting of CABG Associated with: • Increased risk of MI and stroke • GI perforation and bleeding

Opiate Agonists

Universal prescribing alerts:

- The pharmacokinetic profiles of opiate agents differ significantly. Use the specific "opiate" conversion guidelines when prescribing or recommending a different opiate product.
- Do not crush, chew, or dissolve extended-release formulations. The rapid release and absorption can cause a potentially fatal overdose.
- May cause urinary retention; use caution in patients predisposed to complications (i.e., BPH)
- Serious, life-threatening, or fatal respiratory depression may occur with use of all opiates. Monitor for respiratory depression, especially during initiation or following a dose increase.
- Opioid analgesics may cause pooling of blood in the extremities by decreasing peripheral vascular resistance resulting in decreased venous return and pulmonary venous pressure. This action causes blood to move from the central to peripheral circulation, which can worsen certain medical conditions (i.e., those with pulmonary edema)
- Accidental exposure/consumption can result in fatal overdose. Opiates may also cause seizures; use care and caution
- Avoid activities that require mental alertness or coordination. Cholinergic side effects of these agents may cause bradycardia and syncope. Avoid abrupt discontinuation after prolonged use
- Opiate agonists increase the tone of the biliary tract and may cause spasms (especially in the sphincter of Oddi) increasing biliary tract pressure. Plasma amylase and lipase concentrations have been reported to increase to 2 to 15 times the normal values. Use caution in patients with biliary tract disease such as acute pancreatitis or who are undergoing biliary tract surgery.
- Use caution in patients with adrenal insufficiency (i.e., Addison's disease), hypothyroidism, or myxedema. Such patients may be at increased risk of adverse events. Opioids inhibit the secretion of adrenocorticotropic hormone (ACTH), cortisol, and luteinizing hormone (LH); however, the thyroid stimulating hormone may be either stimulated or inhibited by opioids. Rarely, adrenal insufficiency has been reported in association with opioid use.
- Chronic opioid use may lead to symptoms of hypogonadism (with signs or symptoms of androgen deficiency), resulting from changes in the hypothalamic-pituitary-gonadal axis. Monitor patients for symptoms of opioid-induced endocrinopathy, particularly those receiving a daily dose equivalent to 100 mg or more of morphine.
- Opiates are DEA-controlled substances. Opioid agonists are associated with a significant abuse potential and risk of addiction in patients who either obtain these agents appropriately as a prescribed drug or illicitly. The risk of addiction in any individual is unknown however patients with a family history of substance abuse or underlying mental illness are at greater risk.
- Ingestion of alcohol or consumption of that contained in prescription or non-prescription medications, during therapy must be avoided. Avoid use of any concomitant substance that contributes additional CNS and respiratory depression.

Drug Name	FDA-Approved Indications	Adult Dosage Range	Precautions and Clinical Pearls
Generic Name Codeine ■ (BL) (PD)	Pain	**Usual oral dose:** 15 to 60 mg every 4 hours as needed (MDD: 360 mg per day)	• American Pain Society recommends an initial dose of 30 to 60 mg for adults with moderate pain • Medication clearance may be reduced in patients with renal impairment, but no specific dosage adjustments are necessary per manufacturer • Seizures have been reported at normal doses Associated with • Increased mortality in certain populations who are extensive metabolizers; may increase their risk of death (see age-specific PI) • All related universal opiate prescribing alerts
Generic Name Fentanyl citrate **Brand Name** Abstral Actiq Duragesic Fentora Ionsys Lazanda Subsys ▲ □ ■ (BL) (PD)	Cancer pain Severe pain General anesthesia Postoperative pain Regional anesthesia	**Usual transdermal dose:** Based on current oral opiate analgesic dose **Usual oral dose:** SL lozenge: 200 to 400 mcg every 4 hours as needed SL spray: 100 to 200 mcg every 4 hours as needed Buccal film: 200 mcg every 2 hours as needed Buccal tablet: 100 -200 mcg every 4 hours as needed **Usual intranasal dose:** 100 mcg every 2 hours as needed Numerous formulations (including parenteral) are available; confirm formulation and associated dose prior to administration	Associated with: • Transmucosal products available only through the TIRF REMS ACCESS program, a restricted distribution program involving outpatients, prescribers who prescribe to outpatients, pharmacies (inpatient and outpatient), and distributor-required enrollment; see the PI for details • Do not convert patients on a microgram-per-microgram basis from one fentanyl product to another fentanyl product; the substitution of one fentanyl product for another fentanyl product may result in a fatal overdose • IV and IM formulations are available: patient-specific dosing is based on indication and duration of therapy • Contraindication for any use of transmucosal and nasal fentanyl or transdermal patch as an as-needed analgesic, in the management of acute or postoperative pain, or in patients who are opioid nontolerant; monitor closely for respiratory depression during use, particularly during initiation of therapy or after dose increases • Exposure of application site and surrounding area to direct external heat sources (i.e., heating pads, electric blankets, heat or tanning lamps, sunbathing, hot tubs) may increase fentanyl absorption and has resulted in fatalities; closely monitor patients who experience fever or increase in core body temperature • Certain drug interactions may require dose adjustment or avoidance of some combinations • Requires experienced clinician who is knowledgeable in the use of this agent and specialized care setting • All related universal opiate prescribing alerts

Drug Name	FDA-Approved Indications	Adult Dosage Range	Precautions and Clinical Pearls
Generic Name Hydrocodone **Brand Name** Hysingla ER Zohydro ER ▲ ■ ■ QT BL	Severe chronic pain	Dose varies depending on product selected **Illustrative oral dose:** 10 mg every 12 hours	• Monitor hepatic or renal function; may require dose adjustments in patients with impairment • Available in multiple combination products; see the individual product for indications, dosing, and brand name • Seizures have been reported Contraindications: • Use of extended release products in GI obstruction, difficulty swallowing or patients at high risk with conditions that predispose to choking. Associated with: • Instruct patients not to consume alcoholic beverages or use prescription or nonprescription products that contain alcohol while taking Zohydro ER; the co-ingestion of alcohol with Zohydro ER may result in increased plasma levels and a potentially fatal overdose • Certain drug interactions may require dose adjustment or avoidance of some combinations • All related universal opiate prescribing alerts
Generic Name Hydromorphone **Brand Name** Dilaudid Dilaudid-HP Exalgo ▲ ■ ■ BL	Pain	**Usual oral dose (tablets):** 2 to 4 mg every 4 to 6 hours as needed **Usual parenteral dose:** IV: 0.2 to 1 mg every 2 to 3 hours as needed	• Additional formulations are available for IM/SQ and rectal administration Associated with: • Do not confuse high-potency hydromorphone with standard parenteral formulations or other opioids • Monitor for renal and hepatic impairment; dose adjustments may be warranted if they occur • All related universal opiate prescribing alerts
Generic Name Levorphanol **Brand Name** Levo-Dromoran ■ BL	Moderate to severe acute pain Chronic pain	**Usual oral dose:** 2 mg every 6 to 8 hours as needed	• There is no optimal or maximum dose for use in chronic pain; the appropriate dose is one that relieves pain without causing unmanageable side effects • Parenteral formulations are available (SQ and IM) • Seizures have been reported Associated with: • Severe CNS and respiratory depression • Drug interactions may require dose adjustments or avoidance of certain drug combinations • All related universal opiate prescribing alerts

Generic Name Meperidine **Brand Name** Demerol ■ (BL) (PD)	Anesthesia Obstetric pain Pain	**Usual dose:** Oral/IM/SQ: 50 to 150 mg every 3 to 4 hours as needed	• Avoid use in patients with renal impairment due to increased risk of neurotoxicity • Dose reduction with the oral formulation is necessary in patients with hepatic impairment Associated with: • Drug interactions may require dose adjustments or avoidance of certain drug combinations • Severe CNS and respiratory depression • All related universal opiate prescribing alerts
Generic Name Methadone **Brand Name** Dolophine Others ■ (BL) (QT)	Drug detoxification Pain Opioid abuse	**Usual oral dose for pain:** 2.5 mg every 8 to 12 hours in the opioid-naive patient; titrate to pain relief	• Oral concentrate solution is for oral administration only; do not give via IV administration • Dose adjustments may be required in hepatic and renal impairment; no specific recommendations are available Associated with: • QTc prolongation and serious arrhythmias: closely monitor for changes in cardiac rhythm during initiation and dosage increases • Accidental consumption can result in fatal overdose • Methadone should be dispensed only by hospitals, community pharmacies, and maintenance programs approved by the FDA and designated state authorities to treat narcotic addiction in detoxification or maintenance programs • Requires experienced clinician who is knowledgeable in the use of this agent and specialized care setting • All related universal opiate prescribing alerts
Generic Name Morphine **Brand Name** MS Contin Duramorph Infumorph 200 Infumorph 500 Kadian ▲ ■ ■ (PD)	Chronic pain	**Usual oral dose:** 10 to 30 mg every 4 hours as needed **Usual parenteral doses:** IM/SQ: 5 to 10 mg every 4 hours as needed IV: 2.5 to 5 mg every 3 to 4 hours	• Do not use the product if the injectable solution contains a precipitate • Dose adjustments may be required in hepatic and renal impairment; no specific recommendations are available • Epidural and intrathecal administration is available for specific formulations; refer to PI for details (preservative-free products must be used) Associated with: • Observe patients for at least 24 hours after the initial intrathecal or epidural dose; ensure naloxone injection and resuscitative equipment are available in case of life-threatening side effects • In case of accidental contact of Infumorph or Duramorph, rinse the skin with water immediately; take measures in a hospital or clinic to limit diversion • Improper substitution of Infumorph for regular Duramorph is associated with risk: likely to result in serious overdose • Infumorph: not recommended for single-dose IV, IM, or subcutaneous administration • All related universal opiate prescribing alerts

Drug Name	FDA-Approved Indications	Adult Dosage Range	Precautions and Clinical Pearls
Generic Name Oxycodone **Brand Name** Oxycontin Oxaydo Roxicodone ■ ■ (BL) (PD)	Chronic pain	Dose varies depending on product selected **Illustrative oral dose:** IR: 5 to 15 mg every 4 to 6 hours as needed ER: 10 mg every 12 hours	• Available in multiple combination products; see the individual product for indications, dosing, and brand name • All related universal opiate prescribing alerts Associated with: • Certain drug interactions may require dose adjustment or avoidance of some combinations • Take extra care when prescribing and administering oxycodone oral solution to avoid dosing errors due to confusion between milligram and milliliter, and other oxycodone solutions with different concentrations, which could result in accidental overdose and death • Monitor for renal and hepatic impairment; dose adjustments may be warranted if they occur • Discontinue all other around-the-clock opioid drugs upon initiation of oxycodone extended-release tablets.
Generic Name Oxymorphone **Brand Name** Opana Opana ER ▲ ■ ■ (BL)	Anesthesia Anxiety Pain Premedication for procedures	**Usual oral dose:** IR: 5 to 10 mg every 4 to 6 hours as needed ER: 5 mg every 12 hours **Usual parenteral dose:** IM/SQ dose: 1 to 1.5 mg; may repeat every 4 to 6 hours as needed IV dose: 0.5 mg every 4 to 6 hours as needed	Contraindications: • Moderate to severe hepatic impairment • Injectable oxymorphone in patients with upper airway obstruction and in the treatment of patients with pulmonary edema secondary to a chemical respiratory irritant. Associated with: • Need to educate that the recreational ingestion of alcohol or consumption of that contained in prescription or non-prescription medications, during therapy must be avoided. • All related universal opiate prescribing alerts
Generic Name Remifentanil **Brand Name** Ultiva (BL) (PD) (GD)	General anesthesia Postoperative pain	**Usual parenteral dose for analgesia during monitored surgery care:** IV: 0.5 to 1 mcg/kg per dose administered over 30 to 60 seconds given 90 seconds before local anesthetic	• Dose based on ideal body weight in obese patients • Use caution in patients with adrenal insufficiency (i.e., Addison's disease), hypothyroidism, or myxedema Contraindications: • Epidural and intrathecal administration Associated with: • All related universal opiate prescribing alerts
Generic Name Sufentanil citrate **Brand Name** Sufenta ■ (BL) (PD)	Anesthesia of labor General anesthesia	**Usual parenteral dose for severe pain during general anesthesia:** IV: 1 to 2 mcg/kg given as 10 to 25 mcg increments or as a continuous infusion	• Use lean body weight to determine dose in obese patients Associated with: • Severe CNS and respiratory depression • All related universal opiate prescribing alerts

Generic Name Tapentadol **Brand Name** Nucynta Nucynta ER ▪ ■	Diabetic peripheral neuropathy Acute pain	**Usual oral dose:** IR: 50 to 100 mg every 4 to 6 hours as needed (MDD: 600 mg per day) ER: 50 mg twice daily	• Monitor for renal and hepatic impairment; dose adjustments may be warranted if they occur • Reserve higher doses for opiate tolerant (non-naïve) patients as defined as those taking, for a minimum of 1 week: 60 mg or greater of oral morphine daily, 30 mg or greater oral oxycodone daily, 8 mg or greater of oral hydromorphone daily, 25 mg or greater of oral oxymorphone daily, or an equivalent dose of another opioid Associated with • Dose adjustments may be required and certain drug combinations may be contraindicated (i.e., those that may result in additive norepinephrine and/or serotonin concentrations). • Extended-release formulation is intended only for patients requiring continuous, around-the-clock opioid analgesia for an extended period of time and requires an experienced clinician who is knowledgeable in the use of long-acting opioids for the management of chronic pain. • All related universal opiate prescribing alerts
Generic Name Tramadol **Brand Name** Ultram Ultram ED Rybix orally disintegrating tablets (ODT) Others ▲ ▪ ■ (BL)	Dental pain Chronic pain	**Usual oral dose for rapid analgesia ODT tablets:** After initial dose of 50 mg and titration of 50 mg dose increase every 3 days: IR: 50 mg 4 times per day (every 6 hours) Alternatively may give: ER: 100 mg daily	• Report signs of depression or worsening depression; report signs of serotonin syndrome • Monitor for renal and hepatic impairment; dose adjustments may be warranted if they occur • Avoid ER formulation in severe hepatic or renal disease • Avoid in patients with underlying mental health disorders; suicidal ideation has been reported Associated with: • All related universal opiate prescribing alerts • Drug interactions may require dose adjustment or avoidance of certain drugs (increased risk of seizures, cardiovascular events and serotonin syndrome)

Opiate Partial Agonists

Universal prescribing alerts:

- Avoid activities that require mental alertness or coordination.
- Are subject to all the same universal prescribing alerts as opiate agonists; refer to information in that section above.

Drug Name	FDA-Approved Indications	Adult Dosage Range	Precautions and Clinical Pearls
Generic Name Buprenorphine **Brand Name** Belbuca Buprenex Butrans ■ ■ QT BL PD	Chronic pain Opiate agonist dependence and withdrawal	**Usual parenteral dose for pain:** IM/IV: 0.3 mg every 6 to 8 hours as needed **Usual transmucosal dose:** 75 mcg once daily, or every 12 hours if tolerated, placed against the inside of the cheek; may increase to 150 mcg every 12 hours after 4 days if needed **Usual transdermal dose:** 5 mcg per hour patch every 7 days	• Transdermal and buccal buprenorphine should be reserved for patients in whom there is no alternative treatment option • May precipitate withdrawal in someone receiving opiates • Requires experienced clinician who is knowledgeable in the use of this agent • Available in multiple combination products; see the individual product for indications, dosing, and brand name Associated with: • Intramuscular administration or other routes of deep insertion of buprenorphine (i.e., implant) may result in rare but serious neural or vascular injury • Exposure of application site and surrounding area to direct external heat sources (i.e., heating pads, electric blankets, heat or tanning lamps, sunbathing, hot tubs) may increase absorption and has resulted in overdose; closely monitor patients who experience fever or increase in core body temperature • All related universal opiate prescribing alerts
Generic Name Butorphanol **Brand Name** Stadol ▲ ■ ■ GD	**Common indications for use:** Anesthesia Pain Premedication for procedure	**Usual parenteral dose:** IM: 1 to 4 mg every 3 to 4 hours as needed IV: 0.5 to 2 mg every 3 to 4 hours as needed **Usual intranasal dose:** 1 spray (1 mg) in 1 nostril; may repeat in 3 to 4 hours	• Nasal spray must be primed initially and again if not used for more than 48 hours • Nasal spray may cause nasal congestion, epistaxis, pharyngitis, upper respiratory infections, or an unpleasant taste • Monitor for renal and hepatic impairment; dose adjustments may be warranted if they occur • May precipitate withdrawal in opiate users Associated with: • All related universal opiate prescribing alerts
Generic Name Nalbuphine ■	**Common indications for use:** General anesthesia Pain Preoperative and postoperative analgesia	**Usual parenteral dose for 70 kg patient:** IM/IV/SQ: 10 mg every 3 to 6 hours as needed	• Patient may experience nausea, vomiting, fatigue, or sweating • Weight-based dosing; refer to PI for further details • Report signs and symptoms of new-onset or worsening depression or psychiatric symptoms; report signs or symptoms of serotonin syndrome • Rotate subcutaneous injection sites • Has a ceiling effect for respiratory depression, where doses greater than 30 mg do not produce further respiratory depression in the absence of other CNS depressant agents. Associated with: • All related universal opiate prescribing alerts

Generic Name Pentazocine **Brand Name** Talwin ▲ ■ (BL) (PD)	**Common indications for use:** Analgesic General anesthesia induction	Dose varies depending on combination product selected **Illustrative parenteral doses:** IM/IV/SQ: 30 mg every 3 to 4 hours; do not exceed 30 mg per dose IV and 60 mg per dose IM/SQ	• Rotate subcutaneous injection sites (IM administration is preferred whenever possible) • Rare but serious dermatologic reactions have been reported (Stevens-Johnson syndrome, toxic epidermal necrolysis); report rash to healthcare provider immediately • May cause CNS excitation and hypertension through their respective effects on catecholamines • Drug interactions may require dose adjustment or avoidance of certain drug combinations. Associated with: • All related universal opiate prescribing alerts

Miscellaneous Analgesic and Antipyretic Agents

Drug Name	FDA-Approved Indications	Adult Dosage Range	Precautions and Clinical Pearls
Generic Name Acetaminophen **Brand Name** Tylenol Acephen ■ (PD)	Fever Pain	Dose varies depending on combination product selected **Illustrative oral dose regular tablets:** 650 mg every 4 to 6 hours ER: 1300 mg every 8 hours **Usual rectal dose:** 650 mg every 4 to 6 hours **Usual parenteral dose:** IV: patients weighing 50 kg or more: 650 mg every 4 hours or 1000 mg every 6 hours (MDD: 4 g per day)	• Monitor for renal and hepatic impairment; dose adjustments may be warranted if they occur • MDD is 4000 mg per day; hepatic injury may occur at lower dosages • Available in multiple combination products; see the individual product for indications, dosing, and brand name • Caution: use with other acetaminophen-containing products and with other hepatotoxic substances (i.e., alcohol) • Tobacco smoking may potentially increase the risk for acetaminophen-induced hepatotoxicity during overdose Associated with: • Acute, potentially fatal, liver failure
Generic Name Salicylamide	Analgesic Antipyretic	Safety and efficacy of dose not determined	• Used in combination with both aspirin and caffeine in over-the-counter (OTC) pain products Associated with: • Universal prescribing alerts for salicylate agents, refer to that section for further detail

Drug Name	FDA-Approved Indications	Adult Dosage Range	Precautions and Clinical Pearls
Generic Name Ziconotide **Brand Name** Prialt ■	Chronic pain	**Usual intrathecal dose:** 0.1 mcg per hour with slow dose titration every 2 to 3 days up to a maximum of 0.8 mcg per hour (MDD: 19.2 mcg per day)	• Side effects: dizziness, fatigue, diarrhea, lack of appetite • Seizures have been reported Associated with: • Contraindication in patients with psychiatric symptoms • May cause neurologic impairment
Antimigraine agents	Refer to the Antimigraine Agents section.		
Gabapentin	Refer to the Anticonvulsant Agents section.		
Fibromyalgia Agents			
Drug Name	FDA-Approved Indications	Adult Dosage Range	Precautions and Clinical Pearls
Generic Name Milnacipran **Brand Name** Savella Savella Titration Pack ▲ ■	Management of fibromyalgia	**Usual oral dose:** 50 mg twice daily (MDD: 100 mg twice daily)	• Dose escalation should be titrated over 7 days based on individual response; gradually taper to discontinue • Seizures and hyponatremia have been reported • Not recommended in severe renal impairment • May alter urethral resistance and worsen symptoms in patients predisposed to complications (i.e., BPH) • Food may improve tolerability • Monitor blood pressure, heart rate, and signs and symptoms of suicide ideation (e.g., anxiety, depression, clinical worsening, behavior changes) • Certain drug interactions may require dose adjustment or avoidance of some combinations • May increase intraocular pressure Associated with: • Suicidality and antidepressant drugs • Refer to PI for age-specific warnings
Duloxetine	Refer to the Psychotherapeutic Agents section.		
Pregabalin	Refer to the Anticonvulsant Agents section.		
Anti-gout Agents			
Drug Name	FDA-Approved Indications	Adult Dosage Range	Precautions and Clinical Pearls
Generic Name Allopurinol	**Common indications for use:** Gout	**Usual oral dose for gout:** 100 mg once daily, increased by 100 mg weekly until	• Periodic liver-function tests are recommended during the initial stages of allopurinol treatment for patients with hepatic disease. • Reversible hepatotoxicity has been reported

Brand Name Aloprim Zyloprim ▲ (PD)	Nephrolithiasis Hyperuricemia	serum urate concentrations decrease to 6 mg/dL or less, or until reaching a MDD of 800 mg per day	• The risk of hepatotoxicity increases in patients who also have renal impairment. • Patients may experience an initial exacerbation of pain until uric acid levels are decreased
Generic Name Colchicine **Brand Name** Colcrys Mitigare ▲ (BL) (PD) (GD)	**Common indications for use:** Gout	**Usual oral dose for the treatment of gouty flares:** 0.6 mg once or twice daily. Do not exceed 1.2 mg per day	• Specific recommendations for patients undergoing dialysis; refer to PI • May cause myelosuppression and increased risk of infection and bleeding Contraindications: • Dose adjustments may be needed in renal and hepatic impairment under certain conditions, refer to PI • Drug interactions may require dose adjustment or avoidance of certain drug combinations
Generic Name Febuxostat **Brand Name** Uloric	Gout	**Usual oral dose:** 40 mg per day; may increase dose to 80 mg if uric acid not less than 6 mg/dL after 2 weeks (MDD: 120 mg per day)	• Do not use if patients have asymptomatic hyperuricemia • Liver function abnormalities possible; report any signs and symptoms of liver failure to healthcare provider immediately Associated with: • Drug reaction/rash with eosinophilia and systemic symptoms (DRESS) • Potential increased risk of heart failure in patients with preexisting cardiovascular disease and/or risk factors

Opioid Antagonists

Universal prescribing alerts:

- Opiate antagonists have a higher affinity for the opiate receptors in the brain compared to opiates. When used concurrently with an opiate, the antagonists will block the effects of the opiate.
- When these medications are administered and a patient has opioids in his or her system, the antagonists can induce immediate withdrawal symptoms. Adverse effects of these medications are predominantly signs or symptoms of opioid withdrawal (nausea, vomiting, flu-like symptoms, piloerection, and diaphoresis).
- If these medications are used to help manage opioid abstinence or prevent a relapse, the patient should be opiate free when therapy is initiated. The washout period for opiates is 3 to 6 days after the last use of a short-acting opioid or 7 to 10 days after the last use of a long-acting opioid.

Drug Name	FDA-Approved Indications	Adult Dosage Range	Precautions and Clinical Pearls
Generic Name Naloxone **Brand Name** Narcan Evzio (PD)	Opiate overdose Reversal of opiate activity	Dose varies depending on combination product selected **Illustrative parenteral (IV/IM/SQ) and intranasal doses:** 0.4 mg/mL; repeat every 2 to 3 minutes if needed	• Seek medical care immediately if used for opioid overdose • May cause injection-site reactions • Available in multiple combination products; see the individual product for indications, dosing, and brand name

Drug Name	FDA-Approved Indications	Adult Dosage Range	Precautions and Clinical Pearls
Generic Name Naltrexone **Brand Name** ReVia Vivitrol (BL)	Alcohol dependence Opioid dependence	Dose varies depending on combination product selected **Usual oral dose for maintenance treatment alcohol dependence:** 50 mg daily **Usual parenteral dose:** IM: 380 mg every 4 weeks	• May cause injection-site reactions. Administer parenteral doses only as IM • May require dose adjustment in renal and/or hepatic impairment; no specific recommendations available. • May cause hepatocellular injury; reverses after medication discontinuation • Avoid activities that require mental alertness or coordination • May cause abdominal pain, diarrhea, loss of appetite, nausea, and vomiting • May be used to prevent or decrease the desire for alcohol to promote abstinence • Patients should not be actively drinking alcohol at the time of initial Vivitrol administration • Pretreatment with oral naltrexone is not required before using Vivitrol

Anticonvulsant Agents

Barbiturates

Universal prescribing alerts:

- Medications should be discontinued gradually to avoid precipitating withdrawal (and potential seizures).
- Sedation is a common side effect, but tolerance typically develops with continued use.
- Irritability and hyperactivity can occur in children, and agitation and confusion in the elderly.
- Changes in mood should be monitored and reported, especially increases in depressive symptoms or suicidal ideation.
- Barbiturates are controlled substances and have an abuse and addictive potential.
- Avoid activities that require mental alertness or coordination.
- Barbiturates should be given cautiously to patients with hypertension, hypotension, pulmonary disease, cardiac disease, or other hemodynamically-unstable state.
- Some of these agents are DEA-controlled substances; refer to DEA schedules to confirm.

Drug Name	FDA-Approved Indications	Adult Dosage Range	Precautions and Clinical Pearls
Generic Name Mephobarbital **Brand Name** Mebaral ▲ (BL) (PD)	Sedative Prophylactic management of tonic–clonic (grand mal) seizures and absence (petit mal) seizures	**Usual oral dose:** 200 to 600 mg daily, taken as a single dose or in divided doses	• Initiate with a small dose and then gradually increase daily over a period of 4 or 5 days • Reserved as a replacement drug for patients who must be discontinued from phenobarbital due to its excessive drowsiness • Paradoxical reactions, such as agitation and hyperactivity, may occur in patients with acute pain • Specific recommendations for patients undergoing dialysis, refer to PI • Use with caution in hepatic impairment and disease • Osteopenia and osteoporosis reported with long-term use • Monitor behavior, including new-onset suicidality • This drug should be taken when seizures typically occur (i.e., take at night if seizures occur mostly at night) Contraindications: • Manifest or latent porphyria

Generic Name Phenobarbital ▲ BL PD	**Common indications for use:** Management of generalized tonic–clonic (grand mal), status epilepticus, and partial seizures Sedative-hypnotic	**Usual dose for maintenance treatment partial seizures:** IV/IM/Oral: 1 to 3 mg/kg per day given in 1 to 2 divided doses; gradually titrate dosage based on patient response and serum concentrations	• Subcutaneous administration is not recommended • Increase intake of vitamin D and calcium; may cause decrease in calcium • Certain drug interactions may require dose adjustment or avoidance of some combinations • Reserve IV administration only for emergency Contraindications: • Hepatic impairment • Dyspnea/airway obstruction • Porphyria • Intra-arterial administration
Generic Name Primidone **Brand Name** Mysoline ▲ BL PD	Management of grand mal, psychomotor, and focal seizures	**Usual oral dose:** 750 to 1500 mg per day in divided doses 3 to 4 times per day (MDD: 2 g per day)	• Dose escalation taper required; lower starting doses for patients who have not received prior treatment • Supplement with prophylactic doses of folic acid and cyanocobalamin • Certain drug interactions may require dose adjustment or avoidance of some combinations • Use caution in renal and hepatic impairment • Skin reactions can precede potentially fatal hypersensitivity reactions; exfoliative dermatitis has been reported • Specific recommendations for patients undergoing dialysis, refer to PI Contraindications: • Porphyria
Methohexital	Refer to the Anxiolytic, Sedative, and Hypnotic Agents section.		

Benzodiazepines

Universal prescribing alerts:

- All benzodiazepines are associated with a black box warning to avoid coadministration with other CNS depressants.
- Benzodiazepines cause drowsiness and lethargy, but tolerance develops with chronic use.
- Concomitant use with other CNS depressants can worsen drowsiness, lethargy, and CNS depression.
- Administering the medication in divided doses throughout the day can reduce the severity of these side effects.
- Aggression, hyperactivity, irritability, difficulty concentrating, and other behavioral changes can occur in children.
- Monitor for changes in mood, including depressive symptoms and suicidal ideation.
- Taper the medication prior to its discontinuation after chronic therapy; otherwise, seizures may occur.
- Benzodiazepines are controlled substances and have an abuse and addictive potential.
- Avoid activities that require mental alertness or coordination.

Drug Name	FDA-Approved Indications	Adult Dosage Range	Precautions and Clinical Pearls
Generic Name Clobazam **Brand Name** Onfi ■ (BL) (PD) ■	Lennox-Gastaut syndrome: adjunctive treatment of seizures	**Usual oral dose:** Patients weighing 30 kg or more: 20 mg twice daily (starting dose 5 mg twice daily with gradual increase to 20 mg per dose by day 14)	• Dose should be titrated according to patient tolerability and response • Ethanol: concomitant administration may increase the bioavailability of clobazam by 50% • Monitor: respiratory and mental status/suicidality Associated with: • Certain drug interactions may require dose adjustment or avoidance of some combinations • May cause respiratory suppression
Generic Name Clonazepam **Brand Name** Klonopin ■ (BL) (PD)	Panic disorder Seizure disorder	**Usual oral dose for panic:** 0.25 mg twice daily to 1 mg per day (MDD: 4 mg per day)	• Certain drug interactions may require dose adjustment or avoidance of some combinations Contraindications: • Significant liver disease • Acute narrow-angle glaucoma
Clorazepate	Refer to the Anxiolytic, Sedative, and Hypnotic Agents section.		
Diazepam	Refer to the Anxiolytic, Sedative, and Hypnotic Agents section.		
Lorazepam	Refer to the Anxiolytic, Sedative, and Hypnotic Agents section.		

Hydantoins

Universal prescribing alerts:

- Monitor patients for changes in mood, increased depressive symptoms, and suicidal ideation.
- Watch for drug interactions due to hepatic enzyme inhibition and induction.
- Monitor CBC, hepatic function, and serum concentration (if applicable).
- Rare but serious dermatologic reactions (i.e., Stevens-Johnson syndrome and toxic epidermal necrolysis) have been reported with use.
- Avoid activities that require mental alertness or coordination.
- May cause gingival hyperplasia and osteopenia/osteomalacia.
- Monitor patients for signs of hypothyroidism; may alter circulating thyroid hormone.
- May decrease acetylcholine receptor sensitivity; this action may exacerbate symptoms of myasthenia gravis.

Drug Name	FDA-Approved Indications	Adult Dosage Range	Precautions and Clinical Pearls
Generic Name Ethotoin **Brand Name** Peganone (BL) (PD)	Generalized tonic–clonic or complex partial seizures	**Usual oral dose:** 2 to 3 g per day in divided doses	• Administer after food to decrease GI distress • Administer in 4 to 6 divided doses daily • Certain drug interactions may require dose adjustment or avoidance of some combinations • May cause gingival hyperplasia; ensure good oral hygiene and dental check-ups • Supplement folic acid; may cause folate deficiency megaloblastic anemia • Osteopenia and osteomalacia have been reported Contraindications: • Hepatic abnormalities • Hematologic disorders • Monitor: complete blood count (CBC) and urinalysis (upon initiation of therapy and monthly for several months)
Generic Name Fosphenytoin **Brand Name** Cerebyx ■ (BL) (PD)	Control of generalized tonic–clonic status epilepticus Prevention and treatment of seizures occurring during neurosurgery	**Usual parenteral dose:** IV: Loading dose: 15 to 20 mg PE/kg administered at 100 to 150 mg PE/min Follow loading dose with maintenance doses of either fosphenytoin or phenytoin	• Dose, concentration, and infusion rates for fosphenytoin are expressed as phenytoin equivalents (PE) • Fosphenytoin should always be prescribed and dispensed in phenytoin equivalents; fosphenytoin 1.5 mg is equivalent to phenytoin 1 mg and is referred to as 1 mg PE; this is a prodrug of phenytoin • Certain drug interactions may require dose adjustment or avoidance of some combinations; refer to PI for additional ethnic and genetic variation adjustments • Side effects: dry mouth, nausea, vomiting, fatigue, headache • Monitor: continuous blood pressure, ECG, and respiratory function monitoring with loading dose and for 10 to 20 minutes following infusion • Monitor: vital signs, CBC, hepatic function tests, plasma phenytoin concentration; plasma concentrations should not be measured until conversion to phenytoin is complete, approximately 2 hours after an IV infusion or approximately 4 hours after an IM injection • Use caution in renal and hepatic impairment Contraindications: • Sinus bradycardia • Sinoatrial block • Second- and third-degree atrioventricular (AV) block • Adams-Stokes syndrome Associated with: • Cardiovascular risk associated with rapid infusion rates

Drug Name	FDA-Approved Indications	Adult Dosage Range	Precautions and Clinical Pearls
Generic Name Phenytoin **Brand Name** Dilantin Infatabs Dilantin Phenytek Phenytoin Infatabs ■ (PD)	Control of generalized tonic–clonic and complex partial (psychomotor, temporal lobe) seizures Prevention and treatment of seizures occurring during or following neurosurgery	**Usual parenteral dose:** IV: Loading dose: 10 to 20 mg/kg at a maximum rate of 50 mg per minute **Usual oral maintenance dose:** 100 mg every 6 to 8 hours	• Dosage adjustments and closer serum monitoring may be necessary when switching dosage forms; refer to PI for additional ethnic and genetic variation adjustments • Acute use of ethanol inhibits metabolism of phenytoin and may increase CNS depression; chronic use of ethanol stimulates metabolism of phenytoin • Side effects: dry mouth, nausea, vomiting, fatigue, headache and gingival hyperplasia (gum overgrowth) • May need to supplement with vitamin D • Hypocalcemia has been reported in patients taking prolonged high-dose therapy • Certain drug interactions may require dose adjustment or avoidance of some combinations • Monitor: CBC, liver function, suicidality • Monitor plasma phenytoin concentrations; trough concentrations are generally recommended for routine monitoring; monitoring free (i.e., unbound) phenytoin levels may be helpful in patients with severe renal impairment • Injection site reactions have been reported ("purple glove syndrome") • IV monitoring: continuous cardiac monitoring (rate, rhythm, blood pressure) and observation during administration recommended Contraindications: • Sinus bradycardia • Sinoatrial block • Second- and third-degree heart block • Adams-Stokes syndrome Associated with: • Cardiovascular risk associated with rapid IV infusion

Succinimides

Universal prescribing alerts:

- Avoid activities that require mental alertness or coordination.
- Changes in mood should be monitored and reported, especially increases in depressive symptoms or suicidal ideation.
- Monitor: CBC (dyscrasias have been reported), hepatic function tests, urinalysis; changes in mood or symptoms of suicidality.
- The use of succinimide anticonvulsants has been associated with the development of systemic lupus erythematosus (SLE).

Drug Name	FDA-Approved Indications	Adult Dosage Range	Precautions and Clinical Pearls
Generic Name Ethosuximide **Brand Name** Zarontin (BL) (PD)	Management of absence (petit mal) seizures	**Usual oral dose:** 500 to 1500 mg per day in divided doses	• Target dose to achieve therapeutic range • Increase dietary intake of folate • Taper dosage slowly when discontinuing • Monitor: seizure frequency, trough serum concentrations, platelets, and signs of rash • Hepatic dysfunction has been reported • Monitor renal function potentially fatal nephrotic syndromes have been reported • May exacerbate intermittent porphyria • Certain drug interactions may require dose adjustment or avoidance of some combinations
Generic Name Methsuximide **Brand Name** Celontin (BL) (PD)	Control of absence (petit mal) seizures that are refractory to other drugs	**Usual oral dose:** 1200 mg per day in 2 to 4 divided doses	• Target dose to achieve therapeutic range • Taper dosage slowly when initiating or discontinuing • Certain drug interactions may require dose adjustment or avoidance of some combinations • Use caution in hepatic impairment • May exacerbate intermittent porphyria

Miscellaneous Anticonvulsant Agents

Universal prescribing alerts:

- Monitor for changes in mood or symptoms of suicidality.
- Slowly titrate doses during medication initiation and discontinuation.
- Rare but serious dermatologic reactions may occur (i.e., Stevens-Johnson syndrome); monitor for signs and symptoms of skin reactions.
- Avoid activities that require mental alertness or coordination.

Drug Name	FDA-Approved Indications	Adult Dosage Range	Precautions and Clinical Pearls
Generic Name Carbamazepine	Partial seizures with complex symptomology Mixed seizure patterns Trigeminal neuralgia Glossopharyngeal neuralgia	**Usual oral dose for seizure:** Initial: 200 mg twice per day up to 1600 mg per day in divided doses (recommended dose escalation is 200 mg in weekly increments)	• Dosage must be adjusted according to patient's response and serum concentration • Tablets should be administered in 2 to 3 divided doses per day; suspension should be administered 4 times per day • Take with a large amount of water or food to decrease the risk of GI upset • Certain drug interactions may require dose adjustment or avoidance of some combinations • Observe patient for excessive sedation

Drug Name	FDA-Approved Indications	Adult Dosage Range	Precautions and Clinical Pearls
Brand Name Carbatrol Epitol Equetro Tegretol Tegretol-XR ■ (BL) (PD)	Acute manic or mixed episodes associated with bipolar disorder		• Monitor: CBC with platelet count and differential, reticulocytes, serum iron, lipid panel, LFTs, urinalysis, blood urea nitrogen (BUN), serum carbamazepine levels, thyroid function tests, serum sodium and ophthalmic exams • Has been associated with serious rash (sometimes life-threatening) including Stevens Johnson; patients are also at increased risk for sunburn; avoid sun and use appropriate precautions Contraindications: • Bone marrow depression Associated with: • Increased risk of dermatologic side effects in patients with HLA-B*1502; patients with Asian ancestry are at increased risk and should receive HLA-B*1502 genotype screening prior to therapy initiation • Aplastic anemia and agranulocytosis have been reported
Generic Name Eslicarbazepine **Brand Name** Aptiom ▲ (BL)	Partial-onset seizures (monotherapy or adjunct therapy)	**Usual oral dose:** 800 to 1600 mg daily	• Do not use with oxcarbazepine • Monitor: LFTs, serum sodium and chloride, symptoms of CNS depression (dizziness, gait disturbances, somnolence), visual changes
Generic Name Ezogabine **Brand Name** Potiga ▲ ■ ■ (GD)	Partial-onset seizures Adjunctive treatment for partial-onset seizures in patients who have responded inadequately to several alternative treatments and for whom the benefits outweigh the risk of retinal abnormalities and potential decline in visual acuity	**Usual oral dose:** 200 to 400 mg 3 times per day (MDD: 1200 mg per day)	• Gradually reduce dose over at least 3 weeks unless safety concerns require abrupt withdrawal • Monitor: seizures; electrolytes, bilirubin, QT interval, renal and hepatic function; urologic symptoms • Observe for excessive sedation, confusion, psychotic symptoms, and hallucinations; changes in mood or symptoms of suicidality; skin discoloration around the lips, nail beds of fingers or toes, face, and legs • Perform ophthalmic exams at baseline and 6-month intervals; fluorescein angiograms, optical coherence tomography, perimetry, and electroretinograms may also be considered • Certain drug interactions may require dose adjustment or avoidance of some combinations Associated with: • Retinal abnormalities and potential vision loss
Generic Name Felbamate	Monotherapy or adjunctive therapy in the treatment of partial seizures (with and without generalization)	**Usual oral dose:** 1200 to 3600 mg per day in 3 to 4 divided doses	• Not indicated for use as first-line treatment • Monitor: serum levels of concomitant anticonvulsant therapy; obtain transaminases (AST, ALT) levels before initiation of therapy and regularly thereafter • Obtain hematologic evaluations before therapy begins, frequently during therapy, and for a significant period after discontinuation

Brand Name Felbatol ■ (BL) (PD)	Adjunctive therapy in the treatment of partial and generalized seizures associated with Lennox-Gastaut syndrome		• Monitor for changes in mood or symptoms of suicidality • Certain drug interactions may require dose adjustment or avoidance of some combinations • May be administered with or without food • Shake suspension prior to use Contraindications: • Hepatic dysfunction • History of any blood dyscrasia Associated with: • Aplastic anemia • Acute liver failure
Generic Name Gabapentin **Brand Name** Gralise Gralise Starter Neurontin ▲ (BL) (PD)	**Common indications for use:** Postherpetic neuralgia Seizures, partial onset (excluding Gralise): as adjunctive therapy in the treatment of partial seizures with and without secondary generalization	**Usual dose for seizures:** 900 to 1800 mg per day administered in 3 divided doses	• Gralise should be taken with food • Formulations are not interchangeable; refer to PI for product details • Monitor for renal and hepatic impairment; dose adjustments may be warranted if they occur • Avoid extended release formulations in patients with severe renal impairment • Monitor serum levels of concomitant anticonvulsant therapy • See PI for age-specific indications
Generic Name Lacosamide **Brand Name** Vimpat ▲ ■ (BL)	Partial-onset seizures: monotherapy or adjunctive therapy in the treatment of partial-onset seizures	**Usual dose:** Monotherapy: Oral/IV: 150 to 200 mg twice daily Adjunctive therapy: Oral/IV: 100 to 200 mg twice daily (MDD: 400 mg per day)	• Administer loading doses under medical supervision because of the increased incidence of CNS adverse reactions • Certain drug interactions may require dose adjustment or avoidance of some combinations • Dose adjustment required in patients with mild to moderate hepatic impairment • Monitor: patients with conduction problems, sodium channelopathies, and concomitant medications that prolong PR interval or severe cardiac disease; these patients should have ECG tracing prior to the start of therapy and when at steady state • Monitor patients closely during IV infusions; cases of bradycardia and AV block have occurred during infusions • Monitor for changes in mood or symptoms of suicidality

Drug Name	FDA-Approved Indications	Adult Dosage Range	Precautions and Clinical Pearls
Generic Name Lamotrigine **Brand Name** Lamictal ■ ■ (BL) (PD)	Bipolar I disorder (IR only) Epilepsy	**Illustrative oral dose for seizures:** IR: 225 to 375 mg per day in 2 divided doses ER: 300 to 400 mg once daily	• Dose titration is available in specific starter regimens for patients concomitantly taking enzyme-inducing antiepileptics, valproic acid, or polypharmacy • Certain drug interactions may require dose adjustment or avoidance of some combinations • If the medication is discontinued for more than 5 half-lives (approximately 5 days for monotherapy; approximately 2 days if used with enzyme-inducing antiepileptic drugs), it may require titrating with the initial schedule • Monitor: serum levels of concurrent anticonvulsants, LFTs, renal function, hypersensitivity reactions (especially rash), seizure frequency and duration, changes in mood or symptoms of suicidality, signs/symptoms of aseptic meningitis Associated with: • Serious skin rashes (Stevens-Johnson syndrome, toxic epidermal necrolysis)
Generic Name Levetiracetam **Brand Name** Keppra Keppra XR Roweepra Spritam ▲ (BL) (PD)	Myoclonic seizures: adjunctive therapy in the treatment of myoclonic seizures in adults and adolescents 12 years and older with juvenile myoclonic epilepsy Partial-onset seizures Primary generalized tonic–clonic seizures	**Illustrative dose:** Oral/IV: 1500 mg twice daily	• Monitor renal function; dose adjustment is required for patients with renal impairment • Monitor CNS depression: impaired coordination, ataxia, abnormal gait, weakness, fatigue, dizziness, somnolence • Monitor psychiatric and behavioral symptoms: aggression, agitation, anger, anxiety, apathy, confusion, depersonalization, depression, emotional lability, hostility, hyperkinesias, irritability, nervousness, neurosis, suicidal thoughts, personality disorder
Generic Name Magnesium sulfate **Brand Name** Epsom Salt ▲ (PD)	Laxative for the relief of occasional constipation (OTC labeling) Treatment and prevention of hypomagnesemia Prevention and treatment of seizures in severe pre-eclampsia or eclampsia Pediatric acute nephritis Cardiac arrhythmias (ventricular tachycardia/fibrillation) caused by hypomagnesemia Soaking aid for minor cuts and bruises (OTC labeling)	No optimal dosing regimen for treatment of seizures	• In case of IV rapid administration, monitor ECG, vital signs, and deep tendon reflexes • Monitor magnesium concentrations if frequent or prolonged dosing is required, particularly in patients with renal dysfunction, calcium, and potassium concentrations • Monitor renal function • Magnesium sulfate and elemental magnesium dosing equivalency information is available in the PI Contraindications: • Heart block; myocardial damage

Generic Name Oxcarbazepine **Brand Name** Oxtellar XR Trileptal ▲ (BL) (PD)	Partial seizures Monotherapy or adjunctive therapy in the treatment of partial seizures (IR) Adjunctive therapy in the treatment of partial seizures (ER)	**Illustrative oral dose for adjunct treatment:** ER: 1200 to 2400 mg once per day	• Thyroid function tests; may depress serum T4 without affecting T3 levels or thyroid-stimulating hormone (TSH) • May cause hyponatremia • Monitor: seizure frequency; serum sodium (particularly during first 3 months of therapy), thyroid function tests and CBC, behavioral changes, symptoms of CNS depression and suicidality, serum levels of concomitant antiepileptic drugs during titration as necessary • Certain drug interactions may require dose adjustment or avoidance of some combinations
Generic Name Perampanel **Brand Name** Fycompa ▲ ■ ■ (PD)	Partial-onset seizures (adjunct) Primary generalized tonic–clonic seizures (adjunct)	**Usual oral dose:** 8 to 12 mg per day at bedtime	• Monitor renal and hepatic function; dose adjustment is required for patients with renal or hepatic impairment • Certain drug interactions may require dose adjustment or avoidance of some combinations • Monitor seizure frequency • Monitor suicidality during therapy and for at least 1 month after discontinuation • Monitor weight Associated with: • Serious or life-threatening psychiatric and behavioral adverse effects
Generic Name Pregabalin **Brand Name** Lyrica ▲ (BL)	Management of neuropathic pain associated with diabetic peripheral neuropathy or with spinal cord injury Management of postherpetic neuralgia Adjunctive therapy for partial-onset seizure disorder Management of fibromyalgia	**Usual oral dose for seizures and/or neuropathic pain:** 150 mg per day in divided doses (MDD: 600 mg per day)	• Monitor renal function; dose adjustment is required for patients with renal impairment • Monitor: measures of efficacy (pain intensity/seizure frequency); degree of sedation; symptoms of myopathy or ocular disturbance; weight gain/edema; skin integrity (in patients with diabetes); suicidality • DEA-controlled substance
Generic Name Rufinamide **Brand Name** Banzel (QT) (BL) (PD)	Lennox-Gastaut syndrome: adjunctive treatment of seizures associated with this syndrome	**Usual oral dose:** 400 to 800 mg per day (MDD: 3200 mg per day in divided doses)	• Take with food • Monitor: seizures (frequency and duration); serum levels of concurrent anticonvulsants; suicidality; rash (may indicate multiorgan hypersensitivity reactions) • Certain drug interactions may require dose adjustment or avoidance of some combinations • See PI for age-specific indications for use Contraindications: • Familial short QT syndrome

Drug Name	FDA-Approved Indications	Adult Dosage Range	Precautions and Clinical Pearls
Generic Name Tiagabine **Brand Name** Gabitril (BL) (PD)	Partial seizures: adjunct therapy	**Illustrative oral dose:** 32 to 56 mg per day	• Target trough concentration of 50–250 nmol/L has been suggested • Administer with food • Not recommended for use in patients with severe hepatic impairment • Monitor: seizure frequency, LFTs (periodically), suicidality • Do not use a loading dose, rapid titration, or large dose increments • Certain drug interactions may require dose adjustment or avoidance of some combinations • See PI for age-specific indications for use
Generic Name Topiramate **Brand Name** Qudexy XR Topamax Topamax Sprinkle Trokendi XR ▲ (PD)	Epilepsy Monotherapy: partial-onset or primary generalized tonic–clonic seizures Adjunctive therapy: partial-onset seizures, primary generalized tonic–clonic seizures, or seizures associated with Lennox-Gastaut syndrome Migraine (IR only)	**Usual oral dose for adjunctive therapy:** IR: 200 mg twice daily ER: 400 mg once daily	• Ketogenic diet may increase the possibility of acidosis and kidney stones; use extreme caution in patients with renal impairment • Monitor: seizure frequency; hydration status; electrolytes and serum creatinine; symptoms of acute and long-term acidosis; ammonia level in patients with unexplained lethargy, vomiting, or mental status changes; intraocular pressure; suicidality; weight and eating behaviors; increased bleeding has been reported in some patients • Altered temperature regulation has been reported with use; stay well hydrated and avoid extreme temperatures Contraindications: • Extended release: recent alcohol use (within 6 hours prior to and 6 hours after administration) • Certain drug interactions may require dose adjustment or avoidance of some combinations (i.e., metabolic acidosis with concomitant use of metformin)
Generic Name Valproate/divalproex **Brand Name** Depakene Depakote Depakote ER Stavzor ■ (BL)	Complex partial seizures; simple and complex absence seizures Adjunct therapy in patients with multiple seizure types that include absence seizures Mania associated with bipolar disorder Migraine prophylaxis	**Usual oral dose:** 10 to 15 mg/kg per day (500 to 2000 mg per day; MDD: 60 mg/kg per day) **Usual IV dose:** Equivalent to the total oral daily dose	• Divide doses higher than 250 mg per day and increase dose slowly to minimize GI upset • Take with food • Side effects: headache, nausea, vomiting, dizziness, fatigue, constipation, diarrhea, abdominal pain, weight changes, hair loss • Monitor: liver enzymes, prothrombin time (PT)/partial thromboplastin time (PTT), serum ammonia, suicidality, motor and cognitive function, CBC with platelets, thyroid function • Certain drug interactions may require dose adjustment or avoidance of some combinations Associated with: • Hepatic failure • Specific alerts for women of childbearing age • Pancreatitis

Generic Name Vigabatrin **Brand Name** Sabril ▲ ■ (BL) (PD)	Refractory complex partial seizures (adjunct)	**Usual oral dose:** 1.5 g twice daily	• Available only through SHARE: a special restricted program under a risk evaluation and mitigation strategy • Reserved for patients who have inadequately responded to several alternative antiepileptic medications • Monitor: ophthalmologic examination at baseline and per guidelines available in the package insert • Monitor for excessive sedation and changes to hemoglobin and hematocrit Associated with: • Permanent bilateral concentric visual field constriction and blindness • Requires experienced clinician who is knowledgeable in the use of this agent and specialized-care setting
Generic Name Zonisamide **Brand Name** Zonegran (BL)	Partial seizures (adjunct)	**Usual oral dose:** 100 to 400 mg per day	• Monitor: metabolic profile, serum creatinine, BUN, serum bicarbonate, suicidality, decreased sweating, elevated body temperature • Side effects: asthenia, headache, lack of appetite, diarrhea, insomnia • Certain drug interactions may require dose adjustment or avoidance of some combinations
Acetazolamide	Refer to the Eye, Ear, Nose, and Throat Preparations chapter.		

Psychotherapeutic Agents

Antidepressant Agents

Monoamine Oxidase Inhibitors

Universal prescribing alerts:

- Use antidepressants with caution in patients with underlying cardiovascular disease or any condition (including concurrent medications that cause same adverse effect) that increases the risk of a prolonged QTc interval.
- The FDA labeling of all antidepressants carry a black box warning for suicidality.
- Monitor blood glucose; blood pressure and heart rate; diet and weight; and mood, suicidal ideation, or unusual behavior (especially during the initial months of therapy or when doses are increased or decreased). Additional monitoring may be warranted based on the patient's specific medical conditions.
- Avoid tyramine-rich foods and concurrent use of sympathomimetics (and other drugs with MAOI-like actions). Numerous serious drug interactions have been noted.
- At least 2 weeks should elapse between the discontinuation of other serotoninergic agents. Specific agents, such as fluoxetine, may require longer periods prior to their initiation.
- Universal prescribing alerts for all CNS depressants include: These medications may cause drowsiness or dizziness, so patients should use caution while driving or operating machinery until the effects of the drug are known.

Drug Name	FDA-Approved Indications	Adult Dosage Range	Precautions and Clinical Pearls
Generic Name Phenelzine **Brand Name** Nardil ■ (GD)	Depression	**Usual oral dose:** 60 to 90 mg per day	• May alter insulin sensitivity; monitor blood glucose in patients with diabetes Contraindications: • Congestive heart failure • Pheochromocytoma • Abnormal LFTs or history of hepatic disease • Renal disease or severe renal disease/impairment • Should not undergo elective surgery requiring general anesthesia; refer to PI for further detail
Generic Name Tranylcypromine **Brand Name** Parnate ■	Depression	**Usual oral dose:** 30 mg per day in 2 divided doses (MDD: 60 mg per day)	• Anticholinergic universal prescribing alerts apply Contraindications: • Cardiovascular disease (including hypertension) • Cerebrovascular defect • History of headache • History of hepatic disease or abnormal LFTs • Pheochromocytoma
Rasagiline	Refer to the Antiparkinsonian Agents section.		
Selegiline	Refer to the Antiparkinsonian Agents section.		
Selective Serotonin–Norepinephrine Reuptake Inhibitors			
Universal prescribing alerts: • The FDA labels of all antidepressants carry a black box warning for suicidality. • Monitor blood glucose; blood pressure and heart rate (QTc); diet and weight; and mood, suicidal ideation, or unusual behavior (especially during the initial months of therapy or when doses are increased or decreased). • Additional monitoring may be warranted based on the patient's specific medical conditions (i.e., increased bleeding risk) and intraocular pressure in those patients with baseline elevations or a history of glaucoma. • Hyponatremia has occurred during treatment with serotonergic antidepressants and may be the result of the syndrome of inappropriate antidiuretic hormone secretion (SIADH). • Use SNRIs with caution in patients with underlying cardiovascular disease or any condition (including concurrent use of medications that cause the same adverse effect) that increases the risk of prolonged QTc. • All CNS depressants may cause drowsiness or dizziness. Patients should use caution while driving or operating machinery until the effects of the drug are known. Numerous serious drug interactions have been noted. • Platelet aggregation may be impaired by serotonin and serotonin norepinephrine reuptake inhibitors (SSRIs, SNRIs) due to platelet serotonin depletion, possibly increasing the risk of a bleeding complication (i.e., gastrointestinal bleeding, hematomas, hemorrhage). Concurrent use of other medications (or other patient specific factors) that enhance bleeding potential may increase this risk. Patients should be instructed to promptly report any bleeding events to their healthcare professional.			

- Avoid concurrent serotonergic agents to reduce risk of serotonin syndrome.
- When discontinuing these agents, dose should be tapered to avoid withdrawal syndrome.

Drug Name	FDA-Approved Indications	Adult Dosage Range	Precautions and Clinical Pearls
Generic Name Desvenlafaxine **Brand Name** Pristiq Khedezla ▲ ■ ■ (BL)	Major depressive disorder	**Usual oral dose:** 50 mg once daily	• Administer at approximately the same time each day, with or without food • Drug interactions may require dose adjustment or avoidance of certain drug combinations • May interfere with urine detection of phencyclidine and amphetamine (false-positive) • Monitor: renal function for dosing purposes; lipid panel (i.e., total cholesterol, low-density lipoprotein [LDL], triglycerides)
Generic Name Duloxetine **Brand Name** Cymbalta Irenka ■ (BL) (PD)	Major depressive disorder Diabetic peripheral neuropathic pain Fibromyalgia (except Irenka) Generalized anxiety disorder Chronic musculoskeletal pain OA	**Usual oral dose:** 20 mg twice daily; may increase dose to 30 mg twice daily or give 60 mg once daily (MDD: 120 mg daily)	• Administer without regard to meals • Use with caution in patients where weight loss is undesirable (i.e., anorexia) • Do not sprinkle contents on chocolate pudding • Monitor: creatinine, BUN, transaminases • Consider adherence when deciding on once or twice daily dose options • Do not use in patients with severe renal impairment (i.e., CrCl less than 30 mL/min) • Not recommended for use in patients with hepatic impairment • May cause urinary retention and orthostatic hypotension Contraindications: • Uncontrolled closed-angle glaucoma
Generic Name Levomilnacipran **Brand Name** Fetzima Fetzima Titration ▲ ■ (BL)	Major depressive disorder	**Usual oral dose:** 20 mg once daily; may increase dose by 40 mg per day no sooner than every 2 days based on patient's response (MDD: 120 mg per day)	• Administer with or without food at approximately the same time each day • Drug interactions may require dose adjustment or avoidance of certain drug combinations • Avoid alcohol: ethanol may accelerate drug release by interacting with extended-release properties • Avoid use in patients undergoing dialysis and in those prone to obstructive urinary disorders • Seizures have been reported Contraindications: • Uncontrolled closed-angle glaucoma

Drug Name	FDA-Approved Indications	Adult Dosage Range	Precautions and Clinical Pearls
Generic Name Venlafaxine **Brand Name** Effexor XR ▲ ■ QT ■ BL	Major depressive disorder Generalized anxiety disorder Panic disorder Social anxiety disorder	Dosage varies on indication for use and formulation prescribed **Usual oral dose for depression:** IR tablets: 75 mg per day, administered in 2 or 3 divided doses; may increase by 75 mg per day no sooner than every 4 days as tolerated; usual dosage: 75 to 225 mg per day XR: 75 mg once daily; may increase to no more than 75 mg per day no sooner than every 4 days as tolerated; usual dosage: 75 to 225 mg per day (some patients may require a 37.5 mg starting dose)	• Administer with food • Contents of ER capsules may be mixed in applesauce and swallowed immediately without chewing • Administer the XR formulation in the morning or evening at the same time each day; many indications for use are specific to the XR formulation • May interfere with urine detection of phencyclidine and amphetamine (false-positives) • May cause increase in heart rate, blood pressure elevated cholesterol or hyponatremia • Patients may be switched to the XR formulation at the nearest equivalent dose to the IR formulation (mg per day) • Maximum dose limits are higher for hospitalized patients
Milnacipran	Refer to the Analgesic and Antipyretic Agents section.		
Selective Serotonin Reuptake Inhibitors			

Universal prescribing alerts:

- The FDA labeling of all antidepressants carry a black box warning for suicidality.
- All CNS depressants may cause drowsiness or dizziness. Patients should use caution while driving or operating machinery until the effects of the drug are known. Numerous serious drug interactions have been noted.
- Monitor blood glucose, blood pressure and heart rate (QTc); diet and weight; and mood, suicide ideation, or unusual behavior (especially during the initial months of therapy or when doses are increased or decreased). Additional monitoring may be warranted based on the patient's specific medical conditions (i.e., increased bleeding risk), seizures, and intraocular pressure in those patients with baseline elevations or a history of glaucoma.
- Use SSRIs with caution in patients with underlying cardiovascular disease or any condition (including concurrent use of medications that cause the same adverse effect) that increases the risk of prolonged QTc.
- Use caution in patients with closed-angle glaucoma. The pupillary dilation that can occur with antidepressants may precipitate a closed-angle glaucoma attack in certain predisposed patients.
- Consider more frequent monitoring of bone density during long-term use of an SSRI; osteopenia/osteoporosis has been reported.
- Avoid concurrent serotonergic agents to reduce risk of serotonin syndrome.

- Hyponatremia has occurred during treatment with serotonergic antidepressants and may be the result of the SIADH.
- Platelet aggregation may be impaired by serotonin and serotonin norepinephrine reuptake inhibitors (SSRIs, SNRIs) due to platelet serotonin depletion, possibly increasing the risk of a bleeding complication (i.e., gastrointestinal bleeding, hematomas, hemorrhage). Concurrent use of other medications (or other patient-specific factors) that enhance bleeding potential may increase this risk. Patients should be instructed to promptly report any bleeding events to the practitioner.
- When discontinuing these agents, dose should be tapered to avoid withdrawal syndrome.

Drug Name	FDA-Approved Indications	Adult Dosage Range	Precautions and Clinical Pearls
Generic Name Citalopram **Brand Name** Celexa ■ ■ QT BL PD GD	Depression	**Usual oral dose for depression in adults less than 60 years old:** 20 mg once daily; may increase to maximum dose of 40 mg per day	• Doses greater than 40 mg daily are not recommended due to the risk of QTc prolongation • May be administered without regard to food • GI side effects are usually transient and will stop after 1 to 2 weeks of use • Monitor: signs of hyponatremia (has been infrequently reported), increased bleeding times, and sexual dysfunction • Monitor: ECG; patients are at increased risk for QT-prolonging effects if they have certain conditions • Certain drug interactions may require dose adjustment or avoidance of some combinations; refer to PI for additional ethnic and genetic variation adjustments
Generic Name Escitalopram **Brand Name** Lexapro ■ ■ QT BL PD GD	Major depressive disorder Generalized anxiety disorder	**Usual oral dose for depression:** 10 mg once daily; dose may be increased to a maximum of 20 mg once daily after at least 1 week	• May be taken with or without food • Escitalopram is the active enantiomer of citalopram • Specific guidelines for dosage adjustments of escitalopram in patients with severe renal impairment are not available; however, there is potential for reduced clearance and escitalopram should be dosed cautiously
Generic Name Fluoxetine **Brand Name** Prozac Sarafem ■ QT BL PD GD	Major depressive disorder Bulimia nervosa Obsessive–compulsive disorder Premenstrual dysphoric disorder Panic disorder Bipolar depression (in combination with olanzapine)	**Usual oral dose for depression:** Initial: 20 mg per day; may increase after several weeks if inadequate response (MDD: 80 mg per day) Lower doses have been used for initial treatment; goal dose varies based on indication for use	• The elimination half-life of fluoxetine is prolonged in patients with hepatic impairment • Available in numerous dosage formulations, including a once-weekly dosage • Patients maintained on 20 mg per day may be changed to the 90 mg once-weekly formulation • When converting to the once-weekly dose formulation, begin 7 days after the last daily dose

Drug Name	FDA-Approved Indications	Adult Dosage Range	Precautions and Clinical Pearls
Generic Name Fluvoxamine ■ QT BL PD	Obsessive–compulsive disorder	**Usual oral dose:** IR: 50 mg once daily at bedtime; may be increased in 50-mg increments at 4- to 7-day intervals, as tolerated; usual dose range: 100 to 300 mg per day (MDD: 300 mg per day) ER: 100 mg once daily at bedtime; may be increased in 50-mg increments at intervals of at least 1 week; usual dosage range: 100 to 300 mg per day (MDD: 300 mg per day)	• May be administered with or without food • Administer total daily doses greater than 100 mg per day in divided doses; if the doses are unequal, give the larger dose at bedtime • Lower doses may be required for patients with hepatic impairment; however, no specific recommendations are available • Cigarette smoking increases the metabolism of fluvoxamine by 25% and may decrease the effectiveness of this agent • Drug interactions may require dose adjustment or avoidance of certain drug combinations
Generic Name Paroxetine **Brand Name** Brisdelle Paxil Pexeva ▲ ■ ■ BL PD GD	Major depressive disorder Generalized anxiety disorder Obsessive–compulsive disorder Panic disorder Post-traumatic stress disorder Premenstrual dysphoric disorder Social anxiety disorder Vasomotor symptoms of menopause	**Usual oral dose for depression:** 20 mg once daily; increase if needed by 10 mg per day increments of no less than weekly (MDD: 50 mg per day) Paxil CR: 25 mg once daily; increase if needed by 12.5 mg per day increments of no less than weekly (MDD: 62.5 mg per day)	• May be taken without regard to meals, preferably in the morning • Formulation-specific indications for use (e.g., Brisdelle for hot flashes) • Anticholinergic universal prescribing alerts are associated with this agent • Monitor for sedation
Generic Name Sertraline **Brand Name** Zoloft ■ BL PD	Major depressive disorder Obsessive–compulsive disorder Panic disorder Post-traumatic stress disorder Premenstrual dysphoric disorder Social anxiety disorder	**Usual oral dose for depression:** Initial: 50 mg per day; may increase daily dose, at intervals of not less than 1 week, to a maximum of 200 mg per day	• Administer once daily either in the morning or in the evening; if somnolence is noted, administer at bedtime • May interfere with urine detection of benzodiazepines (false-positive) • Certain drug interactions may require dose adjustment or avoidance of some combinations • Use caution in patients with diabetes. Decreased blood glucose and increase insulin sensitivity has been reported (dose adjustments of hypoglycemics may be necessary)

Serotonin Modulators

Universal prescribing alerts:

- The FDA labeling of all antidepressants carry a black box warning for suicidality.
- Monitor blood glucose; blood pressure and heart rate (QTc); diet and weight; and mood, suicidal ideation, or unusual behavior (especially during the initial months of therapy or when doses are increased or decreased).
- Use serotonin modulators with caution in patients with underlying cardiovascular disease or any condition (including concurrent use of medications that cause the same adverse effect) that increases the risk of prolonged QTc.
- All CNS depressants may cause drowsiness or dizziness. Patients should use caution while driving or operating machinery until the effects of the drug are known. Seizure threshold may be lowered and numerous serious drug interactions have been reported.
- Use caution in patients with glaucoma; antidepressants may precipitate a closed-angle glaucoma attack in certain patients
- Certain drug interactions may require dose adjustment or avoidance of some combinations.
- Hyponatremia has occurred during treatment with serotonergic antidepressants and may be the result of the SIADH.
- Avoid concurrent serotonergic agents to reduce risk of serotonin syndrome.
- When discontinuing these agents, dose should be tapered to avoid withdrawal syndrome.

Drug Name	FDA-Approved Indications	Adult Dosage Range	Precautions and Clinical Pearls
Generic Name Nefazodone ■ GD	Major depressive disorder	**Usual oral dose:** 100 mg twice daily	• Increase in increments of 100 to 200 mg per day at weekly intervals as tolerated and needed • Seizures have been reported • Avoid in patients with hepatic impairment or who may be at higher risk of hepatic impairment Associated with: • Hepatotoxicity and hepatic failure • Age-specific contraindication; refer to PI
Generic Name Trazodone **Brand Name** Oleptro ■ QT PD	Major depressive disorder	**Usual oral dose:** IR: 150 mg per day in divided doses; may increase by 50 mg per day every 3 to 4 days (MDD: 400 mg per day) ER: 150 mg once daily at bedtime; may increase by 75 mg per day every 3 days (MDD: 375 mg per day)	• IR tablet: dosing after meals may decrease lightheadedness and postural hypotension • ER: take on an empty stomach; swallow whole or as a half-tablet without food • Among the more sedating antidepressants, but has few anticholinergic effects • May interfere with urine detection of amphetamine/methamphetamine (false-positive) • Higher maximum doses may be used for inpatients under direct medical supervision • Patients with hepatic impairment may require lower doses; however, no specific recommendations are available

Drug Name	FDA-Approved Indications	Adult Dosage Range	Precautions and Clinical Pearls
Generic Name Vilazodone **Brand Name** Viibryd ■	Major depressive disorder	**Usual oral dose:** 10 mg once daily for 7 days, then increase to 20 mg once daily; may increase up to 40 mg once daily after a minimum of 7 days based on response and tolerability (MDD: 40 mg per day)	• Administer with food to improve absorption • Gradual taper is recommended for all antidepressant discontinuations; however, the manufacturer recommends a specific taper for vilazodone • Drug interactions may require dose adjustments or avoidance of certain drug combinations
Generic Name Vortioxetine **Brand Name** Trintellix ■	Major depressive disorder	**Usual oral dose:** 10 mg once daily; increase to 20 mg once daily as tolerated; consider 5 mg once daily for patients who do not tolerate higher doses (MDD: 20 mg per day)	• Administer without regard to meals • Certain drug interactions may require dose adjustment or avoidance of some combinations; refer to PI for additional ethnic and genetic variation adjustments
Tricyclic Antidepressants and Other Norepinephrine-Reuptake Inhibitors			
Universal prescribing alerts: • The FDA labeling of all antidepressants carry a black box warning for suicidality. • Monitor: blood pressure and heart rate (QTc); diet and weight; and mood, suicidal ideation, or unusual behavior (especially during the initial months of therapy or when doses are increased or decreased). • Additional monitoring may be warranted based on the patient's specific medical conditions (i.e., increased bleeding risk). LFTs should be performed and drug discontinuation considered if there is persistent elevation of liver enzymes. • Use TCAs with caution in patients with underlying cardiovascular disease, cardiac conduction defects, or any condition (including concurrent use of medications that cause the same adverse effect) that increases the risk of prolonged QTc leading to complete cardiac collapse and sudden death. Use with caution in patients with cardiac conditions (some contraindications exist). Obtain a baseline ECG in older adults and patients with a cardiac history. Cigarette smoking may decrease the effectiveness of some TCAs. • Contraindications include patients in the acute recovery phase following myocardial infarction. • All CNS depressants may cause drowsiness or dizziness. Patients should use caution while driving or operating machinery until the effects of the drug are known. Numerous serious drug interactions have been noted. • Due to the potential anticholinergic side effects of TCAs (e.g., dry eyes, constipation, worsening of benign prostatic hyperplasia [BPH], glaucoma, reduced sweating and temperature regulation), use standard anticholinergic precautions in patients with conditions that can be worsened with these side effects. • Patients may experience greater sun sensitivity when taking TCAs and should be counseled on precautions during treatment. • Blood dyscrasias have been reported with TCAs, so use these agents cautiously in patients who are predisposed to or have current hematologic disease. • TCAs may increase the risk of seizure and hypertensive episodes; they may require temporary discontinuation prior to elective surgery or injection of radiocontrast, for example. • Use with caution in patients with diabetes and monitor their glucose levels closely; TCAs may increase or decrease serum glucose. • Certain drug interactions may require dose adjustment or avoidance of some combinations. There are suggested therapeutic plasma concentration ranges for most TCAs. Plasma concentration monitoring should be considered in patients with an inadequate response or excessive adverse effects. • TCAs may worsen extrapyramidal symptoms (EPS) and involuntary movements, which appear to be similar to tardive dyskinesia, can occur.			

Drug Name	FDA-Approved Indications	Adult Dosage Range	Precautions and Clinical Pearls
Generic Name Amitriptyline **Brand Name** Elavil ■ QT BL PD GD	Depression	**Usual oral dose:** 75 mg per day in divided doses or 50 to 100 mg at bedtime (MDD: 150 mg per day)	• Administer higher doses preferably in the late afternoon or at bedtime to minimize daytime sedation • Use with caution in patients with hepatic impairment, who may require lower doses; discontinue with persistent elevation of LFTs • Higher doses may be used for hospitalized inpatients • Use standard anticholinergic precautions • May cause sun sensitivity • Amitriptyline is metabolized to nortriptyline • May administer without regard to meals
Generic Name Amoxapine **Brand Name** Asendin ■ QT BL GD	Depression	**Usual oral dose:** 50 mg administered 2 to 3 times per day; doses may be increased to 100 mg by the end of the first week based on response and tolerability; doses greater than 300 mg daily should be divided (MDD: 400 mg per day)	• Higher doses may be used for hospitalized inpatients • Dosages greater than 300 mg per day should be given in divided doses and should be used only if lower doses have been ineffective for at least 2 weeks • Use caution in patients with hepatic impairment • May precipitate psychotic symptoms in some individuals • May be administered without regard to meals • The entire daily dose may be administered at one time, preferably at bedtime, provided the dose does not exceed 300 mg • Movement disorder assessment is recommended prior to the first dose and then every 3 to 6 months thereafter
Generic Name Clomipramine **Brand Name** Anafranil ■ QT BL PD	Obsessive–compulsive disorder	**Usual oral dose:** 25 mg per day; may gradually increase as tolerated over the first 2 weeks to approximately 100 mg daily in divided doses; may further increase the dose over the next several weeks up to a maximum of 250 mg per day	• During titration, may divide doses and administer with meals to decrease gastrointestinal side effects • After titration, may administer total daily dose at bedtime to decrease daytime sedation • Monitor for increased glucose; may interfere with urine detection of methadone (false-positive) • Agranulocytosis has been reported, though it is rare • Patients with hepatic impairment may require lower doses; however, no specific recommendation is available
Generic Name Desipramine **Brand Name** Norpramin ■ BL GD	Depression	**Usual oral dose:** 50 to 75 mg once daily or in divided doses; increase dose based on tolerance and response up to 100 to 200 mg once daily	• Patients may experience excitation or stimulation; in such cases, administer as a single morning dose or divided dose • Higher doses may be used for hospitalized inpatients • May interfere with urine detection of amphetamines/methamphetamines (false-positive) • Patients with hepatic impairment may require lower doses; however, no specific recommendation is available • Active metabolite of imipramine

Drug Name	FDA-Approved Indications	Adult Dosage Range	Precautions and Clinical Pearls
Generic Name Doxepin **Brand Name** Silenor Zonalon □ ■ QT BL	Depression Anxiety Insomnia (Silenor only) Eczematous dermatitis (Zonalon topical only)	**Usual oral dose for depression:** 75 mg as a single dose at bedtime or in divided doses; gradually increase dose based on response and tolerability to a usual dose of 100 to 300 mg per day Silenor: maximum dose is 6 mg per day	• Administer the total daily dosage in divided doses or on a once-daily dosage schedule • Higher doses may be used for hospitalized patients • If the once-daily schedule is employed, the maximum recommended dose is 150 mg once daily at bedtime • Silenor should not be taken during or within 3 hours of a meal • Patients with hepatic impairment may require lower doses (though no specific recommendation is available Contraindications: • In patients predisposed to urinary retention (e.g., bladder obstruction, BPH or renal disease) • Use of doxepin cream in patients with severe BPH due to the presence of significant plasma levels after topical application of the drug
Generic Name Imipramine **Brand Name** Tofranil ■ QT PD GD	Depression Enuresis	**Usual oral dose:** Initial: 75 mg per day; may increase gradually to 150 mg per day; may be given in divided doses or as a single bedtime dose (MDD: 200 mg per day)	• Higher doses may be used for hospitalized inpatients • Imipramine is metabolized to desipramine, its active metabolite • Patients with hepatic impairment may require lower doses (though no specific recommendation is available)
Generic Name Maprotiline ■ BL PD	Major depressive disorder Anxiety	**Usual oral dose:** 75 mg once daily or in divided doses; increase gradually in 25 mg increments after 2 weeks based on response and tolerability up to a maximum dose of 150 mg per day	• Higher initial and maximum doses may be considered for use in severely depressed hospitalized patients • Lower dosages are recommended for adults older than 60 years to lessen adverse effects • Patients with hepatic impairment may require lower doses (though no specific recommendation is available) Contraindications: • Patients at increased risk of seizure
Generic Name Nortriptyline **Brand Name** Pamelor □ ■ QT BL PD	Depression	**Usual oral dose:** 25 to 50 mg per day as a single or divided dose; adjust dose based on response and tolerability up to a maximum dose of 150 mg per day	• Total daily doses may be given once daily • Use caution in patients with hepatic impairment

Drug Name	FDA-Approved Indications	Adult Dosage Range	Precautions and Clinical Pearls
Generic Name Protriptyline **Brand Name** Vivactil ■ QT BL PD GD	Depression	**Usual oral dose:** 5 to 10 mg per day divided into doses given 3 to 4 times per day; gradually increase dose based on response and tolerability up to a maximum dose of 60 mg per day	• Do not exceed 40 mg for the initial dose • Administer the larger portion of the daily dose (and increases in dosage) in the morning • Protriptyline is more likely to cause activation versus sedation • Patients with hepatic impairment may require lower doses (though no specific recommendation is available)
Generic Name Trimipramine **Brand Name** Surmontil ■ BL PD GD	Depression	**Usual oral dose:** 75 mg in divided doses, with gradual increases to 150 mg, up to a maximum dose of 200 mg per day	• Administer without regard to food • Administer initial doses in divided doses • Administer maintenance doses as a single dose at bedtime • Use caution in patients with hepatic impairment; if the drug must be used in such patients, a lower initial dosage and cautious titration are recommended • Higher initial and maximum doses may be considered for use in severely depressed, hospitalized patients
Miscellaneous Antidepressant Agents			
Drug Name	**FDA-Approved Indications**	**Adult Dosage Range**	**Precautions and Clinical Pearls**
Generic Name Bupropion **Brand Name** Aplenzin Buproban Wellbutrin Zyban ■ BL PD ■	Major depressive disorder Seasonal affective disorder Smoking cessation	**Usual oral dose:** IR: 100 mg 3 times per day (MDD: 450 mg per day) XL: 150 mg twice daily (MDD: 400 mg per day)	• Do not use in patients with seizure disorders, history of anorexia, or history of bulimia • May cause seizures and/or anorexia in patients undergoing abrupt discontinuation of alcohol or sedatives • May cause CNS stimulation • May elevate blood pressure (monitor)
Generic Name Mirtazapine **Brand Name** Remeron ▲ ■ ■	Major depressive disorder	**Usual oral dose:** 15 to 45 mg per day	• Akathisia or psychomotor restlessness most often occurs in the first few weeks of treatment • May cause anticholinergic effects; use with caution in patients with conditions worsened by this action • Hematologic side effects have been reported; monitor for these effects • Bone fractures have been associated with antidepressant treatment • May increase serum cholesterol and triglyceride levels • May cause hyponatremia • May cause mild pupillary dilation, which can lead to narrow-angle glaucoma in susceptible individuals • Use with caution in patients with hepatic impairment, renal dysfunction, or seizure disorders

Antipsychotic Agents

Second-Generation (Atypical) Agents

Universal prescribing alerts:

- The FDA labeling of all antipsychotic agents carry a black box warning: Elderly patients with dementia-related psychosis who are treated with antipsychotic drugs are at an increased risk of death. These agents are not approved for the treatment of patients with dementia-related psychosis.
- The FDA labeling of some antipsychotic agents carry a black box warning for increased risk of suicidal thinking and behavior in certain patients with major depressive disorder and psychiatric disorders.
- Agents in this category have been associated with QT prolongation and torsades de pointes. Use caution in patients with cardiac disease or other conditions that may increase the risk of QT prolongation, including cardiac arrhythmias, congenital long QT syndrome, heart failure, bradycardia, myocardial infarction, hypertension, coronary artery disease, hypomagnesemia, hypokalemia, hypocalcemia, or in patients receiving medications known to prolong the QT interval or cause electrolyte imbalances. Females, elderly patients, patients with diabetes, thyroid disease, malnutrition, alcoholism, or hepatic disease may also be at increased risk for QT prolongation. It is recommended that electrolyte imbalances be corrected prior to initiation of agents that affect the QT interval. Because QT prolongation can occur following an overdose, an electrocardiogram should be obtained in cases of overdose. Even though all these agents are associated with some level of QTc risk, the QTc warning symbol has been added when the manufacturer has emphasized this risk in the PI.
- Several medications in this category have been associated with weight gain and metabolic syndrome. The greatest risk is with clozapine and olanzapine. Aripiprazole, ziprasidone, and many of other newer SGAs have been associated with a lower risk.
- Monitoring of blood glucose, LFTs, neurologic function, serum cholesterol profile, and weight is recommended.
- Antipsychotic agents may lower seizure threshold; use caution in patients at higher risk. Use these medications with caution in patients taking concurrent benzodiazepines, sleep medications, and medications that lower the seizure threshold.
- Antipsychotics have been reported to disrupt the body's ability to reduce core body temperature (i.e., thermoregulatory processes), which is likely due to effects within the hypothalamus predisposing patients to hyperthermia. Patients receiving antipsychotic agents should be advised of conditions that contribute to an elevation in core body temperature (e.g., strenuous exercise, ambient temperature increase, or dehydration).
- Antipsychotic agents have been associated with esophageal dysmotility and aspiration, increasing the incidence of aspiration pneumonia in certain patient populations.
- A syndrome of potentially irreversible, involuntary, dyskinetic movements may develop in patients treated with antipsychotic drugs, although the incidence of this occurrence is less commonly reported with second generation agents. Monitoring of abnormal involuntary movement scale (AIMS) assessment is recommended. Also monitor for signs and symptoms of neuroleptic malignant syndrome (NMS).
- Use caution in patients with hematological disease because leukopenia, neutropenia, and agranulocytosis have been associated with antipsychotic use. A history of drug-induced dyscrasia or preexisting low white blood cell (WBC) count may increase the risk of developing these adverse effects. Patients with clinically significant neutropenia should be closely monitored for fever and infection, and discontinuation of the antipsychotic should be considered if a clinically significant decline in WBC occurs without a clear cause.
- A rare but potentially fatal DRESS has been reported with the use of some SGAs (olanzapine and ziprasidone) and requires urgent discontinuation of agent and emergency intervention.

Drug Name	FDA-Approved Indications	Adult Dosage Range	Precautions and Clinical Pearls
Generic Name Aripiprazole **Brand Name** Abilify Abilify Maintena Aristada ■ QT BL PD	**Common indications for use:** Schizophrenia Irritability associated with autistic disorder Bipolar disorder Major depressive disorder Tourette syndrome	**Usual oral dose for schizophrenia:** 10 to 30 mg per day (MDD: 30 mg per day) **Usual parenteral dose:** Long-acting injection (LAI) dose based on oral regimen. Refer to PI for conversion and usual IM dose.	• Certain drug interactions may require dose adjustment or avoidance of some combinations • Impulse control symptoms have been reported • Administer without regard to meals • The extended-release IM injection should be administered in the deltoid or gluteal muscle • Use with caution in patients with hematologic disease. as hematologic effects have been associated with aripiprazole's use

		Recommended dosing frequency of LAI: Aristada: every 4 to 6 weeks Maintena: every 4 weeks	• Monitor patients on antidiabetic agents for worsening glycemic control • Drug interactions may require dose adjustment or avoidance of certain drug combinations • Aristada and Maintena are LAI • LAI requires previous use of oral agent; refer to PI for details on oral challenge to rule out allergy, oral overlap, storage, and reconstitution (if applicable)
Generic Name Asenapine **Brand Name** Saphris ■ QT BL	Bipolar disorder Schizophrenia	**Usual oral dose for schizophrenia:** 5 to 10 mg sublingually twice daily (MDD: 20 mg per day)	• Patient should not eat or drink for 10 minutes after administration • Associated vasodilation may result in additive effects during concurrent use of antihypertensive drugs • Monitor patients on antidiabetic agents for worsening glycemic control • Tongue soreness has been reported with use of this sublingual formulation
Generic Name Brexpiprazole **Brand Name** Rexulti ▲ ■ ■ BL	Schizophrenia Major depressive disorder	**Usual oral dose as depression adjunct:** 0.5 to 1 mg per day **Usual oral dose for schizophrenia:** 1 to 4 mg per day (MDD: 4 mg per day)	• Long half-life: may be an advantage for nonadherent patients • Drug interactions may require dose adjustment or avoidance of certain drug combinations
Generic Name Cariprazine **Brand Name** Vraylar ■ BL	Schizophrenia Bipolar I disorder	**Usual oral dose for schizophrenia:** 1.5 to 6 mg per day (MDD: 6 mg per day)	• Use is not recommended in patients with severe hepatic or renal impairment • Drug interactions may require dose adjustment of avoidance of certain drug combinations

Drug Name	FDA-Approved Indications	Adult Dosage Range	Precautions and Clinical Pearls
Generic Name Clozapine **Brand Name** Clozaril FazaClo Versacloz ■ QT BL	Treatment-resistant schizophrenia Suicidal behavior in schizophrenia or schizoaffective disorder	**Usual oral dose:** 12.5 to 450 mg per day in divided doses (MDD: 900 mg per day)	• Patient, prescriber, and pharmacy must all be registered in the clozapine REMS program • Routine blood monitoring is required at a frequency based on patient's clinical status and duration of use • Dose must be titrated upon initiation of therapy and when resuming therapy after a disruption in dosing of 48 to 72 hours due to risk of respiratory depression and seizures • Change in smoking status affects clinical efficacy and therapeutic results • Drug interactions may require dose adjustment or avoidance of certain drug combinations Associated with: • Severe neutropenia/agranulocytosis: can lead to serious infection and death; monitor absolute neutrophil count (ANC) prior to and during treatment; monitor for symptoms of agranulocytosis and infection. • Seizures: risk is dose related; significantly increases with daily doses of more than 600 mg • Myocarditis and cardiomyopathy may be fatal; discontinue and obtain cardiac evaluation if findings suggest these cardiac reactions • May cause QT prolongation, torsades de pointes, ventricular arrhythmias, cardiac arrest, sudden death, orthostatic hypotension, bradycardia, syncope • Monitor: AIMS assessment, blood glucose, CBC with differential, LFTs, neurologic function, serum cholesterol profile, ANC, and weight • High risk of weight gain and metabolic syndrome • Anticholinergic properties can lead to severe constipation; however, patients often experience concurrent hypersalivation (sialorrhea) • May be administered orally without regard to meals
Generic Name Iloperidone **Brand Name** Fanapt Fanapt Titration Pack ■ QT BL	Schizophrenia	**Usual oral dose:** Initial: 1 mg twice daily Maintenance: 6 to 12 mg twice daily (MDD: 24 mg per day)	• Use with caution in patients with hematologic disease • Abrupt discontinuation is not recommended • May be administered without regard to meals • Monitoring of AIMS assessment is recommended • Use is not recommended in patients with severe hepatic impairment • Drug interactions may require dose adjustment or avoidance of certain drug combinations

Generic Name Lurasidone **Brand Name** Latuda BL	Schizophrenia Depression/bipolar I disorder	**Usual oral dose range for schizophrenia:** 40 to 60 mg per day (MDD: 160 mg per day)	• Must be taken with food (minimum 350 calories) • May cause missed menses • Monitor: renal and hepatic function; may require dose adjustments • Certain drug interactions may require dose adjustment or avoidance of some combinations
Generic Name Olanzapine **Brand Name** Zyprexa Zyprexa Zydis (ODT) Zyprexa Relprevv QT BL PD GD	Schizophrenia Acute or mixed episodes of bipolar mania Bipolar disorder Treatment-resistant bipolar depression (in combination with fluoxetine)	**Usual oral dose for schizophrenia:** 2.5 to 20 mg per day (MDD: 20 mg per day) **Usual parenteral dose:** IR (short acting): 10 to 30 mg every 2 to 4 hours (MDD: 30 mg per day) Long-acting injection (LAI) dose based on oral regimen. Refer to PI for conversion and usual IM dose. Recommended dosing frequency of LAI: every 2 to 4 weeks	• Patient, prescriber, and pharmacy registration in the Relprevv REMS program is required • High risk of weight gain and metabolic syndrome • Higher serum concentrations may be experienced in Japanese Asian patients • Change in smoking status affects clinical efficacy and therapeutic results • Anticholinergic prescribing alerts associated with use • LAI requires previous use of oral agent; refer to PI for details on oral challenge to rule out allergy, oral overlap (not required for olanzapine), storage, and reconstitution (if applicable) Associated with: • Post-injection sedation (including coma) and delirium following administration of Zyprexa Relprevv; a 3-hour observation period is required following each Zyprexa Relprevv dose
Generic Name Paliperidone **Brand Name** Invega Invega Sustenna Invega Trinza QT BL PD	Schizophrenia Schizoaffective disorder	**Usual oral dose for schizophrenia:** 6 mg per day (MDD: 12 mg per day) **Usual parenteral dose:** Long-acting injection (LAI) dose based on oral regimen; refer to PI for conversion and usual IM dose Recommended dosing frequency of LAI: Sustenna: every month Trinza: every 3 months	• Monitor for orthostatic hypotension • Certain drug interactions may require dose adjustment or avoidance of some combinations • May see tablet shell in feces • LAI requires previous use of oral agent; refer to PI for details on oral challenge to rule out allergy, oral overlap (not required for paliperidone), storage, and reconstitution (if applicable); Trinza requires previous use of Sustenna

Drug Name	FDA-Approved Indications	Adult Dosage Range	Precautions and Clinical Pearls
Generic Name Quetiapine **Brand Name** Seroquel Seroquel XR. QT BL PD GD	Schizophrenia Bipolar I disorder Major depressive disorder, adjunctive therapy (XR only)	**Usual oral dose for schizophrenia:** IR: 150 to 750 mg per day (MDD: 750 mg per day) ER: 400 to 800 mg per day (MDD: 800 mg per day)	• Monitor hepatic function; dose adjustment may be warranted • Associated with metabolic changes, including hyperglycemia, dyslipidemia, and weight gain • Use with caution in patients with known cardiovascular disease (CVD) • Risk of hypotension: monitor blood pressure • Use with caution in individuals with preexisting leukopenia, neutropenia, or agranulocytosis • Monitor: neurologic and ophthalmic function
Generic Name Risperidone **Brand Name** Risperdal Risperdal Consta Risperdal M-Tab QT BL PD GD	Schizophrenia Bipolar disorder Irritability/aggression associated with autistic disorder	**Usual oral dose for schizophrenia:** 0.5 to 6 mg per day (MDD: 6 mg per day) **Usual parenteral dose:** Long-acting injection (LAI) dose based on oral regimen; refer to PI for conversion and usual IM dose Recommended dosing frequency of LAI: Consta: every 2 weeks	• Monitor hepatic function; dose adjustment may be warranted • Use with caution in patients with known CVD • Risk of hypotension: monitor ECG • Use with caution in individuals with preexisting leukopenia, neutropenia. or agranulocytosis • Tardive dyskinesia has been reported with use of risperidone, especially at higher doses • Hyperprolactinemia may occur and persist throughout treatment, resulting in an increased risk for gynecomastia, galactorrhea, and osteoporosis • LAI requires previous use of oral agent; refer to PI for details on oral challenge to rule out allergy, oral overlap, storage, and reconstitution (if applicable)
Generic Name Ziprasidone **Brand Name** Geodon QT BL	Schizophrenia Bipolar disorder Acute agitation in schizophrenia (IM only)	**Usual oral dose for schizophrenia:** 20 to 80 mg twice daily (MDD: 160 mg per day) **Usual parenteral dose for acute agitation:** IM (short acting): 10 mg every 2 hours or 20 mg every 4 hours (MDD: 40 mg per day)	• Use with caution in patients with known CVD • Risk of hypotension • Closely monitor patients with a history of leukopenia, neutropenia, and agranulocytosis • Must be taken with food (at least 500 kcal)

First-Generation (Conventional/Typical) Agents

Universal prescribing alerts:

- The FDA labeling of all antipsychotic agents carry a black box warning: Elderly patients with dementia-related psychosis who are treated with antipsychotic drugs are at an increased risk of death. These agents are not approved for the treatment of patients with dementia-related psychosis.
- The FDA labeling of some antipsychotic agents carry a black box warning for increased risk of suicidal thinking and behavior in certain patients with major depressive disorder and psychiatric disorders.

- Agents in this category have been associated with QT prolongation and torsades de pointes. Use caution in patients with cardiac disease or other conditions that may increase the risk of QT prolongation including cardiac arrhythmias, congenital long QT syndrome, heart failure, bradycardia, myocardial infarction, hypertension, coronary artery disease, hypomagnesemia, hypokalemia, hypocalcemia, or in patients receiving medications known to prolong the QT interval or cause electrolyte imbalances. Females, elderly patients, patients with diabetes, thyroid disease, malnutrition, alcoholism, or hepatic disease may also be at increased risk for QT prolongation. It is recommended that electrolyte imbalances be corrected prior to initiation of agents that affect the QT interval. Because QT prolongation can occur following an overdose, an electrocardiogram should be obtained in cases of overdose.
- A syndrome of potentially irreversible, involuntary, dyskinetic movements may develop in patients treated with antipsychotic drugs. Monitoring of abnormal involuntary movement using the AIMS assessment is recommended. Also monitor for signs and symptoms of NMS.
- Use these medications with caution in patients taking concurrent benzodiazepines, sleep medications, and medications that lower the seizure threshold. Antipsychotic agents may lower seizure threshold, use caution in patients at higher risk.
- Antipsychotics have been reported to disrupt the body's ability to reduce core body temperature (i.e., thermoregulatory processes) likely due to effects within the hypothalamus predisposing patients to hyperthermia. Patients receiving antipsychotic agents should be advised of conditions that contribute to an elevation in core body temperature (e.g., strenuous exercise, ambient temperature increase, or dehydration).
- Antipsychotic agents have been associated with esophageal dysmotility and aspiration, increasing the incidence of aspiration pneumonia in certain patient populations.

First-Generation (Conventional/Typical) Agents: Butyrophenones

Drug Name	FDA-Approved Indications	Adult Dosage Range	Precautions and Clinical Pearls
Generic Name Haloperidol **Brand Name** Haldol Haldol Decanoate ■ QT BL PD GD	**Common indications for use:** Schizophrenia Psychotic disorders Tourette disorder Behavior disorders Hyperactivity	**Usual oral dose for schizophrenia:** 5 mg 2 to 3 times per day **Usual parenteral dose:** IM (short acting): 2 to 5 mg; may repeat dose at 1 hour intervals not to exceed maximum 20 mg per day Long-acting injection (LAI) dose based on oral regimen. Refer to PI for conversion and usual IM dose. Recommended dosing frequency of LAI: Decanoate: every 4 weeks	• Use with caution in patients with severe preexisting cardiovascular disorders • Tardive dyskinesia may occur with chronic use; patients should report any EPS • Potentially fatal NMS may occur • May increase risk of seizures, rapid mood fluctuation, and bronchopneumonia • Avoid activities requiring mental alertness • May impair heat regulation • May exhibit anticholinergic effects • Advise against sudden discontinuation • Avoid concomitant use of alcohol • LAI requires previous use of oral agent; refer to PI for details on oral challenge to rule out allergy, oral overlap, storage, and reconstitution (if applicable) Contraindications: • Use in patients who are in a coma or who exhibit severe toxic CNS depression • Haloperidol lactate (short acting) is not FDA approved for IV use. This administration route has been associated with QT prolongation and torsade de pointes • Use in patients with Parkinson's disease

First-Generation (Conventional/Typical) Agents: Phenothiazines

Universal prescribing alerts:

- These agents are associated with significant anticholinergic effects; refer to universal prescribing alerts in the Autonomic Agents chapter.
- Patients should avoid exposure to sunlight (UV) including the use of tanning beds; patients should follow accepted UV-protective practices when exposed.

Drug Name	FDA-Approved Indications	Adult Dosage Range	Precautions and Clinical Pearls
Generic Name Chlorpromazine ■ QT BL PD GD	**Common indications for use:** Schizophrenia and psychotic disorders Bipolar disorder Nausea/vomiting Tetanus Porphyria Hiccups	**Usual oral dose for schizophrenia:** 200 to 400 mg per day **Usual parenteral dose:** IM: 200 to 800 mg per day in divided doses every 4 to 6 hours (initial 25 mg dose with gradual dose increase over several days is recommended)	• Can cause significant orthostatic hypotension and increased risk of falls, especially with IM injectable • IM: inject slowly, deep into upper outer quadrant of buttock • Do not administer subcutaneously; IV administration is limited to surgery only • Avoid skin contact with solution; may cause contact dermatitis • Smoking status may influence drug effects • Certain drug interactions may require dose adjustment or avoidance of some combinations • May cause false-positive pregnancy test as well as false-positives for phenylketonuria, amylase, uroporphyrins, and urobilinogen • Monitor ophthalmic function • May cause skin discoloration Contraindications: • Use in patients who are in a coma or who exhibit severe toxic CNS depression; avoid additional CNS depressants (e.g., alcohol, barbiturates, opioids)
Generic Name Fluphenazine **Brand Name** Prolixin Prolixin Decanoate ■ QT BL PD GD	Management of manifestations of psychotic disorders and schizophrenia	**Usual oral dose for schizophrenia:** 2.5 to 10 mg per day in divided doses **Usual parenteral dose:** IM (short acting): 2.5 to 10 mg per day in divided doses at 6 to 8 hour intervals Long-acting injection (LAI) dose based on oral regimen; refer to PI for conversion and usual IM dose Recommended dosing frequency of LAI: Decanoate: every 2 to 4 weeks	• The oral liquid concentrate should be diluted immediately prior to administration • Only the decanoate formulation may be administered subcutaneously • Do not prepare bulk dilutions or store bulk dilutions • Monitor ophthalmic function screening • Monitor closely for hypotension; initiate at lower doses and taper the dosage slowly when discontinuing the medication, especially when using parenteral formulations • Certain drug interactions may require dose adjustment or avoidance of certain drug combinations • Smoking status may influence drug effects • LAI requires previous use of oral agent; refer to PI for details on oral challenge to rule out allergy, oral overlap, storage, and reconstitution (if applicable) Contraindications: • Age contraindication for decanoate; refer to PI • Severe CNS depression and coma • Subcortical brain damage • Patients receiving large doses of hypnotics • Blood dyscrasias • Hepatic disease

Generic Name Perphenazine ■ (BL)	Treatment of schizophrenia Severe nausea and vomiting	**Usual oral dose for schizophrenia:** 4 to 8 mg 3 times per day (MDD: 24 mg per day)	• Certain drug interactions may require dose adjustment or avoidance of some combinations • Monitor ophthalmic function • Monitor blood pressure; may cause orthostatic hypotension; initiate at lower doses and taper the dosage slowly when discontinuing the medication • Available in a combination of products, refer to PI • Smoking status may influence drug effects Contraindications: • Severe CNS depression • Subcortical brain damage • Bone marrow suppression • Blood dyscrasias • Liver damage
Generic Name Prochlorperazine **Brand Name** Compazine Compro ■ (QT) (BL) (PD)	Severe nausea and vomiting Psychotic disorders, including schizophrenia and anxiety	**Usual oral dose for severe nausea and vomiting:** 5 to 10 mg administered 3 to 4 times per day; doses up to 150 mg per day may be required **Usual parenteral dose for severe nausea and vomiting:** IM: 10 to 20 mg; repeat every 1 to 4 hours Alternative doses and routes of administration are available for additional indications (i.e., rectal and IV dosing); refer to PI	• Not recommended as an antipsychotic due to its inferior efficacy compared to other phenothiazines • IM: inject deep into the outer quadrant of the buttock • Increase dietary intake of riboflavin • Avoid skin contact with injection solution; contact dermatitis has occurred • False-positives for pregnancy and phenylketonuria have been reported • Monitor: blood pressure and heart rate, fluid balance, and for dehydration; during IV administration continuously monitor BP and HR • Monitor: seizures, especially in patients with known seizure disorder • Monitor: excessive sedation, neuromuscular malignant syndrome, autonomic instability, anticholinergic effects, EPS Contraindications: • Age contraindication for use; refer to PI • Coma or presence of large amounts of CNS depressants (e.g., alcohol, opioids, barbiturates) • Postoperative management of nausea/vomiting for certain patients

Drug Name	FDA-Approved Indications	Adult Dosage Range	Precautions and Clinical Pearls
Generic Name Thioridazine ■ QT BL PD	Schizophrenia	**Usual oral dose:** 200 to 800 mg in 2 to 4 divided doses (MDD: 800 mg per day)	• Certain drug interactions may require dose adjustment or avoidance of some combinations • Reserved for the management of symptoms in patients with schizophrenia who have failed trials of at least two other antipsychotic agents due to its risks of cardiac arrhythmias • Smoking status may influence drug effects • May interfere with urine detection of methadone and phencyclidine (false-positives) • Review and monitor ophthalmic function • Assess for CNS depression/level of sedation • Monitor AIMS for signs of tardive dyskinesia and Parkinsonism • Initiate at lower doses and taper the dosage slowly when discontinuing the medication due to risk of orthostatic hypotension • Use caution in hepatic impairment Contraindications: • Severe CNS depression • Severe hypertensive/hypotensive heart disease • Coma Associated with: • Contraindication for patients with QT prolongation
Generic Name Trifluoperazine ■ QT BL PD	Schizophrenia Nonpsychotic anxiety	**Usual oral dose for schizophrenia:** 15 or 20 mg per day in divided doses; some patients may require up to 40 mg per day	• Phenothiazines may produce false-positive tests for phenylketonuria • Certain drug interactions may require dose adjustment or avoidance of some combinations • Assess mental status; vital signs (as clinically indicated); weight, height, BMI, and waist circumference; CBC; and electrolytes and liver function, blood glucose, lipid panel • Monitor ophthalmic function • Initiate at lower doses and taper the dosage slowly when discontinuing the medication • Assess for EPS, suicidal ideation, sedation, NMS, and CNS changes • Smoking status may influence drug effects Contraindications: • Comatose or greatly depressed states due to CNS depressants • Bone marrow suppression and blood dyscrasias • Hepatic disease

First-Generation (Conventional/Typical) Agents: Thioxanthenes

Universal prescribing alerts:

- Thioxanthenes carry a high risk for tardive dyskinesia, especially in women and older adults.

Drug Name	FDA-Approved Indications	Adult Dosage Range	Precautions and Clinical Pearls
Generic Name Thiothixene ■ QT BL	Schizophrenia	**Usual oral dose:** 15 to 30 mg per day (MDD: 60 mg per day)	• Certain drug interactions may require dose adjustment or avoidance of some combinations • May cause false-positive pregnancy test • Monitor for signs of worsening psychosis, extrapyramidal side effects, drug-induced Parkinsonism, tardive dyskinesia, and acute dystonia • Monitor for excess sedation, orthostatic hypotension, and anticholinergic side effects • Titrate dosage upon initiation and taper upon discontinuation Contraindications: • Severe CNS depression and coma • Circulatory collapse • Blood dyscrasias

Miscellaneous Antipsychotic Agents

Drug Name	FDA-Approved Indications	Adult Dosage Range	Precautions and Clinical Pearls
Generic Name Loxapine **Brand Name** Adasuve ■ BL	Schizophrenia Agitation associated with schizophrenia or bipolar disorder (inhalation only)	**Usual oral dose for schizophrenia:** 60 to 100 mg day in single dose or divided 2 times daily (MDD: 250 mg per day) **Usual inhalation dose:** 10 mg once daily	• Registration in REMS program is required to distribute, dispense, and administer the Adasuve inhalation • Certain drug interactions may require dose adjustment or avoidance of some combinations • False-positive tests for phenylketonuria, amylase, uroporphyrins, and urobilinogen are possible • Monitor vital signs, ECG, signs of anticholinergic side effects, orthostatic hypotension, and EPS • Dosing should be titrated slowly with initiation and discontinuation • Monitor for signs of tardive dyskinesia and NMS Contraindications: • Oral: severe drug-induced CNS depression; coma • Inhalation: current diagnosis or history of asthma, COPD, or other lung disease associated with bronchospasm; acute respiratory symptoms or signs (e.g., wheezing); current use of medications to treat airway disease; history of bronchospasm following loxapine treatment Associated with: • Bronchospasm

Drug Name	FDA-Approved Indications	Adult Dosage Range	Precautions and Clinical Pearls
Generic Name Molindone ■ (BL)	Schizophrenia	**Illustrative oral dose for schizophrenia:** 5 to 25 mg in divided doses 3 to 4 times per day; up to 225 mg per day may be required	• Monitor ophthalmic function Contraindications: • Severe CNS depression • Coma
Generic Name Pimozide **Brand Name** Orap (QT) (BL) (PD) (GD)	Tourette disorder in patients who have failed to respond satisfactorily to standard treatment	**Usual oral dose:** 1 to 2 mg per day in divided doses, then increase dosage as needed every other day (MDD: 10 mg per day or 0.2 mg/kg per day, whichever is less)	• If therapy requires exceeding a dose of 4 mg per day, hepatic metabolism genotyping/phenotyping should be performed ("poor metabolizers" should not receive doses in excess of 4 mg per day) • Hyperprolactinemia may occur and persist throughout treatment, resulting in an increased risk for gynecomastia, galactorrhea, and osteoporosis • Monitor ophthalmic function and blood pressure at the beginning of therapy and periodically throughout • Perform ECG at baseline and periodically during therapy (especially during dosage adjustment) • Initiate at lower doses and decrease the dosage slowly when discontinuing the medication Contraindications: • Severe toxic CNS depression and coma • Congenital long QT syndrome and/or history of cardiac arrhythmias • Certain drug interactions may require dose adjustment or avoidance of some combinations; refer to PI for additional ethnic and genetic variation adjustments • Hypokalemia or hypomagnesemia

Anorexigenic Agents and Respiratory and CNS Stimulants

Amphetamines

Universal prescribing alerts:

- Dose medications in the morning and early in the day to avoid sleep disturbance. Do not administer at bedtime.
- Contraindications include advanced arteriosclerosis, symptomatic cardiovascular disease, moderate to severe hypertension, hyperthyroidism, agitated states, history of drug abuse, and use during or within 14 days of MAOI therapy.
- Amphetamines are considered stimulant medications and are associated with peripheral vasculopathy, including Raynaud's phenomenon. Worsening of peripheral vascular disease is likely and the effects on circulation have been observed in all age groups at doses considered to be within therapeutic range.
- Amphetamine may precipitate motor or phonetic tics in those with Tourette syndrome and may increase ocular pressure and visual disturbances.

- Obtain the patient's baseline weight, height, and vital signs. Assess for development of weight loss, hypertension, and tachycardia. Growth can be stalled in children and adolescents; monitor their height and weight. Assess for mood for swings or depression, irritability, sleep disturbance, cardiac arrhythmias, or signs of abuse. Obtain periodic urine toxicology screening for verification of compliance.
- Amphetamine may cause hypercortisolism, as amphetamines can cause a significant increase in plasma corticosteroid concentrations (the elevation is greatest in the evening). Use caution, may lower seizure threshold.
- Both hepatic disease and renal impairment may inhibit the elimination of amphetamines and result in prolonged exposures.
- Medications should be tapered prior to discontinuation, especially after chronic use.
- Amphetamine serum levels may be reduced if taken with acidic food, juices, or vitamin C.
- These agents are DEA-scheduled-controlled substances.

Drug Name	FDA-Approved Indications	Adult Dosage Range	Precautions and Clinical Pearls
Generic Name Amphetamine **Brand Name** Evekeo Adzenys XR-ODT Dyanavel XR suspension ■ (BL) (PD)	ADHD Exogenous obesity (IR only) Narcolepsy (IR only)	Dose varies depending on product selected **Illustrative oral dose for ADHD:** IR tablet: 5 mg twice per day (MDD: 60 mg per day) XR ODT: 12.5 mg per day XR suspension: 2.5 to 5 mg per day (MDD: 20 mg per day)	• Use an oral dosing syringe when dosing the suspension • Shake the suspension well prior to administration • Administer with or without food; for exogenous obesity, administer 30 to 60 minutes before meals • Administer the first dose on awakening; administer additional doses at intervals of 4 to 6 hours; avoid late-evening dosing • Amphetamine serum levels may be reduced if taken with acidic food, juices, or vitamin C • Adderall is a mixture of amphetamine and dextroamphetamine • Available as multiple products that are not interchangeable. See the individual product for indications, dosing, and brand name. Associated with: • Contraindication for use in patients with history of substance abuse (including alcoholism)
Generic Name Benzphetamine **Brand Name** Regimex	Obesity (short-term adjunct)	**Usual oral dose:** 25 to 50 mg per day (MDD: 50 mg 3 times per day)	• Doses should be individualized based on patient response • Indications for obese patients is specific to BMI and presence of other risk factors such as hypertension, diabetes, and/or dyslipidemia; refer to PI • Amphetamines may elevate plasma corticosteroid levels and interfere with urinary steroid determinations • Certain drug interactions may require dose adjustment or avoidance of some combinations Contraindications: • Cardiac disease, glaucoma, cardiac disease, hyperthyroidism and substance abuse

Drug Name	FDA-Approved Indications	Adult Dosage Range	Precautions and Clinical Pearls
Generic Name Dextroamphetamine **Brand Name** Dexedrine Spansule DextroStat Dexedrine ProCentra Zenzedi ■ (PD)	ADHD Narcolepsy	**Usual oral dose for ADHD:** IR: 5 mg once or twice daily (MDD: 40 mg per day) **Usual oral dose for narcolepsy:** ER: 10 mg per day (MDD: 60 mg per day)	• Abrupt discontinuation following high doses or prolonged use may result in withdrawal symptoms • Formulations are specific to indication and age of patient and thus are not all interchangeable; refer to PI • Adderall is a mixture of amphetamine and dextroamphetamine Contraindications: • Cardiac disease, glaucoma, cardiac disease, hyperthyroidism and substance abuse
Generic Name Lisdexamfetamine **Brand Name** Vyvanse ▲ ■ (PD)	ADHD Binge eating disorder	**Usual oral dose:** 30 mg per day each morning (MDD: 70 mg per day)	• Amphetamines may elevate plasma corticosteroid levels and interfere with urinary steroid determinations • Avoid doses later than noon to avoid insomnia • Priapism has been reported
Generic Name Methamphetamine **Brand Name** Desoxyn ■ (PD)	ADHD Exogenous obesity	**Illustrative oral dose for ADHD:** 5 mg once or twice daily (MDD: 20 to 25 mg per day)	• For obesity, administer 30 minutes before each meal • Certain drug interactions may require dose adjustment or avoidance of some combinations Contraindications: • Cardiac disease, glaucoma, cardiac disease, hyperthyroidism and substance abuse
Anorexigenic Agents			
Universal prescribing alerts: • Individualize therapy to achieve a response with the lowest effective dose. • Anorexigenic agents are recommended only for obese patients with a body mass index of 30 kg/m^2 or greater, or 27 kg/m^2 or greater in the presence of other risk factors such as hypertension, diabetes, and/or dyslipidemia or a high waist circumference. • Doses should not be administered in the evening or at bedtime. • Monitoring should include a baseline cardiac evaluation (for preexisting valvular heart disease and pulmonary hypertension); an echocardiogram during therapy; weight, waist circumference, and blood pressure; and renal function (especially in elderly patients). • Contraindications include advanced arteriosclerosis, severe hypertension, pulmonary hypertension, hyperthyroidism, glaucoma, agitated states, history of drug abuse, during or within 14 days of MAO inhibitor therapy, and concurrent use of other anorectic agents.			

Amphetamine Derivatives

Drug Name	FDA-Approved Indications	Adult Dosage Range	Precautions and Clinical Pearls
Generic Name Diethylpropion **Brand Name** Tenuate	Obesity (short-term adjunct)	**Usual oral dose:** IR: 25 mg 3 times per day CR: 75 mg daily at midmorning	• Controlled-release formulation: do not crush tablet; administer at midmorning • DEA-controlled substance
Generic Name Phendimetrazine	Obesity (short-term)	**Usual oral dose:** 105 mg per day	• Administer 30 to 60 minutes before the morning meal • DEA-controlled substance
Brand Name Phentermine **Brand Name** Adipex-P Suprenza	Obesity (short-term adjunct)	Dose varies depending on product selected **Illustrative oral dose:** 15 to 37.5 mg per day	• Capsules, tablets: administer before breakfast or 1 to 2 hours after breakfast; tablets may be divided in half and dose may be given in 2 divided doses • Orally disintegrating tablets (Suprenza): with dry hands, place tablet on the tongue and allow to dissolve; then swallow with or without water • Certain drug interactions may require dose adjustment or avoidance of some combinations • DEA-controlled substance • Available in multiple combination products; see the individual product for indications, dosing, and brand name

Selective Serotonin Receptor Agonists

Drug Name	FDA-Approved Indications	Adult Dosage Range	Precautions and Clinical Pearls
Generic Name Lorcaserin **Brand Name** Belviq ▲	Chronic weight management	**Usual oral dose:** 10 mg twice daily	• Evaluate response by week 12; if patient has not lost 5% or more of baseline body weight, discontinue therapy • Used as an adjunct to a reduced-calorie diet and increased physical activity in patients with either an initial BMI greater than or equal to 30 kg/m^2 or an initial BMI greater than or equal to 27 kg/m^2 and at least one weight-related comorbid condition • Certain drug interactions may require dose adjustment or avoidance of some combinations • Monitor: weight and waist circumference; CBC, blood glucose, prolactin levels (if galactorrhea or gynecomastia occurs) • Monitor: depression or suicidal thoughts/behavior; signs and symptoms of serotonin syndrome/NMS–like reaction; signs and symptoms of valvular heart disease (dyspnea, dependent edema)

Respiratory and Other Central Nervous System Stimulants			
Universal prescribing alerts: • Do not use in patients with marked anxiety, glaucoma, motor tics, or a family history or diagnosis of Tourette syndrome. • Do not use in patients with preexisting structural heart abnormalities or other serious cardiac problems. Use with caution in patients with hypertension or other cardiac diseases that might be exacerbated by an increase in blood pressure or heart rate. Patients should be evaluated for cardiac disease prior to initiation of therapy. • Do not use these stimulants during or within 14 days of MAO inhibitor therapy. • Priapism has been reported. Patients who develop priapism should discontinue therapy and seek immediate medical attention. • Respiratory and CNS stimulants may exacerbate symptoms of behavior and thought disorders. Use with caution in patients with preexisting psychiatric disorders. • These agents may lower the seizure threshold. Use with caution in patients with a seizure disorder.			
Drug Name	**FDA-Approved Indications**	**Adult Dosage Range**	**Precautions and Clinical Pearls**
Generic Name Ammonia spirit, aromatic	Fainting	**Usual inhaled dose:** 1 crushed ampule or opened bottle of solution	• Use with caution in patients with asthma, bronchitis, emphysema, or other chronic respiratory disease • Use with caution in patients with ocular diseases
Generic Name Caffeine/caffeine and sodium benzoate **Brand Name** Tablets: NoDoz Keep Alert Stay Awake Vivarin Oral solution: Cafcit Parenteral injection: Cafcit Caffeine Citrate Caffeine and Sodium Benzoate (GD)	Acute respiratory depression Stimulant	**Usual oral dose:** 100 to 200 mg per dose **Usual parenteral dose:** IM/IV: 250 mg once, may repeat as needed (MDD: 2500 mg per day)	• Avoid use in patients with symptomatic cardiac arrhythmias, anxiety, agitation, or tremor • Use with caution in patients with seizure disorder • Certain drug interactions may require dose adjustment or avoidance of some combinations

Generic Name Dexmethylphenidate **Brand Name** Focalin Focalin XR ■ (PD)	ADHD	**Usual oral dose:** IR: 2.5 mg twice daily (MDD: 20 mg per day) ER: 10 mg once daily (MDD: 40 mg per day)	• May be associated with peripheral vasculopathy; monitor for signs of digital changes • Has been associated with difficulty with accommodation and blurred vision • DEA-controlled substance
Generic Name Doxapram **Brand Name** Dopram	Respiratory stimulant	**Usual parenteral dose:** IV bolus: 0.5 to 1 mg/kg; may repeat (maximum cumulative dose: 2 mg/kg) IV infusion: 5 mg/min (maximum cumulative dose: 4 mg/kg)	• Use with caution in patients with hepatic or renal impairment • If the patient has received inhaled anesthesia known to sensitize the myocardium to catecholamines, avoid use of doxapram until the anesthetic has been eliminated
Generic Name Methylphenidate **Brand Name** Ritalin LA Aptensio XR Metadate CD Ritalin Concerta Metadate ER Ritalin SR Methylin Quillivant XR Daytrana ■ (PD)	ADHD Narcolepsy	**Illustrative oral dose for ADHD:** IR: 5 mg twice daily (MDD: 60 mg in 2 to 3 divided doses) ER (Concerta): 18 to 36 mg per day each morning (MDD: 72 mg per day) **Usual transdermal dose:** 10 to 30 mg per day	• Administer 30 to 45 minutes before meals • Permanent loss of skin color may result with use of the Daytrana patch at and around the application site as well as at distant sites; monitor for signs of skin depigmentation • May be associated with peripheral vasculopathy; monitor for signs of digital changes • Priapism has been reported; patients who develop priapism should discontinue therapy and seek immediate medical attention • Has been associated with difficulty with accommodation and blurred vision • DEA-controlled substance
Theophylline	Refer to the Smooth Muscle Relaxants chapter.		

Wakefulness-Promoting Agents

Universal prescribing alerts:

- Serious and life-threatening rashes—including Stevens-Johnson syndrome, toxic epidermal necrolysis, and drug rash with eosinophilia and systemic symptoms—have been reported. Discontinue use at the first sign of a rash.
- Do not use these agents in patients with a history of left ventricular hypertrophy or mitral valve prolapse. Use with caution in patients with a history of myocardial infarction or angina.
- Wakefulness-promoting agents may cause CNS depression. Patients should use caution when performing tasks that require mental alertness.
- Use with caution in patients with hepatic impairment. Dosage reductions are recommended for patients with severe impairment.
- Use with caution in patients with renal impairment.
- Use with caution in patients with a history of a psychiatric disorder. Discontinue therapy if psychiatric symptoms develop.
- Use with caution in patients with Tourette syndrome; may exacerbate symptoms.
- Use with caution in patients taking certain hepatic enzyme inhibitors and inducers; it may be necessary to adjust the dosage.

Drug Name	FDA-Approved Indications	Adult Dosage Range	Precautions and Clinical Pearls
Generic Name Armodafinil **Brand Name** Nuvigil ■ (BL)	Narcolepsy Obstructive sleep apnea Shift-work disorder	**Usual oral dose for narcolepsy:** 150 to 250 mg per day each morning	• Certain drug interactions may require dose adjustment or avoidance of some combinations • DEA-controlled substance
Generic Name Modafinil **Brand Name** Provigil ▲ ■ (BL)	Narcolepsy Obstructive sleep apnea Shift-work disorder	**Usual oral dose for narcolepsy:** 200 mg per day each morning (MDD: 400 mg per day)	• DEA-controlled substance

Miscellaneous Central Nervous System Stimulants

Drug Name	FDA-Approved Indications	Adult Dosage Range	Precautions and Clinical Pearls
Generic Name Acamprosate ▲	Alcohol abstinence	**Usual oral dose:** 666 mg 3 times per day A lower dose may be effective in some patients	• Treatment should be initiated as soon as possible following the period of alcohol withdrawal when the patient has achieved abstinence and should be maintained if the patient relapses • Abstinence is required for initiation of treatment; however, treatment should be continued in the event of a relapse • May be administered without regard to meals • Monitor: alcohol abstinence; symptoms of depression or suicidal thinking; renal function Contraindications: • Severe renal impairment (CrCl less than or equal to 30 mL/min)

Generic Name Atomoxetine **Brand Name** Strattera ■ ■ (PD)	ADHD	**Usual oral dose:** 40 to 80 mg per day as either a single daily dose or 2 evenly divided doses in the morning and late afternoon/early evening; may increase to 100 mg per day in 2 to 4 additional weeks to achieve optimal response (MDD: 100 mg per day)	• May be discontinued without the need for a tapering dose • Swallow capsule whole; if opened accidentally, wash the hands immediately and do not touch the eyes (product is an ocular irritant) • Administer with or without food as a single daily dose in the morning or as two evenly divided doses in morning and late afternoon/early evening • Certain drug interactions may require dose adjustment or avoidance of some combinations • Patients who are known to be poor metabolizers: initial dose is 40 mg per day; if the patient tolerates the therapy but has an inadequate response, may increase after minimum of 4 weeks to 80 mg per day • Thoroughly evaluate patients for cardiovascular risk; monitor heart rate and blood pressure, and consider obtaining ECG prior to initiation • Monitor patient growth (height/weight gain), attention, hyperactivity, anxiety, and worsening of aggressive behavior or hostility • Monitor blood pressure and pulse: baseline and following dose increases, and periodically during treatment Contraindications: • Narrow-angle glaucoma • Current or past history of pheochromocytoma • Severe cardiac or vascular disorders in which the condition would be expected to deteriorate with clinically important increases in blood pressure Associated with: • Suicidal ideation in certain patients
Generic Name Dextromethorphan and quinidine **Brand Name** Nuedexta (QT)	Pseudobulbar affect	**Usual oral dose:** Dextromethorphan 20 mg/quinidine 10 mg once daily for 7 days, then increase to twice daily (every 12 hours) thereafter; reassess patient periodically to determine if continued use is necessary	• May be administered with or without food • Administer twice-daily doses every 12 hours • Patients should avoid consuming grapefruit juice • Monitor: QT interval at baseline and 3 to 4 hours after the first dose in patients at risk for QTc prolongation • Monitor: potassium and magnesium prior to and during therapy • Monitor: CBC, liver and renal function tests • Periodically assess risk factors for arrhythmias during treatment • Periodically reassess the need for treatment: spontaneous improvement of pseudobulbar affect may occur • Monitor: worsening myasthenia gravis or other sensitive conditions due to anticholinergic effects Contraindications: • Prolonged QT interval • Congenital QT syndrome • History of torsade de pointes, heart failure, or complete atrioventricular (AV) block without an implanted pacemaker or at high risk of complete AV block

Drug Name	FDA-Approved Indications	Adult Dosage Range	Precautions and Clinical Pearls
Generic Name Flumazenil ■ (PD)	Reverses sedative effects of the benzodiazepines used in conscious sedation and general anesthesia Benzodiazepine overdose	**Illustrative parenteral dose:** IV: Initial dose: 0.2 mg over 15 seconds Repeat doses if desired level of consciousness is not obtained, 0.2 mg may be repeated at 1-minute intervals (maximum: 4 doses) Maximum total cumulative dose: 1 mg	• Avoid alcohol for the first 24 hours after administration or as long as the effects of benzodiazepines exist • Specific administration guidelines available in the PI • Monitor: return of sedation, respiratory depression, and other residual effects of benzodiazepines for at least 2 hours and until the patient is stable and resedation is unlikely Contraindications: • Patients given benzodiazepines for control of potentially life-threatening conditions (e.g., control of intracranial pressure or status epilepticus) • Patients who are showing signs of serious cyclic-antidepressant overdose Associated with: • Seizures
Generic Name Memantine **Brand Name** Namenda Namenda Titration Pak Namenda XR Namenda XR Titration Pack ▲	Alzheimer's disease	**Usual oral dose:** IR: Initial: 5 mg per day; increase dose by 5 mg per day to a target dose of 20 mg per day (specific dose titrations are recommended in the PI) ER: Initial: 7 mg once daily; increase dose by 7 mg per day to a target maximum dose of 28 mg once daily	• Administer without regard to meals • Certain drug interactions may require dose adjustment or avoidance of some combinations • Monitor for hypertension, CNS changes, rash, cognitive function, periodic ophthalmic exam, and constipation on a regular basis throughout therapy • Wait at least 1 week between dosage changes • Doses higher than 5 mg per day should be given in 2 divided doses • If treatment is interrupted for longer than several days, the treatment may need to be restarted at a lower dose and retitrated

Generic Name Riluzole **Brand Name** Rilutek	Amyotrophic lateral sclerosis (ALS)	**Usual oral dose:** 50 mg every 12 hours	• Riluzole can extend survival or time to tracheostomy • Higher daily doses are not associated with increased benefits, but adverse events are increased • Administer at the same time each day, at least 1 hour before or 2 hours after a meal • Certain drug interactions may require dose adjustment or avoidance of some combinations • Consuming charbroiled food may increase riluzole elimination • Smoking status may influence drug effects • A high-fat meal decreases absorption of riluzole and peak blood levels by 45% • Monitor serum aminotransferases including ALT levels before and during therapy. Maximum increases in serum ALT usually occur within 3 months after the start of therapy and are usually transient when less than 5 times the upper limit of normal. Discontinue therapy if ALT levels are 5 or more times the upper limit of normal or if jaundice develops.
Generic Name Sodium oxybate **Brand Name** Xyrem ■ ■	Excessive daytime sleepiness/cataplexy	**Illustrative oral dose:** Initial: 2.25 g at bedtime after the patient is in bed, and 2.25 g 2.5 to 4 hours later (4.5 g per night); titrate to effect; usual effective dosage range: 6 to 9 g per night	• Take on an empty stomach; separate the last meal (or food) and the first dose by 2 hours or longer; try to take at a similar time each day • Has a high sodium content • The patient should lie down immediately after taking the dose and should remain in bed • Sodium oxybate oral solution is available only to prescribers and patients enrolled in the Xyrem REMS Program and is dispensed to the patient only by the central pharmacy, which is specially certified • Patients must be seen at least every 3 months; prescriptions can be written for a maximum of 3 months (the first prescription may be written for only a 1-month supply) • Monitor: emergence of depression or suicidality; anxiety, confusion, or other behavior abnormalities; drug abuse, misuse, and addiction • DEA-controlled substance Contraindications: • Concomitant use with ethanol or sedative-hypnotic agents • Succinic semialdehyde dehydrogenase deficiency Associated with: • CNS depression • Misuse and abuse • Restricted access

Drug Name	FDA-Approved Indications	Adult Dosage Range	Precautions and Clinical Pearls
Generic Name Tetrabenazine **Brand Name** Xenazine ■	Chorea associated with Huntington disease	**Usual oral dose:** Initial: 12.5 mg once daily in the morning; may increase to 12.5 mg twice daily after 1 week Dosage may be increased by 12.5 mg per day at weekly intervals Daily doses higher than 37.5 mg should be divided into 3 doses Maximum single dose: 25 mg	• May administer without regard to meals • Available only through specialty pharmacies • Monitor: improvement in movement disorder; signs and/or symptoms of depression or suicidal ideation; signs and symptoms of NMS; orthostatic blood pressure • Certain drug interactions may require dose adjustment or avoidance of some combinations • Patients requiring more than 50 mg per day: perform genotyping to evaluate metabolizer status Contraindications: • Hepatic impairment • Patients who are actively suicidal or who have inadequately treated depression Associated with: • Depression • Suicidality
Guanfacine	Refer to the Cardiovascular Agents chapter.		

Anxiolytic, Sedative, and Hypnotic Agents

Barbiturates

Universal prescribing alerts:

- Barbiturates are controlled substances due to their high abuse potential. Alcohol not only increases the risk of lethal overdose, but it also diminishes the anticonvulsant effects of these agents.
- Osteomalacia, osteopenia, and osteoporosis have been reported with long-term therapy (patients using barbiturates who have end-stage renal disease are at higher risk).
- Barbiturates can cause severe and potentially fatal reactions that are preceded by skin eruptions. Hypersensitivity reactions to anticonvulsants may present as various organ system problems, including cardiac, hematologic, hepatic, renal, and dermatologic.
- Barbiturates can stimulate the activity of enzymes such as ALA synthetase, increasing porphyrin precursors, enhancing porphyrin synthesis, and potentially exacerbating porphyria. Use is contraindicated in patients with this disease.
- These agents should be discontinued gradually to avoid the possibility of precipitating withdrawal.
- Limit barbiturates to short-term use only for insomnia; their efficacy for sleep induction and maintenance is lost after 14 days.
- The CNS depressant effects of these agents may contribute to mental status changes; monitor closely.

Drug Name	FDA-Approved Indications	Adult Dosage Range	Precautions and Clinical Pearls
Generic Name Amobarbital **Brand Name** Amytal Sodium (BL) (PD)	Hypnotic in short-term treatment of insomnia Reduce anxiety and provide sedation preoperatively Tonic clonic seizures	**Illustrative parenteral dose for insomnia:** IM: 65 mg at bedtime	• Stability and compatibility information is available in the PI • Certain drug interactions may require dose adjustment or avoidance of some combinations • IV administration is indication specific, refer to PI • Monitor: vital signs and cardiac function during IV administration; renal and hepatic function with prolonged therapy • DEA-controlled substance Contraindications: • History of manifest or latent porphyria • Marked liver function impairment • Marked respiratory disease in which dyspnea or obstruction is evident
Generic Name Butabarbital **Brand Name** Butisol Sodium (BL) (PD) (GD)	Anxiety Insomnia Sedative Hypnotic	**Illustrative oral dose for anxiety:** 15 to 30 mg 3 to 4 times per day	• Rate of absorption is increased if given as a solution on an empty stomach • Paradoxical reactions, such as agitation and hyperactivity may occur in patients with acute pain • Avoid in severe hepatic impairment (hepatic coma/encephalophy) • Monitor: renal and hepatic function • DEA-controlled substance Contraindications: • In patients with manifest or latent porphyria
Generic Name Mephobarbital **Brand Name** Mebaral (BL) (PD)	Sedative Anxiety Seizures Prophylactic epilepsy	**Usual oral dose for anxiety:** 32 to 100 mg 3 or 4 times daily	• Shares the toxic potential of the barbiturates; the usual precautions of barbiturate administration should be observed when used • Use caution in patients with myasthenia gravis and myxedema • Paradoxical reactions, such as agitation and hyperactivity may occur in patients with acute pain • DEA-controlled substance Contraindications: • In patients with manifest or latent porphyria

Drug Name	FDA-Approved Indications	Adult Dosage Range	Precautions and Clinical Pearls
Generic Name Pentobarbital **Brand Name** Nembutal BL PD	Sedative-hypnotic Insomnia Status epilepticus (refractory)	**Usual parenteral dose for sedation:** IM: 150 to 200 mg	• Adjust the dose based on the patient's age, weight, and condition • Use caution in renal and hepatic impairment; specific dose adjustments are not available • When mixed with an acidic solution, a precipitate may form; use only a clear solution • Certain drug interactions may require dose adjustment or avoidance of some combinations • Monitor: respiratory (oxygenation), cardiovascular, and CNS status; cardiac monitor; blood pressure • Additional monitoring may be required for specific patients; refer to PI • DEA-controlled substance Contraindications: • In patients with manifest or latent porphyria
Generic Name Phenobarbital **Brand Name** Luminal ▲ BL PD	Management of generalized tonic–clonic (grand mal), status epilepticus, and partial seizures Sedative-hypnotic Insomnia	**Usual oral dose for sedation and anxiety:** 30 to 120 mg in 2 to 3 divided doses **Illustrative parenteral dose for preoperative anxiety:** IV/IM: 100 to 200 mg 60 to 90 minutes before surgery	• Causes a loss of vitamin D due to malabsorption; increase intake of foods rich in vitamin D • Certain drug interactions may require dose adjustment or avoidance of some combinations • Interferes with assays for lactate dehydrogenase (LDH) • Monitor: phenobarbital serum concentrations, mental status, CBC, LFTs, seizure activity • Specific recommendations for patients undergoing dialysis, refer to PI • DEA-controlled substance Contraindications: • Marked hepatic impairment • Dyspnea/airway obstruction • Porphyria • Intra-arterial administration
Generic Name Secobarbital **Brand Name** Seconal BL PD	Preanesthetic agent Short-term treatment of insomnia	**Usual oral dose for insomnia:** 100 mg at bedtime	• Certain drug interactions may require dose adjustment or avoidance of some combinations • Monitor: blood pressure, heart rate, respiratory rate, CNS status, liver function, renal function • DEA-controlled substance Contraindications: • Marked hepatic impairment • Dyspnea or airway obstruction • Porphyria

Benzodiazepines

Universal prescribing alerts:

- Should be avoided in patients with pulmonary disease if possible. Additionally, avoid coadministration with other CNS depressants, especially opioids, unless no other alternatives are available. Coadministration with other CNS depressants (including alcohol) may cause death. The FDA has issued a black box warning alerting patients and prescribers of this serious risk.
- Avoid use in patients with respiratory depression including severe chronic obstructive pulmonary disease (COPD) or sleep apnea. Death has been reported in patients with severe pulmonary disease shortly after the initiation of benzodiazepines.
- Benzodiazepines are controlled substances due to their high abuse potential.
- These agents should be discontinued gradually to avoid the possibility of precipitating withdrawal (which may include seizures).
- Benzodiazepines may cause loss of coordination, paradoxical reactions and cognitive impairment that may worsen symptoms of Parkinson's disease. These agents may also exacerbate acute intermittent porphyria.
- Benzodiazepines are contraindicated in patients with acute closed-angle glaucoma but may be used in patients with open-angle glaucoma who are receiving appropriate therapy (contraindication alerts were included in the drug grid for specific agents where manufacturer emphasized this risk).
- Patients with hepatic dysfunction should use only lorazepam, oxazepam, or temazepam (LOT), because these agents are not extensively metabolized by the liver and have less risk of accumulating to toxic levels in such patients.
- Benzodiazepines may be associated with complex sleep behaviors. Monitor for and report behavioral changes (i.e., suicidal ideation).
- Patients should avoid tasks requiring alertness or coordination.
- Anterograde amnesia may occur with any short-acting benzodiazepine if given in sufficient doses.

Drug Name	FDA-Approved Indications	Adult Dosage Range	Precautions and Clinical Pearls
Generic Name Alprazolam **Brand Name** Xanax Xanax XR Alprazolam Alprazolam XR Intensol ■ ■ (BL) (PD) (GD)	General anxiety disorder Short-term relief of symptoms of anxiety Panic disorder, with or without agoraphobia Anxiety associated with depression	**Usual oral dose for panic disorder:** IR/ODT/solution: Initial: 0.5 mg 3 times per day; titrate dose upward every 3 to 4 days (usual MDD: 4 mg per day) Alternatively may give: ER: 3 to 6 mg per day	• Periodic reassessment and consideration of dosage reduction are recommended • Titrate doses upward carefully for patients requiring doses more than 4 mg per day • Certain drug interactions may require dose adjustment or avoidance of some combinations • Monitor: respiratory and cardiovascular status • DEA-controlled substance Contraindications: • Narrow-angle glaucoma
Generic Name Chlordiazepoxide ▲ ■ (BL) (PD) (GD)	Management of anxiety disorder or the short-term relief of symptoms of anxiety Withdrawal symptoms of acute alcoholism Preoperative apprehension and anxiety	**Illustrative oral dose for mild to moderate anxiety:** 5 to 10 mg 3 to 4 times per day	• Monitor: respiratory and cardiovascular status (including orthostasis); mental status; periodic blood counts and LFTs; if used for ethanol withdrawal, signs and symptoms of ethanol withdrawal • Certain drug interactions may require dose adjustment or avoidance of some combinations • DEA-controlled substance

Drug Name	FDA-Approved Indications	Adult Dosage Range	Precautions and Clinical Pearls
Generic Name Clorazepate **Brand Name** Tranxene-T ■ (BL) (PD) (GD)	Generalized anxiety disorder Management of ethanol withdrawal Adjunct anticonvulsant in management of partial seizures	**Usual oral dose for anxiety:** 7.5 to 15 mg 2 to 4 times per day	• Certain drug interactions may require dose adjustment or avoidance of some combinations • Requires acid for active drug to be absorbed • Test interactions: decreased hematocrit; abnormal liver and renal function tests • Monitor: respiratory and cardiovascular status, excess CNS depression; suicidality • DEA-controlled substance Contraindications: • Closed (narrow) angle glaucoma
Generic Name Diazepam **Brand Name** Valium Diazepam Intensol Diastat AcuDial ■ (BL) (PD) (GD)	**Common indications for use:** Management of anxiety disorders Ethanol withdrawal symptoms Skeletal muscle relaxant Treatment of convulsive disorders Preoperative or preprocedural sedation and amnesia	**Usual dose for anxiety:** Oral/IM/IV: 2 to 10 mg 2 to 4 times per day as needed	• Certain drug interactions may require dose adjustment or avoidance of some combinations • False-negative urinary glucose determinations may occur when using Clinistix or Diastix • Absorption may be decreased if taken with food • Maintain adequate hydration, unless fluid restricted • Monitor: respiratory, cardiovascular, and mental status; check for orthostasis • Use caution in renal and hepatic impairment; dose adjustments may be necessary, though no specific recommendations are available • Smoking cessation may result in a reduced clearance of metabolites, despite use of nicotine replacement • DEA-controlled substance Contraindications: • Myasthenia gravis • Severe respiratory insufficiency • Severe hepatic insufficiency • Sleep apnea syndrome • Acute narrow-angle glaucoma
Generic Name Estazolam **Brand Name** Prosom ■ (BL) (PD)	Short-term management of insomnia	**Usual oral dose for insomnia:** 1 mg at bedtime; some patients may require 2 mg	• Certain drug interactions may require dose adjustment or avoidance of some combinations • Monitor: respiratory and cardiovascular status; CBC and urinalysis periodically during prolonged use • Dosage adjustments may be needed for patients with renal and/or hepatic impairment • DEA-controlled substance

Generic Name Flurazepam ▲ ■ (BL) (GD)	Insomnia	**Usual oral dose for insomnia:** 15 to 30 mg at bedtime	• Certain drug interactions may require dose adjustment or avoidance of some combinations • Monitor: daytime alertness; respiratory rate; behavior profile • DEA-controlled substance
Generic Name Lorazepam **Brand Name** Ativan Lorazepam Intensol ■ (BL) (PD) (GD)	Anxiety Insomnia Anesthesia premedication (parenteral) Status epilepticus (parenteral) Anesthesia premedication (sublingual)	**Usual oral dose for anxiety:** Initial: 2 to 3 mg per day in 2 to 3 divided doses; usual dose: 2 to 6 mg per day in divided doses Daily dose may vary from 1 to 10 mg per day	• IV administration issues: do not exceed 2 mg/min or 0.05 mg/kg over 2 to 5 minutes; monitor IV site during administration; avoid intra-arterial administration; avoid extravasation; IM/IV doses are indication specific • Monitor: respiratory and cardiovascular status • Relatively safer to use in patients with hepatic dysfunction (undergoes conjugative metabolism as opposed to oxidative metabolism) with careful clinical monitoring versus other benzodiazepines • May require dose adjustments in severe renal impairment; no dose recommendations are available • DEA-controlled substance Contraindications: • Acute narrow-angle glaucoma • Sleep apnea (parenteral) • Intra-arterial injection of parenteral formulation • Severe respiratory insufficiency (except during mechanical ventilation)
Generic Name Midazolam ▲ ■ (BL) (PD) (GD)	**Common indications for use:** Anxiety Preoperative sedation Moderate sedation prior to diagnostic or radiographic procedures ICU sedation (continuous infusion) Induction and maintenance of general anesthesia	**Usual parenteral dose for preoperative anxiety:** IM: 0.07 to 0.08 mg/kg 30 to 60 minutes prior to surgery procedure (approximately 5 mg for average adult) Alternatively may give: IV: 1 to 5 mg given over a 2-minute period just prior to surgery	• Individualize dose based on the patient's age, underlying diseases, and concurrent medications; reductions of as much as 50% are needed in certain patients • IV stability and compatibility information is available in the PI • Use caution in renal and hepatic impairment; no specific hepatic dose adjustments is available • Certain drug interactions may require dose adjustment or avoidance of some combinations • Monitor: respiratory and cardiovascular status; a blood pressure monitor is required during IV administration • DEA-controlled substance Contraindications: • Closed-angle glaucoma • Epidural or intrathecal administration Associated with: • Respiratory depression • Requires experienced clinician who is knowledgeable in the use of this agent and specialized care setting

Drug Name	FDA-Approved Indications	Adult Dosage Range	Precautions and Clinical Pearls
Generic Name Oxazepam ■ (BL) (PD) (GD)	Management of anxiety disorders, including anxiety associated with depression Management of ethanol withdrawal	**Usual oral dose for anxiety:** 10 to 15 mg 3 to 4 times per day	• Monitor respiratory and cardiovascular status • Metabolized by glucuronidation to inactive metabolites; may be relatively safer than other benzodiazepines for patients with hepatic impairment; monitor patient's clinical status • DEA-controlled substance
Generic Name Quazepam **Brand Name** Doral ■ (BL)	Insomnia	**Usual oral dose:** 7.5 to 15 mg at bedtime	• Long half life • Monitor respiratory and cardiovascular status with use • Recommended for short-term treatment of insomnia (i.e., 7 to 10 days) • DEA-controlled substance
Generic Name Temazepam **Brand Name** Restoril ■ (BL) (GD)	Insomnia	**Usual oral dose for insomnia:** 15 to 30 mg at bedtime Some patients may respond to 7.5 mg for transient insomnia	• Certain drug interactions may require dose adjustment or avoidance of some combinations • Monitor: respiratory and cardiovascular status • Recommended for short-term treatment of insomnia • Metabolized by glucuronidation to inactive metabolites; may be relatively safer than other benzodiazepines for patients with hepatic impairment; monitor patient's clinical status • DEA-controlled substance
Generic Name Triazolam **Brand Name** Halcion ■ (BL) (GD)	Insomnia	**Usual oral dose for insomnia:** 0.25 mg at bedtime 0.125 mg at bedtime may be sufficient in some patients, such as those with low body weight (MDD: 0.5 mg per day)	• Certain drug interactions may require dose adjustment or avoidance of some combinations; if the patient consumes grapefruit, keep its use consistent • Short-term (generally 7 to 10 days) treatment of insomnia • Use caution in renal and hepatic impairment • Administer on an empty stomach; do not take with a meal or immediately after a meal • Onset of action is rapid; the patient should take immediately before bedtime • DEA-controlled substance
Clonazepam	Refer to the Anticonvulsant Agents section.		
Miscellaneous Anxiolytic, Sedative, and Hypnotic Agents			
Universal prescribing alerts: • These agents may cause CNS depression. Patients should exercise caution when performing tasks that require mental alertness or coordination.			

Drug Name	FDA-Approved Indications	Adult Dosage Range	Precautions and Clinical Pearls
Generic Name Buspirone (BL)	Generalized anxiety disorder	**Usual oral dose:** 15 to 30 mg per day administered in 2 to 3 divided doses; dosage should not exceed maximum dose of 60 mg per day	• May be taken with or without food, but must be consistent • Certain drug interactions may require dose adjustment or avoidance of some combination • Avoid consuming large quantities of grapefruit juice • The presence of buspirone may result in a false-positive on a urinary assay for metanephrine/catecholamine • Take on a scheduled basis; not to be used only "as needed" for anxiety • Avoid use in severe renal and/or hepatic disease
Generic Name Dexmedetomidine **Brand Name** Precedex ■ (GD)	Intensive care unit sedation Procedural sedation	**Usual parenteral dose for sedation:** IV: Initial: Loading infusion of 1 mcg/kg over 10 minutes, followed by a maintenance infusion of 0.2 to 0.7 mcg/kg per hour	• High-alert medication; errors have occurred due to misinterpretation of dosing information; maintenance dose expressed as mcg/kg per hour • Adjust rate to desired level of sedation; titration no more frequently than every 30 minutes may reduce the incidence of hypotension • Certain drug interactions may require dose adjustment or avoidance of some combinations • Use caution in renal and hepatic impairment; consider dose reductions although no specific recommendations are available • Use of additional agents with amnestic properties (e.g., benzodiazepines) may be necessary • Stability and compatibility information is available in the PI • Monitor: level of sedation; heart rate, respiration, rhythm, and blood pressure; pain control
Generic Name Droperidol ■ (QT) (BL) (PD)	Prevention and/or treatment of nausea and vomiting from surgical and diagnostic procedures	**Usual parenteral dose:** IV: 0.625 to 1.25 mg administered at the end of surgery	• Stability and compatibility information is available in the PI • Monitor: QT prolongation and vital signs; serum magnesium and potassium; mental status and AIMS score • Observe for dystonias, extrapyramidal side effects, and temperature changes; may exacerbate Parkinsonian symptoms • Seizures have been reported Associated with: • Contraindication for use in patients with known or suspected QT prolongation, including congenital long QT syndrome • Arrhythmias, QT prolongation, and torsades de pointes, including some fatal cases, have been reported

Drug Name	FDA-Approved Indications	Adult Dosage Range	Precautions and Clinical Pearls
Generic Name Eszopiclone **Brand Name** Lunesta ■ (BL) (GD)	Insomnia	**Usual oral dose:** 1 to 2 mg immediately before bedtime; may be increased up to maximum dose of 3 mg per day	• Certain drug interactions may require dose adjustment or avoidance of some combinations • Avoid taking after a heavy meal; may delay onset (empty stomach is preferred) • Daytime function may be impaired in patients taking higher doses (2 or 3 mg) • Patients taking this medication are at increased risk for complex sleep behaviors and hazardous sleep-related activities. Monitor and report any usual changes in behavior (i.e., suicidal ideation or depression) • May cause respiratory depression; use care in high-risk patients with preexisting respiratory disorders • DEA-controlled substance
Generic Name Hydroxyzine **Brand Name** Vistaril ▲ (BL) (PD) (QT)	Pruritus Antiemetic Anxiety Atopic dermatitis Urticaria Sedation induction	Dose is dependent on indication for use and patient's clinical response **Illustrative oral dose for anxiety:** 50 mg 3 to 4 times per day as needed **Usual parenteral dose for anxiety:** IM: 50 to 100 mg; may repeat every 6 to 8 hours as needed	• Subject to all universal anticholinergic prescribing alerts and warnings • May increase anticholinergic effects; use with caution in patients with narrow-angle glaucoma, prostatic hypertrophy, or urinary obstruction • Use with other CNS depressants or alcohol may intensify sedative effects; use with caution in patients taking these agents • Use caution in hepatic impairment; no specific dose recommendation is available Contraindications: • Subcutaneous, IV, and intra-arterial administration • QT prolongation has been reported; contraindicated in patients with risk of QT prolongation/torsades
Generic Name Meprobamate ▲ (BL) (PD)	Anxiety disorders	**Usual oral dose:** 1200 to 1600 mg per day in 3 to 4 divided doses, up to 2400 mg per day	• Effects may be potentiated when used with other sedative drugs or ethanol • Monitor mental status; avoid abrupt discontinuation • Seizures and suicidal ideation have been reported • Use caution in hepatic disease; no specific recommendations are available • DEA-controlled substance Contraindications: • Acute intermittent porphyria can be exacerbated by therapy with this agent
Generic Name Promethazine **Brand Name** Phenadoz Phenergan Promethegan ▲ ■ (BL) (PD) (GD)	Allergic conditions Antiemetic Motion sickness Sedative Adjunct to postoperative analgesia/anesthesia	**Usual oral and rectal dose for allergic pruritis:** 25 mg at bedtime **or** 12.5 mg before meals and at bedtime (range: 6.25 to 12.5 mg 3 times per day)	• IV administration is not the preferred route; severe tissue damage may occur • Certain drug interactions may require dose adjustment or avoidance of some combinations • May interfere with urine detection of amphetamine/methamphetamine (false-positive); alters the flare response in intradermal allergen tests; hCG-based pregnancy tests may result in false-negatives or false-positives • Extravasation management: if extravasation occurs, stop the infusion immediately and follow the guidelines for management available in the PI • Subject to all anticholinergic prescribing alerts and warnings

		Illustrative parenteral dose: IM: 12.5 to 50 mg per dose	Contraindications: • Coma • Treatment of lower respiratory tract symptoms, including asthma • Intra-arterial or subcutaneous administration Associated with: • Increased risk in certain populations and potential to cause serious tissue injury (injection) • Age-specific contraindication for use, refer to PI
Generic Name Ramelteon **Brand Name** Rozerem BL	Insomnia	**Usual oral dose:** 8 mg within 30 minutes of bedtime	• Do not administer with a high-fat meal • Swallow tablet whole; do not break • Monitor for CNS changes, abnormal thinking, and behavior changes (avoid if there is seizure disorder) • Decreased testosterone and increased prolactin have been reported during use • Avoid use in patients with severe hepatic impairment • Patients taking this medication are at increased risk for complex sleep behaviors and hazardous sleep-related activities • Certain drug interactions may require dose adjustment or avoidance of some combinations Contraindications: • History of angioedema
Generic Name Suvorexant **Brand Name** Belsomra BL	Insomnia	**Usual oral dose:** 10 mg within 30 minutes of bedtime (MDD: 20 mg per day)	• May cause abnormal thinking and behavioral changes • Patients taking this medication are at increased risk for complex sleep behaviors and hazardous sleep-related activities. Monitor for CNS changes, abnormal thinking, and behavior changes • Drug interactions may require dose adjustments or avoidance of certain drug combinations • Must take when there is at least 7 hours of planned sleep • Use is not recommended in patients with severe hepatic impairment • DEA-controlled substance Contraindications: • Narcolepsy

Drug Name	FDA-Approved Indications	Adult Dosage Range	Precautions and Clinical Pearls
Generic Name Tasimelteon **Brand Name** Hetlioz (BL)	Non-24-hour sleep–wake disorder	**Usual oral dose:** 20 mg once daily at the same time each night before bedtime	• Effects may not become apparent for weeks or months due to differences in circadian rhythms • Decreased testosterone and increased prolactin has been reported • Tobacco smoking reduces the efficacy of this drug • Administer without food; take at the same time every night before bedtime; swallow capsule whole • Avoid or limit ethanol when taking • Monitor for CNS changes, abnormal thinking, and behavior changes • Certain drug interactions may require dose adjustment or avoidance of some combinations
Generic Name Zaleplon **Brand Name** Sonata ■ (BL) (GD)	Insomnia	**Usual oral dose:** 10 mg immediately before bedtime (range: 5 to 20 mg)	• Recommended only for short-term use • Administer immediately before bedtime or when the patient is in bed and cannot fall asleep • Avoid taking with or after a heavy, high-fat meal; reduces absorption • Patients taking this medication are at increased risk for complex sleep behaviors and hazardous sleep-related activities. Monitor for CNS changes, abnormal thinking, and behavior changes • Certain drug interactions may require dose adjustment or avoidance of some combinations • Not recommended in cases of hepatic impairment • Monitor: daytime alertness; respiratory rate (in patients with compromised respiration); behavior profile; tolerance, abuse, and dependence • DEA-controlled substance
Generic Name Zolpidem **Brand Name** Ambien Ambien CR Edluar Intermezzo Zolpimist ■ (BL) (GD)	Insomnia Products have specific indications for trouble falling asleep or returning to sleep in the middle of the night; refer to PI	**Usual oral dose:** IR tablet, oral spray: 5 mg (females) or 5 to 10 mg (males) immediately before bedtime (MDD: 10 mg per day) ER tablet: 6.25 mg (females) or 6.25 to 12.5 mg (males) immediately before bedtime (MDD: 12.5 mg per day)	• The lowest effective dose should be used; higher doses may be more likely to impair the patient's next-morning activities • Ingest immediately before bedtime due to its rapid onset of action • Regardless of dosage form, do not administer with or immediately after a meal • Certain drug interactions may require dose adjustment or avoidance of some combinations • Patients taking this medication are at increased risk for complex sleep behaviors and hazardous sleep-related activities; monitor for CNS changes, abnormal thinking, and behavior changes • Use caution or avoid in patients with respiratory disease • Monitor: daytime alertness; fall risk; respiratory rate; behavior profile; tolerance, abuse, and dependence • Reevaluate if insomnia persists after 7 to 10 days of use • DEA-controlled substance • Drug is available in multiple dosage formulations and administration vehicles; refer to PI for dosing (formulations are not interchangeable)

Drug Name	FDA-Approved Indications	Adult Dosage Range	Precautions and Clinical Pearls
Diphenhydramine	Refer to the Antihistamine Agents chapter.		
Doxylamine	Refer to the Antihistamine Agents chapter.		
Fospropofol	Refer to the Miscellaneous General Anesthetic Agents section.		
Propofol	Refer to the Miscellaneous General Anesthetic Agents section.		
General Anesthetic Agentes			
Barbiturates			
Drug Name	**FDA-Approved Indications**	**Adult Dosage Range**	**Precautions and Clinical Pearls**
Generic Name Methohexital **Brand Name** Brevital Sodium ■ (PD)	Induction of anesthesia Procedural sedation	**Usual parenteral dose:** IV: Induction: 1 to 1.5 mg/kg	• Stability and compatibility information is available in the PI • Caution in cases of adrenal insufficiency (Addison's disease), renal disease, myxedema, severe anemia or other disease that can potentiate the hypnotic effects • Use cautiously in patients with extreme obesity • Monitor: respiratory, cardiovascular (including blood pressure), and CNS status; monitor for CNS changes, abnormal thinking, and behavior changes • DEA-controlled substance Contraindications: • Patients in whom general anesthesia is contraindicated • Porphyria Associated with: • Requires experienced clinician who is knowledgeable in the use of this agent and specialized care setting (able to provide continuous monitoring of respiratory and cardiac function)
Miscellaneous General Anesthetics Agents			
Drug Name	**FDA-Approved Indications**	**Adult Dosage Range**	**Precautions and Clinical Pearls**
Generic Name Etomidate **Brand Name** Amidate	Induction/maintenance of general anesthesia	**Usual parenteral dose for the induction of anesthesia:** IV: 0.2 to 0.6 mg/kg over 30 to 60 seconds Maintenance of anesthesia: 10 to 20 mcg/kg/min	• Prolonged infusion is not recommended • Leads to reduced plasma cortisol and aldosterone levels • May induce cardiac depression • Use caution in patients with renal and hepatic impairment; dose adjustment may be needed although no specific recommendations are available

Drug Name	FDA-Approved Indications	Adult Dosage Range	Precautions and Clinical Pearls
Generic Name Fospropofol **Brand Name** Lusedra	Monitored anesthesia care in adults undergoing diagnostic or therapeutic procedures	**Illustrative parenteral dose for patients weighing 61 to 89 kg:** IV bolus initial dose: 6.5 mg/kg (maximum: 577.5 mg) Supplemental doses: 1.6 mg/kg (maximum: 140 mg; 25% of the initial dose) as needed to achieve the required level of sedation	• Prodrug of propofol • Administer supplemental oxygen to all patients • Do not mix fospropofol disodium with other fluids or therapeutic agents prior to administration • Flush the infusion line before and after administration as directed by manufacturer; refer to PI • Weight-based dosing for all patients, refer to PI • May cause the loss of spontaneous respiration and hypoxemia; avoid use in high-risk patients
Generic Name Propofol **Brand Name** Diprivan Fresenius Propoven (PD) (GD)	Induction of anesthesia Maintenance of anesthesia in patients Monitored anesthesia care sedation during procedures Sedation in intubated, mechanically ventilated ICU patients	**Illustrative parenteral dose (age < 55 years):** IV: 2 to 2.5 mg/kg (administer in approximately 40-mg dose increments every 10 seconds until onset of induction)	• Review age-specific dosing information in the PI prior to use; dose must be individualized based on total body weight and titrated to the desired clinical effect • High-alert medication: heightened risk of causing significant patient harm when used in error • Wait at least 3 to 5 minutes between dosage adjustments to clinically assess drug effects • Increase doses in patients with chronic alcoholism • Refer to stability and compatibility information in PI • May cause the loss of spontaneous respiration and hypoxemia; avoid use in high-risk patients • Certain drug interactions may require dose adjustment or avoidance of some combinations (i.e., with opioids) • Requires experienced clinician who is knowledgeable in the use of this agent and specialized care setting (able to provide continuous monitoring of respiratory and cardiac function) • Management: zinc replacement therapy may be needed for those at risk of zinc deficiency

Antimanic Agents

Drug Name	FDA-Approved Indications	Adult Dosage Range	Precautions and Clinical Pearls
Generic Name Lithium salts **Brand Name** Lithobid ■	Bipolar disorder (episode or maintenance)	Dose is dependent on indication for use, formulation selected, and patient's clinical response	• Caution: lithium toxicity, Brugada syndrome, chronic lithium therapy, comorbid infection, diarrhea, geriatric patients, hypothyroidism, pregnancy, renal function, sodium depletion, sweating, and dehydration • Avoid activities requiring mental alertness • May cause diarrhea, nausea, ataxia, and hand tremor

		Optimal response can usually be established and maintained with 600 mg orally 3 times per day; this dose will typically produce an effective lithium serum concentration in the range of 1 to 1.5 mEq/L	• Instruct patient to discontinue therapy if signs of toxicity occur; counsel to seek emergency assistance with development of lightheadedness, palpitations, or shortness of breath • Advise patient to maintain adequate fluid intake • Multiple drug–drug interactions have been identified for lithium salts • A lower initial dosage for the first few days may minimize intolerance; adjust every 3 to 4 days to achieve target concentration • A definitive maximum dosage has not been established
Aripiprazole	Refer to the Psychotherapeutic Agents section.		
Asenapine	Refer to the Psychotherapeutic Agents section.		
Carbamazepine	Refer to the Anticonvulsant Agents section.		
Cariprazine	Refer to the Psychotherapeutic Agents section.		
Lamotrigine	Refer to the Anticonvulsant Agents section.		
Lurasidone	Refer to the Psychotherapeutic Agents section.		
Olanzapine	Refer to the Psychotherapeutic Agents section.		
Quetiapine	Refer to the Psychotherapeutic Agents section.		
Risperidone	Refer to the Psychotherapeutic Agents section.		
Valproate/divalproex	Refer to the Anticonvulsant Agents section.		
Ziprasidone	Refer to the Psychotherapeutic Agents section.		

Antimigraine Agents

Selective Serotonin Agonists

Universal prescribing alerts:

- Antimigraine agents may cause CNS depression. Patients should use caution when performing tasks that require mental alertness.
- Do not use within 24 hours of another 5HT1 agonist (or serotonergic agents such as MAO inhibitors), ergotamine derivatives, or ergotamine-containing medications. Concomitant administration may cause serotonin syndrome.
- Coronary artery vasospasm, ischemia, myocardial infarction, ventricular tachycardia or fibrillation, cardiac arrest, and death have been reported (these agents are therefore contraindicated in patients with these conditions or are at high risk). Monitor for symptoms suggesting angina following dosing. These agents are also contraindicated for use in patients with peripheral vascular disease, including but not limited to ischemic bowel disease.
- Cerebral/subarachnoid hemorrhage, stroke, hypertension, hypertensive crisis, peripheral vascular ischemia, and colonic ischemia have been reported.

Drug Name	FDA-Approved Indications	Adult Dosage Range	Precautions and Clinical Pearls
Generic Name Almotriptan **Brand Name** Axert ▲ ■	Migraine	**Usual oral dose:** 6.25 to 12.5 mg for one dose; may repeat after 2 hours (MDD: 25 mg per day)	• Almotriptan contains a sulfonyl group, which is structurally different from a sulfonamide; however, use caution in patients with a sulfonamide allergy • Certain drug interactions may require dose adjustment or avoidance of some combinations
Generic Name Eletriptan **Brand Name** Relpax	Migraine	**Usual oral dose:** 20 to 40 mg for one dose; may repeat after 2 hours (MDD: 80 mg per day)	• Use not recommended for patients with severe hepatic impairment • Certain drug interactions may require dose adjustment or avoidance of some combinations
Generic Name Frovatriptan **Brand Name** Frova	Migraine	**Usual oral dose:** 2.5 mg for one dose; may repeat after 2 hours (MDD: 7.5 mg per day)	• Use with caution in patients with severe hepatic impairment • Drug (or its metabolites) may bind to the melanin of the eye; visual disturbances have been reported with prolonged use
Generic Name Naratriptan **Brand Name** Amerge ▲ ■	Migraine	**Usual oral dose:** 1 to 2.5 mg for one dose; may repeat after 4 hours (MDD: 5 mg per hour)	• Do not use in patients with severe renal impairment (CrCl less than15 mL/min) or severe hepatic impairment • Take without regard to food (with plenty of fluids)
Generic Name Rizatriptan **Brand Name** Maxalt Maxalt-MLT (PD)	Migraine	**Usual oral dose:** 5 to 10 mg for one dose; may repeat after 2 hours (MDD: 30 mg per day)	• Use with caution in patients with hepatic impairment and patients undergoing dialysis • Certain drug interactions may require dose adjustment or avoidance of some combinations • Swallow oral tablets whole with liquid and allow orally disintegrating tablets to dissolve on tongue; may take without regard to food

Generic Name Sumatriptan **Brand Name** Imitrex Sumavel DosePro Alsuma Zecuity ■	Migraine Cluster headache	**Usual oral dose:** 25 to 100 mg for one dose; may repeat after 2 hours (MDD: 200 mg per day) **Usual intranasal dose:** 5 to 20 mg in one nostril; may repeat after 2 hours (MDD: 40 mg per day) **Usual subcutaneous dose:** 6 mg for one dose; may repeat after 1 hour (MDD: 12 mg per day) **Usual transdermal dose:** One patch (6.5 mg) for one dose; may apply a second patch after 2 hours (MDD: 2 patches per day)	• Use of oral, intranasal, transdermal, and Alsuma and Imitrex injectables is contraindicated in patients with severe hepatic impairment; Sumavel is not recommended in patients with severe hepatic impairment (products are not interchangeable; refer to PI for indications and prescribing directions prior to use) • Seizures in patients have been reported after sumatriptan administration; use with caution in patients with a seizure disorder • Allergic contact dermatitis may occur with use of the transdermal patch; discontinue if allergic contact dermatitis is suspected
Generic Name Zolmitriptan **Brand Name** Zomig Zomig ZMT ■ (PD)	Migraine	**Usual oral dose:** 1.25 to 2.5 mg; may repeat in 2 hours (MDD: 10 mg per day) **Usual intranasal dose:** 2.5 mg; may repeat in 2 hours (MDD: 10 mg per day)	• Use with caution in patients with hepatic impairment • Dosage reduction is recommended in patients with moderate to severe hepatic impairment • Use of the orally disintegrating tablets or nasal inhalation is not recommended in patients with moderate to severe hepatic impairment • Oral tablets may be divided into half, however, orally disintegrating tablets must be placed on tongue whole and dissolved; may be taken without regard to food
Miscellaneous Antimigraine Agents			
Acetaminophen	Refer to the Analgesic and Antipyretic Agents section.		
Butorphanol	Refer to the Analgesic and Antipyretic Agents section.		
Caffeine and sodium benzoate	Refer to the Anorexigenic Agents and Respiratory and CNS Stimulants section.		

Miscellaneous Antimigraine Agents	
Dihydroergotamine	Refer to the Autonomic Agents chapter.
Ergotamine	Refer to the Autonomic Agents chapter.
Ketoprofen	Refer to the Analgesic and Antipyretic Agents section.
Opiate agonists	Refer to the Analgesic and Antipyretic Agents section.
Propranolol	Refer to the Cardiovascular Agents chapter.
Salicylates	Refer to the Analgesic and Antipyretic Agents section.
Timolol	Refer to the Cardiovascular Agents chapter.
Topiramate	Refer to the Anticonvulsant Agents section.
Valproate/divalproex	Refer to the Anticonvulsant Agents section.

Antiparkinsonian Agents

Adamantanes

Drug Name	FDA-Approved Indications	Adult Dosage Range	Precautions and Clinical Pearls
Generic Name Amantadine GD	Influenza A virus Parkinsonism Drug-induced extrapyramidal reaction	**Usual oral dose for Parkinsonism:** 100 mg twice daily	• Avoid abrupt discontinuation due to withdrawal syndrome • Use with caution in patients with angle-closure glaucoma, congestive heart failure, advanced age, epilepsy, melanoma, significant psychiatric disorders, or suicidal ideation • May cause diminished mental alertness, anticholinergic symptoms, blurred vision, compulsive behavior, and NMS • Do not drink alcohol while taking this drug • Monitor for CNS change (i.e., behavioral changes) • Seizures have been reported • Specific recommendations for patients undergoing dialysis • Recurrent eczema or rash can be aggravated with use • Monitor routinely for melanoma

Anticholinergic Agents

Universal prescribing alerts:

- Anticholinergic agents are better tolerated in younger patients. Use with caution in patients older than 65 years.
- Medications with anticholinergic properties are associated with an increased risk of falls, cognitive impairment, constipation, dry mouth, urinary retention, and dry eyes.
- Use extreme caution when giving these medications with other agents with anticholinergic properties.
- Use with caution in patients with narrow-angle glaucoma, benign prostate hyperplasia, or cardiac arrhythmias.
- Patients should avoid alcohol consumption while taking these agents.
- Although these agents can be used to reduce EPS, it is important to note that antiparkinsonism agents do not alleviate the symptoms of tardive dyskinesia, and in some instances may aggravate them; use caution.
- Anticholinergic may exacerbate dementia symptoms and should be avoided in patients with dementia.
- Impairment of heat regulation can lead to potentially fatal hyperthermia.

Drug Name	FDA-Approved Indications	Adult Dosage Range	Precautions and Clinical Pearls
Generic Name Benztropine **Brand Name** Cogentin BL GD	Parkinsonism (adjunct therapy) Drug-induced EPS	**Usual dose for drug induced EPS:** IV/IM/Oral: 1 to 4 mg or once or twice daily	• May cause muscle weakness, mental confusion with excitement, visual hallucinations, urinary retention, dysuria, tachycardia, or rash • Patients should avoid activities requiring mental alertness or coordination • Report sudden muscle weakness or stiffness Contraindications: • Use in patients with dementia
Generic Name Trihexyphenidyl BL	Parkinsonism (adjunct therapy) Drug-induced extrapyramidal disorders	**Illustrative oral dose for Parkinsonism:** IR: 1 to 10 mg per day in 3 to 4 divided doses ER: 5 to 10 mg per day in 2 divided doses 12 hours apart	• May cause mental confusion with excitement, visual hallucinations, dysuria, hypertension, obstructive disease of the GI or genitourinary system, or severe nausea/vomiting • Patients should avoid activities requiring mental alertness or coordination • Caution in hepatic and renal impairment; no specific dose recommendations are available • Avoid abrupt discontinuation due to risks of withdrawal symptoms, NMS, and exacerbation of Parkinsonian symptoms • Patients should be educated on the signs of a significant allergic or untoward reaction
Diphenhydramine	Refer to the Antihistamine Agents chapter.		
Orphenadrine	Refer to the Autonomic Agents chapter.		

Catechol-*O*-Methyltransferase Inhibitors

Universal prescribing alerts:

- COMT inhibitors are ineffective as monotherapy for managing Parkinsonian symptoms. They are useful only as adjunct treatment in patients receiving dopamine replacement therapy.
- Do not use concurrently with nonselective MAO inhibitors.
- Do not use in patients with major psychosis disorders due to the risk of exacerbating psychosis.
- Use of COMT inhibitors has been associated with hallucinations, abnormal thinking, compulsive or psychotic-like behaviors, and loss of impulse control. It may be necessary to adjust the dosage to avoid these side effects.
- Somnolence and falling asleep while engaged in activities have been reported. Patients should be evaluated for risks that may exacerbate these symptoms, such as concomitant use of sedating medications or sleep disorders. Monitor for drowsiness or sleepiness.
- New-onset or exacerbation of preexisting dyskinesia may occur when COMT inhibitors are used concurrently with levodopa.
- Use of these medications has been associated with a syndrome resembling NMS upon abrupt withdrawal. Gradual dosage reduction is recommended when discontinuing therapy.
- COMT inhibitors may cause orthostatic hypotension and syncope. Use with caution in patients at risk of hypotension.
- COMT inhibitors may cause severe rhabdomyolysis.
- Use with caution in patients with lower gastrointestinal disease or an increased risk of dehydration. These medications have been associated with delayed development of diarrhea.

Drug Name	FDA-Approved Indications	Adult Dosage Range	Precautions and Clinical Pearls
Generic Name Entacapone **Brand Name** Comtan	Parkinson's disease (adjunct to levodopa/carbidopa to treat end-of-dose "wearing-off")	**Usual oral dose for Parkinson's disease:** 200 mg up to 8 times per day (MDD: 1600 mg per day)	• Use with caution in patients with hepatic impairment or biliary obstruction • This medication (and other dopamine potentiators) has been linked to the exacerbation of impulse control disorders and high-risk behaviors; monitor CNS effects • Hypotension and syncope have been reported • Highly protein-bound drug; use caution when giving entacapone with other highly protein-bound drugs • Also available in a combination product with levodopa/carbidopa (Stalevo) • Monitor skin for melanoma; patients with Parkinson's appear to be at higher risk
Generic Name Tolcapone **Brand Name** Tasmar ■	Parkinson's disease (adjunct to levodopa/carbidopa)	**Usual oral dose:** 100 to 200 mg 3 times per day	• Do not initiate in patients with clinical evidence of liver disease or with two transaminase values greater than the upper limit of normal • Only for patients also receiving carbidopa and levodopa; discontinue tolcapone if clinical improvement does not occur within 3 weeks, regardless of dose • A patient-signed consent form acknowledging the risks of hepatic injury should be obtained by the treating prescriber • Use with caution in patients with severe renal impairment Associated with: • Risk of hepatotoxicity: fatal liver injury has been reported with use • Use only in patients who are experiencing inadequate symptom control or who are not candidates for other available treatments

Dopamine Precursors			
Drug Name	**FDA-Approved Indications**	**Adult Dosage Range**	**Precautions and Clinical Pearls**
Generic Name Levodopa/carbidopa **Brand Name** Sinemet Sinemet CR Duopa Rytary	Parkinson's disease Post-encephalitic Parkinsonism Symptomatic Parkinsonism following carbon monoxide intoxication or manganese intoxication	**Usual oral dose for Parkinson's disease:** IR: Carbidopa 25 mg/ levodopa 100 mg 3 times per day ER: Carbidopa 50 mg/ levodopa 200 mg twice daily As disease progresses, patients may require as much as 1000 to 1500 mg per day of levodopa for symptom management	• Use with extreme caution in patients with psychiatric disorders due to risk of exacerbating psychosis; monitor for depression and suicidal tendencies • Abnormal thinking and behavioral changes have been reported • May cause or exacerbate dyskinesia; dosage reduction may be necessary because of this effect • Somnolence and falling asleep while engaged in activities have been reported; monitor for drowsiness or sleepiness • Has been associated with a syndrome resembling NMS upon abrupt withdrawal; gradual dosage reduction is recommended when discontinuing therapy • Monitor for signs and symptoms of postural hypotension; use with caution in patients with hypotension • Use with caution in patients with severe cardiovascular disease, endocrine disease, open-angle glaucoma, peptic ulcer disease, hepatic impairment, renal impairment, seizure disorder, or respiratory disease • Monitor patients for peripheral neuropathy Contraindications: • History of melanoma • Closed-angle glaucoma • Specific drug interactions that may require dose adjustments or avoidance of certain drug combinations

Dopamine Receptor Agonists

Ergot-Derived Dopamine Receptor Agonists

Universal prescribing alerts:

- Ergot derivatives may cause CNS depression. Patients should use caution when performing tasks that require mental alertness.
- These agents may cause auditory or visual hallucinations. Symptoms may persist for several weeks following the medication's discontinuation.
- These agents have been associated with compulsive behaviors, loss of impulse control, hypersexuality, and aggression. Dose reduction or discontinuation generally reverses these behaviors.
- Do not use ergot derivatives in patients with uncontrolled hypertension, history of valve disorder, or history of a pulmonary, pericardial, or retroperitoneal fibrotic disorder.

Drug Name	FDA-Approved Indications	Adult Dosage Range	Precautions and Clinical Pearls
Generic Name Bromocriptine **Brand Name** Cycloset Parlodel (PD)	Acromegaly Hyperprolactinemia Parkinson's disease Type 2 diabetes mellitus (adjunct to diet and exercise)	Dose is dependent on indication for use, formulation selected, and patient's clinical response **Illustrative oral dose for hyperprolactinemia:** Initial: 1.25 to 2.5 mg per day Maintenance: 20 to 30 mg per day (MDD: 100 mg per day)	• Has been associated with fibrotic valve thickening • Has been associated with hypertension, seizures, myocardial infarction, and stroke; discontinue if hypertension, severe or unremitting headache, or evidence of CNS toxicity develops • May cause pleural, pulmonary, or retroperitoneal fibrosis and constrictive pericarditis; discontinue if fibrotic changes are noted; may cause pleural and pericardial effusions • Increased gastric secretions and fatal GI bleeding have been reported; avoid use in high-risk patients • Use caution in patients with underlying psychiatric conditions • Has been associated with a syndrome resembling NMS upon abrupt withdrawal; gradual dosage reduction is recommended when discontinuing therapy • Certain drug interactions may require dose adjustment or avoidance of some combinations Contraindications: • Patients with syncopal migraine (also known as basilar/hemiplegic migraine or basilar-type migraine) • Uncontrolled hypertension
Generic Name Cabergoline	Hyperprolactinemia	**Usual oral dose:** 0.25 mg twice weekly (maximum: 1 mg twice weekly) Titrate doses gradually (refer to PI)	• Use with caution in patients with severe hepatic impairment, renal insufficiency, peptic ulcer disease, or Raynaud syndrome • Depression and impulsivity has been reported; monitor for behavioral changes • Prior to initiating and throughout treatment, an ECG should be performed to assess the risk of cardiac valvulopathy, discontinue cabergoline if an ECG reveals signs of valvulopathy • Initial doses greater than 1 mg may cause orthostatic hypotension Contraindications: • Avoid in patients with uncontrolled hypertension and use caution in patients taking antihypertensive agents • History of pulmonary, pericardial, cardiac valvular, or retroperitoneal fibrotic disorders

Non-Ergot-Derived Dopamine Receptor Agonists

Drug Name	FDA-Approved Indications	Adult Dosage Range	Precautions and Clinical Pearls
Generic Name Apomorphine **Brand Name** Apokyn ▲ QT	Parkinson's disease (adjunct for relief of hypomobility "off" episodes)	**Usual parenteral dose:** SQ: initial test dose 2 mg If patient tolerates test dose and responds: Starting dose: 2 mg as needed; may increase dose in 1-mg increments every few days (maximum dose: 6 mg per injection) If patient tolerates but does not respond to 2-mg test dose: Second test dose: 4 mg (MDD: 20 mg per day)	• Certain drug interactions may require dose adjustment or avoidance of some combinations • For subcutaneous use only (not IV) • Derivative of morphine; should not be used in patients with decreased alertness, gag reflex or respiratory depression, seizures, seizure disorder, unconsciousness or coma; monitor CNS for behavioral changes • Should be administered in the abdomen, upper arm, or upper leg; rotate sites (to avoid skin reactions) • Taper dosage slowly when discontinuing • Monitor: supine and standing blood pressure and pulse before and after each test dose; refer to PI for details • Monitor: signs and symptoms of orthostatic hypotension; drowsiness or sleepiness; mental status and behavioral changes; periodic skin examinations; nausea and vomiting; dyskinesias; and excessive sedation or somnolence • Avoid use (or use extreme caution) in patients with cardiac decompensation, cerebrovascular disease, or a susceptibility to nausea or vomiting. • Begin antiemetic therapy 3 days prior to initiation and continue for 2 months before reassessing need • Avoid use of antidopaminergic antiemetic drugs such as promethazine
Generic Name Pramipexole **Brand Name** Mirapex Mirapex ER ▲	Parkinson's disease Restless legs syndrome (IR only)	**Usual oral dose for RLS:** IR: 0.125 mg once daily 2 to 3 hours before bedtime; increase gradually every 4 to 7 days up to 0.5 mg per nightly dose **Usual oral dose for Parkinson's disease:** ER initial: 0.375 mg once daily (maximum: 4.5 mg once daily)	• Retitration of dose should be considered for any significant interruption in therapy • Administer with food to decrease nausea • Dosage should be increased to achieve a maximum therapeutic effect, balanced against the side effects of dyskinesia, hallucinations, somnolence, and dry mouth • Taper dosage slowly when discontinuing • Monitor: blood pressure and heart rate (especially during dose escalation); body weight changes; CNS depression; fall risk; behavior changes (compulsive behaviors); periodic skin examinations • Increase doses gradually not more frequently than every 4 to 7 days

Drug Name	FDA-Approved Indications	Adult Dosage Range	Precautions and Clinical Pearls
Generic Name Ropinirole **Brand Name** Requip Requip XL ▲	Parkinson's disease Restless legs syndrome (IR only)	**Usual oral dose for Parkinson's disease:** IR initial dose: 0.25 mg 3 times per day gradually increase dose up to 8 mg per dose (maximum: 24 mg per day)	• Interruption in therapy may warrant retitration • Administer without regard to meals • Do not crush, split, or chew extended-release tablets • Certain drug interactions may require dose adjustment or avoidance of some combinations • Titrate dosage slowly when increasing doses or discontinuing ropinirole; refer to PI for specific guidelines • Monitor: blood pressure (orthostatic); daytime alertness; CNS depression; fall risk; behavior changes (e.g., compulsive behavior) • Specific recommendations for patients undergoing dialysis • Cigarette smoking may decrease the effectiveness of this agent
Generic Name Rotigotine **Brand Name** Neupro	Parkinson's disease Restless legs syndrome	**Usual transdermal dose for Parkinson's disease:** Apply 1 patch (2 mg per 24 hours) once daily; may increase by 2 mg per 24 hours weekly, based on clinical response and tolerability Lowest effective dose: 4 mg per 24 hours MDD: 6 mg per 24 hours	• Transdermal patch contains metal (e.g., aluminum); remove patch prior to magnetic resonance imaging (MRI) or cardioversion • Higher strength patches are available for patients requiring dose increases • Taper dosage slowly when discontinuing; do not discontinue abruptly • Monitor: blood pressure (including orthostatic); daytime alertness; periodic skin evaluations (melanoma development)

Monoamine Oxidase B Inhibitors

Universal prescribing alerts:

- Use caution in patients with underlying cardiovascular disease or any condition (including concurrent use of medications that cause the same adverse effects) that increases the risk of prolonged QTc.
- Avoid tyramine-rich foods and concurrent use of sympathomimetics (and other drugs with MAOI-like actions). Numerous serious drug interactions have been noted.
- At least 2 weeks should elapse between the discontinuation of other serotonergic agents and beginning of MAO-B inhibitor use; specific agents such as fluoxetine require longer periods prior to their initiation.
- All medications with CNS depressant effects may cause drowsiness or dizziness. Patients should use caution while driving or operating machinery until the effects of the drug are known.
- Monitor blood pressure and heart rate; diet, weight, and blood glucose; and mood, mental status, suicidal ideation, and unusual (impulsive or other) behavior (especially during the initial months of therapy or when doses are increased or decreased).
- Use cautiously in patients with peptic ulcer disease due to possible reactivation of ulcers. This effect is believed to be caused by stimulation of the histamine receptors in the stomach or by the inhibition of MAO in the stomach, preventing the breakdown of gastric histamine.

Drug Name	FDA-Approved Indications	Adult Dosage Range	Precautions and Clinical Pearls
Generic Name Rasagiline **Brand Name** Azilect ■	Parkinson's disease	Dose is dependent on indication for use and patient's clinical response **Usual oral dose as monotherapy or adjunctive therapy of Parkinson's disease (not including levodopa):** 1 mg once daily (MDD: 1 mg per day)	• Certain drug interactions may require dose adjustment or avoidance of some combinations • When added to existing levodopa therapy, a dose reduction of levodopa may be required to avoid exacerbation of dyskinesias • Tyramine alert: concurrent ingestion of foods rich in tyramine, dopamine, tyrosine, phenylalanine, tryptophan, or caffeine may cause sudden and severe high blood pressure (hypertensive crisis or serotonin syndrome)
Generic Name Selegiline **Brand Name** Eldepryl Emsam (patch) Zelapar ■	Parkinson's disease (adjunct to dopamine replacement) Major depressive disorder (patch only)	**Usual oral dose for Parkinson's disease:** 5 mg twice daily with breakfast and lunch **Usual transdermal dose for depression:** Initial: 6 mg per 24 hour patch at the same time each day (rotate application sites). Increase dose at intervals no less than every 2 weeks if needed up to max 12 mg per 24 hours	• Caution patients against eating foods high in tyramine • The Emsam patch is indicated only for depression; its label carries a black box warning for suicidality (as is the case for all antidepressants) • Tyramine alert: tyramine-containing foods/beverages/dietary supplements should be avoided beginning on the first day of selegiline 9 mg per 24 hour or 12 mg per 24-hour treatment.

Chapter 8

Electrolytic, Caloric, and Water Balance Agents

Authors: **Tammie Lee Demler, PharmD, BS Pharm, MBA, RPh, BCPP and Charlene Meyer, PharmD**

Editor: **Claudia Lee, RPh, MD**

Learning Objectives

- Identify current pharmacologic agents that are appropriate for each condition/diagnosis.
- Recommend optimal pharmacologic interventions based on patient-specific characteristics.
- Provide appropriate patient-specific counseling points and optimal overall medication management.

Key Terms: Electrolytic, caloric, and water balance agents; acidifying agents; alkalinizing agents; ammonia detoxicants; replacement preparations; ion-removing agents; calcium removing agents; potassium removing agents; phosphate removing agents; diuretic agents; loop diuretics; osmotic diuretics; potassium-sparing; thiazide and thiazide-like diuretics; vasopressin antagonists; irrigating solutions; uricosuric agents; caloric agents

Overview of Electrolytic, Caloric, and Water Balance Agents

Electrolytes

It is estimated that approximately 60% of the human body's weight consists of water. Approximately 30% of this water is found outside of the cells (extracellular), while the remaining 70% is found within the cells (intracellular). Electrolytes are dissociated ions that are dissolved in the body's water. Positive ions are called cations; negative ions are called anions. Together, cations and anions balance each other out to support homeostasis.

Electrolytes are electrically charged particles found in the blood, plasma, urine, and other fluids that are essential for critical bodily functions including, but not limited to, fluid balance, nerve integrity, and muscle function. Sodium, potassium, calcium, chlorine, magnesium, and phosphate are all examples of electrolytes found in fluids, supplements, and foods. The balance of electrolytes is constantly fluctuating based on shifting fluid levels in the body; however, significant changes (i.e., deficiency or excess) of electrolytes can disrupt the overall balance and functioning of the body and may result in death without prompt intervention.

In a healthy patient, electrolytes exist within a "normal" range. In contrast, when a person has a disease, is in shock, or is exposed to medications that can alter electrolytes, an imbalance may develop. Low values can be increased to normal levels by supplementation of the specific electrolyte; if they are dangerously low, intravenous (IV) therapy may be necessary. High electrolyte levels can be decreased to the normal range by a number of mechanisms, including the use of certain medications that bind electrolytes and promote their excretion. If a medication is the cause of the imbalance, changing the medication or decreasing the dose of the offending agent may be the only solution. In patients with end-stage renal disease (ESRD), dialysis is often the only way to filter out (or "remove") excessive electrolytes.

Most medications will not alter the tonicity (i.e., the concentration of electrolytes in solution). One key exception is parenteral (IV) medications, which can be altered to become isotonic. *Isotonic* means the osmolality is the same as that of physiological body fluids. Both sodium chloride 0.9% and dextrose 5% are isotonic and, therefore, are typically used as diluents for intravenous drug administration. Hypertonic solutions have a high osmolality and can cause damage by drawing out water from the inside of cells, whereas hypotonic solutions have a low osmolality and drive water into the cells, which can cause cells to rupture. The tonicity of a solution affects not only parenteral administration of that solution, but also medications that target mucous membranes, such as ophthalmic solutions, for which hypertonic and hypotonic solutions can cause irritation.

The kidney filters plasma, so it is a major site of action for diuretic medications and is vital in maintaining overall homeostasis. The proximal tubule filters most of the sodium chloride and water out of the plasma. The thin descending loop of the kidney is highly permeable to water, which makes it an ideal site to increase excretion by promoting diuresis in conditions such as edema. The thick ascending loop aids in reabsorbing sodium chloride, with the remaining sodium chloride being reabsorbed in the distal tubule. The distal tubule is also the major site of action for antidiuretic hormone (ADH), also called vasopressin. In the presence of vasopressin, aquaporin water channels are created to reabsorb water. Aldosterone is another important hormone that acts on the distal tubule and the collecting duct to reabsorb sodium and water. The onset of action of aldosterone is approximately 1 hour. Thus, it is delayed compared to other mechanisms to control sodium and water reabsorption. The last segment of the nephron, the collecting duct, can make slight changes to reabsorption or in acid-base balance.

Caloric Balance

A calorie is a unit of energy that fuels the body to carry out both the basic necessities of life and activities pursued during the day. Patients in the hospital or with severe debilitating diseases often need additional support to obtain the necessary calories to heal and maintain health. If the patient has a functional gastrointestinal tract but cannot or does not desire to eat, a nasogastric tube can be used to provide the essential nutritional calories. In situations where the gut is unusable for an extended period of time, such as obstruction or inflammation, total parenteral nutrition (TPN) is used.

TPN is given through a central line and contains a high concentration of ingredients, which can damage peripheral veins due to phlebitis. TPN delivered through a peripheral line must have a lower osmolality to be safe for the patient. The three main components of TPN are amino acids, dextrose, and lipids, all of which provide different calories per gram of substance. Amino acids provide protein, dextrose provides glucose, and lipids provide fats. Lipids cannot be used if the patient has an egg allergy, as they are sourced from eggs. TPN also contains electrolytes, vitamins, and minerals whose amounts are tailored to the patient's individual needs. Insulin can be added to TPN to meet the basal requirements for this hormone.

When calculating the caloric needs of a patient, an estimated energy requirement equation (e.g., the Harris-Benedict equation) is used. Activity level is then determined along with any other special needs. For example, patients with burns require more calories due to the extensive healing process required to overcome these severe injuries. These calculations provide the information needed to construct a TPN solution. Water is then added to ensure optimal fluid intake or restricted if the patient has edema. When preparing a TPN, sterility is crucial, as the patients receiving such nutrition often have compromised immune systems.

Water Balance

Water balance reflects the amount of the water we take in and the amount of water we excrete. Every day, water is excreted through bowel movements, perspiration, and respiration. When the water balance is low, thirst is commonly triggered as a symptom of impending dehydration. The kidney is capable of diluting urine to increase excretion depending on the water balance and changing needs of the body. More water will be needed during periods of exercise or when there are water losses due to illness. Vasopressin also controls water by creating aquaporins that promote water removal. Unfortunately, water balance becomes easily unbalanced with too much water causing edema, pain, difficulty walking, and difficulty breathing and too little water causing dehydration and dryness. Elderly individuals can sometimes lose their sense of thirst and may not be aware when they become dehydrated.

Edema can be treated with diuresis, usually with the pharmacotherapeutic assistance of diuretic medications. When reabsorption of sodium into the nephron is decreased, water will follow the sodium to dilute the concentration of ions. Often, a side effect of diuretics is a low potassium level, a factor that may need to be monitored to ensure the level of this ion does not drop significantly.

To treat dehydration, fluid loss, and overall water deficit, parenteral (IV) fluids are often given. Crystalloids are fluids that contain water, electrolytes, and possibly glucose. They are not equivalent to colloids, which are fluids that consist of blood products, such as albumin. Both crystalloids and colloid fluids are used to replenish water. Which fluid is selected for administration depends on the other conditions of the patient, such as tonicity.

Dextrose, sodium chloride, and lactated Ringer's solutions are all crystalloids. Dextrose is a useful source of free water when sodium levels are high. Normal saline contains 0.9% sodium chloride and is isotonic; it is useful to replenish water without changing the osmolality. Hypotonic and hypertonic saline are also used when appropriate to correct fluid and electrolytes. Lactated Ringer's solution is considered to match normal physiology, but is not as effective at increasing fluids as normal saline.

Colloids, such as albumin, hetastarch, and dextran, are also used to increase fluids. Albumin, the most frequently used colloid, increases intercellular fluids in patients with specific conditions. Although albumin increases intercellular fluid more dramatically than crystalloids do, crystalloids are still preferred for this indication. Maintenance fluids may be needed in the hospital for patients who are unable to take in enough water to balance out the daily loss of water through bodily functions; this water loss can be replaced with parenteral (IV) fluids.

8.1 Acidifying, Alkalinizing, and Ammonia Detoxicant Agents

Although not often used, acidifying agents can help correct metabolic alkalosis or create an acidic pH in the urine. Alkalinizing agents are much more common and can help neutralize stomach acid, correct metabolic acidosis, and treat hyperammonemia. Caution is advised to prevent overcorrection. Ammonia detoxicants aid in the removal of excess ammonia from the blood. Ammonia is a substance that contains nitrogen and hyperammonemia is a metabolic disturbance characterized by an excess of ammonia in the blood. It is a dangerous condition that may lead to encephalopathy and death. Lactulose is one of the most common ammonia detoxicants currently available for use and is also frequently used as a laxative (and these additional indications for use are discussed in the Gastrointestinal Agents chapter).

Acidifying Agents

Ammonium chloride

Alkalinizing Agents

Citrate salts
Sodium bicarbonate
Sodium lactate

Ammonia Detoxicants

Acetohydroxamic acid
Carglumic acid
Lactulose
Sodium phenylacetate and sodium benzoate
Sodium phenylbutyrate

Case Studies and Conclusions

CM is a 54-year-old African American male who is in the hospital due to liver failure. He has a past history that is significant for alcoholism with relapse. CM is diagnosed with hepatic encephalopathy, which is now causing hyperammonemia. He is lethargic and incoherent in speech. His skin and the whites of his eyes are yellow. The family is distraught and begins asking you questions.

1. Which medication can be used to treat CM's hyperammonemia?
   a. Sodium phenylbutyrate
   b. Sodium phenylacetate/sodium benzoate
   c. Carglumic acid
   d. Sodium bicarbonate

Answer B is correct. Sodium phenylacetate/sodium benzoate is indicated for acute hyperammonemia. Carglumic acid is used for urea cycle disorder treatment, and sodium phenylbutyrate is indicated for chronic hyperammonemia. Sodium bicarbonate is not used to correct ammonia levels.

2. Which medication can be given to improve CM's encephalopathy?
   a. Lactulose
   b. Carglumic acid
   c. Acetohydroxamic acid
   d. Ammonia detoxicant

Answer A is correct. Lactulose is indicated for systemic hepatic encephalopathy and improves cognition.

8.2 Replacement and Removal Agents

Ion-Removing Agents

When patients have low electrolyte levels, the deficient electrolytes can easily be replaced by giving the electrically charged particle that they are lacking in a stable salt form. These preparations come in various forms, including oral solid tablets, chewable tablets, parenteral (IV) solutions, and powders. Sometimes such an imbalance occurs due to a lack of the electrolyte in the diet or due to a disease state, such as lack of calcium in osteoporosis. When providing supplementation, the provider should be careful not to overcorrect the balance. Hetastarch and hydroxyethyl starch are not often used, but are beneficial parenteral choices when a patient has experienced a large blood loss. Often, however, the goal is to replenish fluid volume, which can be done in more cost-effective and less risky ways.

The medications called binders work by binding to specific ions and removing them from the circulation in the body. These agents can be administered to prevent complications, such as using cellulose sodium phosphate to prevent kidney stones caused by calcium buildup, or using sodium polystyrene sulfonate to help remove potassium ions when the kidney is not working properly. Each removal agent comes with its own unique precautions.

Replacement Preparations

Calcium salts
Dextran
Electrolyte solutions
Hetastarch/hydroxyethyl starch
Potassium supplements
Sodium chloride

Ion-Removing Agents

Calcium-Removing Agents

Cellulose sodium phosphate

Potassium-Removing Agents

Sodium polystyrene sulfonate

Phosphate-Removing Agents

Ferric citrate
Lanthanum
Sevelamer
Sucroferric oxyhydroxide
Calcium salts *(see also the Replacement Preparations section)*

Other Ion-Removing Agents

Prussian blue

Case Studies and Conclusions

FW is a 61-year-old female who is on dialysis. Her labs are significant for Ca: 11.5 mg/dL (9.2 to 11mg/dL), K: **4.2 mEq/L** (3.8 to 5 mEq/L), and phosphate: **5.1 mg/dL** (2.3 to 4.7mg/dL). She is currently on levothyroxine 125 mcg per day for hypothyroidism. FW also has a history of dysphagia and has trouble swallowing large tablets and capsules; she prefers to have a smaller pill burden.

1. Which medication would you recommend giving FW to lower her phosphate level?
   a. Lanthanum
   b. Sevelamer
   c. Sucroferric oxyhydroxide
   d. Calcium acetate

Answer A is correct. Sevelamer is also an appropriate choice; however, it involves a high pill burden and does not come in chewable tablets as lanthanum does. Calcium acetate is not appropriate due to the patient's already high calcium levels. Sucroferric oxyhydroxide is contraindicated with levothyroxine use.

2. Which one of the following characteristics is true of sevelamer?
   a. Will raise cholesterol levels
   b. Will bind fat-soluble vitamins
   c. Is available only for parenteral administration
   d. Has aluminum in the formulation

Answer B is correct. Sevelamer lowers total cholesterol, is available for oral administration, and has no aluminum or calcium in the formulation but it does bind fat soluble vitamins. Aluminum products can cause toxicity and are not preferred.

AD is a 75-year-old female patient who asks you about calcium. Her doctor told her to buy over-the-counter (OTC) calcium supplements and she is confused about the many different products available. AD tells you that she likes to take all of her medications first thing in the morning and does not like to eat breakfast.

1. What calcium supplement do you recommend?
   a. Calcium citrate
   b. Calcium carbonate
   c. Calcium gluconate
   d. Calcium chloride

Answer A is correct. Calcium citrate, although usually a bit costlier, does not require stomach acid for absorption and can be taken without food. Calcium carbonate requires food to be most effective. Calcium gluconate and calcium chloride are available as parenteral (IV) solutions only.

8.3 Diuretic Agents

All diuretics promote diuresis by acting on the nephron of the kidney. As such, these agents are not effective in—and should not be used in—patients with severe kidney failure. The location within the nephron where the agent acts determines the potency of the agent. Diuretics of different classes can be combined to increase diuresis. Loop diuretics act in the loop of Henle and because of their significant capacity for diuresis, are used mainly for edema. Osmotic agents draw the water content from the nephron into the collecting duct and are optimal agents to be combined with loop diuretics for increased effect. Potassium-sparing diuretics are important because they are the only class that provides diuresis while also preventing potassium loss from the body. These agents are helpful in patients with low potassium, high blood pressure, or heart failure. Thiazide diuretics work in the distal tubule by inhibiting reabsorption of sodium chloride to draw water into the collecting duct. They are first-line therapies for reducing blood pressure and tend to be more effective compared to angiotensin-converting enzyme (ACE) inhibitors and angiotensin-receptor blockers (ARBs) in African Americans. Thiazide-like diuretics also work in the distal tubule, albeit through a slightly different mechanism. Vasopressin antagonists are helpful to increase free water removal without affecting electrolytes such as sodium. The role of diuretics in the overall management of cardiovascular conditions is guided by consensus recommendations and current evidence-based medicine. Clinicians should be vigilant in staying current with updates and changes to these guidelines, which often may require combinations of different agents to optimize overall diuresis. Additionally, patients should be encouraged to implement lifestyle changes such as increased exercise and a heart healthy diet and to avoid use of OTC medications that can complicate the management of hypertension (such as oral decongestants, etc.).

Loop Diuretics

Bumetanide
Ethacrynic acid
Furosemide
Torsemide

Osmotic Diuretics

Mannitol
Urea *(see also the Other Skin and Mucous Membrane Agents section in the Skin and Mucous Membrane Agents chapter)*

Potassium-Sparing Diuretics

Amiloride
Triamterene
Eplerenone *(see also the Renin–Angiotensin–Aldosterone System Inhibitors section in the Cardiovasular Agents chapter)*
Spironolactone *(see also the Renin–Angiotensin–Aldosterone System Inhibitors section in the Cardiovasular Agents chapter)*

Thiazide Diuretics

Bendroflumethiazide
Chlorothiazide
Hydrochlorothiazide
Methylclothiazide

Thiazide-like Diuretics

Chlorthalidone
Indapamide
Metolazone

Vasopressin Antagonists

Conivaptan
Tolvaptan

Case Studies and Conclusions

WM is a 35-year-old African American female who is being seen for hypertension. She is currently on lisinopril, which is causing a dry cough. She would like to try another medication, but she has a high deductible insurance and cannot afford expensive medication.

1. Which medication do you recommend for WM?

   a. Hydrochlorothiazide
   b. Valsartan
   c. Furosemide
   d. Triamterene

Answer A is correct. Thiazide diuretics are especially effective in African Americans. Valsartan, although it treats hypertension and does not cause cough, is an ARB and will be more expensive than a thiazide. Furosemide is used for edema. Triamterene is not a first-line therapy for hypertension, but can be used in combination with a thiazide for increased potency.

You have recommended hydrochlorothiazide 25 mg at bedtime to WM. She calls to complain of having to urinate during the night.

2. What do you recommend?

   a. Discontinue hydrochlorothiazide and add valsartan
   b. Decrease the hydrochlorothiazide dose by half
   c. Discontinue hydrochlorothiazide and add amlodipine
   d. Take hydrochlorothiazide in the morning

Answer D is correct. By taking hydrochlorothiazide in the morning, WM will not have to urinate during the night, as the effect of the medication wanes over the day. Hydrochlorothiazide does not need to be discontinued if it is working to lower blood pressure, and decreasing the dose may not be needed if WM takes the medication in the morning.

JD is a 57-year-old African American male who is in the hospital for heart failure exacerbation. He currently is on lisinopril 10 mg daily, metoprolol XR 100 mg daily, and atorvastatin 80 mg daily. He is classified as having Class II heart failure and is experiencing hypokalemia. The doctor also notices edema in his legs with pitting edema 2+.

1. Which medication(s) do you recommend to add to JD's heart failure regimen to improve his clinical status?

   a. Hydralazine and isosorbide dinitrate
   b. Spironolactone
   c. Chlorthalidone
   d. Tolvaptan

Answer B is correct. Spironolactone is a potassium-sparing diuretic and is also an appropriate agent to use in heart failure Classes II–IV to decrease morbidity and mortality. Hydralazine and isosorbide dinitrate do not replace potassium (but are also limited in use for African Americans with Class III–IV heart failure only). Chlorthalidone and tolvaptan do not retain potassium (and are not indicated for decreasing heart failure morbidity and mortality).

2. Which medication do you recommend for JD's edema?

   a. Bumetanide 20 mg
   b. Furosemide 20 mg
   c. Triamterene 40 mg
   d. Chlorthalidone 25 mg

Answer B is correct. Loop diuretics are potent agents used to decrease edema and thus are recommended as first-line therapy. Bumetanide is appropriate; however, the dose given in answer A is above the maximum of 10 mg. The dose of chlorthalidone 25 mg is too low to improve edema. The triamterene dose of 40 mg is also too low.

JD is still experiencing edema after several days of increasing his furosemide dose. Currently, he is on furosemide 200 mg every 8 hours.

3. What do you recommend?

   a. Increase furosemide to 300 mg every 8 hours
   b. Add bumetanide 1 mg every 6 hours
   c. Add metolazone 2.5 mg a half-hour before furosemide
   d. Add hydrochlorothiazide 12.5 mg a half-hour before furosemide

Answer C is correct. The maximum total dose of furosemide is 600 mg, which JD is currently at. Adding bumetanide, another loop diuretic, would not increase diuresis. Instead, a diuretic with a different mechanism should be added to the regimen. Hydrochlorothiazide dosing should be at least 25 mg. Metolazone is a thiazide-like diuretic that will increase the efficacy of furosemide if taken a half-hour before furosemide administration.

8.4 Irrigating Solutions and Other Physiologic Agents

Irrigating solutions are used for a variety of purposes, but—as their name implies—are generally intended to wash an area or flush out a body cavity. Often, irrigating solutions are sterile and must contain no pyogenic material. This consideration is especially important for peritoneal dialysis solutions and irrigations for surgeries. Lactated Ringer's solution, sodium chloride, and sterile water are used when the body is depleted of fluid. Depending on the osmolality and water deficit, patients may receive IV bags over several hours.

Irrigating Solutions

Acetic acid
Glycine
Lactated Ringer's solution
Sodium chloride
Sterile water

Uricosuric Agents

Uricosuric agents are used as second-line agents for prophylaxis in gout attacks or when contraindications exist for the first-line agents. These agents prevent reabsorption of urate in the kidneys and generally should not be used in patients with poor kidney function. They should also not be used in patients with acute gout, as their clinical effect is somewhat delayed. The anti-gout xanthine oxidase inhibitors allopurinol, febuxostat, and colchicine are discussed in detail in the Central Nervous System chapter.

Uricosuric Agents

Probenecid

Caloric Agents

As discussed earlier, caloric agents are used primarily in TPN administration. Amino acid, dextrose, and fats make up the backbone of TPN; TPN may also include electrolytes depending on the patient's specific needs. TPN must be individualized and certain ingredients must be avoided in certain patients, such as patients with egg allergy who must avoid fat emulsion. There are specific criteria that are necessary to justify the use of TPN, for example, in cases when the GI system cannot be used for an extended period of time or when other treatments, such as chemotherapy, cause GI complications. In general, length of stay in the hospital exclusively is not a factor nor is nausea/vomiting alone enough to indicate TPN use.

Caloric Agents

Amino acid injection
Dextrose
Fat emulsions
Invert sugars

Case Studies and Conclusions

JT is an 87-year-old white male who has been in the intensive care unit (ICU) for 7 days due to failure to thrive. He has a significant past history of Crohn's disease, hepatic disease, hypertension, and diabetes. He has a severe egg allergy. JT's code status is DNR (do not resuscitate). His status has been declining, as he has experienced constant vomiting and diarrhea when he eats and has complained of stomach pains for the last 3 days. His Crohn's disease symptoms are now severe, and JT can no longer keep food down. The dieticians and provider feel it is time to start TPN.

1. Which of the following is a proper TPN indication for JT?

   a. Hospital stay of 7 days or longer in the ICU
   b. Nausea and vomiting for 3 days
   c. Current chemotherapy that prevents gastrointestinal (GI) transit
   d. Severe Crohn's disease with complications

Answer D is correct. Length of stay in the hospital is not a factor and nausea/vomiting alone is not enough to indicate TPN use. Chemotherapy with GI complications is an indication for TPN; however, JT is not on chemotherapy at this time. TPN is indicated in case of bowel obstruction or when the GI system cannot be used for an extended period of time.

2. Which of the following TPN ingredients is contraindicated for JT?

   a. Fat emulsions
   b. Dextrose solution
   c. Calcium gluconate
   d. Sodium acetate

Answer A is correct. Fat emulsions cannot be used in patients with egg allergy. Dextrose is needed to provide energy and is used cautiously in patients with diabetes.

PJ is a 45-year-old male who recently had his second gout attack within 6 months. He drinks at least 1 or 2 beers daily and consumes carbonated beverages daily. He is reluctant to change his diet to improve his symptoms. Today his urate level came back as 7.3 mg/dL (the goal is less than 6 mg/dL). Currently, PJ is on allopurinol 400 mg twice daily and is finishing a steroid taper. He also has a significant history of uncontrolled hypertension, obesity, and diabetes.

1. Which medication do you recommend adding to PJ's gout prophylaxis regimen?

   a. Chlorthalidone
   b. Probenecid
   c. Hydrochlorothiazide
   d. Sulfinpyrazone

Answer B is correct. Chlorthalidone and hydrochlorothiazide are both thiazide diuretics, which can exacerbate gout and clinically diuretics are not warranted in this patient for this condition. Sulfinpyrazone, although an old treatment for gout, is no longer available in the United States and is not recommended therapy per American College of Rheumatology guidelines.

PJ is also getting over the common cold and wants a recommendation for treating his nasal congestion.

2. What do you recommend?

   a. Pseudoephedrine (Sudafed)
   b. Guaifenesin with Dextromethorphan
   c. Ocean nasal spray (normal saline solution)
   d. All of these agents are appropriate

Answer C is correct. Sudafed should not be used in patients with uncontrolled hypertension. Guaifenesin with Dextromethorphan are unnecessary interventions for nasal congestion. Combinations of products should be avoided unless the products target specific symptoms and in this case the patient is only experiencing nasal congestion. Ocean nasal spray is sodium chloride that irrigates the nose and helps with congestion and does not complicate other disease states.

Tips from the Field

1. Patients with kidney disease will be among the more common patients you deal with when it comes to fluid replacements and need for ion-removing agents. Due to the potentially serious outcomes of elevations of potassium, phosphate and calcium—regaining control of these concentrations and values is critical. See the following table for a quick review of some of the key electrolytes discussed in this chapter.

Electrolyte	Normal Range	Critical Range	Pearls
Sodium (NaCl)	136–142 mEq/L	Higher than 160 mEq/L Lower than 120 mEq/L	• Used to evaluate overall fluid status • Maintains electric potential of transmembranes • The faster the change the more dangerous the complications
Potassium (KCl)	3.8–5 mEq/L	Higher than 7 mEq/L Lower than 2.5 mEq/L	• Acute change more dangerous than chronic shifts • Responsible for acid–base and fluid balance • Controls excitability of muscle and nervous tissue
Calcium (Ca)	9.2–11 mg/dL	Higher than 14 mg/dL Lower than 7 mg/dL	• Regulates endocrine functions and bone metabolism • Preserves cellular membranes, blood coagulation and neuromuscular activity • The faster the change the more dangerous the complications
Phosphate (PO4)	2.3–4.7 mg/dL	Higher than 8 mg/dL Lower than 1 mg/dL	• Regulates bone and cellular membrane integrity, acid–base, and calcium balance • The faster the change the more dangerous the complications • Seen frequently in renal failure

2. Patients with kidney disease are frequently in need of phosphate binders such as sevelamer and the impact of the potential decrease in absorption of fat soluble vitamins must be considered. Vitamins A, D, E and K are the fat-soluble vitamins.

3. Diuretics regimens frequently require combination therapy to improve the magnitude of diuresis—and clinicians should be cautious because some brand name antihypertensive products may include a diuretic agent. Before adding a supplemental diuretic to any antihypertensive regimen, verify the medication the patient is already taking in a brand name form.

4. Patients who are at highest risk of developing sudden metabolic changes, such as metabolic or respiratory acidosis, are those who have rapid increases in potassium (i.e., as a result of using potassium-sparing diuretics) and those who are debilitated, severely ill, or who have uncontrolled diabetes or cardiovascular disease. Patients at higher risk of acid–base imbalances should have correction before receiving diuretics.

5. Potassium supplements: solid dosage forms of potassium salts (especially sustained-release solid oral dosage forms) are contraindicated in patients in whom there is a risk of delayed passage through the GI tract. Patients who are at higher risk of this delayed passage are those with peptic ulcer disease, gastroparesis, GI or esophageal obstruction, esophageal stricture, or ileus because of the significant potential for gastrointestinal irritation, esophageal stricture, ulceration, and potential perforation.

6. Liquid preparations offer an alternative to solid potassium supplements for patients who should not receive oral solid dosage forms.

Tammie Lee and Jacque

Bibliography

Alpers DH, Stenson WF, Taylor BE, Bier DM. *Manual of Nutritional Therapeutics.* 5th ed. Philadelphia, PA: Lippincott Williams & Wilkins; 2008.

American Geriatrics Society. 2015 updated Beers criteria for potentially inappropriate medication use in older adults. *J Am Geriatr Soc.* 2015;63:2227-2246.

Khanna D, FitzGerald JD, Khanna PP, et al. 2012 American College of Rheumatology guidelines for management of gout. Part 1: systematic nonpharmacologic and pharmacologic therapeutic approaches to hyperuricemia. *Arthritis Care Res.* 2012;64(10):1431-1446.

McEvoy GK, ed. *AHFS: Drug Information.* Bethesda, MD: American Society of Health-System Pharmacists; 2016.

PDR. Triamterene: drug summary. http://www.pdr.net/drug-summary/Dyrenium-triamterene-615. Accessed January 20, 2017.

Prestige (Lebanon). Diet and exercise. November 1, 2015. http://www.pressreader.com/lebanon/prestige-lebanon/20151101/282467117764282/TextView. Accessed December 20, 2016.

Sterns RH, Palmer B. Fluid, electrolyte, and acid–base disturbances. *NephSAP.* 2003;2:3-8.

Yancy CW, Jessup M, Bozkurt B, et al. 2013 ACCF/AHA guideline for the management of heart failure: a report of the American College of Cardiology Foundation/American Heart Association Task Force on Practice Guidelines. *J Am Coll Cardiol.* 2013;62(16):e147-e239.

Symbols

- ▲ Renal impairment: Dose adjustment is recommended.
- □ Hepatic impairment: Dose adjustment is recommended.
- ■ Black box warning exists for this drug.
- (QT) QTc prolongation effects have been reported.
- (BL) Beers list criteria (avoid in elderly).
- (PD) FDA-approved pediatric doses are available.
- (GD) FDA-approved geriatric doses are available.
- See primary body system.

Electrolytic, Caloric, and Water Balance Agents

Universal prescribing alerts:

- Known serious hypersensitivity to the specific drug or any other component of the product/formulation selected warrants a contraindication for its use.
- Adverse reactions associated with the use of some **electrolytic, caloric, and water balance agents** include dizziness, drowsiness, vertigo, or fatigue; these agents may also impair the ability to perform tasks requiring mental alertness. Caution should always be recommended when using any new drug for the first time, when there is a dose change, and for continued use of known offending agents.
- Doses expressed here are for usual adult dosage ranges only. "Geriatric doses" are assumed to be the same as the adult doses unless otherwise noted with a symbol. When pediatric dosing is available, a symbol will guide the reader to additional prescribing references. Refer to real-time prescribing references for these age-specific doses.
- Use of electrolytic, caloric, and water balance agents in pregnancy is based on weighing clinical risk versus benefit; safety concerns are not represented in this grid. Refer to the package insert (PI) for more information. Clinicians should continue to provide education about the reproductive risks of any medication and offer risk-reduction strategies (which may include contraceptive use) to women of childbearing age and understand that these reproductive risks may also extend to males. Other medications may decrease the effectiveness of oral contraceptives. Where necessary, an alternative means of birth control should be explored.
- Brand names are provided for those products still available on the market. Due to the ever-changing product availability, refer to Food and Drug Administration (FDA) resources to confirm the actual brands available. This drug summary is for educational purposes only. Prescribing decisions should be based on real-time comprehensive drug databases that are updated on a regular basis.

Acidifying, Alkalinizing, and Ammonia Detoxicant Agents

Acidifying Agents

Drug Name	FDA-Approved Indications	Adult Dosage Range	Precautions and Clinical Pearls
Generic Name Ammonium chloride	**Common indication for use:** Treatment of hypochloremic states or metabolic alkalosis	**Dosing must be individualized** May calculate dose via the chloride-deficit method (refer to PI) and 50% of calculated dose can be administered then reevaluate need for further treatment	• Ammonia toxicity: monitor closely for signs and symptoms of ammonia toxicity, including pallor, diaphoresis, altered breathing, bradycardia, arrhythmias, retching, twitching, seizure, and coma • Consider use in patients who cannot receive sodium chloride and who do not have end-stage hepatic disease Contraindications: • Severe renal or hepatic impairment

Alkalinizing Agents

Drug Name	FDA-Approved Indications	Adult Dosage Range	Precautions and Clinical Pearls
Generic Name Citrate salts	Alkalization of urine Correction of metabolic acidosis Neutralization of gastric acid	Dose depends on type of citrate acids; most likely to be determined by sodium or potassium content	• For contraindications and cautions, refer to the specific citrate salt for more details
Generic Name Sodium bicarbonate	**Common indications for use:** Alkalization of urine Management of metabolic acidosis Treatment of hyperkalemia Management of overdose of tricyclic acids and aspirin	Dose varies with indication for use and patient's clinical response **Illustrative oral dose for urine alkalization:** Initial: 48 mEq (4 g), then 12 to 24 mEq (1 to 2 g) every 4 hours; dose should be titrated to desired urinary pH	• Parenteral (IV) doses for metabolic acidosis should be based on specific weight-based formulas and the desired increase in serum HCO_3^- (mEq/L); refer to PI Contraindications: • Alkalosis • Hypernatremia • Severe pulmonary edema • Hypocalcemia • Unknown abdominal pain
Generic Name Sodium lactate	Prevention and treatment of mild to moderate metabolic acidosis Alkalization of urine	Dose varies with indication for use and patient's clinical response **Usual parenteral dose:** IV: depends on degree of acidosis	Contraindications: • Hypernatremia • Fluid retention • Lactic acidosis

Ammonia Detoxicants

Drug Name	FDA-Approved Indications	Adult Dosage Range	Precautions and Clinical Pearls
Generic Name Acetohydroxamic acid ▲ (PD)	Adjunct treatment of urea-splitting urinary infection	**Usual oral dose:** 250 mg 3 to 4 times per day, for a total dose of 10 to 15 mg/kg per day (MDD: 1500 mg)	• May cause bone marrow suppression, hemolytic anemia, hepatotoxicity, and/or rash • Monitor hematologic and liver functions • Patients should limit or avoid alcohol use during therapy Contraindications: • Infection of non-urease-producing organisms • Poor renal function: serum creatinine more than 2.5 mg/dL and/or creatinine clearance (CrCl) less than 20 mL per minute
Generic Name Carglumic acid	Adjunct treatment of acute/chronic hyperammonemia due to deficiency of *N*-acetylglutamate synthetase (NAGS)	**Usual oral dose acute:** 100 to 250 mg/kg per day divided in 2 to 4 doses (rounded to the nearest 100 mg); titrate to age-appropriate plasma ammonia levels	• Monitor serum ammonia levels and physical symptoms of hyperammonemia such as confusion, vomiting, seizures, and memory impairment • Titrate to appropriate normal plasma ammonia levels for patients based on specific patient factors

Drug Name	FDA-Approved Indications	Adult Dosage Range	Precautions and Clinical Pearls
Generic Name Lactulose **Brand Name** Constulose Enulose Generlac Kristalose (PD)	Treatment of constipation Prevention and treatment of portal-systemic encephalopathy (including hepatic precoma and coma)	**Usual oral dose for constipation:** 10 to 20 g per day (15 to 30 mL); may increase to 40 g per day (60 mL) if necessary	• Although very little lactulose is absorbed systemically, it should be used with caution in diabetes mellitus patients due to its sugar content • If using for greater than 6 months: monitor serum electrolytes (potassium, chloride, carbon dioxide) periodically in older adults and debilitated patients • To improve flavor, may mix solution with water, milk, fruit juice, or carbonated citrus beverage or may be administered on an empty stomach for more rapid results
Generic Name Sodium phenylacetate and sodium benzoate **Brand Name** Ammonul (PD)	Adjunct treatment of acute hyperammonemia and associated encephalopathy in patients with urea-cycle enzyme deficiencies	**Usual parenteral dose** IV: 55 mL/m^2 co-administered with arginine	• Patients may experience extravasation (infuse via central line only), fluid overload (discontinue if severe), gastrointestinal effects (premedicate with antiemetics), hypokalemia (monitor plasma potassium), and neurotoxicity (discontinue if severe) • Any condition in which hypernatremia or edema is of concern might be at particular risk for adverse events (i.e., heart failure, etc.) • May increase risk of seizures • Use caution in renal and hepatic impairment
Generic Name Sodium phenylbutyrate **Brand Name** Buphenyl (PD)	Adjunctive therapy in the chronic management of patients with urea-cycle disorder involving deficiencies of carbamoylphosphate synthetase, ornithine transcarbamylase (OTC), or argininosuccinic acid synthetase (AAS)	**Usual oral dose:** Powder or tablet: 9.9 to 13 g/m^2 per day, administered in equally divided amounts with each meal or feeding, 3 to 6 times daily (MDD: 20 g per day)	• Use caution in renal and hepatic impairment • Initiate carefully in patients who are being treated with corticosteroid therapy; corticosteroids may cause the breakdown of body protein and increase plasma ammonia levels • Any condition in which hypernatremia or edema is of concern might be at particular risk for adverse events (i.e., heart failure, etc.)

Replacement and Removal Agents

Replacement Preparations

Drug Name	FDA-Approved Indications	Adult Dosage Range	Precautions and Clinical Pearls
Generic Name Calcium salts	Supplemental therapy for postmenopausal females	Dose varies with indication for use, formulation selected, and patient's clinical response **Dose depends on the type of calcium salt:** Oral: acetate, carbonate, citrate, gluconate, lactate, or phosphate salt IV: chloride or gluconate salt	• Monitor serum calcium concentrations frequently • Monitor ECG if given IV (gluconate and chloride are only parenteral formulations available) • Most calcium salt forms require stomach acid and food for best absorption (except citrate which can be taken without regard to food and stomach acid) Contraindications: • Ventricular fibrillation • Hypercalcemia • Hypophosphatemia • Renal calculi

Generic Name Dextran 40 LMD in D_5W; LMD in NaCl	Blood volume expander used in treatment of shock or impending shock when blood or blood products are not available	Dose is based on patient's clinical status; for appropriate dose, refer to PI	• Certain dextran concentrations can prolong bleeding time through interference with platelet function, although Dextran 40 appears to have little effect on bleeding time at the recommended dosage; use caution in high-risk patients (and avoid IM injections) • Can increase blood loss because of increased perfusion pressure and improved microcirculatory flow. • Ensure adequate fluid; renal failure is possible in severe dehydration because of increased urine viscosity and specific gravity Contraindications: • Contraindicated in patients with renal disease accompanied by severe oliguria or anuria, and in patients with pulmonary edema; may cause fluid overload
Generic Name Electrolyte solutions	Water and electrolyte imbalances	Dose varies with indication for use, formulation selected, and patient's clinical response (including fluid, electrolyte, acid–base, and glucose balance)	• Monitor for fluid and electrolyte imbalances • Supplement as necessary • Monitor serum glucose when using solutions containing dextrose due to an increased risk of hyperglycemia in patients with diabetes
Generic Name Hetastarch Hydroxyethyl starch **Brand Name** Hespan ▲ ■	Granulocyte yield increase Hypovolemia	**Usual parenteral dose for plasma volume expansion:** IV: 500 to 1000 mL (up to 1500 mL daily) not to exceed 20 mL/kg per day	• Avoid use in patients with preexisting renal dysfunction and use caution in patients at risk of developing heart failure and pulmonary edema • Use caution in hepatic impairment Contraindications: • Renal failure with oliguria or anuria • Use in patients with preexisting coagulopathy or bleeding disorder (may prolong clotting times) • Intracranial bleeding Associated with: • Need to avoid use in critically ill adult patients, including those with sepsis
Generic Name Potassium supplements	**Common indications for use:** Hypokalemia Acute myocardial infarction (AMI) Arrhythmias	**Usual oral dose:** Daily dosage greater than 20 mEq should be divided into multiple doses as opposed to a single dose **Usual parenteral dose:** IV: given only in patients with adequate urine flow; must be administered slowly—do not exceed a rate of 20 mEq per hour	• Monitor ECG and plasma potassium concentrations closely during IV administration of potassium, especially for rate of administration greater than 20 mEq per hour • Administer oral formulations with water or milk after meals to prevent GI upset • Avoid certain formulations (i.e., sustained release tablets) in patients with delayed GI passage/motility; refer to Tips from the Field for further recommendations Contraindications: • Hyperkalemia • Severe renal impairment

Drug Name	FDA-Approved Indications	Adult Dosage Range	Precautions and Clinical Pearls
Generic Name Sodium chloride	**Common indications for use:** Hyponatremia Hypovolemia	Dose varies with indication for use, formulation selected, and patient's clinical response **Usual parenteral dose:** IV: calculated and based on laboratory values (mEq)	• Oral formulations are available • Monitor serum sodium and renal function • Avoid correcting hyponatremia too quickly; recommendations to increase by no more than 10 to 12 mEq/L in the first 24 hours and 18 mEq/L in the first 48 hours; an even slower rate of correction may be appropriate in certain patients; refer to PI Contraindications: • Hypertonic uterus • Hypernatremia • Fluid retention
Ion-Removing Agents			
Calcium-Removing Agents			
Drug Name	**FDA-Approved Indications**	**Adult Dosage Range**	**Precautions and Clinical Pearls**
Generic Name Cellulose sodium phosphate	Hypercalcemia	Dose varies with indication for use, formulation selected, and patient's clinical response Individualized based on 24-hour urinary calcium excretion	Contraindications: • Primary or secondary hyperparathyroidism • Hypomagnesemia • Bone disease • Hypocalcemia • Enteric hyperoxaluria
Potassium-Removing Agents			
Drug Name	**FDA-Approved Indications**	**Adult Dosage Range**	**Precautions and Clinical Pearls**
Generic Name Sodium polystyrene sulfonate **Brand Name** Kayexalate (PD)	Hyperkalemia	**Usual oral dose:** 15 g given 1 to 4 times per day Rectal: 30 to 50 g every 6 hours	• Monitor ECG; monitor for hypokalemia • Separate from other medications; may bind and decrease absorption of other drugs • 15 g dose is approximately 4 level teaspoons of the powder mixed in water or 60 ml of the commercially available suspension • Refer to PI for recommendations for administration • Intestinal necrosis has been reported; avoid in patients who may be at higher risk • Has delayed effect, not intended for urgent treatment Contraindications: • Hypokalemia • Obstructive bowel disease • Reduced gut motility

Phosphate-Removing Agents

Drug Name	FDA-Approved Indications	Adult Dosage Range	Precautions and Clinical Pearls
Generic Name Ferric citrate **Brand Name** Auryxia	Hyperphosphatemia	**Usual oral dose:** 2 to 3 tablets daily (MDD: 12 tablets)	• Monitor serum phosphorus, serum iron, ferritin, and transferrin saturation; adjust dosages as needed • Give with meals Contraindications: • Iron overload syndrome
Generic Name Lanthanum **Brand Name** Fosrenol	Hyperphosphatemia	**Usual oral dose:** Initial: 1500 mg daily, divided and taken with or immediately after meals **Usual dosage range:** 1500 to 3000 mg per day; doses of up to 4500 mg have been evaluated	• Increases of 750 mg daily every 2 to 3 weeks are suggested as needed to reduce the serum phosphate level to less than 6 mg/dL (1.92 mmol/L) • Monitor serum calcium and phosphorus • May offer advantage of smaller pill burden (and option of chewable tablets) when compared to sevelamer • Chew tablets; do not swallow intact tablets • Separate from other medications; may bind and decrease absorption of other drugs Contraindications: • Bowel obstruction
Generic Name Sevelamer **Brand Name** Renagel Renvela	Reduction or control of serum phosphorus in patients with chronic kidney disease on hemodialysis	**Usual oral dose:** 800 to 1600 mg 3 times per day with meals	• Base initial dose on serum phosphorus levels • Maintenance dose adjustment based on serum phosphorus concentration (goal less than 5.5 mg/dL to normal range) • Usual dose is based on patients not taking a phosphate binder; refer to PI for additional dosing recommendations for patients who *are* taking a phosphate binder • Monitor serum calcium and phosphorus • Separate from other medications; may bind (and may also decrease absorption of fat soluble vitamins) Contraindications: • Bowel obstruction

Drug Name	FDA-Approved Indications	Adult Dosage Range	Precautions and Clinical Pearls
Generic Name Sucroferric oxyhydroxide **Brand Name** Velphoro Venofer (PD)	**Common indications for use:** Hyperphosphatemia Anemia	**Usual oral dose:** 1.5 to 2 g daily, divided in 3 doses with meals; increase as needed to achieve serum phosphorus of no more than 5.5 mg/dL	• Monitor serum phosphorus levels • Maintenance dose adjustment based on serum phosphorus concentration (goal less than 5.5 mg/dL to normal range) • Use caution in patients with preexisting hypotension or disease states exacerbated by hypotension • Use caution in hepatic impairment • Do not administer to patients with iron overload • IV dosing is available (not for use IM or SQ) • Requires experienced clinician who is knowledgeable in the use of this agent and specialized care setting • Drug interactions require dose adjustments or avoidance of certain drug combinations (i.e., the absorption of thyroid supplementation may be greatly reduced); refer to PI for additional details
Calcium salts	Refer to the Replacement Preparations section.		
Other Ion-Removing Agents			
Drug Name	FDA-Approved Indications	Adult Dosage Range	Precautions and Clinical Pearls
Generic Name Prussian blue **Brand Name** Radiogardase (PD)	Treatment of known or suspected internal contamination with radioactive cesium and/or radioactive or nonradioactive thallium to increase their rates of elimination	**Usual oral dose:** 3 g given 3 times per day	• Even when treatment cannot be started right away, patients should be given the drug as soon as it becomes available; treatment is still effective even after time has elapsed since exposure • Typical treatment duration is 30 days or more • Base the duration of therapy on weakly radioactivity measurements in the urine and feces • Discontinue when radiation levels are at acceptable levels • Monitor bowel movements, complete blood count (CBC) with differential, platelets, and electrolytes

Diuretic Agents

Loop Diuretics

Universal prescribing alert:

- Loop diuretics can impair glucose tolerance resulting in hyperglycemia; use caution in patients with diabetes.
- May reduce clearance of uric acid, patients with gout or hyperuricemia can have exacerbations of their disease.
- May cause hypokalemia and other electrolyte imbalances. Loop diuretics may induce metabolic alkalosis associated with hypokalemia and hypochloremia; this acid–base imbalance may effectively be treated with potassium chloride replacement.
- May precipitate acute urinary retention due to the increased production and retention of urine; monitor and use caution.
- All diuretics should be used with caution in patients with hepatic disease because minor alterations of fluid and electrolyte balance may precipitate hepatic coma and extra care is advised for patients with acute MI because excessive diuresis may precipitate shock.

Drug Name	FDA-Approved Indications	Adult Dosage Range	Precautions and Clinical Pearls
Generic Name Bumetanide **Brand Name** Bumex ▲ ■ (BL)	Management of edema secondary to heart failure or hepatic or renal disease (including nephrotic syndrome)	**Usual oral dose:** 0.5 to 2 mg per day. May administer multiple daily doses at 4- to 5-hour intervals if response is not adequate (MDD: 10 mg) **Usual parenteral dose:** IM/IV: 0.5 to 1 mg per dose; may repeat in 2 to 3 hours for up to 2 doses if response is not adequate (MDD: 10 mg)	• Use with caution in patients with renal insufficiency, cirrhosis, or ascites • Monitoring: blood pressure, serum electrolytes, renal function, fluid status (weight and I&O) • Avoid in patients with acute MI due to potential for diuresis precipitated shock • Tinnitus and ototoxicity have been reported • Pancreatitis has been reported Contraindications: • Anuria • Hepatic encephalopathy and coma Associated with: • Profound diuresis with water and electrolyte depletion and imbalance
Generic Name Ethacrynic acid **Brand Name** Edecrin (BL)	**Common indications for use:** Management of edema associated with congestive heart failure (HF) Hepatic cirrhosis or renal disease Short-term management of ascites due to malignancy	**Usual oral dose for edema associated with HF:** 50 to 100 mg in 1 or 2 divided doses; may titrate the dose up at 25- to 50-mg increments at intervals of several days to maximum dose of 400 mg per day **Usual parenteral dose:** IV: initial 50 mg and if needed, may repeat dose in 2 to 4 hours	• Monitor BP, renal function, serum electrolytes, hearing, weight, and fluid status • Use caution in renal and hepatic impairment • Has been reported to activate or exacerbate systemic lupus erythematosus (SLE) Contraindications: • Anuria • History of watery diarrhea caused by this product
Generic Name Furosemide **Brand Name** Lasix (BL) (PD)	Management of edema associated with heart failure (HF) and hepatic or renal disease Acute pulmonary edema Treatment of hypertension	**Usual oral dose for edema associated with HF:** Initial: 20 to 80 mg; may repeat dose in 6 to 8 hours. May titrate the dose up at 20 to 40 mg increments up to MDD of 600 mg **Usual parenteral dose:** IM/IV: 20 to 40 mg; may titrate the dose up at 20-mg increments	• Monitor intake and outgo (I&O) and weight in patients within inpatient settings • Monitoring: blood pressure, orthostasis and serum electrolytes, renal function, and hearing • Use caution in patients with hearing impairment • Exacerbation of SLE has been reported with use • Use caution when using high dose (i.e., 80 mg or more) in patients with thyroid disease due to potential inhibition of the binding of thyroid hormones and overall decreased concentration in total thyroid hormone Contraindications: • Anuria

Drug Name	FDA-Approved Indications	Adult Dosage Range	Precautions and Clinical Pearls
Generic Name Torsemide **Brand Name** Demadex (BL)	Management of heart failure and hepatic or renal disease (including chronic renal failure) Treatment of hypertension	Dose varies with indication for use, formulation selected, and patient's clinical response **Illustrative dose for edema associated with HF:** Initial oral/IV: 10 to 20 mg once daily; may increase gradually by doubling dose until the desired diuretic response is obtained (MDD: 200 mg)	• IV and oral dosing are equivalent • Antihypertensive doses are generally lower than those for the management of heart failure • Drug interactions may require dose adjustment Contraindications: • Anuria

Osmotic Diuretics

Universal prescribing alerts:

- May precipitate acute urinary retention due to the increased production and retention of urine; monitor and use caution.
- All diuretics should be used with caution in patients with hepatic disease because minor alterations of fluid and electrolyte balance may precipitate hepatic coma and extra care is advised for patients with acute MI because excessive diuresis may precipitate shock.

Drug Name	FDA-Approved Indications	Adult Dosage Range	Precautions and Clinical Pearls
Generic Name Mannitol ■ (BL)	**Common indications for use:** Adjunctive treatment of edema Induces urinary excretion of toxic substances Irrigation in transurethral surgical procedures	**Usual parenteral dose for edema:** IV: after the initial test dose administer mannitol 10% to 20% via continuous infusion at a rate of 25 to 75 mL per hour	• Used to potentiate diuresis in patients with edema • Intravenous loop diuretics should be given prior to mannitol administration. • Monitor cardiovascular status, urine output, serum electrolytes, serum osmolarity, renal function, and fluid intake during use • Specific warnings are associated with indication for use; refer to PI for complete list of warnings Contraindications: • Anuria
Generic Name Urea	Hyperkeratotic conditions	**Usual topical dose:** Apply 1 to 3 times per day	• Although therapeutically categorized as a diuretic, urea is now limited to topical use • May cause sun sensitivity • Avoid contact with eyes, lips, and mucous membranes • Refer to the Skin and Mucous Membrane Agents chapter; it is therapeutically listed as a diuretic but only approved for use in United States as a topical agent

Potassium-Sparing Diuretics

Universal prescribing alerts

- May precipitate acute urinary retention due to the increased production and retention of urine; monitor and use caution
- All diuretics should be used with caution in patients with hepatic disease because minor alterations of fluid and electrolyte balance may precipitate hepatic coma and extra care is advised for patients with acute MI because excessive diuresis may precipitate shock.
- Debilitated or severely ill patients in whom respiratory acidosis or metabolic acidosis may occur require close monitoring of the acid–base status.

Drug Name	FDA-Approved Indications	Adult Dosage Range	Precautions and Clinical Pearls
Generic Name Amiloride **Brand Name** Midamor ▲ ■ (BL)	Heart failure or hypertension	**Usual oral dose:** Initial: 5 to 10 mg once daily; may increase to 20 mg daily if necessary	• Monitoring: I&O, daily weights, blood pressure, serum electrolytes, renal function, and signs and symptoms of hyperkalemia Contraindications: • Anuria, acute or chronic renal impairment and insufficiency, or evidence of diabetic nephropathy Associated with: • Absolute contraindication for use in patients with hyperkalemia (serum potassium levels greater than 5.5 mEq/L)
Generic Name Triamterene **Brand Name** Dyrenium ▲ ■ (BL)	Edema: associated with congestive heart failure, cirrhosis of the liver, and the nephrotic syndrome; also steroid-induced edema, idiopathic edema, and edema due to secondary hyperaldosteronism	**Usual oral dose for edema:** 100 to 300 mg daily in 1 to 2 divided doses (MDD: 300 mg) **Recommended adjustments for renal impairment:** CrCl greater than 50 mL per minute: no dosage adjustment necessary	Contraindications: • Severe renal impairment or progressive kidney disease • Severe hepatic disease may warrant dose adjustment however no specific recommendation is available Associated with: • Absolute contraindication for use in patients with hyperkalemia (serum potassium levels greater than 5.5 mEq/L)
Eplerenone	Refer to the Cardiovascular Agents chapter.		
Spironolactone	Refer to the Cardiovascular Agents chapter.		

Thiazide Diuretics

Universal prescribing alerts:

- Thiazides may cause sun sensitivity; use appropriate precautions.
- Thiazides and related diuretics have been reported to cause pancreatitis and therefore should be used with caution in patients with a history of pancreatitis.
- Thiazide diuretics are generally considered not effective in severe renal impairment and/or in patients undergoing dialysis.
- Thiazides have been reported to exacerbate SLE.
- May reduce clearance of uric acid, patients with gout or hyperuricemia can have exacerbations of their disease.
- May precipitate acute urinary retention due to the increased production and retention of urine; monitor and use caution.
- All diuretics should be used with caution in patients with hepatic disease because minor alterations of fluid and electrolyte balance may precipitate hepatic coma and extra care is advised for patients with acute MI because excessive diuresis may precipitate shock.
- Debilitated or severely ill patients in whom respiratory acidosis or metabolic acidosis may occur require close monitoring of the acid–base status.

Drug Name	FDA-Approved Indications	Adult Dosage Range	Precautions and Clinical Pearls
Generic Name Bendroflumethiazide **Brand Name** Corzide ▲ ■ (BL)	Hypertension (combination product should not be used for initial therapy)	Initial: bendroflume-thiazide 5 mg (with nadolol 40 mg) once daily; may increase to bendroflumethiazide 5 mg (with nadolol 80 mg) once daily if needed	• May be administered with or without meals • Only available in combination with nadolol in the United States Contraindications: • Anuria • Review beta blocking agents in the Cardiovascular Agents chapter for nadolol's complete list of precautions and contraindications Associated with: • Need to not abruptly withdraw medication that contains a beta blocking agent
Generic Name Chlorothiazide **Brand Name** Diuril Sodium Diuril (BL) (PD)	Management of hypertension Adjunctive treatment of edema	**Usual oral dose for edema:** 500 to 1000 mg daily, divided in 1 to 2 doses **Usual parenteral dose for edema:** IV: 500 to 1000 mg once or twice daily	• Monitoring: I&O, daily weights, blood pressure, serum electrolytes, and renal function • Parenteral administration should be reserved for patients unable to take oral medication or for emergency situations • Do not give by IM or SQ administration; extravasation must be avoided during IV administration to prevent tissue necrosis Contraindications: • Anuria
Generic Name Hydrochlorothiazide **Brand Name** Microzide ▲ (BL) (PD) (GD)	**Common indications for use:** Edema Hypertension	**Usual oral dose for edema:** 25 to 100 mg per day in 1 to 2 divided doses	• Monitoring: I&O, daily weights, blood pressure, serum electrolytes, and renal function • Lower doses may be used for hypertension • Many patients respond to intermittent therapy (i.e., every other day or 3 days each week) when used for edema Contraindications: • Anuria

Generic Name Methyclothiazide (BL)	Edema Hypertension	**Usual oral dose for edema:** 2.5 to 10 mg per day	• Monitoring: blood pressure, weight, serum electrolytes, blood urea nitrogen (BUN), and creatinine • Doses for edema may also be given once every other day, or once per day for 3 to 5 days per week depending on the patient's clinical status • The maximum effective single dose is 10 mg and higher single doses do not typically result in greater diuretic effects, and therefore are not recommended Contraindications: • Anuria

Thiazide-like Diuretics

Universal prescribing alerts:

- May precipitate acute urinary retention due to the increased production and retention of urine; monitor and use caution.
- All diuretics should be used with caution in patients with hepatic disease because minor alterations of fluid and electrolyte balance may precipitate hepatic coma and extra care is advised for patients with acute MI because excessive diuresis may precipitate shock.
- Thiazide–like diuretics are generally considered not effective in severe renal impairment and/or in patients undergoing dialysis.
- Thiazide-like diuretics have been reported to exacerbate SLE.
- May reduce clearance of uric acid, patients with gout or hyperuricemia can have exacerbations of their disease.
- May cause sun sensitivity; use appropriate precautions.

Drug Name	FDA-Approved Indications	Adult Dosage Range	Precautions and Clinical Pearls
Generic Name Chlorthalidone **Brand Name** Thalitone (BL) (PD)	Hypertension Edema associated with heart failure, renal dysfunction, hepatic cirrhosis, or corticosteroid and estrogen therapy	**Illustrative oral dose for edema:** 50 to 100 mg per day or on alternative days (MDD: 200 mg)	• Monitoring: blood pressure, weight, serum electrolytes, BUN, and creatinine • Lower doses may be used for hypertension Contraindications: • Anuria
Generic Name Indapamide (BL)	Heart failure Hypertension	**Usual oral dose for edema associated with HF:** Initial: 2.5 mg once per day; if inadequate response, may increase dose to 5 mg daily after 1 week if needed	• Consider adding another antihypertensive and decreasing the dose if response is not adequate • May require lower doses for other indications (such as hypertension); refer to PI Contraindications: • Anuria

Drug Name	FDA-Approved Indications	Adult Dosage Range	Precautions and Clinical Pearls
Generic Name Metolazone **Brand Name** Zaroxolyn (BL) (PD)	Edema (in renal diseases, including nephrotic syndrome and states of diminished renal function) Hypertension	**Usual oral dose for edema:** Initial: 5 to 10 mg once daily; if needed may titrate up to 20 mg per day	• Electrolyte disturbances: Severe hypokalemia and/or hyponatremia can occur rapidly following initial doses. Hypercalcemia, hypochloremic alkalosis, and hypomagnesemia can also occur. • Hypersensitivity reactions, including angioedema and bronchospasm, have been reported • Renal effects: azotemia and oliguria may occur Contraindications: • Anuria
Vasopressin Agents			
Universal prescribing alerts: • Use care to initiate/re-initiate the use of these agents in facilities where serum sodium concentrations can be closely monitored. Too rapid correction can cause osmotic demyelination resulting in dysarthria, dysphagia, lethargy, changes in affect, seizures, coma, and death.			
Drug Name	**FDA-Approved Indications**	**Adult Dosage Range**	**Precautions and Clinical Pearls**
Generic Name Conivaptan **Brand Name** Vaprisol ■	Treatment of euvolemic and hypervolemic hyponatremia in hospitalized patients	**Illustrative parenteral dose for hyponatremia:** Initial: 20 mg loading dose followed by a maintenance dose of 20 mg continuous infusion over 24 hours The total duration of infusion (after the loading dose) should not exceed 4 days	• Monitoring: blood pressure, weight, serum electrolytes, BUN, urine output, and creatinine • Not intended to treat patients with HF and not recommended in patients with severe renal impairment • Administer loading dose over 30 minutes • Drug interactions may require dose adjustments or avoidance of certain drug combinations • Following the initial day of treatment, may be administered for an additional 1 to 3 days as a continuous infusion of 20 mg per day (if serum sodium goal is not attained, may titrate up to 40 mg per day via continuous infusion) Contraindications: • Anuria • Hypovolemic hyponatremia
Generic Name Tolvaptan **Brand Name** Samsca ■	Hypervolemic and euvolemic hyponatremia (serum sodium less than 125 mEq/L or less marked hyponatremia that is symptomatic and resistant to fluid restriction)	**Usual oral dose:** Initial: 15 mg once daily; after at least 24 hours, may increase to 30 mg once daily to a maximum of 60 mg once daily (titrating dose at intervals of 24 hours or greater based on desired serum sodium values)	• Avoid fluid restriction during the first 24 hours of therapy • Not intended to urgently prevent or to treat serious neurological symptoms • Do not use for more than 30 days (hepatotoxicity) • May be administered without regard to meals • Drug interactions may require dose adjustments or avoidance of certain combinations (i.e., grapefruit juice) Contraindications: • Anuria Associated with: • Serious (sometimes fatal) liver injury; avoid use in patients with hepatic disease or at high risk of injury

Irrigating Solutions and Other Physiologic Agents

Irrigating Solutions

Drug Name	FDA-Approved Indications	Adult Dosage Range	Precautions and Clinical Pearls
Generic Name Acetic acid	Periodic irrigation of indwelling catheters Irrigation of the bladder	**Periodic irrigation of an indwelling urinary:** Use 0.25% acetic acid for continuous irrigation at a rate approximately equal to urine flow; usually 500 to 1500 mL per 24 hours	• Bladder irritation: use of irrigation in patients with mucosal lesions of urinary bladder may cause irritation; open lesions of the bladder mucosa may result in systemic acidosis from absorption • Not for internal intake or IV infusion
Glycine Ringer's Sodium chloride Sterile water			

Uricosuric Agents

Drug Name	FDA-Approved Indications	Adult Dosage Range	Precautions and Clinical Pearls
Generic Name Probenecid **Brand Name** (BL) (PD)	Hyperuricemia associated with gout or gouty arthritis Prolongation and elevation of beta-lactam plasma levels	**Illustrative oral dose for hyperuricemia with gout:** 250 mg twice daily for 1 week; may increase to 500 mg twice daily; if needed, may increase to a maximum of 2 g per day	• Not for use in acute attacks or conditions in which uric acid can increase acutely (i.e., tumor lysis syndrome) • If serum uric acid levels are within normal limits and gout attacks have been absent for 6 months, daily dosage may be reduced by 500 mg every 6 months • May increase dosage in 500 mg increments every 4 weeks • Avoid use in severe renal impairment • May cause GI adverse effects; avoid in patients at high risk (i.e., those with peptic ulcer disease) Contraindications: • Use in patients with blood dyscrasias or hematologic disease • Use in patients with uric acid kidney stones (nephrolithiasis)

Caloric Agents

Drug Name	FDA-Approved Indications	Adult Dosage Range	Precautions and Clinical Pearls
Generic Name Amino acid injections **Brand Name** PROSOL (many others)	Prevents nitrogen loss	Dose varies with indication for use, formulation selected, and patient's clinical response Individualized according to the patient's clinical status and individualized medical needs	• Intended for use in a pharmacy admixture program and is restricted to the preparation of admixtures for intravenous use • Central vein infusion should be considered when amino acid solutions are to be mixed with hypertonic dextrose for the purpose of protein synthesis in patients requiring long-term parenteral nutrition (or those with hypercatabolic or depleted states)

Drug Name	FDA-Approved Indications	Adult Dosage Range	Precautions and Clinical Pearls
Generic Name Dextrose	**Common indications for use:** Hypoglycemia Nutritional supplementation	**Usual oral dose:** 4 to 20 g as a single dose; repeat as necessary **Usual parenteral dose:** IV: 10 to 25 g; repeat as needed	• Repeat dosing as required to normalize blood glucose • Recurrent symptoms of hypoglycemia should be evaluated for medical cause Contraindications: • Diabetic coma • Delirium tremens • Severe dehydration • Glucose-galactose malabsorption syndrome
Generic Name Fat emulsions **Brand Name** Intralipid (many others)	Source of calories and essential fatty acids	Dose varies with indication for use, formulation selected, and patient's clinical response Individualized according to the patient	• Used as a component in TPN • Source of calories and essential fatty acids for patients requiring parenteral nutrition for extended periods of time (usually for more than 5 days) and as a source of essential fatty acids for prevention of Essential Fatty Acid Deficiency (EFAD) • Must follow specific recommendations for order of mixing with other TPN ingredients to maintain appropriate pH balance • Bladder pain, difficult but frequent urge to urinate, burning, painful urination (bloody or cloudy urine), chills, fever, nausea, and vomiting have been reported
Generic Name Invert sugars	Source of calories and water for hydration	Dose varies with indication for use, formulation selected, and patient's clinical response **Usual parenteral dose:** Administer 1 to 3 L of 10% solution intravenously daily	• Invert sugar is a caloric agent consisting of an equimolar carbohydrate mixture of dextrose and fructose (and therefore shares similar actions to that of both dextrose and fructose) • Any advantage over dextrose results from the presence of fructose (each gram of invert sugar provides approximately 4 calories) • Commercially available products are available in combination with electrolytes for IV administration and may can additional inert ingredients; refer to specific manufacturer's PI

Chapter 9

Respiratory Tract Agents

Author: **Wayne H. Grant, PharmD, MBA**

Editor: **Margaret A. Huwer, PharmD**

Learning Objectives

- Identify current pharmacologic agents that are appropriate for each condition/diagnosis.
- Recommend optimal pharmacologic interventions based on patient-specific characteristics.
- Provide appropriate patient-specific counseling points and optimal overall medication management.

Key Terms: Respiratory tract agents, antitussives, opioids, centrally acting antitussives, non-opioids, peripherally acting antitussives, anti-inflammatory agents, leukotriene modifiers, mast cell stabilizers, transmembrane conductance regulator modulators, expectorants, mucolytic agents, phosphodiesterase type 4 inhibitors, miscellaneous respiratory agents, pulmonary surfactants, vasodilating agents, monoclonal antibodies, antifibrotic agents

Overview of Respiratory Tract Agents

Over the past 50 years, treatment of respiratory disorders has been limited and has mainly consisted of antibiotics for infections, potassium iodide as a mucus thinner, and ephedrine and theophylline for bronchodilation. Today's armamentarium of medications applies greater understanding of these diseases and targets the turgid lung.

Pulmonary disease is differentiated based on the phase in which it occurs: acute or chronic. Often these phases will overlap. This differentiation is important, as the drug therapy may be different in selection, dosage, or delivery depending on the phase(s) the patient is experiencing. When respiratory disease is present, the lung's anatomic sites elicit physiologic responses that are detrimental to the patient. Drug therapy is initiated in respiratory tract disorders to improve pulmonary function. Although the advancement of therapies has significantly improved morbidity, a corresponding decline in mortality has not occurred.

Pharmacology of Respiratory Tract Agents

Although pharmacotherapy—meaning the right choice of pharmaceutical agent for the right condition for the right person based on evidence—is imperative, this section will explore the pharmacology of the various respiratory tract medications using a categorical approach, rather than a therapeutic approach. This consideration is important because many drug choices are administered despite the lack of evidence demonstrating their effectiveness.

The goals of care for respiratory disorders involve controlling triggers; decreasing dyspnea, exacerbations, and hospitalizations; and improving exercise tolerance—with the ultimate goal being an enhanced quality of life. The medication choices are only beneficial when combined with lifestyle modifications. Chronic obstructive pulmonary disease (COPD) is an insidious disease and may be seen years to decades after lifestyle modifications are made.

The broad categories of treatments for respiratory tract disorders include symptom relievers, disease modifiers, and palliative enhancers. Such therapies may include anticholinergics, antitussives, anti-inflammatory agents, $beta_2$ agonists, expectorant/mucolytic agents, methylxanthines, and phosphodiesterase 4 inhibitors, among others. Because the pharmacologic management of respiratory disease requires a multiagent approach, it is recommended that the reader review the discussion of autonomic agents before answering the case questions at the end of this chapter.

The impact of respiratory disease has a significant history, with various descriptions of chronic obstructive pulmonary disease reported as early as 1814. In 1846, spirometry was introduced and provided an objective mechanism for the diagnosis of COPD. It would not be until many years later that a comprehensive textbook, *Pulmonary Emphysema*, gave treatment recommendations to the clinician. The past 50 years have been characterized by the greatest understanding of these diseases and their associated drug interventions.

A number of guidelines are available for treatment of respiratory disease. In 1993, a committee formed that was tasked with categorizing lung disease and its management; from this committee's consensus came the National Heart, Lung and Blood Institute (NHLBI)'s lung division, which set out to create a national initiative to focus on the diagnosis, treatment, and research of COPD. Eight years later, the NHLBI began working internationally with the World Health Organization (WHO) to establish the Global Initiative for Obstructive Lung Disease (GOLD), which ultimately classified COPD based on the severity of disease. This collaboration gave rise to a structured format that is a living document, changing as new physiological, pathological, and pharmacologic findings occur.

In January 2016, the GOLD initiative published its latest consensus report, which includes an enhanced focus on symptoms, risk factors, laboratory monitoring, and comorbidities to aid clinicians with the assessment and progression of COPD. Unique to this update was the identification of asthma-COPD overlap syndrome. A December 2015 update defines COPD as "a common preventable and treatable disease, [which] is characterized by persistent airflow limitation that is usually progressive and associated with an enhanced chronic inflammatory response in the airways and the lung to noxious particles or gases. Exacerbations and comorbidities contribute to the overall severity in individual patients."

Other respiratory disorders, such as asthma and cystic fibrosis, also share a long history, significant morbidity, and drug therapy that are described in this chapter. The complexity of the respiratory system is often underestimated, along with its contribution to total overall health. All too often, the pervasive nature of this system in regard to overall health does not become evident until disease affects it. The respiratory system is organized as a series of hollow structures. Air passively enters the nasal or oral cavities, moves past the larynx and into the trachea, and follows a bifurcated path into the individual lungs. Within the lungs, air continues onward through the bronchi and bronchioles, finally settling in the alveoli, where oxygen and carbon dioxide exchange occurs with the circulatory system.

Pathogenesis and Pathophysiology

COPD is a restrictive disease and includes both chronic bronchitis and emphysema. The classic presentation of chronic bronchitis includes a productive cough for longer than 3 months that is observed in two contiguous years. Disease progression may lead to hypercapnia and pulmonary artery vasoconstriction, both of which may trigger right-sided heart failure. Emphysema presents with permanently enlarged airspaces distal to the bronchioles, leading to fibrotic tissue replacement and decreased elasticity. As cardiac output is increasingly affected by this progression, tissues are not perfused with adequate amounts of oxygen, which leads to fatigue and muscle wasting as patients become deconditioned.

Asthma, although restrictive in nature, presents as spasms of the bronchi that affect respirations. Asthma attacks are precipitated by triggers such as allergens or environmental irritants. These attacks can be lethal if not recognized quickly. However, prompt treatment will reverse the attack, and respiratory status will return to baseline in the majority of people. The immune system's mediators of these attacks are $CD4^+$ T lymphocytes and eosinophils. In contrast, the mediators for COPD are $CD8^+$ T lymphocytes, macrophages, and neutrophils. Targeting these mediators can aid in the management of the various types of COPD.

The insidious onset of COPD is multifactorial in nature and includes external insults such as smoking or allergens that enter the pulmonary tract. Airflow may be limited by air trapping, inflammation, gas exchange abnormalities, and mucus hypersecretion. The negative impact of these events requires drug intervention to maximize pulmonary function.

9.1 Antitussive Agents

The presentation of a chronic cough often brings patients into the general healthcare arena. In 2013, approximately 25 million prescriptions were issued for cough. The impact of cough on quality of life requires a multilayered treatment approach that varies based on how advanced the pulmonary disease is. The use of antitussives may help mitigate intermittent or breakthrough cough, but evaluation of the pulmonary condition is required to stabilize the disease and, potentially, eliminate or decrease the incidence of the cough.

Cough is produced by a complex cascade of responses to the inhalation of a foreign substance, such as smoke, allergens, or various chemicals. The removal of these substances is imperative to eliminate or reduce the cough. This can be accomplished through cessation of contact with the external stimuli and the expectoration of internal irritants through forceful expulsion of air from the lungs (i.e., coughing). Afferent vagus nerves richly innervate the aerodigestive tract and travel to the medulla or cough center where a cough is elicited—a process referred to as the cough reflex arc.

While numerous medications to treat cough are available, other potential drug targets that remain under investigation and are the subject of therapies not approved by the Food and Drug Administration (FDA). Conceptually, cough arises through the stimulation of the afferent branches of the vagus nerve. Approaches to alter these pathways are similar to those associated with neuropathic pain disorders. Thus, the promise of cough control is parallel in concept to pain control.

The pharmacology of gamma-aminobutyric acid (GABA) analogues includes agonistic activity at the GABA site as well as additional effects on various neurohormones. One example of such a drug is gabapentin, which targets the brain stem and specifically, the medulla, in response to airway irritation; this effect is hypothesized to be a benefit in decreasing cough. Future consideration of use of these analogues as cough suppressants would require the FDA to also take into account their adverse effects profiles, which may include lethargy, sedation and peripheral edema.

Specific treatments of a cough are stratified based on the specific diagnosis. Clinicians will often use antitussives empirically until the patient seeks a pulmonary specialist. Empiric treatment may include centrally and peripherally acting pharmacologic categories. Central-acting antitussives work directly on the cough reflex arc in the medulla, thereby suppressing the cough and include the opiate antitussive agents and dextromethorphan. Codeine's ability to temper a cough reflects this agent's direct action on the medulla through its binding to mu receptors. With an onset of action of 30 to 60 minutes and duration of effect of 4 to 6 hours, codeine can be useful for treating upper respiratory cough syndrome (postnasal drip) associated with allergens or viral or bacterial illnesses. Approximately 10% of the U.S. population might not respond, however, due to a genetically based inability to convert codeine to its active form in the liver.

Adverse drug reactions (ADRs) within the central nervous system, such as dizziness, drowsiness, and headache, are the most commonly seen side effects of codeine use. Given that this agent interacts with the mu receptor, gastrointestinal (GI) adverse reactions, including constipation, abdominal pain, and nausea, can occur. Dosing variations of opiates are implemented at the lowest dose and titrated up to response or intolerable side effects.

Morphine exhibits similar efficacy and toxicity to that of codeine. Clinically, morphine is not used often for a cough; rather, patients enrolled into hospice or palliative care programs may have morphine prescribed for both cough and dyspnea. Pharmacologically, morphine has a direct effect on the mu receptors, as well as on kappa and delta receptors. The manifestation of this combined drug-induced action is evident in both the spinal cord and the brain stem, leading to a blockade of pain perception. This complex cascade affects numerous neurohormones and neurotransmitters. The end effects are biochemically broad in distribution, as are the adverse reactions experienced by the patient.

Central nervous system adverse reactions are common with morphine use and may include dizziness, drowsiness, and slurred speech. Morphine can cause histamine release, which may be temporary or prolonged, depending on dose and frequency. This histamine release can lead to flushing, redness, and other dermatologic manifestations. It is important to differentiate this type of response from a type I hypersensitivity response; the latter may include life-threating reactions such as angioedema and dyspnea or even more serious reactions resulting in death.

Identifying any adverse response to morphine is important for clinicians in order to distinguish a true drug allergy from drug intolerance. This understanding will allow for other choices in the opioid class to be considered for use in a particular patient. Other ADRs may potentially include constipation, insomnia, dry mouth, and restlessness.

Although its chemical structure is similar to that of morphine, hydromorphone should not be confused with the metabolites of morphine. Hydromorphone is a hydrophilic compound and is often prescribed for intravenous (IV), epidural, or intrathecal use. Because it possesses no renally excreted active metabolites, hydromorphone is the drug of choice when the patient's glomerular filtration (i.e., renal function) is compromised. Its pharmacologic activity in reducing cough is due to its direct effect on the medulla. However, hydromorphone is rarely used by itself, but rather in combination cough preparations.

Hydromorphone does not induce the same degree of histamine release seen with morphine, so dermatologic effects are rarely observed with its use. This property, in addition to its lack of active metabolites, makes hydromorphone a plausible alternative to morphine. Hydromorphone works on the same receptors as morphine (mu, kappa, and delta) and demonstrates the same adverse-effect profile, which may include dry mouth, sedation, and constipation. The potent mu activity of hydromorphone results in lower dosage requirements compared to those of generally recognized equivalent doses of morphine.

Similar in chemical structure to the opioids, but unique in pharmacology, dextromethorphan lacks the opioid-like activity of morphine. However, it possesses antitussive effects owing to its blockade of cough impulses arising from the medulla. Dextromethorphan can also inhibit serotonin receptors, leading to the undesirable adverse reaction called serotonin syndrome (SS). SS can present with agitation, confusion, myoclonus, shivering, and tachycardia.

Use of dextromethorphan at high doses has been associated with abuse reactions, leading to distortions of speech, out-of-body experiences, and visual hallucinations. At the usual prescribed doses, confusion, irritability, and excitement may occur.

Diphenhydramine is a histamine (H_1) antagonist with anticholinergic activity. When it is used as a cough suppressant, this agent may worsen the irritation, as it can dry mucous membranes. Thus, the therapeutic use of diphenhydramine in respiratory disorders is questionable. Additionally, due to a number of serious injuries and overdoses associated with this agent, the Nonprescription Drug Advisory Committee and the Pediatric Advisory Committee of the Food and Drug Administration has recommended that combination cough and cold preparations (including those containing diphenhydramine) be avoided in patients younger than 2 years of age and used with caution patients older than age 2. Avoidance of diphenhydramine is recommended as part of the geriatric guidelines often referred to as the Beers list. Overall, the use of diphenhydramine should be limited.

Chemically related to tetracaine, procaine, and cocaine, benzonatate is speculated to produce its effects through inhibition of pulmonary stretch receptors, and thus is considered a peripherally acting antitussive. This mechanism is thought to exist based on the ability of topical anesthetic agents to inhibit voltage-gated sodium channels. Benzonatate is a local anesthetic, so it should not be chewed or dissolved; because the dysphagia and oropharyngeal anesthesia produced by these routes of administration may result in bronchospasm, laryngospasm, choking, or a compromised airway. Patients must be instructed to swallow capsules whole, and those who are predisposed to swallowing impairments should avoid use of this agent.

Beta agonists, anticholinergics, and glucocorticoids are other medications that play a significant role in respiratory regimens; these agents are discussed in other chapters in greater detail. Clinicians using these medications for respiratory conditions should refer to the latest treatment guidelines and real-time medication information databases prior to prescribing them.

Antitussive Agents

Benzonatate
Dextromethorphan
Codeine *(see also the Analgesic and Antipyretic Agents section in the Central Nervous System Agents chapter)*
Diphenhydramine *(see also the First-Generation Antihistamine Agents section in the Antihistamine Agents chapter)*
Hydrocodone *(see also the Analgesic and Antipyretic Agents section in the Central Nervous System Agents chapter)*

Case Studies and Conclusions

SJ is a 17-year-old white female with a 3-day history of dyspnea, fever, and frequent cough with a past medical history of asthma. She presents to the urgent care clinic with her mother. The mother states that SJ's cough has been ongoing for 1 week and she has been medicating her with dextromethorphan polistirex (30 mg/5 mL) once a day. The mother is concerned that giving the dextromethorphan will cause SJ to become addicted to it. Additionally, the cough medicine helped for only the first few days. After the advanced practice nurse (APN) assesses SJ at the clinic, she determines that SJ has community-acquired pneumonia (CAP), which requires an antibiotic for treatment, and she prescribes azithromycin. SJ has no drug allergies and is currently on no other medications or supplements.

1. Which of the following regimens should the APN recommend for SJ's cough?
   a. Dextromethorphan polistirex: 30 mg/5 mL by mouth every 12 hours as needed for cough
   b. Albuterol metered-dose inhaler (MDI): inhale 2 puffs every 6 hours until cough subsides
   c. Morphine sulfate 5 mg/5 mL: 5 mL by mouth every 4 hours as needed for cough
   d. Hydromorphone: 2 mg by mouth every 6 hours as needed for cough

Answer B is correct. Short-term use of short-acting beta agonists may be prescribed when bronchospasms are caused by bacterial—or, more often, viral—infections.

2. What should the APN tell the mother regarding the use of dextromethorphan?
   a. Dextromethorphan has addictive potential and should be avoided.
   b. Dextromethorphan is the same as morphine and is associated with the same adverse drug reactions.
   c. Dextromethorphan is preferred over diphenhydramine for cough, as it does not have the profound drying and sedative adverse reactions associated with diphenhydramine.
   d. Benzonatate has a well-established ability to produce superior clinical outcomes and should be used instead of dextromethorphan.

Answer C is correct. Diphenhydramine is a histamine (H_1) antagonist with anticholinergic activity. When it is used as a cough suppressant, this agent may worsen the irritation by drying out the mucous membranes.

SJ's mother was concerned with using the dextromethorphan because she had heard that it can cause serotonin sickness (SS).

3. How should the APN address this concern?
   a. If the patient is on a selective serotonin reuptake inhibitor (SSRI), there is a potential for SS to occur if the SSRI is taken together with dextromethorphan.
   b. Dextromethorphan is an SSRI and, therefore, should not be used for cough.
   c. Dextromethorphan has a high addictive potential, and SSRIs may help with the addiction.
   d. SS is a fallacy.

Answer A is correct. Dextromethorphan can inhibit serotonin receptors, leading to the untoward adverse reaction called serotonin syndrome. SS can present with agitation, confusion, myoclonus, shivering, and tachycardia.

SJ responded well to the antibiotic and additional therapy, but she still has a nagging cough. SJ asked her mother to contact the APN and request a medication to stop this cough.

4. Which question(s) should the APN ask?
   a. How many days has SJ been off the antibiotic?
   b. Describe the cough: Is it wet or dry?
   c. What is the frequency of the cough?
   d. All of the above are correct.

Answer D is correct. The clinician must assess whether the continued cough represents an antimicrobial treatment failure or a nonproductive cough. A wet cough is wet and a dry cough may indicate different pathologies, as may the frequency of the cough.

5. What should the APN recommend for SJ, assuming azithromycin was started 10 days ago?
   a. Continue the albuterol MDI treatments.
   b. Stop the albuterol MDI treatments and start morphine 5 mg/5 mL by mouth every 4 hours as needed for cough.
   c. Stop the albuterol MDI treatments and start benzonatate 100 mg by mouth daily.
   d. Stop the albuterol MDI treatments and start dextromethorphan polistirex 30 mg/5 mL by mouth every 12 hours as needed for cough.

Answer A is correct. Short-term use of short-acting beta agonists may be implemented when bronchospasms are caused by bacterial (or, more often, viral) infections.

6. If the APN chose to start this patient on codeine phosphate-guaifenesin solution 10 mg–100 mg/5 mL, what should the APN tell SJ?
   a. This medication is for short-term use.
   b. If this medication does not help, contact me, so I can increase the dose.
   c. If this medication causes constipation, call me for a recommendation. If this medication causes abdominal pain, take it with food.
   d. This medication does not cause drowsiness.
   e. Both A and C are correct.

Answer E is correct. Short-term use of an opioid may be indicated for symptom management, but long-term use is not. As codeine interacts with mu receptors, gastrointestinal adverse reactions, including constipation, abdominal, pain and nausea, can occur.

9.2 Anti-inflammatory Agents

Many respiratory disorders are well known to be associated with inflammation. The symptoms of inflammation can be treated by a number of medications; however, targeting the core issue of inflammation remains the gold standard of treatment for many conditions. Because inflammation can be suppressed via multiple mechanisms, the FDA has approved multiple drug targets for therapeutic resolution, including those addressed by the agents described in this section.

Leukotriene Modifiers

Bronchospasms occur in patients with asthma as the stimulus interacts with arachidonic acid (AA), which is broken down by 5-lipoxygenase (5-LO) to various leukotrienes. These leukotrienes are further metabolized to cysteinyl leukotrienes (cysLTs) and leukotriene B4 (LTB4). The cysLTs are known to cause the rhinosinusitis and smooth-muscle bronchospasm seen in asthma. Attempts to block cysLT led to the discovery of zafirlukast and montelukast, both of which antagonize cysLT. Zileuton was the first drug developed that blocked 5-LO, thereby inhibiting the cysLTs and LTB4.

All leukotriene modifiers are well tolerated. Adverse drug reactions such as elevated transaminases, dyspepsia, headache, and eosinophilia should be monitored. In postmarketing surveillance, montelukast was found to have the potential for producing suicidal ideation, suicide, and changes in behavior and mood, although these adverse drug events (ADEs) are controversial.

Leukotriene Modifiers

Montelukast
Zafirlukast
Zileutron

Mast Cell Stabilizers

As described earlier in this chapter, the complexity of the body's responses to (and clinical outcomes from), the reaction-provoking stimuli are various and multimodal. The deterioration of mast cells is one facet of the body's response to allergens or other external stimuli. During acute exacerbations, mast cell degradation can lead to acute bronchoconstriction through an immunoglobulin E (IgE)-dependent mechanism. This process, along with the release of histamine, leukotrienes, and other chemicals, leads to the symptoms experienced by asthmatics.

The use of cromolyn sodium as a treatment for asthma, rhinitis, and conjunctivitis can help stabilize or prevent the rupture of mast cells, thereby decreasing the overall impact of the various stimuli on bronchial muscle or nasopharyngeal tissue. Patients with aspirin-induced bronchospasm may respond best to cromolyn sodium, as this agent does not produce the negative complications that may be seen with other therapies such as acetaminophen, ketorolac, and tartrazine. Of importance, cromolyn sodium must be continually used during the time of exposure or prior to exposure to environments that might induce the destruction of mast cells. Therefore, adherence to the prescribed frequency is required, since the lack of adherence will result in drug failure.

Mast Cell Stabilizers

Cromolyn

Inhaled Corticosteroids

Anti-inflammatory agents represent another common approach to medication therapy for respiratory conditions; although not primarily covered in this section, they must be included in the discussion of the overall management of respiratory disease (refer to the Hormones and Synthetic Substitutes chapter for more detail). These agents are best separated into inhaled corticosteroids (ICS) and oral corticosteroids. Inhaled corticosteroids are produced in multiple individual or combination products. The treatment of asthma often requires the use of bronchodilating beta agonists (both short-and long-acting), bronchodilating anticholinergic agents, and/or ICS. Short-acting beta agonists (SABAs) may be used for intermittent dosing or immediate-relief dosing; however, if the patient is having symptoms most days, the use of ICS is warranted, such as when the patient has exercise-induced asthma (EIA). More persistent asthma will require the use of long-acting beta agonists (LABAs), ICS, and possibly leukotriene modifiers or monoclonal antibodies.

Inhaled corticosteroids may be used in patients with a high risk of COPD exacerbation. Nevertheless, their use in COPD remains controversial, as the ADRs associated with their use may outweigh their benefits.

The ability of ICS therapy to decrease symptoms and improve quality of life derives from a complex mechanism of action. Ultimately, ICS reduce the inflammatory response that was provoked by the allergen or environmental irritants. The currently available agents all provide the same clinical outcomes, although their side effect profiles differ.

Compared to the oral corticosteroids, ICS have a low potential for causing systemic effects, including hypothalamic-pituitary-adrenal (HPA) suppression. These drugs are deposited in the oropharyngeal region, which may lead to hoarseness and dysphonia. These ADRs can be minimized with proper mouth and throat care after ICS administration, including rinsing and expelling and/or rinsing and swallowing with water. Although rare, systemic ADRs can be seen with high dosing of ICS.

Oral Corticosteroids

Use of oral corticosteroids should be limited, as they can cause numerous ADRs. Most concerning is their potential impact on the HPA axis. Suppression of the HPA axis can lead to weight loss and fatigue. Myopathy induced by steroids may lead to functional loss of muscle and negatively impact respiratory function.

Case Studies and Conclusions

NM is a 23-year-old white female with a history of exercise-induced asthma. She runs 7 days a week, on a year-round basis. The EIA affects her only during her runs.

1. What is the best therapy for EIA?
   a. Dextromethorphan polistirex 30 mg/5 mL by mouth every 12 hours as needed for cough
   b. Ivacaftor 150 mg by mouth every 12 hours
   c. Cromolyn sodium 20 mg via nebulization 4 times daily
   d. Mometasone dry powder 1 actuation by mouth daily

Answer D is correct. If the patient is having symptoms most days, the use of ICS is warranted; this includes conditions such as with EIA.

2. Which of the following therapies may be helpful if NM has seasonal allergies and EIA?
   a. Montelukast 10 mg by mouth daily
   b. Ivacaftor 150 mg by mouth every 12 hours
   c. Roflumilast 500 mcg by mouth daily
   d. Salmeterol 50 mcg, 1 inhalation at least 30 minutes prior to exercise

Answer A is correct. Bronchospasms occur in persons with asthma when the stimulus interacts with arachidonic acid. AA is broken down by 5-lipoxygenase to various leukotrienes. These leukotrienes are further metabolized to cysteinyl leukotrienes and leukotriene B4. The cysLTs are known to cause the rhinosinusitis and smooth-muscle bronchospasms seen in asthma. The blocking of cysLT resulted in the discovery of zafirlukast and montelukast, both of which antagonize cysLT.

3. Which one of the following drugs has been associated with suicidal thoughts?
   a. Montelukast
   b. Diphenhydramine
   c. Cromolyn
   d. Ambrisentan

Answer A is correct. Postmarketing surveillance revealed that montelukast has the potential to produce suicidal ideation, suicide, and changes in behavior and mood, although these ADEs are controversial.

9.3 Cystic Fibrosis Transmembrane Conductance Regulatory Modulators

Cystic fibrosis (CF) is caused by mutations in a single gene called the cystic fibrosis transmembrane conductance regulator (CFTR), which produce a host of clinical symptoms. Although pulmonary congestion symptoms are the most common manifestations, the involvement of other exocrine structures—such as the pancreas, liver, intestines, and sweat glands—is equally concerning. Treatment of CF focuses on the direct modification of CFTR and is specific to the gene's abnormalities. Two drugs are available, ivacaftor and ivacaftor plus lumacaftor, which are indicated based on the gene-specific abnormality. Ultimately, these agents improve the sodium and water exchange within the various tissues by decreasing the viscosity of the secretions.

For the clinician, an important issue with these agents is the multiple drug interactions associated with them. It is also necessary to evaluate their administration specific to the timing of the CFTR modulators.

Cystic Fibrosis Transmembrane Conductance Regulatory Modulators

Ivacaftor

Case Studies and Conclusions

DG is a 19-year-old African American male who presents with his father to the emergency department (ED) with increased symptoms of dyspnea. DG's history of present illness (HPI) reveals cystic fibrosis since birth. During the review of DG's history with the father, you attempt to assess adherence to the medications based on the responses from the father.

1. Which of the following medications directly targets the gene mutations found in patients with cystic fibrosis?
   a. Prednisolone
   b. Ivacaftor
   c. Budesonide
   d. Dornase alfa

Answer B is correct. Treatment of CF focuses on direct modification of CFTR and is specific to the gene's abnormalities. Two drugs are available, ivacaftor and ivacaftor plus lumacaftor, which are indicated based on the gene-specific abnormality. Ultimately, these agents improve the sodium and water exchange within the various tissues by decreasing the viscosity of the secretions.

2. When considering prescribing the drugs used to target the gene mutations present in CF, which of the following issues must clinicians assess prior to initiating therapy?
   a. Environmental hazards
   b. Ability to swallow
   c. Drug interactions
   d. Weight

Answer C is correct. An important consideration for the prescribing clinician is the multiple drug interactions that may occur with CTFR-targeting drugs and the necessity to evaluate their administration specific to the timing of the CFTR modulators.

TT is a 52-year-old white male who presents to his primary care physician with a chief complaint of shortness of breath. He works in construction and finds himself winded more often than not. A smoker since the age of 15, TT now smokes 10 cigarettes per day. The primary care physician sends TT for spirometry testing, which reveals that his FEV/FVC is 50%. Concerned with this result, the physician refers to the guidelines and prescribes therapy.

1. Which guidelines would be most helpful to TT's physician?
   a. Chest
   b. American Heart Association (AHA)/American College of Cardiology (ACC)
   c. GOLD
   d. *DSM-V*

Answer C is correct. The Global Initiative for Obstructive Lung Disease (GOLD) classified COPD based on the severity of the disease. This collaboration gave rise to a structured format for what is a living document, with the guidelines changing as new physiological, pathological, and pharmacologic findings occur.

2. The promotion of smoking cessation is mandatory. In addition, the type of drug therapy most pharmacologically beneficial to TT would be which of the following?
   a. SABAs and LABAs (short- and long-acting beta agonists)
   b. Montelukast (brand or generic, based on patient preference)
   c. SAMAs and LAMAs (short- and long-acting muscarinic antagonists)
   d. Both A and C are correct.

Answer D is correct. The backbone of treatment for obstructive pulmonary disorders is the combination of beta agonists and anticholinergics (antimuscarinic antagonists). The chapter on autonomic agents provides a more comprehensive discussion of these drugs.

3. Which of the following agents does not have any bronchodilator pharmacology?
   a. Albuterol
   b. Ipratropium
   c. Salmeterol
   d. Roflumilast

Answer D is correct. Roflumilast and its active metabolite, roflumilast *N*-oxide, are selective inhibitors of phosphodiesterase 4, a major cyclic AMP metabolizing enzyme in the lung. Although its mechanism is not well defined, roflumilast is thought to exert its therapeutic effect by increasing intracellular cyclic AMP in lung cells, thereby decreasing inflammation. Roflumilast will be discussed in greater detail in a later section of this chapter.

9.4 Expectorants and Mucolytic Agents

The role of mucoactive agents is defined by their ability to induce cough or increase secretions (expectorants), thin mucus (mucolytics), or aid in the movement of mucus (mucokinetic). As part of our innate defenses, mucus is protective in nature, as it sequesters and transports out inhaled toxins. In diseases such as COPD, the insults of external toxins overwhelm the body's mucus-clearing ability. As mucus increases and its movement slows, it becomes an area ripe for potential bacterial growth. This slowed movement, along with the increase in the inflammatory response, contributes to the overall symptom of dyspnea.

The pharmacology of the various agents drives the treatment decision. An agent used most commonly to increase the production of secretions, facilitating the removal of cold-, flu-, and allergy-associated mucous, is guaifenesin. There are few data that demonstrate guaifenesin improves lung function and even fewer data that provide an understanding of the mechanism by which this effect may be achieved, if it occurs at all.

In addition to the FDA-approved mucolytics described here, clinicians may use potassium iodide, acetylcysteine, and cromolyn sodium on an off-label basis for this purpose. Historically, the most commonly used potassium iodide preparation was iodopropylidene glycerol, which was removed from the U.S. market. Various preparations of potassium iodide are available, but they must be used with care as they are not indicated if patients have an iodine allergy or other thyroid conditions. *N*-acetylcysteine (NAC) is the most commonly used mucolytic and, therefore, is included in this chapter. This agent breaks down mucus, decreasing its viscosity and allowing for easier physical expulsion or mechanical suction of this substance. This process often presents with an offensive "rotten egg" smell due to the breakdown of the disulfide bonds in the mucus.

Dornase alfa is a mucolytic most often used in patients with cystic fibrosis (CF) and, more recently, with patients with non-CF disorders. DNase is an enzyme produced in the salivary glands and pancreas that decreases the thickened or viscosity of sputum; dornase alfa is a recombinant human DNase used to augment the body's natural mucolytic processes.

Expectorants

Guaifenesin

Mucolytic Agents

Acetylcysteine
Dornase alfa

Case Studies and Conclusions

TG is a 45-year-old Hispanic female who presents to her family physician with a chief complaint of dyspnea, coughing, and increased throat mucus. Upon review of systems and physical examination, TG is found to be a 1 pack-per-day smoker for the past 30 years, but has had only intermittent episodes of shortness of breath. She has no drug allergies but has hypothyroidism.

1. Which of the following mucolytics will NOT thin TG's throat congestion?
   a. Guaifenesin
   b. Potassium iodide
   c. Acetylcysteine
   d. Cromolyn sodium

Answer A is correct. Guaifenesin is most commonly used to increase the production of secretions due to flu, cold, and allergy (not that caused by cigarette smoking).

2. Which one of the following may have the smell of "rotten eggs"?
   a. Guaifenesin
   b. Potassium iodide
   c. Acetylcysteine
   d. Cromolyn sodium

Answer C is correct. *N*-acetylcysteine (NAC) is the most commonly used mucolytic. It breaks down mucus, decreasing its viscosity; this allows for easier physical expulsion or mechanical suction of the mucus. This process often presents with an offensive "rotten egg" smell due to the breakdown of the disulfide bonds in the mucus.

3. Which of the following should NOT be recommend to TG?
   a. Dornase alfa
   b. Potassium iodide
   c. Acetylcysteine
   d. Cromolyn sodium
   e. Both A and B are correct.

Answer E is correct. The potassium iodide preparation consisted of iodopropylidene glycerol, which was removed from the U.S. market. Dornase alfa is more typically indicated for cystic fibrosis.

4. Health literacy considerations require clinicians to assess the how well their patients understand their medications with regard to use, dosing, frequency, duration, and adverse events. Regarding the mucolytic, dornase alfa, which one of the following statements is INCORRECT?
   a. Dornase alfa must be taken daily.
   b. Dornase alfa is used when pulmonary function is less than 40%.
   c. Dornase alfa increases the viscosity of secretions.
   d. Dornase alfa does not alter the mutated genes associated with CF.

Answer C is correct. DNase is an enzyme produced in the salivary glands and pancreas that decreases the thickened or viscosity of sputum.

WD is an 85-year-old Asian American male who, while visiting his son and daughter-in-law, finds that he is coming down with a cold. WD goes to the pharmacy to sift through the many bottles of cough and cold medications, attempting to find something that may make him feel better. Frustrated, he goes to the pharmacy counter and speaks with the pharmacist.

1. If the patient has a nonproductive cough and feelings of congestion, which of the following medications might you recommend?
   a. Guaifenesin
   b. Potassium iodide
   c. Acetylcysteine
   d. Cromolyn sodium

Answer A is correct. Guaifenesin is most commonly used to increase production of secretions; however, it does not suppress cough. If the patient does not find relief from increased secretions, he may be advised to consider using a cough suppressant (such as dextromethorphan) and seeking evaluation by a clinician to rule out a more serious cause of cough.

2. How should you explain the function of an expectorant?
   a. It aids in the discontinued production of secretions.
   b. It aids in thickening of secretions.
   c. It aids in increasing secretions.
   d. It aids when genetic mutations exist.

Answer C is correct. An expectorant increases the production of secretions.

3. Guaifenesin has well-established evidence of its benefit as an expectorant, so a solid evidence-based recommendation can be made for its use to improve lung function.
   a. True
   b. False

Answer B is correct. There are few data that show guaifenesin improves lung function.

9.5 Phosphodiesterase Type 4 Inhibitors and Miscellaneous Respiratory Agents

Phosphodiesterase Type 4 Inhibitors

The pharmacology of the phosphodiesterase type 4 (PDE4) inhibitor class of medications is specific to one commercially available product, roflumilast. Roflumilast and its active metabolite, roflumilast *N*-oxide, are selective inhibitors of PDE, a major cyclic AMP-metabolizing enzyme in the lung. Although its mechanism of action is not well defined, this agent is thought to exert its therapeutic effect by increasing intracellular cyclic AMP in lung cells, thereby decreasing inflammation. The most common ADRs associated with roflumilast are headache, weight loss, and diarrhea.

Phosphodiesterase Type 4 Inhibitors

Roflumilast

Pulmonary Surfactants

Calfactant, poractant alfa, and beractant are natural surfactants used in the treatment of neonatal respiratory distress syndrome (RDS). Although the use of these agents is currently limited to pediatric patients (and thus not a focus for this text), the novel mechanism of action of causing decreased surface tension of the lungs, allowing for alveolar function to be maintained, and leading to normalization of oxygenation is notable. Prominent ADRs include cardiovascular and additional pulmonary complications. These surfactants are administered via the endotracheal route.

Pulmonary Surfactants

Beractant
Poractant alfa

Vasodilating Agents and Miscellaneous Respiratory Agents

Consideration of cardiovascular disorders when patients already have respiratory disorders is important, although that is not the intention of this chapter. Pulmonary hypertension (PH) is a hemodynamic abnormality that affects the right side of the heart, but it presents with symptoms such as dyspnea, fatigue, dizziness, and cough. Various pathologies may also compromise the lungs, such as pulmonary fibrosis and thrombosis, that lead to mechanical compression and distortion of pulmonary vessels.

Algorithms guiding treatment of pulmonary hypertension differentiate between patients based on their vasodilator-positive versus vasodilator-negative responses. If a vasodilator-positive response is observed, the drug of choice is an oral calcium-channel blocker. If a negative response occurs, the use of prostanoid, endothelin receptor antagonists, or phosphodiesterase type 5 (PDE5) inhibitors is recommended.

The oral calcium-channel blockers used to treat pulmonary hypertension are amlodipine, diltiazem, and nifedipine. Pharmacologically, these agents benefit patients with PH by blocking calcium channels on the smooth muscle within the pulmonary artery, leading to vasodilation and decreased pressure and symptoms. Typical adverse reactions to these drugs include peripheral edema, headache, and gastrointestinal symptoms such as constipation.

For negative responders, treatment is initiated with a single drug therapy and progresses to combination therapy as the disease worsens. PDE5 inhibitors such as sildenafil and tadalafil are used to treat pulmonary hypertension, but they should not be considered if the patient is on nitrate therapy, as an exaggerated hypotensive response has led to deaths in such cases. These agents are discussed in greater detail in the Cardiovascular Agents chapter.

The endothelin receptor antagonists (ERAs) are bosentan, ambrisentan, and macitentan. Working on the vascular endothelin cells, the ERAs reverse the vasoconstrictive effects of endothelin. Adverse reactions of concern are fluid retention, peripheral edema, and hepatic toxicity or impairment.

The benefit of prostenoids, such as epoprostenol, treprostinil, and iloprost, derives from their promotion of vasodilation. Pulmonary edema, syncope, and flushing are some of many ADRs observed with these agents.

Riociguat is a soluble guanylate cyclase (sGC) stimulator with dual action involving nitrous oxide and stimulation of sGC that leads to vasodilation and antifibrotic, antiproliferative, and anti-inflammatory effects. Novel in its class, this drug is contraindicated in pregnancy and can be associated with hypotension, headache, dyspepsia, and anemia.

Vasodilating Agents

Ambrisentan
Bosentan

Epoprostenol
Iloprost
Macitentan
Riociguat
Selexipag
Treprostinil

Miscellaneous Respiratory Tract Agents

Omalizumab is a monoclonal antibody indicated for patients with asthma. By inhibiting immunoglobulin E (IgE), omalizumab prevents the binding of IgE to mast cells and basophils, reducing their degradation—and, therefore, the release of mediators that result in an allergic response. Of importance is that omalizumab can cause anaphylaxis by itself, which prompted the FDA to require a black box warning on this agent's label. Other ADRs include malignancy, fever, arthralgia, and parasitic infection. Other agents included in this miscellaneous category are alpha-proteinase inhibitors ([A_1-PI] human). These agents increase a specific protein called alpha 1-antitrypsin or "AAT" that is insufficiently produced in patients with respiratory disease such as emphysema.

Miscellaneous Respiratory Tract Agents

Alpha-Proteinase Inhibitors

Alpha-proteinase inhibitor (human)

Monoclonal Antibodies

Omalizumab

Antifibrotic Agents

Nintedanib is a tyrosine kinase inhibitor indicated for idiopathic pulmonary fibrosis (IPF). Adverse effects that may occur with its use include bleeding, cardiovascular events, and elevations in various hepatic enzymes. Nintedanib must be administered with food and swallowed whole; patients should not crush or chew the medication.

Pirfenidone is an antifibrotic and anti-inflammatory agent used for the treatment of IPF. Its dosing is complex, as increases in doses are done weekly for the first two weeks and then remain constant after day 14. Concerning issues with use of this medication are changes in hepatic enzymes and the potential for photosensitivity reactions to occur. Angioedema has also been noted with pirfenidone. Educating patients on signs and symptoms such as chest tightness, wheezing, blue skin color, and swelling of face and lips is required.

Antifibrotic Agents

Nintedanib
Pirfenidone

Case Studies and Conclusions

LG is an 83-year-old white female who presents to the ED with shortness of breath. After ruling out any cardiovascular complications, LG is sent for a right heart catheterization, which reveals pulmonary hypertension (PH).

1. When considering treatment for PH, what is the first question to ask?
   a. Is the PH vasodilator positive?
   b. Is the PH vasodilator negative?
   c. Is the PH vasodilator neutral?
   d. Both A and B are correct.

Answer D is correct. The algorithm for treatment of pulmonary hypertension differentiates between vasodilator-positive and vasodilator-negative responses. For positive responders, the first-line drug is oral calcium-channel blockers. For negative responders, the use of prostanoids, endothelin receptor antagonists, or phosphodiesterase type 5 inhibitors is recommended.

2. If the PH vasodilator is positive, which of the following drugs is NOT a therapeutic option?
   a. Amlodipine
   b. Diltiazem
   c. Atenolol
   d. Nifedipine

Answer C is correct. Oral calcium-channel blockers used to treat pulmonary hypertension include amlodipine, diltiazem, and nifedipine; atenolol is a beta blocker.

3. If the PH vasodilator is negative, what is (are) the therapeutic option(s)?
   a. Epoprostenol
   b. Sildenafil
   c. Bosentan
   d. All of these medications may be considered.

Answer D is correct. For negative responders, treatment is initiated with a single drug therapy and progresses to combination therapy as the disease worsens. Phosphodiesterase type 5 inhibitors such as sildenafil and tadalafil are used, but they should not be considered if the patient is on nitrate therapy, as an exaggerated hypotensive response has led to deaths. The endothelin receptor antagonists—bosentan, ambrisentan, and macitentan—are used if/when the response to the PDE5 inhibitors is not sufficient.

Tips from the Field

1. The FDA Nonprescription Drug Advisory Committee and the Pediatric Advisory Committee has recommended that nonprescription cough and cold products should not be used in children less than 2 years of age and an official ruling regarding the use of these products in children older than 2 has not yet been announced. Refer to pediatric drug references for additional information (FDA, 2008).
2. The FDA released new recommendations in 2016 requiring a black box warning alerting prescribers to avoid combined use of opioid medicines with other drugs (including benzodiazepines) that depress the central nervous system (CNS) because this could lead to serious adverse effects. It is important to explore alternatives to opiate-containing cough regimens when a patient is taking other CNS depressants.
3. It is critical that patients do not continue to self-medicate with any OTC product when cough lingers or is accompanied by other symptoms that are suggestive of infection or new pulmonary disease.
4. COPD is a disease that has been associated with smoking and is complicated further with continued tobacco dependence. Encourage smoking cessation for all your patients at every encounter. Refer to the Tips from the Field in Chapter 4 to assist in your encouragement of patients who are smokers.

Tammie Lee and Jacque

Bibliography

Aboussouan LS. Role of mucoactive agents in the treatment of COPD. *UpToDate.* December 14, 2015. http://www.uptodate.com/contents/role-of-mucoactive-agents-in-the-treatmentofcopd?source=machineLearning&search=expectorant&selectedTitle=1%7E33§ionRank=1&anchor=H26#H26. Accessed June 2016.

American Geriatrics Society. 2015 updated Beers criteria for potentially inappropriate medication use in older adults. *J Am Geriatr Soc.* 2015;63:2227-2246.

Barnes PJ. Pulmonary pharmacology. In: Brunton LL, Chabner BA, Knollman BC, eds. *Goodman & Gilman's The Pharmacological Basis of Therapeutics*. 12th ed. New York, NY: McGraw-Hill; 2015: 1031-1066. http://accesspharmacy.mhmedical.com/content.aspx?bookid=1613&Sectionid=102161403. Accessed December 11, 2016.

Barnes PJ. Asthma. In: Kasper DL, Fauci AS, Hauser SL, Longo DL, Jameson JL, Loscalzo J, eds. *Harrison's Principles of Internal Medicine*. 19th ed. New York, NY: McGraw-Hill Education; 2015. http://accessmedicine.mhmedical.com/book.aspx?bookid=1130. Accessed December 28, 2016.

Barst RJ, Gibbs JS, Ghofrani HA, et al. Updated evidence-based treatment algorithm in pulmonary arterial hypertension. *J Am Coll Cardiol.* 2009;54:S78-S84.

Barst RJ, Rubin LJ. Pulmonary hypertension. In: Fuster V, Walsh RA, Harrington RA, et al., eds. *Hurst's The Heart.* 13th ed. New York, NY: McGraw-Hill; 2011: 1609-1633.

Bonderman D, Pretsch I, Steringer-Mascherbauer R, et al. Acute hemodynamic effects of riociguat in patients with pulmonary hypertension associated with diastolic heart failure (DILATE-1). *Chest.* 2014:146(5)1274-1285.

Bourdet SV, Williams DM. Chronic obstructive pulmonary disease. In: DiPiro JT, Talbert RL, Yee GC, Matzke GR, Wells BG, Posey LM, eds. *Pharmacotherapy: A Pathophysiologic Approach.* 6th ed. New York, NY: McGraw-Hill; 2005: 554.

Brink DS, Lechner AJ. Development and functional anatomy of the lungs and airways. In: Lechner AJ, Matuschak GM, Brink DS, eds. *Respiratory: An Integrated Approach to Disease.* New York, NY: McGraw-Hill; 2015: 9-22. http://accessmedicine.mhmedical.com/content.aspx?sectionid=105763575&bookid=1623&Resultclick=2&q=anatomy+of+lungs. Accessed December 14, 2016.

Chen S-L, Huang Y-K, Chow L-H, Tao P-L. Dextromethorphan differentially affects opioid antinociception in rats. *Br J Pharmacol.* 2005;144:400-404.

Choby GW, Lee S. Pharmacotherapy for the treatment of asthma: current treatment options and future directions. *Int Forum Allergy Rhinol.* 2015;5(suppl 1):S35-S40.

Elsevier/Gold Standard. List of monographs A-Z. *Clin Pharmacol.* December 13, 2015. http://www.clinicalpharmacology-ip.com/default.aspx. Accessed December 14, 2016.

Evans MS, Maglinger GB, Fletcher AM, Johnson SR. Benzonatate inhibition of voltage-gated sodium currents. *Neuropharmacology.* 2015;101:179-187.

Fleischman RJ, Frazer DG, Daya M, Jui J, Newgard CD. Effectiveness and safety of fentanyl compared with morphine for out-of-hospital analgesia. *Prehosp Emerg Care.* 2010;14(2):167-175.

Food and Drug Administration. Medication guide: daliresp. December 28, 2015. http://www.fda.gov/downloads/Drugs/DrugSafety/UCM286063.pdf. Accessed December 14, 2016.

Genentech. Xolair. December 28, 2015. http://www.gene.com/download/pdf/xolair_prescribing.pdf. Accessed December 14, 2016.

Gerdes JS, Seiberlich W, Sivieri EM, et al. An open label comparison of calfactant and poractant alfa administration traits and impact on neonatal intensive care unit resources. *J Pediatr Pharmacol Therap.* 2006;11(2):92-100.

GeriatricsCareOnline. American Geriatrics Society 2015 updated Beers criteria for potentially inappropriate medication use in older adults. http://geriatricscareonline.org/toc/american-geriatrics-society-updated-beers-criteria-for-potentially-inappropriate-medication-use-in-older-adults/CL001. Accessed December 14, 2016.

Global Initiative for Chronic Obstructive Lung Disease. Global strategy for the diagnosis, management and prevention of COPD. January 2015. http://goldcopd.org/global-strategy-diagnosis-management-prevention-copd-2016. Accessed December 4, 2016.

Global Initiative for Obstructive Lung Disease. Global Initiative for Chronic Obstructive Pulmonary Disease, based on an April 1998 meeting of the National Heart, Lung, and Blood Institute and the World Health Organization. April 1998. http://www.goldcopd.org/uploads/users/files/GOLDWkshp2003Changes.pdf. Accessed December 14, 2016.

Kaplan AG. Applying the wisdom of stepping down inhaled corticosteroids in patients with COPD: a proposed algorithm for clinical practice. *Int J COPD.* 2015;10(1):2535-2548.

Katcher J, Walsh D. Opioid-induced itching: morphine sulfate and hydromorphone hydrochloride. *J Pain Symp Manage.* 1999:17(1);70-72.

Linn KA, Long MT, Pagel PS. "Robo-tripping": dextromethorphan abuse and its anesthetic implications. *Anesthesiol Pain Med.* 2014;4(5). doi: 10.5812/aapm.20990

Maguire JJ, Davenport AP. Endothelin receptors and their antagonists. *Semin Nephrol.* 2015;35(2):125-136.

McGraw-Hill Global Education Holdings. AccessPharmacy. December 2015. http://accesspharmacy.mhmedical.com. Accessed December 14, 2016.

McEvoy GK, ed. *AHFS: Drug Information.* Bethesda, MD: American Society of Health-System Pharmacists; 2016.

Meltzer EO, Chervinsky P, Busse W, et al. Roflumilast for asthma: efficacy findings in placebo-controlled studies. *Pulmon Pharmacol Therap.* 2015;35(suppl):S20-S27.

Nair GB, Ilowite JS. Pharmacologic agents for mucus clearance in bronchiectasis. *Clin Chest Med.* 2012;33:363-370.

Nieman LK. Clinical manifestations of adrenal insufficiency in adults. *UpToDate.* December 13, 2015. http://www.uptodate.com/contents/clinical-manifestations-of-adrenal-insufficiency-in-adults?source=see_link. Accessed December 14, 2016.

Peters-Golden M. Agents affecting the 5-lipoxygenase pathway in the treatment of asthma. *UpToDate.* December 14, 2015. http://www.uptodate.com/contents/agents-affecting-the-5-lipoxygenase-pathway-in-the-treatment-of-asthma?source=preview&search=%2Fcontents%2Fsearch&anchor=H29#H8. Accessed December 14, 2016.

Petty TL. The history of COPD. *Int J COPD.* 2006;1:3-14.

Ryan NM. A review on the efficacy and safety of gabapentin in the treatment of chronic cough. *Exp Opin Pharmacother.* 2015;16:135-145.

Torbic H, Hacobian G. Evaluation of inhaled dornase alfa administration in non-cystic fibrosis patients at a tertiary academic medical center. *J Pharmacy Pract.* 2016;29:480-483.

Treatment of subacute and chronic cough in adults. *UpToDate.* December 18, 2015. http://www.uptodate.com/contents/treatment-of-subacute-and-chronic-cough-in-adults?source=related_link. Accessed December 14, 2016.

U.S. Food & Drug Administration. Public health advisory: FDA recommends that over-the-counter (OTC) cough and cold products not be used for infants and children under 2 years of age. 2008. http://www.fda.gov/NewsEvents/Newsroom/PressAnnouncements/2008/ucm051137.htm. Accessed November 16, 2016.

Voynow JA, Mascarenhas M, Kelly A, Scanlin TF. Cystic fibrosis. In: Grippi MA, Elias JA, Fishman JA, Kotloff RM, Pack AI, Senior RS, eds. *Fishman's Pulmonary Diseases and Disorders.* 5th ed. New York, NY: McGraw Hill: 2015.

Symbols

- ▲ Renal impairment: Dose adjustment is recommended.
- ▢ Hepatic impairment: Dose adjustment is recommended.
- ■ Black box warning exists for this drug.
- (QT) QTc prolongation effects have been reported.
- (BL) Beers list critetia (avoid in elderly).
- (PD) FDA-approved pediatric doses are available.
- (GD) FDA-approved geriatric doses are available.
-  See primary body system.

Respiratory Tract Agents

Universal prescribing alerts:

- Known serious hypersensitivity to the specific drug or any other component of the product/formulation selected warrants a contraindication for its use.
- Adverse reactions associated with the use of some **respiratory tract agents** include dizziness, drowsiness, vertigo, and fatigue; these agents may also impair the ability to perform tasks requiring mental alertness. Caution should always be recommended when using any new drug for the first time, when there is a dose change, and for continued use of known offending agents.
- Doses expressed are for usual adult dosage ranges only. "Geriatric doses" are assumed to be the same as adult doses unless otherwise noted with a symbol. Where pediatric dosing is available, a symbol will guide the reader to additional prescribing references. Refer to real-time references for these age-specific doses.
- Use of **respiratory tract agents** in pregnancy is based on weighing clinical risk versus benefit; safety concerns are not represented in this grid. Refer to the package insert (PI) for more information. Clinicians should continue to provide education about the reproductive risks of any medication and offer risk-reduction strategies (which may include contraceptive use) to women of childbearing age and understand that these reproductive risks may also extend to males. Other medications may decrease the effectiveness of oral contraceptives. Where necessary, an alternative means of birth control should be explored.
- Brand names are provided for those agents still available on the market. Due to the ever-changing product availability, refer to Food and Drug Administration (FDA) resources to confirm the actual brands available. This drug summary is for educational purposes only. Prescribing decisions should be based on real-time comprehensive drug databases that are updated on a regular basis.

Antitussive Agents

Drug Name	FDA-Approved Indications	Adult Dosage Range	Precautions and Clinical Pearls
Generic Name Benzonatate **Brand Name** Tessalon Perles Zonatuss	Nonproductive cough	**Usual oral dose:** 100 mg 3 times per day as needed; may increase to every 6 hours if needed not to exceed the maximum daily dose (MDD) of 600 mg per day	• Swallow whole; pharmacologic action may cause choking if chewed or opened and swallowed • Candy-like appearance; keep out of reach of children • Associated with CNS sedation, mental confusion, visual hallucinations or other bizarre behaviors

Drug Name	FDA-Approved Indications	Adult Dosage Range	Precautions and Clinical Pearls
Generic Name Dextromethorphan **Brand Name** Delsym Robitussin DM (various combination products) (PD)	Cough caused by common cold or inhaled irritants	**Usual oral dose:** IR capsules and syrups: 10 to 20 mg every 4 hours or 15 mg every 6 to 8 hours as needed ER suspension: 60 mg twice daily (not to exceed maximum dose of 120 mg per day)	• Healthcare providers should monitor for problems of abuse or misuse • Patients should notify healthcare provider if their cough does not improve within 7 days • Not to be used for chronic cough • Use caution in patients with hepatic impairment
Codeine	Refer to the Central Nervous System Agents chapter.		
Diphenhydramine	Refer to the Antihistamine Agents chapter.		
Hydrocodone	Refer to the Central Nervous System Agents chapter.		

Anti-inflammatory Agents

Leukotriene Modifiers

Drug Name	FDA-Approved Indications	Adult Dosage Range	Precautions and Clinical Pearls
Generic Name Montelukast **Brand Name** Singulair (PD)	Prophylaxis and chronic treatment of asthma Seasonal and perennial allergic rhinitis Prevention of exercise-induced bronchospasm (EIB)	**Usual oral dose for EIB:** 10 mg daily (2 hours prior to exercise for EIB)	• Watch for eosinophilia and vasculitis • Use caution in patients with hepatic impairment • Patients may experience neuropsychiatric events • Caution patients about potential suicide ideation • Not intended for rescue treatment • Patients who take daily use for asthma should not take extra doses for EIB

Generic Name Zafirlukast **Brand Name** Accolate PD	Chronic treatment and prophylaxis of asthma	**Usual oral dose:** 20 mg twice daily	• Watch for hepatotoxicity, eosinophilia, infections, neuropsychiatric events, and vasculitis (special observation in those with withdrawal of corticosteroids) • Not intended for rescue treatment Contraindications: • Hepatic impairment, including hepatic cirrhosis
Generic Name Zileuton **Brand Name** Zyflo	Prophylaxis and chronic treatment of asthma	**Usual oral dose:** ER: 1200 mg twice daily	• Watch for hepatotoxicity and neuropsychiatric events (monitor liver function tests at baseline and throughout ongoing course and caution patients about potential suicide ideation) • May potentiate sedation and hepatic injury when combined with ethanol • Absorption is improved when administered with food Contraindications: • Active liver disease or transaminase elevations 3 times the upper limit of normal (ULN) or greater

Mast-Cell Stabilizers

Drug Name	FDA-Approved Indications	Adult Dosage Range	Precautions and Clinical Pearls
Generic Name Cromolyn **Brand Name** NasalCrom Opticrom PD	**Common indications for use:** Adjunct in the management of patients with asthma Prevention and treatment of seasonal and perennial allergic rhinitis Treatment of allergic conjunctivitis, vernal keratoconjunctivitis, vernal conjunctivitis, and vernal keratitis	**Usual oral inhalation dose for asthma:** Inhale 2 sprays (800 mcg per spray) 4 times per day at regular intervals **Usual intranasal dose for allergic rhinitis:** 1 spray in each nostril 3 to 4 times per day **Usual ophthalmic dose for allergic conjunctivitis:** 1 to 2 drops into affected eye(s) 4 to 6 times per day	• May take 4 to 6 weeks to see therapeutic effects • Available in various dose forms for administration (solution for nebulization, powder capsules for oral inhalation); oral capsules are available for alternative indications, refer to PI • May experience transient burning or stinging with ophthalmic use • May experience withdrawal symptoms when withdrawing or tapering drug • Dose reductions may be required for hepatic and renal impairment; no specific dose recommendations are available Contraindications: • Acute asthma attacks

Cystic Fibrosis Transmembrane Conductance Regulator Modulators

Drug Name	FDA-Approved Indications	Adult Dosage Range	Precautions and Clinical Pearls
Generic Name Ivacaftor **Brand Name** Kalydeco ▲ ■ (PD)	Cystic fibrosis	**Usual oral dose:** 150 mg every 12 hours	• May cause dizziness • Effective in patients with specific gene expressions • May increase hepatic transaminases (use caution in patients with hepatic disease and impairment) • Monitor for cataracts • Use caution in renal impairment • Drug interactions may require dose adjustments or avoidance of certain drug combinations • Also available in combination with lumacaftor (Orkambi)

Expectorants and Mucolytic Agents

Expectorants

Drug Name	FDA-Approved Indications	Adult Dosage Range	Precautions and Clinical Pearls
Generic Name Guaifenesin **Brand Name** Mucinex (PD)	Cough expectorant	**Usual oral dose:** IR: 200 to 400 mg every 4 hours ER: 600 to 1200 mg every 12 hours MDD: 2.4 g per day	• Do not use for persistent chronic cough; contact the physician if symptoms do not improve within 7 days • Do not use for cough associated with angiotensin-converting-enzym (ACE) inhibitor use or heart failure • Take with 8 oz of water

Mucolytic Agents

Drug Name	FDA-Approved Indications	Adult Dosage Range	Precautions and Clinical Pearls
Generic Name Acetylcysteine **Brand Name** Acetadote Mucomyst (PD) (GD)	**Common indications for use:** Adjunctive therapy in respiratory conditions Antidote for acetaminophen overdose	**Usual inhalation dose of nebulized solution for respiratory conditions:** 1 to 10 mL of 20% solution *or* 2 to 20 mL of 10% solution every 2 to 6 hours	• Increased bronchial secretions may develop after inhalation; use caution in those with impaired gag reflex • Bronchospasm may occur • Oral administration (and cautions) is reserved for alternative indications; refer to PI • Pungent smell (rotten eggs) may be sensed with nebulization

Drug Name	FDA-Approved Indications	Adult Dosage Range	Precautions and Clinical Pearls
Generic Name Dornase alfa **Brand Name** Pulmozyme	Cystic fibrosis	**Usual inhalation dose:** 2.5 mg daily	• If pulmonary function is less than 40% of the normal level, dornase alfa does not significantly reduce the risk of respiratory infection that may require parenteral antibiotics • Must be used with a recommended nebulizer

Phosphodiesterase Type 4 Inhibitors and Miscellaneous Respiratory Agents

Phosphodiesterase Type 4 Inhibitors

Drug Name	FDA-Approved Indications	Adult Dosage Range	Precautions and Clinical Pearls
Generic Name Roflumilast **Brand Name** Daliresp	COPD	**Usual oral dose:** 500 mcg once daily	• Watch for arrhythmias, gastrointestinal side effects, and neuropsychiatric effects • Use with caution in patients with underlying psychiatric conditions: depression, anxiety and suicidal ideation have been reported • Not intended for rescue (not a bronchodilator) • Use in combination with at least one long-acting bronchodilator • Drug interactions may require dose adjustments or avoidance of certain drug combinations Contraindications: • Moderate or severe hepatic impairment (Child-Pugh class B or C)

Pulmonary Surfactants

Beractant	Pediatric use: refer to PI		
Poractant alfa	Pediatric use: refer to PI		

Vasodilating Agents

Drug Name	FDA-Approved Indications	Adult Dosage Range	Precautions and Clinical Pearls
Generic Name Ambrisentan **Brand Name** Letairis ■ (BL)	Pulmonary arterial hypertension	**Usual oral dose:** 5 mg once daily increase to 10 mg as tolerated (MDD: 10 mg per day)	• Watch for fluid retention and peripheral edema • Watch for hematologic changes: use is not recommended in patients with clinically significant anemia • Peripheral and pulmonary edema have been reported with use • May cause an increase in serum liver aminotransferases Contraindications: • Idiopathic pulmonary fibrosis • Severe hepatic impairment

Drug Name	FDA-Approved Indications	Adult Dosage Range	Precautions and Clinical Pearls
Generic Name Bosentan **Brand Name** Tracleer ■ ■ (BL) (PD)	Pulmonary arterial hypertension	**Usual oral dose for patients weighing 40 kg or more:** 62.5 mg twice daily for 4 weeks, then increase to 125 mg twice daily For patients who weigh less than 40 kg: refer to PI	• Use is not recommended in patients with moderate to severe hepatic impairment • Watch for fluid retention and peripheral edema; use caution (or avoid) in patients with heart failure • Watch for hematologic changes: use is not recommended in patients with clinically significant anemia Associated with: • High incidence of transaminase elevations with or without bilirubin and rare cases of unexplained hepatic cirrhosis • Requires experienced clinician who is knowledgeable in the use of this agent and enrolled in Risk Evaluation and Mitigation Strategy (REMS) program
Generic Name Epoprostenol **Brand Name** Flolan Veletri (BL)	Pulmonary arterial hypertension	**Usual parenteral dose:** IV: 2 ng/kg per minute initially, increase dose in increments of 1 to 2 ng/kg per minute at intervals of 15 minutes or longer until dose-limiting side effects occur	• Watch for pulmonary edema, rebound pulmonary hypertension, and effects from vasodilation • Monitor use with antiplatelets, anticoagulants, antihypertensives, digoxin, and thrombolytic agents Contraindications: • Chronic use in patients with heart failure • Chronic use in patients who develop pulmonary edema during dose initiation
Generic Name Iloprost **Brand Name** Ventavis ■	Pulmonary arterial hypertension	**Usual inhalation: dose:** 2.5 mcg per dose initially, increase to 5 mcg per dose 6 to 9 times daily (administer no more often than every 2 hours)	• Watch for pulmonary edema, rebound pulmonary hypertension, and syncope • May cause bronchospasm and syncope • Monitor use with antiplatelets, anticoagulants, antihypertensives, digoxin, and thrombolytic agents • Use caution in patients with hepatic impairment • Dose delivered at the mouthpiece via the I-neb AAD system
Generic Name Macitentan **Brand Name** Opsumit ■ (BL)	Pulmonary arterial hypertension	**Usual oral dose:** 10 mg daily	• Watch for fluid retention and peripheral edema • Possible hematologic effects: do not use in patients with severe anemia • Increases in liver aminotransferases, hepatotoxicity, and liver failure have been reported • Structure or toxicity profile is similar to existing hazardous agents; refer to PI

Generic Name Riociguat **Brand Name** Adempas ■ (BL)	Chronic thromboembolic pulmonary hypertension Pulmonary arterial hypertension	**Usual oral dose:** Initial: 1 mg 3 times per day; may increase by 0.5 mg 3 times per day if systolic blood pressure remains higher than 95 mm Hg and no signs or symptoms of hypotension occur (MDD: 2.5 mg 3 times per day)	• Serious bleeding has been observed • Patient may experience CNS effects • Reduces blood pressure: use with caution in patients with signs of hypotension; use with caution in elderly patients • Structure or toxicity profile is similar to that of existing hazardous agents • Drug interactions may require dose adjustments or avoidance of certain drug combinations • Cigarette smoking reduces the serum concentrations (and effectiveness) of this agent • Not recommended for use in patients with renal and/or hepatic impairment
Generic Name Selexipag **Brand Name** Uptravi ■ (GD)	Pulmonary arterial hypertension	**Usual oral dose:** 200 mcg twice daily (MDD: 1600 mcg twice daily)	• Will likely cause headache • May cause flushing and diarrhea
Generic Name Treprostinil **Brand Name** Orenitram Remodulin Tyvaso ■ (BL) (PD)	Pulmonary arterial hypertension	**Usual inhalation dose:** 18 mcg (3 inhalations) every 4 hours, 4 times per day initially; increase dose to 54 mcg (9 inhalations) 4 times per day as tolerated **Usual oral dose:** 0.25 mg every 12 hours or 0.125 mg every 8 hours; increase dose as needed to reach optimal clinical response	• May increase the risk of bleeding • May produce symptomatic hypotension • May produce rebound pulmonary hypertension • Requires a specific inhalation system • Parenteral dose regimens are available, refer to PI Contraindications: • Use of oral formulation in patients with severe hepatic impairment

Miscellaneous Respiratory Tract Agents			
Alpha-Proteinase Inhibitors			
Drug Name	FDA-Approved Indications	Adult Dosage Range	Precautions and Clinical Pearls
Generic Name Alpha1-proteinase inhibitors (A_1-PI) **Brand Name** Aralast Aralast NP Glassia Prolastin Prolastin-C Zemaira	Alpha$_1$-antitrypsin deficiency	**Usual dose:** IV: 60 mg/kg weekly Inhalation: 100 mg every 12 hours for 1 week	• Not to be used in patients with immunoglobulin A (IgA) deficiency and antibodies to IgA • Designated as an orphan drug for the following indications: cystic fibrosis, graft-versus-host disease, diabetes type 1 with residual beta cell function, bronchiectasis
Monoclonal Antibodies			
Drug Name	FDA-Approved Indications	Adult Dosage Range	Precautions and Clinical Pearls
Generic Name Omalizumab **Brand Name** Xolair ■ (PD) (GD)	Asthma	**Usual parenteral dose:** SQ: dose and frequency based on body weight and pretreatment total IgE serum levels	• Possible agent for eosinophilia and vasculitis • Fever, arthralgias, and rash are possible • Malignant neoplasms have been reported rarely • Total IgE levels remain elevated for up to 1 year following treatment Associated with: • Anaphylaxis
Antifibrotic Agents			
Drug Name	FDA-Approved Indications	Adult Dosage Range	Precautions and Clinical Pearls
Generic Name Nintedanib **Brand Name** Ofev ■	Idiopathic pulmonary fibrosis	**Usual oral dose:** 150 mg every 12 hours	• May increase risk of bleeding and myocardial infarction • GI effects are common and should be treated with supportive care • Cigarette smoking decreases the efficiency of this drug and should be avoided
Generic Name Pirfenidone esbriet	Idiopathic pulmonary fibrosis	**Usual oral dose:** Titrated weekly over 3 weeks from one capsule 3 times per day (801 mg per day) to 3 capsules 3 times per day (2403 mg per day)	• Angioedema has been reported • May impair mental alertness • Take with food to reduce GI upset • Patients will be photosensitive for the first 6 months of treatment • Monitor for weight loss • Cigarette smoking decreases the efficiency of this drug and should be avoided

Chapter 10

Eye, Ear, Nose, and Throat Preparations

Authors: **Tammie Lee Demler, PharmD, BS Pharm, MBA, RPh, BCPP and Charlene Meyer, PharmD**

Editor: **Claudia Lee, RPh, MD**

Learning Objectives

- Identify current pharmacologic agents that are appropriate for each condition/diagnosis.
- Recommend optimal pharmacologic interventions based on patient-specific characteristics.
- Provide appropriate patient-specific counseling points and optimal overall medication management.

Key Terms: Antiallergic agents, anti-infective agents, anti-inflammatory agents, local anesthetic agents, mydriatic agents, mouthwashes and gargles, vasoconstrictors, antiglaucoma agents, alpha-adrenergic agonists, beta-adrenergic blocking agents, carbonic anhydrase inhibitors, miotics, prostaglandin analogues

Overview of Eye, Ear, Nose, and Throat Preparations

The agents covered in this chapter are primarily administered topically as eye, ear, nose, and throat (EENT) preparations. However, these same agents may be administered via oral or inhaled routes when their use involves another body system or when systemic absorption must be optimized. These agents are, consequently, examined in greater detail in chapters devoted to those purposes.

Topical administration provides the opportunity to deliver therapeutic effects while limiting unintended systemic effects. This outcome results from the fact that even though these drug products are administered topically, they are absorbed less (and so have less bioavailability) than if orally ingested or inhaled. For some of the EENT agents, this dosage delivery option allows for bypassing of hepatic first-pass effects, thus representing a creative way of providing an effective alternative medication intervention.

Several cautions must be recognized when using EENT agents. First, because most EENT are products applied topically, patients may be less likely to realize or understand that these products are associated with potentially serious side effects. Consequently, education about side effects and risks is important. Second, older adults and younger children may experience greater topical absorption due to differences in skin thickness and areas of exposure.

Eyes

The eyes are therapeutic targets for treatment for a wide array of conditions. Glaucoma, infection and allergic symptoms are all among the most notable conditions treated with eye drops. Ophthalmic products are formulated to be physiologically similar to natural eye fluids in terms of pH, osmotic balance, and sterility. For this reason, some eye drops may be used in the ear, but ear drops cannot be used in the eye, as they do not share the same physiologic nature of eye fluids. Even though eye products are intended to result in topical action, their systemic absorption may have unintended or exaggerated systemic effects. For example, some glaucoma eye drops are actually members of the same therapeutic category as oral blood pressure medications and, therefore, can affect blood pressure and heart rate. This systemic action can be minimized by instilling drops and then blocking the inner tear duct closest to the nose for a few minutes after installation. Also note that the eye cannot accommodate more than a drop or two before tears are triggered to flush the "foreign" irritant, thereby diluting or eliminating the therapeutic action of the drugs. It is important to be mindful that the sterility of drops may be altered if contact is made with the eye, fingers, or any other nonsterile surface. Even eyes that are not "infected" can contain bacteria that will potentially contaminate the sterility of the drops in use. There are three common types of conjunctivitis (a condition otherwise known as "pink eye"), which is an infection of the layer of the eye covering the sclera. They are bacterial, viral, and allergic. Each diagnosis requires different treatment interventions; however, all but the allergic type should be considered contagious. Experts have significantly differing opinions about the "beyond use" dates of eye drops with some believing that drops should be used for only a limited number of weeks once opened, whereas others support the continued use of these products up to the manufacturer's expiration date. Everyone agrees, however, that antibiotic products should be discarded after the resolution of the infection and that any remaining supply should not be kept for future use.

Eye ointments are intended for use when prolonged tissue contact is required or is more desirable—for example, overnight, when blurring of vision is not a problem. Individuals who wear contact lenses must use caution because these medications are often not compatible with contact lens material and may cause discoloration of the lens. Also, in cases where allergic reactions are experienced, the allergen cannot be removed from the lens; consequently, the lens may no longer be usable. The selection of eye drops can be further individualized by exploring alternative agents for more convenient (less frequent) administration frequency and/or alternative mechanisms of action that can offset negative adverse effects of some drops (such as dryness of the eye) instead of adding artificial tears to provide balance.

Ears

The treatment of acute otitis externa (AOE) is one of the many therapeutic interventions that can be made with the use of otic drops. Treatments have ranged between the use of an antiseptic (such as acetic acid) or an antibacterial (such as an aminoglycoside) or with a steroid plus an antimicrobial versus an antimicrobial alone. There are numerous expert opinions on which agent (or combination of agents) is preferred and once selected, what formulation is safer in the midst of potential tympanic membrane (TM) perforation. Although medical references do not specifically favor a suspension over a solution in the setting of presumed or confirmed TM rupture (or vice versa), some providers will request a suspension instead of a solution to avoid a potentially higher risk of inner ear penetration and thus, ototoxicity. It has also been suggested that suspensions are less likely than solutions to promote the passage of contaminants into the canal. Treatment strategies change over time with updated recommendations and the availability of improved medication options available to us. In the past, ear pain was treated with specific agents that today are not supported for safety and efficacy. For example, in 2016, the FDA announced planned enforcement actions against manufacturers who distribute unapproved prescription otic products labeled to relieve ear pain, infection, and inflammation. There are manufacturers who continue to distribute products intended for the treatment of ear pain, infection, and inflammation despite the warnings from the FDA that ingredients in these products (such as hydrocortisone and benzocaine) have not been fully evaluated for safety and efficacy. These unapproved drug labels often do not disclose that they lack FDA approval and prescribers may be unaware of these concerns. It is imperative that clinicians stay current with guidelines and the availability of FDA-approved products for use.

Nose

The nasal passage is continuous with the oral pharynx, so nasal drops often have an undesirable "taste" that the patient will describe as a negative aspect with use. Nasal products can take the form of drops or sprays. Clearing the nasal passage prior to instillation of drops or liquids is the best way to achieve maximum exposure and therapeutic benefits. It is best for the patient to clear the nose with a gentle blow prior to installation. A gentle inhalation to encourage the penetration of the product is an ideal technique to improve and maximize nasally administered products.

Throat

Topical agents used for pain (anesthetics) may impair the gag reflex, so these medications are best used after eating meals or drinking beverages. Older adults may be at increased risk of choking, so caution is warranted for these products' use in elderly patients. Lidocaine products, if systemically absorbed or swallowed, may also cause changes to heart rate or rhythm. It is important to educate patients when medications should be swished but not swallowed.

10.1 Antiallergic Agents

The pharmacology used to suppress allergy is multifactorial and often employs agents from several different therapeutic categories. Most of the antiallergy products described in this section must be used as scheduled, whether allergic symptoms are present or not, for the duration of treatment. While the mechanisms of action for many of these agents are based on the suppression of the action of histamine, they are not exclusively antihistamines. Those that are antihistamines are still subject to the sedating side effects if any degree of absorption occurs. Stabilization of mast cells is another therapeutic strategy used in this family of medications, preventing the release of chemical mediators responsible for the "typical" allergic symptoms that include inflammation, itching, and irritation.

Antiallergic Agents

Alcaftadine
Azelastine
Bepotastine
Cromolyn
Emedastine
Epinastine
Ketotifen
Lodoxamide
Nedocromil
Olopatadine
Pemirolast

Case Studies and Conclusions

CG is a 24-year-old African American male who is being seen in the doctor's office due to complaints of watery, red, and itchy eyes. His symptoms started when the weather was getting warmer. Last week CG went hiking in the mountains, and his eyes became worse during his adventure. Since CG is busy all the time, he is hoping for a medication that he does not have to carry in his pocket wherever he goes during the day.

1. Which ophthalmic agent do you recommend for CG for his allergic conjunctivitis?
   a. Cromolyn
   b. Ketotifen
   c. Lodoxamide
   d. Emedastine

Answer B is correct. Ketotifen is used 2 to 3 times daily, which is optimal for CG's busy lifestyle. Cromolyn is used 4 to 6 times a day, lodoxamide is used 4 times a day, and emedastine can be used up to 4 times a day for optimal effects.

2. What is the mechanism of action for ketotifen?
   a. Mast cell stabilizer
   b. Selectively inhibits histamine H_1 receptors
   c. Selectively inhibits histamine H_2 receptors
   d. Nonselectively inhibits histamine receptors

Answer B is correct. Histamine H_2 receptors are located in the stomach and are not involved in allergy symptoms.

CG has been using the agent you suggested, but now complains of dry eyes that developed after he started using the medication.

3. What do you recommend?
   a. Add artificial tears to help moisturize his eyes
   b. Discontinue the suggested agent and start loratadine
   c. Discontinue the suggested agent and start nedocromil
   d. Decrease the suggested agent dosage to once a day

Answer C is correct. Adding artificial tears for an adverse effect is polypharmacy—a practice that should be avoided if other medication options are available. Loratadine is a systemic agent that addresses multiple symptoms of allergy; it is not needed when the patient's problem is only allergic conjunctivitis. Ketotifen should be used at least twice a day, so decreasing the frequency of its use may not be enough to relieve CG's symptoms. Nedocromil is used twice a day; as a mast cell stabilizer, it has a different mechanism of action than ketotifen and may provide a more tolerable adverse-effect profile for CG.

NS is a 46-year-old white female who is looking for relief for her runny and itchy nose. She says that this problem is caused by allergies, as it happens only when the pollen count is high. NS prefers not to take oral medications because she feels that she is sensitive to systemic medications.

1. What do you recommend for NS's allergy symptoms?
   a. Loratadine
   b. Olopatadine
   c. Ledoxamide
   d. Cromolyn

Answer D is correct. Cromolyn has very few side effects compared to olopatadine, which can cause ulcers in the nose when used on a long-term basis. Since NS is worried about adverse effects, this medication is the best choice for her. Loratadine acts systemically; ledoxamide is available only for ophthalmic use (not nasal use).

NS asks you about using the agent you suggested for her allergies. She wants to know when to use it.

2. What do you tell her?
   a. Use it every day, all year round
   b. Use it during the summer months
   c. Use it as needed when symptoms appear
   d. Use it only when symptoms are bad

Answer B is correct. NS says her symptoms occur only when pollen counts are high, which would be in the summertime; thus, there is no need for her to use cromolyn year around. By using cromolyn daily instead of as needed or when her symptoms are worse, NS can prevent symptoms from occurring in the first place.

10.2 Anti-infective Agents

EENT antibacterial agents can be susceptible to resistance, as is the case with systemically administered formulations. Clinical response to a topically applied antibiotic may be easier for a patient to assess, with infections generally involving more specific symptoms (e.g., redness, pain). EENT infections can be highly contagious; thus, in cases involving infections such as conjunctivitis, education about hand hygiene and reduced exposure to household contacts is key. Some of the more "classic" antibiotic side effects, such as sun sensitivity with sulfonamides and quinolones and renal effects with aminoglycosides, are nearly nonexistent with topically applied products. Proper aseptic technique is necessary when applying these products to avoid cross-contamination. Overuse or misuse can still contribute to bacterial resistance, however, so these agents should be used only when they are clinically indicated.

Antibacterial Agents

Bacitracin
Besifloxacin

Ciprofloxacin
Doxycycline
Erythromcyin
Gatifloxacin
Gentamicin
Levofloxacin
Minocycline
Moxifloxacin
Neomycin
Ofloxacin
Polymyxin B
Sulfacetamide
Tobramycin

Antifungal Agents

Natamycin

Antiviral Agents

Trifluridine

Miscellaneous Anti-infective Agents

Boric acid
Carbamide peroxide
Chlorhexidine

Case Studies and Conclusions

JB is a 34-year-old male who comes to your office with an uncomplicated ophthalmic infection that he received from his 5-year-old son. His son was prescribed first bacitracin and then ofloxacin a week later after the bacitracin failed to work. The doctor determined JB's infection is likely caused by bacteria.

1. What do you recommend to treat JB's eye infection?
   a. Bacitracin
   b. Ofloxacin
   c. Neomycin, polymyxin B, and hydrocortisone
   d. Natamycin

Answer B is correct. Since bacitracin did not work for JB's son, it will mostly likely not cure his infection either. Adding hydrocortisone when the eye is not inflamed is unnecessary. Natamycin is an antifungal agent, not an antibacterial drug.

2. What should you tell JB about using ophthalmic agents?
   a. Wash your hands before and after using eye drops.
   b. It is okay to touch the eye when it itches.
   c. Many drops can be used at once in one eye.
   d. Ear drops can be used in the eye if necessary.

Answer A is correct. The patient should to avoid touching the eye to ensure the bacteria do not spread to other areas or to other people. The eye is not able to accommodate a large volume of liquid, so it is recommended to use only one or two drops at a time. When using more than one agent, wait 5 minutes in between their applications.

JB calls later and reports that his eyes are doing much better, but now his ear is plugged with wax. He wants a recommendation for a medication to remove the built-up wax.

3. What do you tell him?
   a. Ofloxacin
   b. Zinc sulfate
   c. Gatifloxacin
   d. Carbamide peroxide

Answer D is correct. Carbamide peroxide is the only over-the-counter (OTC) medication of the listed here than can loosen wax in the ear.

10.3 Anti-inflammatory Agents

Topical corticosteroids are very useful in suppressing irritation, inflammation, and allergic symptoms. Due to their local suppressant effects on immunity, patients and prescribers should be aware that their use is associated with increased risk of growth of opportunistic organisms such as yeast (i.e., thrush) and the emergence or worsening of a rash. For a more detailed discussion about corticosteroids, refer to the Hormones and Synthetic Substitutes chapter.

Anti-inflammatory agents may sometimes mask or worsen acute infections. Avoid these medications or use them with caution in patients with latent or active tuberculosis; untreated bacterial, fungal, parasitic, or viral infections; or ocular herpes infection. Reactivation of a viral infection may occur with these agents in such patients.

Many steroidal eye drops are also available as suspensions. Patients should be educated that shaking these products prior to use is required to ensure that the proper dose is administered. As is the case with oral steroids, these products vary in potency, and their selection is based on the prescriber's assessment of the patient's individual needs for the particular strength of action.

The proper administration technique for the concurrent use of eye drops is to use a solution prior to a suspension, with one drop administered at a time. Any additional drops may trigger the eye to naturally tear to flush out the extra fluid, which will dilute the medication effects. In some cases, severe ophthalmic inflammation requires both oral and topical administration.

Corticosteroids

Beclomethasone
Budesonide
Ciclesonide
Dexamethasone
Difluprednate
Flunisolide
Fluocinolone
Fluorometholone
Fluticasone
Hydrocortisone
Loteprednol
Mometasone
Prednisolone
Rimexolone
Triamcinolone

Nonsteroidal Anti-inflammatory Agents

Bromfenac
Flurbiprofen
Ketorolac
Nepafenac

Miscellaneous Anti-inflammatory Agents

Cyclosporine

Case Studies and Conclusions

VC is a 34-year-old female who is suffering from seasonal allergies and is looking for relief. She asks for help to relieve her runny and itchy nose. She has gone through multiple boxes of tissues.

1. Which steroid would be optimal to treat VC's allergy symptoms?
   a. Lotepredenol
   b. Prednisolone
   c. Fluticasone
   d. Dexamethasone

Answer C is correct. Fluticasone is available as a nasal spray and is indicated for nasal allergy symptoms. The remaining agents are intended for administration through the ophthalmic or otic route.

2. What is a common side effect of fluticasone nasal spray that you should counsel VC on?
   a. May cause glaucoma
   b. Can cause nasal dryness
   c. May suppress growth
   d. May cause decreased efficacy of the immune system

Answer B is correct. Fluticasone nasal sprays rarely cause glaucoma and immunosuppression; rather, these adverse effects are more likely to occur with long-term use and with systemic steroids. Suppression of growth is rare with use of nasal products and is in seen in pediatric patients only, not adults.

TC is a 68-year-old white male who just had cataract surgery. His medical history is significant for nonsteroidal anti-inflammatory drug (NSAID) allergy, hypertension, and hypercholesterolemia. His son is with him, and is asking about the postoperative care for his father. He wants to ensure that TC knows how to use the medication when he gets home.

1. Which medication would be best to reduce TC's inflammation?
   a. Rimexolone
   b. Mometasone
   c. Cyclosporine
   d. Ketorolac

Answer A is correct. Rimexolone is approved for postoperative ophthalmic surgery inflammation. Mometasone is not available for ophthalmic use. Cyclosporine is indicated for chronic dry eyes, not for postoperative inflammation. TC has an allergy to NSAIDs, so he should not take ketorolac.

2. How long should you instruct TC's son that his father should use the suggested agent?
   a. Start using the eye drops when TC gets home and continue for 1 week
   b. Use the eye drops in 24 hours and continue for 1 week
   c. Start using eye drops when TC gets home and continue for 2 weeks
   d. Use the eye drops after 24 hours postsurgery and continue for 2 weeks

Answer C is correct. Instruct TC to use 1 to 2 drops in the surgical eye 4 times daily for 2 weeks. Eye drops should be used within 24 hours after surgery and should continue longer than 1 week unless otherwise directed.

10.4 Local Anesthetic, Mydriatic, and Vasoconstrictor Agents

Local Anesthetic Agents

Local anesthetics are used therapeutically for their pain-relieving actions. Although other senses can be involved, these agents primarily cause a reversible block pain sensation. Certain agents can act on specific nerve pathways to provide local anesthetic nerve block while others can achieve muscular paralysis. Some local anesthetics are structurally related to cocaine and the ones described below are available for topical use.

Local Anesthetic Agents

Cocaine
Dyclonine
Proparacaine
Tetracaine
Benzocaine *(see also the Antipruritic and Local Anesthetic Agents section in the Skin and Mucous Membrane Agents chapter)*

Mydriatic Agents

Pupillary dilation that occurs when the eyes are exposed to low light conditions is called mydriasis. This dilation can also be pharmacologically initiated with exogenous sympathetic stimulation when specific drugs are administered and may also be caused by disease or injury. Pupils that have had drug induced mydriasis will remain excessively dilated and will not react with normal pupillary constriction reflexes even when exposed to bright light. The use of pharmacologic mydriatic agents is generally limited to examination of the inner eye (i.e., retina) and surgical interventions. Some of these agents are discussed at greater length elsewhere in this text.

Mydriatic Agents

Atropine
Cyclopentolate
Dipivefrin
Homatropine
Tropicamide
Epinephrine *(see also the Autonomic-Sympathomimetic Adrenergic Agents section in the Autonomic Agents chapter)*
Phenylephrine *(see also the Autonomic-Sympathomimetic Adrenergic Agents section in the Autonomic Agents chapter)*
Scopolamine *(see also the Autonomic-Anticholinergic Agents section in the Autonomic Agents chapter)*

Vasoconstrictors

Vasoconstricting pharmacologic agents cause a narrowing of blood vessels similar to that which occurs naturally when there is a contraction of the muscular wall of small arterioles and larger vessels. The vascular effects of these agents as a target of systemic pharmacotherapy is discussed at length in other chapters within this text (refer to companion drug grid). Because many of these agents are also applied topically to provide relief to eyes, nose, and other mucous membranes that are red, irritated, and swollen through the temporary shrinkage of blood vessels, they are also included in this chapter. Overuse of vasoconstricting agents may result in rebound swelling and redness when the agents are discontinued and during use may deprive target tissues of necessary oxygenation by limiting blood perfusion by constricting vessels supplying blood to extremity tissues.

Vasoconstrictors

Naphazoline
Oxymetazoline
Phenylephrine
Tetrahydrozoline
Epinephrine *(see also the Autonomic-Sympathomimetic Adrenergic Agents section in the Autonomic Agents chapter)*

Mouthwashes and Gargles

Hydrogen peroxide

Case Studies and Conclusions

FI is a 55-year-old male who is asking about the medications that he just picked up from the pharmacy. He currently has walking pneumonia and has been prescribed epinephrine nebulizers. In a month, FI is going on a cruise; he frequently gets seasick, so he was prescribed scopolamine patches. He explains that he is very excited because his son will be joining him. His past history is significant for hypertension, diabetes, and hypothyroidism.

1. What is a common side effect of epinephrine that FI should be concerned about?
   a. May raise blood pressure
   b. May increase intraocular pressure
   c. May worsen his benign prostrate hypertrophy
   d. May worsen his hypothyroidism

Answer A is correct. Epinephrine is a sympathomimetic agent and can increase blood pressure. Since epinephrine will be used for a short time, this patient's blood pressure should be monitored as needed. Although epinephrine may increase intraocular pressure and worsen benign prostrate hypertrophy, FI is not suffering from these conditions. Epinephrine worsens hyperthyroidism, not hypothyroidism.

2. What should you tell FI concerning his scopolamine patch?
   a. Apply the patch behind the ear once a day.
   b. Most people have no reactions to scopolamine.
   c. Scopolamine may cause drowsiness.
   d. Apply the patch only when you feel seasick.

Answer C is correct. Many people experience notable drowsiness from scopolamine, which might impact FI's enjoyment of his vacation, especially if combined with alcohol. The scopolamine patch is applied once every 3 days and should be applied before getting on the boat to prevent seasickness.

TC is a 46-year-old male who is suffering from the common cold. His medical history is significant for hypercholesterolemia and diabetes. He is looking for an over-the-counter (OTC) medication to help with his congestion.

1. Which medication do you recommend for TC's congestion?
   a. Epinephrine
   b. Atropine
   c. Tetrahydrozoline
   d. Oxymetazoline

Answer D is correct. Oxymetazoline comes in an OTC nasal spray and helps relieve congestion. Tetrahydrozoline is for ophthalmic use only. Atropine and epinephrine will not help with congestion.

2. How long should you instruct TC to use the suggested nasal spray?
   a. Until symptoms are gone
   b. For 1 week as needed
   c. For 3 to 5 days as needed
   d. For 2 weeks as needed

Answer C is correct. Using a vasoconstrictor, such as oxymetazoline, for longer than 3 to 5 days can cause rebound congestion and reduced oxygenation to extremity tissues.

10.5 Antiglaucoma Agents

Currently there is no absolute cure for glaucoma. However, there are two main types of treatments for this condition that are intended to lower intraocular pressure, a modifiable risk factor for glaucoma; they include medication and surgery.

There are essentially two types of glaucoma: open-angle and closed-angle. Open-angle glaucoma, which is the most common type of glaucoma, is often treated with prescription eye drops that lower intraocular pressure (IOP) through various pharmacologic mechanisms. These medications can be used as single-agent therapy or sometimes in combination with each other. If eye drops do not lower IOP enough, surgery may be required. Even patients who require surgical intervention may still require eye drops to control IOP. Uncontrolled glaucoma may result in blindness. There are numerous pharmacotherapeutic targets that can be used to provide control that include agents covered more comprehensively in other sections of this text (these include the alpha-adrenergic agonists and beta adrenergic blocking agents). Another drug target includes the influence over carbonic anhydrase, which is a family of enzymes responsible for maintaining acid–base balance in blood and other tissues, and transporting carbon dioxide out of tissues. Carbonic anhydrase inhibitors are a class of agents that suppress the activity of carbonic anhydrase and clinically have been used as antiglaucoma agents, diuretics, antiepileptics, and in the management of mountain sickness among other conditions. Prostaglandins have also been identified as a target of drug therapy. For example, bimatoprost is a structural analog to a specific prostaglandin that increases the outflow of aqueous fluid from the eye and lowers intraocular pressure.

Opposite to the mydriatic agents discussed earlier, miotics (pupillary constrictors) have also been used in the treatment of chronic open-angle glaucoma and acute angle-closure glaucoma. As an illustrative example, the miotic agent, pilocarpine, acts on muscarinic receptors found on the iris sphincter muscle, causing the muscle to contract, resulting in pupil constriction (miosis). Pilocarpine also acts on the ciliary muscle and causes it to contract, ultimately facilitating the rate that aqueous humor leaves the eye and therefore decreasing intraocular pressure.

Alpha-Adrenergic Agonists

Brimonidine

Beta-Adrenergic Blocking Agents

Betaxolol
Levobunolol
Timolol

Carbonic Anhydrase Inhibitors

Acetazolamide
Brinzolamide
Dorzolamide
Methazolamide

Miotics

Acetylcholine
Carbachol
Pilocarpine

Prostaglandin Analogues

Bimatoprost
Latanoprost
Tafluprost
Travoprost

Miscellaneous EENT Agents

Aflibercept
Apraclonidine
Cysteamine
Ocriplasmin
Pegaptanib

Ranibizumab
Unoprostone
Verteporfin

Case Studies and Conclusions

PE is a 62-year-old African American female who was recently diagnosed with open-angle glaucoma. Her past medical history is significant for hypertension, kidney stones, cataracts, and diabetes. She wants to know more about the medication she will be on.

1. What do you recommend for PE as first-line therapy for optimal intraocular pressure–lowering effects?
   a. Latanoprost
   b. Pilocarpine
   c. Acetazolamide
   d. Laser trabeculoplasty

Answer A is correct. Latanoprost is a highly effective agent for reducing intraocular pressure compared to other medications on the market. Pilocarpine should not be used if a patient has cataracts. Acetazolamide is available as an oral agent and should not be used in patients with a history of kidney stones; in general, this medication is not tolerated well. Laser trabeculoplasty is the last-line treatment.

2. What is a common side effect of the agent you suggested that PE should know about?
   a. May decrease heart rate
   b. May increase glucose levels
   c. Can cause fuller eyelashes
   d. May lighten iris pigmentation

Answer C is correct. Decreased heart rate is a side effect of beta blockers, not prostaglandin analogues. Latanoprost does not affect glucose levels and can darken—not lighten—iris pigmentation.

PE calls back and is complaining about her eyelashes. She says they look like spiders and she would like to try a different medication.

3. Which medication(s) do you recommend that has (have) a similar efficacy to latanoprost?
   a. Timolol
   b. Dorzolamide
   c. Timolol and dorzolamide
   d. Travoprost

Answer C is correct. Travoprost is the same drug class as latanoprost and will likely cause the same fuller eyelash adverse effect. Timolol and dorzolamide are not as effective as latanoprost, but together they can more effectively decrease intraocular pressure.

4. Which of the following is a counseling point for the agent(s) that you suggested for PE?
   a. Your vision may become permanently blurry.
   b. It is okay to wear contacts while instilling the eye drops.
   c. This agent may cause your eyes to be sensitive to light.
   d. Use of this agent will commonly will mask the symptoms of low blood sugar.

Answer C is correct. Sensitivity to light is a common side effect of timolol. Vision may become blurry, but only for a few minutes while putting the eye drops in. It is recommended not to wear contacts while putting eye drops in to ensure full absorption of the medication. Beta blockers are known to mask the symptoms of low blood sugar; however, since timolol is an ophthalmic agent and the eye is not highly vascularized, this symptom is rare.

Tips from the Field

Using Drops for Eyes and Ears

1. Read the instructions carefully before you use any medication drops. Storage of drops should generally be at room temperature and away from heat, moisture, and direct light. There may be exceptions to this, so it is important to follow instructions carefully.
2. Pharmaceutically, the differences between ophthalmic products and otic products are that ophthalmic products are sterile and are buffered to a neutral pH. Otherwise, they are identical to their otic family members.
3. Do not use drops if they change color or turn cloudy. Do not use them if they have particles floating in them. Wash your hands before and after you instill drops.
4. Patients using ear drops may be experiencing a painful condition. Suggest that they warm the drops by holding the bottle in their hands for a few minutes, which may make the administration of the drops more comfortable. Suspensions must be shaken prior to use; read directions to verify the proper handling of the product you are using.
5. Position to optimize the penetration of ear drops by tilting the head to one side allowing the affected ear to be exposed. Gently pull and hold the lobe of the ear up and back while gently squeezing the bottle to drop the correct number of drops into the ear and keep head tilted for several minutes to allow the medication to coat and penetrate the ear canal.
6. Ear pain can be extremely uncomfortable and given the limited options of topical FDA-approved medications for use; patients and healthcare providers should explore oral analgesic options to manage pain until the primary condition has resolved (i.e., until antibiotics have resolved the infection causing pain).
7. Decongestants temporarily reduce the swelling of nasal and sinus tissues and provide quick relief to bothersome symptoms often experienced in vasomotor rhinitis. This condition is an inflammation of the nose due to compromised nerve control in the blood vessels located in the nose. Use care not to overuse decongestant medications.

Tammie Lee and Jacque

Bibliography

American Geriatrics Society. 2015 updated Beers criteria for potentially inappropriate medication use in older adults. *J Am Geriatr Soc.* 2015;63:2227-2246.

American Glaucoma Society. FAQs: what is the treatment for glaucoma? http://www.americanglaucomasociety.net/patients/faqs. Accessed June 23, 2016.

American Optometric Association. Glaucoma: how is glaucoma treated? http://www.aoa.org/Glaucoma.xml. Accessed June 23, 2016.

France RC. *Introduction to Sports Medicine and Athletic Training.* 2nd ed. Clifton Park, NY: Delmar, Cengage: 2011.

McEvoy GK, ed. *AHFS: Drug Information.* Bethesda, MD: American Society of Health-System Pharmacists; 2016.

Pfaff JA, Moore GP. Otolaryngology. In: Marx JA, Hockberger RS, Walls RM, eds. *Rosen's Emergency Medicine: Concepts and Clinical Practice.* 8th ed. Philadelphia, PA: Saunders; 2010: 877-887.

Rosenfeld RM, Schwartz SR, Canon CR, et al. Clinical practice guideline: acute otitis externa. *Otolaryngol Head Neck Surg.* 2014; 150(2):161-168.

U.S. Federal Drug Administration. Unapproved prescription ear drop (otic) products: not FDA evaluated for safety, effectiveness, and quality. July 7, 2016. http://www.fda.gov/Safety/MedWatch/SafetyInformation/SafetyAlertsforHumanMedicalProducts/ucm453430.htm. Accessed January 20, 2017.

Symbols

- Renal impairment: Dose adjustment is recommended.
- Hepatic impairment: Dose adjustment is recommended.
- Black box warning exists for this drug.
- QTc prolongation effects have been reported.
- 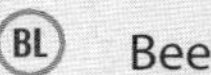 Beers list criteria (avoid in elderly).
- 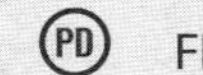 FDA-approved pediatric doses are available.
-  FDA-approved geriatric doses are available.
-  See primary body system.

Eye, Ear, Nose, and Throat Preparations

Universal prescribing alerts:

- Known serious hypersensitivity to the specific drug or any other component of the product/formulation selected warrants a contraindication for its use.
- Although these products are generally applied topically to the affected area, systemic absorption is still possible. Adverse reactions associated with the use of some **eye, ear, nose, and throat (EENT) preparations** may include dizziness, drowsiness, vertigo, and fatigue; these agents may also impair the patient's ability to perform tasks requiring mental alertness. Caution should always be recommended when using any new drug for the first time, when there is a dose change, and for continued use of known offending agents.
- Contact lenses should not be worn during treatment of ophthalmic infections; hearing aids and other devices require assessment when using medications that are instilled into the ear(s) as well. Wash hands before and after instilling drops. After instilling eye drops, wait at least 10 to 15 minutes before inserting contact lenses. Do not touch the tip of the container to any surface, the eyelids, or the surrounding area. If more than one topical ophthalmic drug is being used, administer the drugs at least 5 to 10 minutes apart. Keep the bottle tightly closed when not in use. Educate patients on good ophthalmic installation techniques, which include tilting the head back while instilling drops in the eye, keeping the eye open, and making an effort to wait a few seconds before blinking a few times to make sure the eye is covered with the solution. To reduce unintended topical effects, patients should wipe away excess medication from the skin and should avoid touching the applicator to the eye so as not to contaminate the tip of the applicator.
- Do not keep EENT drops longer than the recommended expiration date (this may be adjusted to less than the manufacturer's "beyond use" date for sterile products after first use). Consult a pharmacist or drug reference for information on the medication's stability.
- Doses expressed are for usual adult dosage ranges only. "Geriatric doses" are assumed to be the same as adult doses unless otherwise noted with a symbol. Where pediatric dosing is available, a symbol will guide the reader to additional prescribing references. Refer to real-time prescribing references for these age-specific doses.
- Use of EENT preparations in pregnancy is based on clinical risk versus benefit; safety concerns are not represented in this grid. Refer to the package insert (PI) for more information. Clinicians should continue to provide education about the reproductive risks of any medication and offer risk-reduction strategies (which may include contraceptive use) to women of childbearing age and understand that these reproductive risks may also extend to males. Other medications may decrease the effectiveness of oral contraceptives. Where necessary, an alternative means of birth control should be explored.
- Brand names are provided for those agents still available on the market. Due to the ever-changing product availability, refer to Food and Drug Administration (FDA) resources to confirm the actual brands available. This drug summary is for educational purposes only. Prescribing decisions should be based on real-time comprehensive drug databases that are updated on a regular basis.

Antiallergic Agents

Universal prescribing alerts:

- The efficacy of many of these agents is improved when used at the scheduled prescribing frequency for symptom prevention; even when symptoms are absent.
- Most often allergic symptoms require the use in both eyes for ophthalmic indications, however the FDA labeling routinely indicates use in affected eye(s).
- These agents should not be used as monotherapy for infection.

Drug Name	FDA-Approved Indications	Adult Dosage Range	Precautions and Clinical Pearls
Generic name Alcaftadine **Brand Name** Lastacaft	Allergic conjunctivitis	**Usual ophthalmic dose:** 0.25% solution: instill 1 drop into affected eye(s) daily	• Most frequent ocular adverse reactions reported: irritation, burning and/or stinging upon instillation, eye redness and eye pruritus • Most frequent non-ocular adverse reactions reported: nasopharyngitis and headache
Generic Name Azelastine (nasal) **Brand Name** Astepro Astelin (PD) **Generic Name** Azelastine (ophthalmic) **Brand Name** Optivar	Allergic rhinitis Allergic conjunctivitis	**Usual intranasal dose:** 1 to 2 sprays (137 mcg/spray) in each nostril twice daily **Usual ophthalmic dose:** 0.05% solution: instill 1 drop into affected eye(s) twice daily	• May cause central nervous system (CNS) depression; patients should use caution when performing tasks that require mental alertness • Use with other CNS depressants or alcohol may intensify the sedative effects; avoid these combinations • May enhance the effect of anticholinergic agents • It may help to blow nose gently prior to use of nasal spray; patients should not blow immediately after administration to allow appropriate exposure to the medication • May cause bitter taste, headache, rhinitis, nasal burning, pharyngitis, epistaxis, sinusitis, paroxysmal sneezing, nausea, and dry mouth • Reprime nasal spray after days of non-use
Generic Name Bepotastine **Brand Name** Bepreve	Allergic conjunctivitis	**Usual ophthalmic dose:** 1.5% solution: instill 1 drop into affected eye(s) twice daily	• May cause mild taste, eye irritation, headache, and nasopharyngitis following instillation

Generic Name Cromolyn **Brand Name** NasalCrom (nasal) Opticrom (ophthalmic)	Allergic rhinitis Vernal keratoconjunctivitis Vernal conjunctivitis Vernal keratitis	**Usual intranasal dose:** 1 spray (5.2 mg per spray) in each nostril 3 to 4 times per day **Usual ophthalmic dose:** 4% solution: instill 1 to 2 drops in affected eye(s) 4 to 6 times per day	• Temporary stinging or burning may occur • May take 2 to 4 weeks before symptomatic relief observed • For best results when using for allergic rhinitis, initiate 1 to 2 weeks before anticipated contact with allergens • NasalCrom available over the counter
Generic Name Emedastine **Brand Name** Emadine	Allergic conjunctivitis	**Usual ophthalmic dose:** 0.05% solution: instill 1 drop in affected eye(s) up to 4 times per day	• May cause some eye burning, irritation, itching, dryness, other eye discomfort, or blurred vision may occur • Headache and a bad taste in the mouth have also been reported
Generic Name Epinastine **Brand Name** Elestat	Allergic conjunctivitis	**Usual ophthalmic dose:** 0.05% solution: instill 1 drop into affected eye(s) twice daily	• Treatment should be continued throughout the period of exposure (i.e., until the pollen season is over or until exposure to the offending allergen is terminated), even when symptoms are absent • Contamination of multidose ophthalmic solutions may cause bacterial keratitis • Ocular adverse reactions reported: burning sensation in the eye, folliculosis, hyperemia, and pruritus. • Non-ocular adverse reactions reported were infection (cold symptoms and upper respiratory infections), rhinitis, headache, sinusitis, increased cough, and pharyngitis
Generic Name Ketotifen **Brand Name** Alaway Zaditor	Allergic conjunctivitis	**Usual ophthalmic dose:** 0.025% solution: instill 1 drop into affected eye(s) twice daily	• Convenient administration schedule over other alternatives that are dosed more frequently throughout the day • Available over the counter • Ocular adverse reactions reported: burning or stinging, conjunctivitis, discharge, dry eyes, eye pain, itching, keratitis, lacrimation disorder, mydriasis, photophobia, and rash • Non-ocular adverse reactions reported: flu syndrome and pharyngitis

Drug Name	FDA-Approved Indications	Adult Dosage Range	Precautions and Clinical Pearls
Generic Name Lodoxamide **Brand Name** Alomide	Vernal keratoconjunctivitis Vernal conjunctivitis Vernal keratitis	**Usual ophthalmic dose:** 0.1% solution: instill 1 or 2 drops into affected eye(s) 4 times day for up to 3 months	• Temporary ocular stinging or burning may occur • Other ocular events reported: ocular itching/pruritus, blurred vision, dry eye, tearing/discharge, hyperemia, crystalline deposits, and foreign body sensation
Generic Name Nedocromil **Brand Name** Alocril	Allergic conjunctivitis	**Usual ophthalmic dose:** 2% solution: instill 1 or 2 drops into both eyes twice daily	• Treatment should be continued throughout the period of exposure (i.e., until the pollen season is over or until exposure to the offending allergen is terminated), even when symptoms are absent • May cause ocular stinging or burning, headache, unpleasant taste, and nasal congestion, eye redness, photophobia, and rhinitis
Generic Name Olopatadine **Brand Name** Patanase (nasal) Pataday(ophthalmic) Patanol (ophthalmic) Pazeo (ophthalmic) (PD)	Allergic rhinitis Allergic conjunctivitis	**Usual intranasal dose:** 2 sprays (665 mcg per spray) in each nostril twice daily **Usual ophthalmic dose Patanol:** 0.1% solution: instill 1 drop into affected eye(s) twice daily at an interval no less than 6 to 8 hours	• Increased risk of developing nasal ulcerations • Use with other CNS depressants or alcohol may cause additive CNS depression • Monitor nasal mucosa periodically for ulcerations or perforations • May cause headache as well as less commonly reported adverse events of: asthenia, blurred vision, burning or stinging, cold syndrome, dry eye, foreign body sensation, hyperemia, hypersensitivity, keratitis, lid edema, nausea, pharyngitis, pruritis, rhinitis, sinusitis, and temporary taste alterations • Prime with no less than 5 pumps prior to first use and reprime if not used within 7 days • The nasal device should be discarded after 240 sprays (enough for 30 days of dosing) even if the container is not completely empty
Generic Name Pemirolast **Brand Name** Alamast	Allergic conjunctivitis	**Usual ophthalmic dose:** 0.1% solution: instill 1 or 2 drops into affected eye(s) 4 times per day	• Symptomatic response to therapy (decreased itching) may be evident within a few days, but frequently requires longer treatment (up to 4 weeks).

Anti-infective Agents

Antibacterial Agents

Universal prescribing alerts:

- Prolonged use of anti-infective agents may result in bacterial or fungal superinfection.
- Use of these agents must be based on infections caused by susceptible bacteria.
- Systemic exposure following topical, otic, or ophthalmic administration is low. However, refer to the Anti-infective Agents chapter for potential systemic side effects reported with oral use of these agents (i.e., tendon inflammation and rupture have occurred with quinolone antibiotics and if experienced with use, topical administration should be discontinued if any tendon pain or inflammation occurs).

Drug Name	FDA-Approved Indications	Adult Dosage Range	Precautions and Clinical Pearls
Generic Name Bacitracin baciguent ophthalmic	Superficial ophthalmic infections	**Usual ophthalmic dose:** Apply a thin film/ribbon to the conjunctival sac(s) of affected eye(s) every 3 to 4 hours for 7 to 10 days	• Anaphylactic reactions have occurred with repeated exposure to bacitracin • Ophthalmic ointment may cause blurry vision; use with care and do not drive or operate machinery during therapy Associated with: • Nephrotoxicity has been reported with systemic use
Generic Name Besifloxacin **Brand Name** Besivance	Bacterial conjunctivitis	**Usual ophthalmic dose:** 0.6% suspension: instill 1 drop into affected eye(s) 3 times per day for 7 days	• Suspension must be shaken prior to use • May cause temporarily blurred vision, eye pain, eye irritation, eye pruritus and headache
Generic Name Ciprofloxacin **Brand Name** Ciloxan (ophthalmic) Cetraxal (otic)	Bacterial conjunctivitis Corneal ulcer Acute otitis externa (AOE)	**Usual ophthalmic dose for bacterial conjunctivitis:** 0.3% solution: instill 1 or 2 drops into the affected eye(s) every 2 hours for 2 days, then every 4 hours for 5 days 0.3% ointment: apply ½-inch ribbon to the conjunctival sac(s) of affected eye(s) 3 times per day for 2 days, then twice daily for 5 days **Usual otic dose AOE:** 0.2% solution: instill into affected ear(s) every 12 hours for 7 days	• May cause local burning or discomfort; formation of white crystalline precipitates, lid margin crusting, foreign body sensation, itching, conjunctival hyperemia, and a bad taste following instillation • Less commonly reported: corneal staining, keratopathy/keratitis, allergic reactions, lid edema, tearing, photophobia, corneal infiltrates, nausea, and decreased vision • The otic solution is for use in the ear only: To minimize the chance of dizziness, warm the container in the hands for at least 1 minute. Have patient lie with the affected ear upward and then the solution should be instilled. This position should be maintained for at least 1 minute to facilitate penetration of the drops into the ear. Repeat, if necessary, for the opposite ear.

Drug Name	FDA-Approved Indications	Adult Dosage Range	Precautions and Clinical Pearls
Generic Name Doxycycline **Brand Name** Atridox	Periodontitis	**Usual subgingival dose:** Depends on size, shape, and number of pockets being treated Total product contains 50 mg of doxycycline (10% in the ATRIGEL® Delivery System)	• This is a subgingival controlled-release product composed of a two-syringe mixing system; Syringe A contains a polymeric formulation and Syringe B contains 50 mg of doxycycline hyclate; refer to PI for details • The use of tetracyclines during tooth development may cause permanent discoloration of the teeth; do not use doxycycline in patients at risk for this age-based adverse effect; refer to PI • Photosensitivity may occur when absorbed systemically; use skin protection and avoid prolonged sunlight exposure
Generic Name Erythromycin	Superficial ocular infections	**Usual ophthalmic dose:** 0.5% ointment: apply ½-inch ribbon into to the conjunctival sac of the affected eye(s) up to 6 times per day	• Ointment may cause temporarily blurred vision
Generic Name Gatifloxacin **Brand Name** Zymaxid	Bacterial conjunctivitis	**Illustrative ophthalmic dose:** 0.5% solution: instill 1 drop into affected eye(s) every 2 hours for 1 day, then 2 to 4 times per day on days 2 through 7 or as otherwise directed	• May cause conjunctival irritation, increased lacrimation, keratitis, papillary conjunctivitis and less commonly: chemosis (swelling/edema), conjunctival hemorrhage, dry eye, eye discharge, eye irritation, eye pain, eyelid edema, headache, red eye, reduced visual acuity and taste alterations • Available in higher strengths; refer to PI for product availability
Generic Name Gentamicin **Brand Name** Genoptic Gentak	Bacterial ophthalmic infections	**Illustrative ophthalmic dose:** 0.3% solution: instill 1 or 2 drops into the affected eye(s) every 4 hours (2 drops every hour for severe infection) 0.3% ointment: apply ½-inch ribbon to the conjunctival sac of the affected eye(s) 2 to 3 times per day or as otherwise directed	• Discontinue use if sensitization occurs • Ointment may cause temporarily blurred vision • May cause ocular burning and irritation upon drug instillation • Nonspecific conjunctivitis, conjunctival epithelial defects, and conjunctival hyperemia have been reported • Other adverse reactions which have occurred rarely are thrombocytopenic purpura, and hallucinations
Generic Name Levofloxacin **Brand Name** Quixin	Bacterial conjunctivitis	**Usual ophthalmic dose:** 0.5% solution: instill 1 or 2 drops every 2 hours for 2 days, then every 4 hours for 5 days	• May cause transient decreased vision, fever, foreign body sensation, headache, transient ocular burning, ocular pain or discomfort, pharyngitis, and photophobia • Other reported reactions reported are lid edema, ocular dryness, and ocular itching.

Generic Name Minocycline **Brand Name** Arestin	Periodontitis	**Usual subgingival dose:** Dose depends on size, shape, and number of pockets being treated Each unit dose cartridge contains the equivalent of 1 mg minocycline	• This is a subgingival sustained-release product containing minocycline microspheres incorporated into a bioresorbable polymer • Product is provided as a dry powder, packaged in a unit-dose cartridge that the oral health care professional removes from its pouch and connects the cartridge to the spring-loaded cartridge handle mechanism to administer the product • The use of tetracyclines during tooth development may cause permanent discoloration of the teeth; do not use minocycline in patients at risk for this age-based adverse effect; refer to PI • Photosensitivity may occur when absorbed systemically; use skin protection and avoid prolonged sunlight exposure • Monitor for signs of oral candidiasis
Generic Name Moxifloxacin **Brand Name** Moxeza Vigamox	Bacterial conjunctivitis	**Usual ophthalmic dose:** Moxeza 0.5% solution: instill 1 drop into the affected eye(s) twice daily for 7 days	• Different brand names may have variable suggested dosing frequencies; refer to PI • Ocular adverse events reported included conjunctivitis, decreased visual acuity, dry eye, keratitis, ocular discomfort, ocular hyperemia and pain, ocular pruritus, subconjunctival hemorrhage, and tearing • Nonocular adverse events reported were fever, increased cough, infection, otitis media, pharyngitis, rash, and rhinitis
Generic Name Neomycin **Brand Name** Neo-Polycin (ophthalmic) Cortimyxin (ophthalmic) Cortisporin (otic)	Superficial ocular infections Ocular inflammatory conditions Otitis externa	**Usual ophthalmic dose:** Solution: instill 1 or 2 drops into the affected eye(s) every 3 to 4 hours Ointment: apply ½-inch ribbon to the conjunctival sac of the affected eye(s) every 3 to 4 hours for 7 to 10 days **Usual otic dose:** Instill 4 drops into the affected ear(s) 3 to 4 times per day (maximum of 10 days unless otherwise directed)	• Neomycin may cause permanent sensorineural hearing loss due to cochlear damage: Limit therapy to 10 days; do not use in patients with a perforated tympanic membrane. • Ocular products are generally available in combination with bacitracin and polymyxin B or hydrocortisone and polymyxin B • Bacterial keratitis may occur with use of topical ophthalmic products in a multiple-dose container • Otic products are generally available in combination with polymyxin B and hydrocortisone • Use care when selecting and administering; available as solution and suspension, which may translate into significant differences in presence of perforation • The otic preparation is for otic use only

Drug Name	FDA-Approved Indications	Adult Dosage Range	Precautions and Clinical Pearls
Generic Name Ofloxacin **Brand Name** Ocuflox (ophthalmic) **Brand Name** Floxin (otic) PD	Bacterial conjunctivitis Corneal ulcer Otitis externa Chronic suppurative otitis media (OM) Acute otitis media	**Usual ophthalmic dose for bacterial conjunctivitis:** 0.3% solution: instill 1 or 2 drops into the affected eye(s) every 2 to 4 hours for 2 days, then 4 times per day for 5 days **Usual otic dose for chronic suppurative OM:** 0.3% solution: instill 10 drops into the affected ear(s) twice daily for 14 days	• Eye drops may cause ocular burning or discomfort, stinging, redness, itching, chemical conjunctivitis/keratitis, ocular/periocular/facial edema, foreign body sensation, photophobia, blurred vision, tearing, dryness, and eye pain • Rare reports of dizziness and nausea • The otic preparation is for use in ear only and the solution should be warmed in hands prior to use • Position patient so affected ear is upward and pump tragus 4 times by pushing inward to facilitate penetration into the middle ear; this position should be maintained for five minutes; repeat, if necessary, for the opposite ear
Generic Name Polymyxin B **Brand Name** Neo-Polycin (ophthalmic) Cortisporin (otic)	Superficial ocular infections Otitis externa	**Usual ophthalmic dose:** Ointment: apply ½-inch ribbon to the conjunctival sac of the affected eye(s) every 3 to 4 hours for 7 to 10 days **Usual otic dose:** Instill 4 drops into the affected ear(s) 3 to 4 times per day (maximum of 10 days)	Ophthalmic: • Often found in combination with bacitracin; bacitracin and neomycin; or bacitracin, neomycin, and hydrocortisone • Bacterial keratitis may occur with use of topical ophthalmic products in multiple-dose containers Otic: • Usually found in combination with neomycin and hydrocortisone • Use care when selecting and administering; available as solution and suspension, which may translate into significant differences in presence of perforation • The otic preparation is for use in the ear only
Generic Name Sulfacetamide **Brand Name** Bleph-10	Bacterial conjunctivitis Trachoma (in addition to systemic treatment)	**Usual ophthalmic dose** 10% solution: instill 1 or 2 drops into the affected eye(s) every 1 to 3 hours **Usual ophthalmic dose:** 10% ointment: apply ½-inch ribbon to the conjunctival sac of the affected eye(s) 4 times per day (every 3 to 4 hours and at bedtime)	• Regardless of the route of administration, discontinue at the first sign of a serious reaction • Agranulocytosis, aplastic anemia, and other blood disorders have been reported • Stevens-Johnsons syndrome, toxic epidermal necrolysis, and other severe dermatologic reactions have been reported • Rare fatalities associated with fulminant hepatic necrosis have been reported • More commonly reported adverse effects include local irritation, stinging and burning (non-specific conjunctivitis, conjunctival hyperemia, and secondary infections have also been reported less commonly)

Drug Name	FDA-Approved Indications	Adult Dosage Range	Precautions and Clinical Pearls
Generic Name Tobramycin **Brand Name** Tobrex	Bacterial conjunctivitis Endophthalmitis Keratitis	**Usual ophthalmic dose** 0.3% solution: instill 1 or 2 drops into the affected eye(s) every 2 to 4 hours 0.3% ointment: apply ½-inch ribbon to the conjunctival sac of the affected eye(s) 2 to 3 times per day	• May cause localized ocular toxicity, including lid itching and swelling, and conjunctival erythema • If topical ocular tobramycin is administered concomitantly with systemic aminoglycoside antibiotics, care should be taken to monitor the total serum concentration • Patients should use the minimum effective dose and apply pressure to lacrimal sac after instillation to decrease systemic absorption of solution • Ointment may cause temporarily blurred vision

Antifungal Agents

Universal prescribing alerts:

- Prolonged use of anti-infective agents may result in bacterial or other opportunistic infections

Drug Name	FDA-Approved Indications	Adult Dosage Range	Precautions and Clinical Pearls
Generic Name Natamycin **Brand Name** Natacyn	Fungal blepharitis Fungal conjunctivitis Fungal keratitis	**Usual ophthalmic dose for fungal blepharitis:** 5% suspension: instill 1 drop into conjunctival sac of the affected eye(s) every 4 to 6 hours	• May cause a change in vision, chest pain, corneal opacity, dyspnea, eye discomfort, eye edema, eye hyperemia, eye irritation, eye pain, foreign body sensation, paresthesia, and tearing • More frequent dosing regimens are available for more serious infections • Shake suspensions prior to use

Antiviral Agents

Drug Name	FDA-Approved Indications	Adult Dosage Range	Precautions and Clinical Pearls
Generic Name Trifluridine **Brand Name** Viroptic	Herpes simplex keratoconjunctivitis Herpes simplex keratitis	**Usual ophthalmic dose:** 1% solution: instill 1 drop into the affected eye(s) every 2 hours (MDD: 9 drops), then every 4 hours for 7 days once re-epithelialization occurs	• Do not exceed 21 days of treatment, as ocular toxicity may occur; if symptoms have not improved within 7 to 14 days, consider an alternative therapy • May cause mild, transient burning or stinging upon instillation, and palpebral edema • Superficial punctate keratopathy, epithelial keratopathy, stromal edema, irritation, keratitis sicca, hyperemia, and increased intraocular pressure have also been rarely reported

Miscellaneous Anti-infective Agents

Drug Name	FDA-Approved Indications	Adult Dosage Range	Precautions and Clinical Pearls
Generic Name Boric acid **Brand Name** Borofax	Ocular irritation	**Usual ophthalmic dose:** Apply ½ filled eyecup as irrigating solution	• Solution for topical application to the eye only. • Patients should apply boric acid irrigating solution to the eye with the aid of an eyecup and should be instructed on how to avoid contamination of the interior surfaces and rim of the eyecup • Discard any solution that shows evidence of contamination (i.e., discolored, cloudy or particles)

Drug Name	FDA-Approved Indications	Adult Dosage Range	Precautions and Clinical Pearls
Generic Name Carbamide peroxide **Brand Name** Cankaid (oral) Debrox (otic) (PD)	Oral irritation and inflammation Cerumen removal	**Usual oral irrigation dose:** 10% oral solution: Apply several drops undiluted to affected area of the mouth 4 times per day (after meals and at bedtime); expectorate after 2 to 3 minutes **Usual otic dose:** 6.5% otic solution: 5 to 10 drops into the affected ear(s) twice daily for 4 days	Oral: • Do not swallow the oral topical solution • Patients should contact their provider if the condition worsens with treatment, or for use lasting longer than 7 days Otic: • Avoid contact of the medication with hearing aids • Patients should contact their provider for use lasting longer than 4 days
Generic Name Chlorhexidine **Brand Name** Peridex	Gingivitis Periodontitis	**Usual oral dose as rinse:** 0.12% oral rinse: swish and expectorate 15 mL twice daily	• Staining of oral surfaces may occur, especially with unremoved plaque or teeth fillings that have rough surfaces; patients with frontal restoration should be advised of potential permanent staining • Formation of calcium salt deposits (calculus) and altered taste perception have been reported • Recommended to rinse undiluted for 30 seconds, morning and evening after tooth brushing • Do not rinse with water or other mouthwashes, brush teeth or eat immediately after using (do not swallow)

Anti-inflammatory Agents

Cortiscosteroids

Universal prescribing alerts:

- Corticosteroids may cause hypercorticism or suppression of the hypothalamic–pituitary–adrenal (HPA) axis, leading to adrenal insufficiency. Do not exceed recommended doses.
- Corticosteroids may mask or worsen acute infections. Avoid or use with caution in patients with latent or active tuberculosis, active herpes infection, or uncontrolled infections. Reactivation of a viral infection may occur.
- Patients prone to developing HPA axis suppression, intracranial hypertension, Cushing's syndrome, and growth suppression should be monitored closely.
- Avoid nasal corticosteroid use in patients with recent nasal septal ulcers, nasal surgery, or nasal trauma until healing has occurred.
- Corticosteroids may increase intraocular pressure, open-angle glaucoma, and cataracts. Use with caution in patients with a history of ocular disease. Chronic users or patients who report visual changes should consider routine eye exams. Monitor intraocular pressure especially if use exceeds 10 days.
- Nasal septal perforation and *Candida albicans* infections of the nose or pharynx may occur. Monitor for adverse nasal effects and periodically examine the nasal mucosa of patients on long-term therapy.
- Refer to the Hormones and Synthetic Substitutes chapter for systematic corticosteroid universal prescribing alerts and additional information.

Drug Name	FDA-Approved Indications	Adult Dosage Range	Precautions and Clinical Pearls
Generic Name Beclomethasone **Brand Name** Qnasl Beconase Beconase AQ PD	Rhinitis Allergic rhinitis	**Usual intranasal dose for rhinitis:** Beconase AQ: 1 to 2 sprays (42 mcg per spray) in each nostril twice daily	• Multiple formulations are available for use; all with different dosing recommendations and instructions for use; refer to PI for product specific details • Priming is required prior to initial use and some products have a dose counter that should be verified prior to and throughout use • In the presence of excessive nasal mucous secretion or edema of the nasal mucosa, use of a nasal vasoconstrictor may be needed during the first 2 to 3 days of therapy in order for the drug to reach the intended site of action • May cause mild nasopharyngeal transient irritation and sneezing headache, nausea, or lightheadedness reported nasal stuffiness, nosebleeds, rhinorrhea, or tearing eyes • Rare cases of ulceration of the nasal mucosa and nasal septum perforation as well as wheezing, cataract formation, increased intraocular pressure have been reported • Altered taste and smell (including loss of these senses) have been reported
Generic Name Budesonide **Brand Name** Rhinocort Rhinocort AQ PD	Rhinitis	**Usual intranasal dose for rhinitis:** Rhinocort AQ: 1 spray (32 mcg per spray) in each nostril once daily; dose may be increased up to maximum dose of 4 sprays per nostril once daily	• As is the case with other topical steroids, clinical improvement may be seen in 1 to 2 days but maximum benefit may take up to 2 weeks (decrease to lowest effective dose after establishing symptom control) • Some patients who do not achieve symptom control at the recommended starting dosage may benefit from an increased dose • Epistaxis, nasal septum perforation, and impaired wound healing have been reported with use
Generic Name Ciclesonide **Brand Name** Omnaris Zetonna	Rhinitis	**Usual intranasal dose rhinitis:** Zetonna nasal spray: 1 spray (32 mcg) in each nostril daily	• Shaking, priming, and repriming prior to use is required • Different formulations have different dosing recommendations; refer to PI for details • May result in a more serious or fatal varicella or measles infection in susceptible patients; prophylactic medications should be considered for patients exposed to either virus • Epistaxis, nasal septum perforation, and impaired wound healing have been reported with use

Drug Name	FDA-Approved Indications	Adult Dosage Range	Precautions and Clinical Pearls
Generic Name Dexamethasone **Brand Name** Maxidex	Allergic conjunctivitis Allergic marginal corneal ulcer Graves' ophthalmopathy Macular edema post retinal vein occlusion Otitis externa	**Usual ophthalmic dose (0.1%):** 1 or 2 drops every hour during the day and every 2 hours at night; gradually reduce to every 4 hours, then 3 to 4 times per day **Usual otic dose:** Use ophthalmic solution: 3 to 4 drops into the affected ear(s) 2 to 3 times per day	• Do not use for ocular infections caused by a virus, *Mycobacterium*, or fungus • Do not administer via the otic route if there is a perforation of an eardrum membrane • May use ophthalmic ointment to external ear • Use with caution in patients with ocular diseases that cause thinning of the cornea or sclera; perforations may occur • Available as an ocular implant (Ozurdex) Contraindications: • Glaucoma with a cup-to-disc ratio of greater than 0.8
Generic Name Difluprednate **Brand Name** Durezol	Uveitis Postoperative ocular inflammation	**Usual ophthalmic dose:** 0.05% emulsion: instill 1 drop into the affected eye(s) 4 times per day for 14 days, taper off	• Do not use for ocular infections caused by a virus, *Mycobacterium*, or fungus • Prolonged use may result in cataract formation • Use with caution in patients with ocular diseases that cause thinning of the cornea or sclera; perforations may occur • Use with extreme caution in patients with a history of ocular herpes simplex; reevaluate after 2 days if symptoms have not improved
Generic Name Flunisolide PD	Allergic rhinitis	**Usual intranasal dose:** 2 sprays (58 mcg) in each nostril twice daily	• May cause nasal burning/stinging, epistaxis, nasal dryness, hoarseness, pharyngitis, increased cough, nausea, smell, and taste alterations
Generic Name Fluocinolone **Brand Name** DermOtic (otic) Iluvien (ocular implants) Retisert (ocular implants)	Chronic eczematous external otitis (EO) Diabetic macular edema Uveitis	**Usual otic dose for EO:** 0.01% oil: instill 5 drops twice daily for 1 or 2 weeks	Ocular implants: • Must be administered by a healthcare professional under aseptic conditions Contraindications for ocular use: • Glaucoma with a cup-to-disc ratio greater than 0.8

Generic Name Fluorometholone **Brand Name** Flarex FML 0.1% FML 0.25%	Allergic conjunctivitis Keratitis Postoperative ocular inflammation Uveitis	**Usual ophthalmic dose** 0.1% suspension: instill 1 drop into affected eye(s) 2 to 4 times per day 0.1% ointment: apply ½-inch ribbon to the conjunctival sac of the affected eye(s) 1 to 3 times per day	• During the initial 24 to 48 hours, the dosing frequency may be increased as per manufacturer; refer to PI • Shake suspension prior to use • Care should be taken not to discontinue therapy prematurely • Prolonged use may result in cataract formation; use with caution in patients after cataract surgery • Perforations may occur with ocular diseases that thin the cornea or sclera Contraindications: • Use in most viral diseases of the cornea and conjunctiva • Use with caution in patients with a history of herpes simplex virus
Generic Name Fluticasone **Brand Name** Flonase (propionate) Veramyst (furoate) BL PD	Allergic rhinitis Perennial nonallergic rhinitis	**Usual intranasal dose:** 2 sprays (50 mcg per spray) in each nostril daily for 1 week, then reduce to 1 or 2 sprays in each nostril as directed	• Use with caution in patients with moderate to severe hepatic impairment (systemic absorption possible) • May cause nasal dryness with prolonged use • Available OTC • Different formulations are available with different dosing recommendations; use care when selecting
Generic Name Hydrocortisone **Brand Name** Cortisporin (ophthalmic) Cortisporin (otic) BL PD	Bacterial conjunctivitis Uveitis Otitis externa	**Usual ophthalmic dose:** Ophthalmic suspension: instill 1 or 2 drops into the affected eye(s) every 3 to 4 hours **Usual ophthalmic dose:** Ophthalmic ointment: Apply ½-inch ribbon to the conjunctival sac of the affected eye(s) 3 to 4 times per day **Usual otic dose:** Suspension or solution: 4 drops 3 to 4 times per day	• Shake suspension prior to use Ophthalmic: • Usually combined with bacitracin, neomycin, and polymyxin B • Perforations of the cornea or sclera may occur with long-term use Otic: • Usually combined with neomycin and polymyxin B • Use care when selecting and administering; available as solution and suspension, which may translate into significant differences in presence of perforation • Prolonged treatments have been associated with the development of Kaposi sarcoma in patients with HIV/AIDS • The otic preparation is for otic use only

Drug Name	FDA-Approved Indications	Adult Dosage Range	Precautions and Clinical Pearls
Generic Name Loteprednol **Brand Name** Alrex Lotemax (BL)	Seasonal allergic conjunctivitis Postoperative ocular inflammation Ophthalmic inflammatory conditions	**Usual ophthalmic dose:** 0.2% suspension: instill drop into affected eye(s) 4 times per day **Usual ophthalmic dose** 0.5 % ointment: apply post surgically as directed	• May mask or worsen secondary ocular infections • Perforations may occur with diseases that cause thinning of the cornea or sclera • Brands differ on strength and dosing directions; refer to PI and select products with care • Shake suspension prior to use
Generic Name Mometasone **Brand Name** Nasonex (BL) (PD)	Allergic rhinitis	**Usual intranasal dose:** 2 sprays (50 mcg per spray) in each nostril daily	• Intranasal mometasone undergoes extensive first-pass metabolism in the liver; use caution in patients with hepatic impairment • Patients who have experienced recent nasal surgery, nasal septal perforation or ulcer, or nasal trauma should not use a nasal corticosteroid until healing has occurred • Shake well prior to use and prime as directed
Generic Name Prednisolone **Brand Name** Omnipred Pred Forte Pred Mild (BL)	Allergic conjunctivitis Corneal injury Ophthalmic inflammatory conditions	**Illustrative ophthalmic dose:** 1% suspension: instill 1 or 2 drops into affected eye(s) 2 to 4 times per day	• Perforations may occur with diseases that cause thinning of the cornea or sclera • Prednisone acetate ophthalmic suspension, varying strengths: 0.12%, 0.125%, or 1% • Shake suspension prior to use
Generic Name Rimexolone **Brand Name** Vexol (BL)	Anterior uveitis Postoperative ocular inflammation	**Usual ophthalmic dose for uveitis:** Instill 1 or 2 drops into the affected eye(s) every hour for 7 days, then every 2 hours for 7 days, then taper off	• Perforations may occur with diseases that cause thinning of the cornea or sclera • Use beginning 24 hours after surgery and continuing through the first 2 weeks of the post-operative period

Generic Name Triamcinolone **Brand Name** Nasacort (nasal) Triesence (ophthalmic) BL PD	Allergic rhinitis Ocular disease Visualization during vitrectomy	**Usual intranasal dose:** 2 sprays (55 mcg per spray) in each nostril daily	• As with other steroidal products, do not use in patients with active ocular herpes simplex • Intravitreal use has been associated with endophthalmitis and visual disturbances • May cause systemic corticosteroid symptoms such as Cushing's syndrome, hyperglycemia, and glycosuria • Intravitreal dosing is available, refer to PI

Nonsteroidal Anti-inflammatory Agents

Universal prescribing alerts:

- Use with caution in patients who report a history of aspirin or NSAID sensitivity.
- Use with caution in patients with diabetes, bleeding disorders, receiving anticoagulants, ocular disease, and rheumatoid arthritis.
- Refer to the analgesics and anti-inflammatory agents in the Central Nervous System Agents chapter for NSAID universal prescribing alerts and additional information.

Drug Name	FDA-Approved Indications	Adult Dosage Range	Precautions and Clinical Pearls
Generic Name Bromfenac **Brand Name** Bromday Prolensa Xibrom	Postoperative ocular inflammation following cataract removal Ocular pain	**Usual ophthalmic dose:** 1 drop into the affected eye(s) once daily beginning 1 day prior to surgery and until 2 weeks after surgery	• Discontinue if signs of corneal epithelial damage occur; may cause a loss of vision • May cause keratitis • Various products contain different concentrations of active ingredient; use care when selecting
Generic Name Flurbiprofen **Brand Name** Ocufen BL	Intraoperative miosis inhibition	**Usual ophthalmic dose:** 0.03% solution: instill 1 drop into the affected eye(s) every 30 minutes, beginning 2 hours prior to surgery, for a total of 4 drops per affected eye	• Patients having bilateral ocular surgery who are using this solution for intraoperative miosis inhibition should use 1 bottle for each eye to avoid the potential for cross-contamination

Drug Name	FDA-Approved Indications	Adult Dosage Range	Precautions and Clinical Pearls
Generic Name Ketorolac **Brand Name** Acular Acuvail (BL)	Allergic conjunctivitis Postoperative inflammation following cataract removal Ocular pain	**Usual ophthalmic dose:** 0.5% solution: instill drop into the affected eye(s) 4 times per day	• Discontinue if signs of corneal epithelial damage occur; may cause a loss of vision • Various products contain different concentrations of active ingredient; use care when selecting • Preservative-free eye solution containers are for single-use only and should be discarded after each use • To avoid the potential for cross-contamination, use one bottle for each eye after bilateral ocular surgery. Do not use the same bottle for both eyes • When using with other ophthalmic products, drops should be administered at least 5 minutes apart
Generic Name Nepafenac **Brand Name** Ilevro Nevanac	Postoperative inflammation following cataract removal Ocular pain	**Usual ophthalmic dose:** 0.3% solution: instill 1 drop into the affected eye(s) daily beginning 1 day prior to surgery and until 2 weeks after surgery; additionally, 1 drop 30 to 120 minutes prior to surgery	• Discontinue if signs of corneal epithelial damage occur; may cause a loss of vision • May cause keratitis • Various products contain different concentrations of active ingredient; use care when selecting

Miscellaneous Anti-inflammatory Agents

Drug Name	FDA-Approved Indications	Adult Dosage Range	Precautions and Clinical Pearls
Generic Name Cyclosporine **Brand Name** Restasis ■	Xerophthalmia associated with keratoconjunctivitis sicca	**Usual ophthalmic dose:** 0.05% solution: instill 1 drop in both eyes every 12 hours	• Prior to use, invert the vial several times to obtain a uniform emulsion • Remove contact lenses prior to instillation of drops; lenses may be reinserted 15 minutes after administration • May be used with artificial tears; allow a 15-minute interval between administration of products • To avoid contamination, do not touch the vial tip to the eyelids or other surfaces Associated with: • Specific cautions when used systemically; refer to PI

Local Anesthetic, Mydriatic, and Vasoconstrictor Agents

Local Anesthetic Agents

Drug Name	FDA-Approved Indications	Adult Dosage Range	Precautions and Clinical Pearls
Generic Name Cocaine	Topical anesthesia (and vasoconstriction) for mucous membranes of the oral, laryngeal, or nasal cavities	**Usual topical dose:** Concentrations of 1% to 10% may be used, with 4% being the most frequently used	• Use only on mucous membranes of the oral, laryngeal, and nasal cavities; do not use on extensive areas of broken skin; monitor vital signs • May apply with cotton applicators, as a spray, or instill directly into the mucous cavity • Dosage depends on the area to be anesthetized, tissue vascularity, technique of anesthesia, and individual patient tolerance • Duration of effect lasts for 30 minutes or longer depending on concentration and vascularity of anesthetized tissue • DEA-controlled substance
Generic Name Dyclonine **Brand Name** Sucrets	Temporary relief of pain associated with oral mucosa	**Usual oral dose:** 1 lozenge every 2 hours as needed (MDD: 10 lozenges per day)	• Allow the lozenge to dissolve slowly in the mouth • May temporarily increase risk of choking; avoid use in patients who are predisposed to this risk
Generic Name Proparacaine **Brand Name** Alcaine	Short corneal and conjunctival procedures	**Usual ophthalmic dose:** 0.5% solution: instill 1 drop in the affected eye(s) every 5 to 10 minutes for 5 to 7 doses	• Prolonged use may result in permanent corneal opacification and visual loss, and is not recommended • Do not use the solution if it is discolored; protect the eye from irritating chemicals, foreign bodies, and blink reflex; use an eye patch if necessary • For topical ophthalmic use only
Generic Name Tetracaine **Brand Name** Altacaine Tetcaine TetraVisc Forte	Short-term (nonsurgical procedures) anesthesia Minor surgical procedures Prolonged surgical procedures	**Illustrative ophthalmic dose for short-term (nonsurgical procedures) anesthesia:** 0.5% solution: instill 1 or 2 drops into the affected eye(s) just prior to evaluation	• For topical ophthalmic use only • Do not use if the solution contains crystals, or is cloudy or discolored • Many warning and contraindications for use for other conditions where systemic anesthetic is required; refer to PI
Benzocaine	Refer to Skin and Mucous Membrane Agents chapter.		

Mydriatic Agents

Universal prescribing alerts:

- To avoid excessive systemic absorption with ophthalmic products, finger pressure should be applied on the lacrimal sac during and for 2 to 3 minutes following application (using sterile technique to reduce risk of infection).

Drug Name	FDA-Approved Indications	Adult Dosage Range	Precautions and Clinical Pearls
Generic Name Atropine BL	**Common indications for use:** Cycloplegia (mydriasis induction) Treatment of iritis	**Usual ophthalmic dose for mydriasis:** 1% solution: instill 1 drop into affected eye(s) 1 hour prior to procedure Alternatively may use: 1% ointment: apply a thin ribbon to conjunctival sac(s) of affected eye(s) up to 3 times daily	• Refer to the Autonomic Agents chapter for universal prescribing alerts for systemic use • Universal prescribing alerts for anticholinergic agents apply when there is systemic absorption • Photophobia and altered night vision have been reported with use; use care and plan accordingly • Ointment may cause blurred vision
Generic Name Cyclopentolate **Brand Name** Cyclogyl PD	Mydriasis Cycloplegia	**Usual ophthalmic dose:** 0.5%, 1%, or 2% solution: instill 1 or 2 drops of solution into affected eye(s) approximately 40 to 50 minutes prior to procedure; may repeat in 5 to 10 minutes if needed	• Heavily pigmented irises may require use of higher strength • Seizures have been reported with topical use (risk increases with higher strength products) Contraindications: • Untreated narrow-angle glaucoma and presence of untreated anatomically narrow angles • Certain patients with history of seizure, refer to PI
Generic Name Dipivefrin **Brand Name** Propine	Glaucoma	**Usual ophthalmic dose:** 0.1% solution: instill 1 drop every 12 hours into the affected eye(s)	• Pro-drug of epinephrine • Discolored or darkened ophthalmic solutions have lost their potency • Use with caution in patients with heart disease and those with in patients with partial or complete loss of the eye lens (aphakia) • Reversible macular edema has been reported with use Contraindications: • Hypersensitivity to epinephrine • Angle-closure glaucoma

Generic Name Homatropine **Brand Name** Homatropaire Isopto Homatropine (PD)	**Common indications for use:** Iritis/iridocyclitis Mydriasis and cycloplegia for refraction Uveitis	**Usual ophthalmic dose for uveitis:** 2% or 5% solution: instill 1 or 2 drops into affected eye(s) every 3 to 4 hours	• Individuals with heavily pigmented irises may require higher dosages • Patients with renal impairment may be at risk of anticholinergic toxicity Contraindications: • Primary glaucoma or tendency toward glaucoma (open and closed angle)
Generic Name Tropicamide **Brand Name** Mydral Mydriacyl	Mydriasis Cycloplegia	**Usual ophthalmic dose:** 0.5% solution: 1 to 2 drops in the affected eye(s) 15 to 20 minutes before exam	• Individuals with heavily pigmented eyes may require higher strength or additional doses • Monitor: ophthalmic exam, intraocular pressure, CNS reactions (especially in pediatric patients
Epinephrine	Refer to the Autonomic Agents chapter.		
Phenylephrine	Refer to the Autonomic Agents chapter.		
Scopolamine	Refer to the Autonomic Agents chapter.		
Vasoconstrictors			
Drug Name	**FDA-Approved Indications**	**Adult Dosage Range**	**Precautions and Clinical Pearls**
Generic Name Naphazoline **Brand Name** AK-Con (ophthamic) Prinvine (nasal)	Decrease in eye redness and nasal congestion	**Usual ophthalmic dose:** 0.1% solution: instill 1 or 2 drops or sprays every 6 hours if needed; therapy should not exceed 3 days **Usual intranasal dose:** 0.05% solution: instill 1 or 2 sprays per nostril every 6 hours as needed; therapy should not exceed 3 days	• May cause sedation and toxicity if inadvertently swallowed • Associated with rebound vasodilation with overuse (and decreased oxygenation to affected tissues) • Use with caution in patients with cardiovascular disease • Drug interactions may require dose adjustment or avoidance of certain combinations • Do not use if the solution changes color or becomes cloudy Contraindications (ophthalmic): • Narrow-angle glaucoma • Anatomically narrow angle

Drug Name	FDA-Approved Indications	Adult Dosage Range	Precautions and Clinical Pearls
Generic Name Oxymetazoline **Brand Name** Afrin (nasal) Visine-LR (ophthalmic) PD	Nasal congestion (nasal) Relief of eye redness (ophthalmic)	**Usual intranasal dose:** 2 or 3 sprays into each nostril twice daily for no longer than 3 days **Usual ophthalmic dose:** 1 or 2 drops in the affected eye(s) every 6 hours as needed or as directed by the healthcare provider for no longer than 3 days	• Associated with rebound vasodilation with overuse (and decreased oxygenation to affected tissues) • Use with caution in patients with cardiovascular disease • Drug interactions may require dose adjustment or avoidance of certain combinations
Generic Name Phenylephrine **Brand Name** Neo-Synephrine and others (nasal) Neofrin and others (ophthalmic) PD	Nasal congestion (nasal) Mydriasis and decongestant effects (ophthalmic)	**Illustrative intranasal dose:** 0.25% to 1% solution: 2 to 3 sprays in each nostril no more than every 4 hours for no more than 3 days **Illustrative opthalmic dose:** 0.12% solution: instill 1 or 2 drops into affected eye(s) up to 4 times daily; not to exceed 3 days of therapy	• Higher doses (i.e., 2.5% and 10%) are available for mydriasis and ophthalmic surgical procedures Contraindications: • Hypertension • Thyrotoxicosis • Specific age ranges
Generic Name Tetrahydrozoline **Brand Name** Tyzine (nasal) Visine (ophthalmic) PD	Nasal congestion Ocular decongestant: relief of red eyes	**Usual intranasal dose:** 0.1% nasal solution: instill 2 to 4 drops or 3 to 4 sprays of solution into each nostril every 3 to 4 hours as needed, no more frequently than every 3 hours **Usual ophthalmic dose:** 0.05% solution: instill 1 to 2 drops into the affected eye(s) up to 4 times per day	• Do not use if the solution changes color or becomes cloudy • Drug interactions may require dose adjustment or avoidance of certain combinations • Monitoring: blood pressure, heart rate, symptom response • Relieves redness of the eye due to minor eye irritation and protects against further irritation; temporarily relieves burning and discomfort from dryness of the eye or exposure to wind and sun Contraindications: • Do not use in specific age groups; refer to PI
Epinephrine	Refer to the Autonomic Agents chapter.		

Mouthwashes and Gargles

Drug Name	FDA-Approved Indications	Adult Dosage Range	Precautions and Clinical Pearls
Generic Name Hydrogen peroxide **Brand Name** Peroxyl (PD)	Removal of oral secretions Mouth, gum, or dental irritation	**Usual dose of oral rinse (1.4%):** Topical: 10 mL swished around mouth over the affected area for at least 1 minute, then spit out; may use up to 4 times per day after meals and at bedtime **Usual dose of oral gel (1.7%):** Topical: Apply several drops to the affected area, allow medication to remain on site for at least 1 minute, then spit out; may use up to 4 times per day after meals and at bedtime	• Should not be used in abscesses • Will bubble in mouth; do not swallow • Repeated use as a mouthwash or gargle may produce irritation of the buccal mucous membrane or "hairy tongue" • Has become less popular given that safer and more effective agents are now available (known to be cytotoxic to healthy cells and granulating tissues, and therefore its use should be limited to no longer than 7 days)

Antiglaucoma Agents

Alpha-Adrenergic Agonists

Universal prescribing alerts:

- To avoid excessive systemic absorption with ophthalmic products, finger pressure should be applied on the lacrimal sac during and for 2 to 3 minutes following application (use sterile technique to prevent infection).

Drug Name	FDA-Approved Indications	Adult Dosage Range	Precautions and Clinical Pearls
Generic Name Brimonidine **Brand Name** Alphagan P	Elevated intraocular pressure (IOP)	**Usual ophthalmic dose:** 0.1%, 0.15%, or 0.2% solution: instill 1 drop in the affected eye(s) 3 times per day (approximately every 8 hours)	• Monitoring: IOP routinely (first month of therapy may not reflect long-term level of IOP reduction) • Topical dosage formulations available also for the treatment of persistent (nontransient) facial erythema of acne rosacea • Refer to the Cardiovascular Agents chapter for complete review of precautions for systemic alpha-adrenergic agonists Contraindications: • Do not use in specific age groups; refer to PI

Beta-Adrenergic Blocking Agents

- Refer to the Cardiovascular Agents chapter for complete review of precautions for systemic beta-adrenergic blocking agents including black box warnings associating use with the development of myocardial ischemia, myocardial infarction, ventricular arrhythmias, or severe hypertension, particularly in patients with preexisting cardiovascular disease when abruptly discontinuing any beta-adrenergic blocking agent.
- To avoid excessive systemic absorption with ophthalmic products, finger pressure should be applied on the lacrimal sac during and for 2 to 3 minutes following application (use sterile technique to prevent infection).

Drug Name	FDA-Approved Indications	Adult Dosage Range	Precautions and Clinical Pearls
Generic Name Betaxolol **Brand Name** Betoptic-S (PD)	Chronic open-angle glaucoma Ocular hypertension	**Usual ophthalmic dose:** 0.5% solution (or 0.25% suspension): Instill 1 drop in the affected eye(s) twice daily (may use 2 drops per dose of the solution)	• Shake suspension well before using. • Monitoring: intraocular pressure (IOP lowering effects may require a few weeks; if IOP is not controlled on this regimen, concomitant therapy with alternative agents should be considered) • Use care when selecting products (0.25% resin-formulated suspension is also available) Contraindications: • Sinus bradycardia • Heart block greater than first-degree (except in patients with a functioning artificial pacemaker) • Cardiogenic shock and uncompensated cardiac failure
Generic Name Levobunolol **Brand Name** Betagan	Glaucoma (open-angle, chronic) Intraocular hypertension	**Usual ophthalmic dose:** 0.25% solution: instill 1 to 2 drops into the affected eye(s) twice daily Alternatively may use 0.5% solution once daily	• For topical ophthalmic use only • Monitoring: intraocular pressure, heart rate, funduscopic exam, visual field testing Contraindications: • Bronchial asthma • Severe chronic obstructive pulmonary disease (COPD) • Sinus bradycardia • Second- or third-degree atrioventricular (AV) block • Overt cardiac failure or cardiogenic shock
Generic Name Timolol **Brand Name** Betimol Istalol Timoptic Timoptic-XE (PD)	Elevated intraocular pressure	**Usual ophthalmic dose:** Gel-forming solution (Timoptic-XE): instill 1 drop (0.25% or 0.5% solution) once daily Standard 0.25% solution: instill 1 drop into the affected eye(s) twice daily; if response is not adequate, increase to 1 drop (0.5% solution) twice daily	• Ophthalmic formulations are for topical ophthalmic use only; multiple formulations available use care when selecting product • Invert closed bottle and shake gel-forming solutions once before use • Monitoring: intraocular pressure (after approximately 4 weeks of therapy) Contraindications: • Bronchial asthma or history of bronchial asthma • Severe COPD • Sinus bradycardia • Second- or third-degree AV block • Overt cardiac failure and cardiogenic shock

Carbonic Anhydrase Inhibitors			
Drug Name	**FDA-Approved Indications**	**Adult Dosage Range**	**Precautions and Clinical Pearls**
Generic Name Acetazolamide **Brand Name** Diamox Sequels ▲ (PD)	**Common indications for use:** Glaucoma Altitude illness Edema	**Illustrative oral dose for chronic simple (open-angle) glaucoma:** 250 mg 1 to 4 times per day or 500 mg extended-release capsule twice daily	• May be administered with food; may cause an alteration in taste, especially for carbonated beverages • Short-acting tablets may be crushed and suspended in cherry or chocolate syrup to disguise the bitter taste of the drug; do not use fruit juices • Alternatively, submerge tablet in 10 mL of hot water and add 10 mL honey or syrup • May cause false-positive results for urinary protein with Albustix, Labstix, Albutest, and Bumintest tests; interferes with high-performance liquid chromatographic (HPLC) theophylline assay and serum uric acid level • Sulfonamide derivatives; may cause sun sensitivity • Monitoring: intraocular pressure; serum electrolytes, CBC with differential Contraindications: • Hepatic disease, insufficiency, or cirrhosis • Severe renal disease or dysfunction • Decreased sodium and/or potassium levels • Adrenocortical insufficiency • Hyperchloremic acidosis • Long-term use in noncongestive angle-closure glaucoma
Generic Name Brinzolamide **Brand Name** Azopt ▲	Ocular hypertension Open-angle glaucoma	**Usual ophthalmic dose:** 1% suspension: instill 1 drop in affected eye(s) 3 times per day	• Shake well before use • Monitoring: intraocular pressure • Not recommended in patients with severe renal impairment • Use caution in patients with hepatic impairment
Generic Name Dorzolamide **Brand Name** Trusopt ▲	Elevated intraocular pressure	**Usual ophthalmic dose:** 2% solution: instill drop in the affected eye(s) 3 times per day	• Monitoring: ophthalmic exams and IOP periodically • Not intended for monotherapy management of closed angle glaucoma • Not recommended for use in patients with renal impairment • Limited to 3-month maximum use in certain age-specific populations; refer to PI

Drug Name	FDA-Approved Indications	Adult Dosage Range	Precautions and Clinical Pearls
Generic Name Methazolamide **Brand Name** Neptazane ▲	Chronic open-angle or secondary glaucoma Short-term therapy of acute angle-closure glaucoma prior to surgery	**Usual oral dose:** 50 to 100 mg 2 to 3 times per day	• Monitoring: CBC and platelet count (baseline and periodically), serum electrolytes (periodically) • Monitor blood pressure prior to beginning therapy and after first few doses, especially in patients on another concomitant diuretic therapy • If the patient has diabetes, blood glucose levels may be elevated; monitor blood sugars closely • Use and teach the patient postural hypotension precautions Contraindications: • Marked kidney or liver dysfunction (and cirrhosis) • Adrenal gland failure • Hyperchloremic acidosis • Hyponatremia and hypokalemia • Long-term treatment of angle-closure glaucoma
Miotics			
Universal prescribing alerts: • To avoid excessive systemic absorption with ophthalmic products, finger pressure should be applied on the lacrimal sac during and for 2 to 3 minutes following application (use sterile technique to prevent infection).			
Drug Name	**FDA-Approved Indications**	**Adult Dosage Range**	**Precautions and Clinical Pearls**
Generic Name Acetylcholine **Brand Name** Miochol-E	Intraocular surgery only; refer to PI	Refer to PI for dosage	• Refer to the Autonomic Agents chapter for universal prescribing alerts and cautions
Generic Name Carbachol **Brand Name** Isopto Carbachol Miostat	Glaucoma Ophthalmic surgery (miosis)	**Usual ophthalmic dose for glaucoma:** 1.5 or 3% solution: instill 1 to 2 drops up to 3 times per day	• Discard unused portion and use sterile technique • Specific surgical administration guidelines are available in the PI • Injectable formulations available for intraocular injection; use care when selecting products • Retinal detachment has been reported in susceptible individuals; use caution Contraindications: • Acute iritis • Acute inflammatory disease of the anterior chamber

Generic Name Pilocarpine **Brand Name** Isopto Carpine Pilopine HS	**Common indication for use:** Glaucoma	**Illustrative ophthalmic dose:** 1% solution: instill or 2 drops into the affected eye(s) up to 4 times per day; adjust the concentration and frequency as required to control elevated intraocular pressure **Usual ophthalmic dose:** 4% gel: apply ½-inch ribbon to the conjunctival sac of the affected eye(s) once daily at bedtime	• If both solution and gel are used, the solution should be applied first, then the gel at least 5 minutes later • Following administration of the solution, apply finger pressure on the lacrimal sac for 1 to 2 minutes • Monitoring: intraocular pressure, funduscopic exam, visual field testing • Multiple concentrations are available; use care when selecting product • Systemic absorption may cause additional side effects; refer to PI if necessary Contraindications: • Acute inflammatory disease of the anterior chamber of the eye • Specific contraindications apply to oral systemic use; refer to PI

Prostaglandin Analogues			
Drug Name	FDA-Approved Indications	Adult Dosage Range	Precautions and Clinical Pearls
Generic Name Bimatoprost **Brand Name** Lumigan Latisse	Elevated intraocular pressure (Lumigan) Hypotrichosis of the eyelashes (Latisse)	**Illustrative ophthalmic dose:** Lumigan solution: instill drop into the affected eye(s) once daily in the evening	• If used with other topical ophthalmic agents, separate administration by at least 5 minutes • Monitoring: intraocular pressure • Multiple concentrations are available; refer to PI when selecting products • May cause photophobia; use care • Systemic absorption may cause additional side effects; refer to PI if necessary Lumigan: • May be used with other eye drops to lower intraocular pressure (0.01 and 0.03% available) Latisse: • Remove make-up and contact lenses prior to application • Apply with the sterile applicator provided only; do not use other brushes or applicators • Do not apply to lower eyelash line • Do not reuse applicators; use a new applicator for the second eye

Drug Name	FDA-Approved Indications	Adult Dosage Range	Precautions and Clinical Pearls
Generic Name Latanoprost **Brand Name** Xalatan	Elevated intraocular pressure	**Usual ophthalmic dose:** 0.005% solution: instill 1 drop in the affected eye(s) once daily in the evening	• Stored in refrigerator prior to use; once open the commercial ophthalmic product (Xalatan) may be stored at room temperature for up to six weeks • May be used with other eye drops to lower IOP • More frequent administration may decrease the IOP-lowering effect • Monitoring: IOP and regularly examine patients who develop increased iris pigmentation • Monitor for blurred vision, burning and stinging, conjunctival hyperemia, foreign body sensation, itching, increased pigmentation of the iris, and punctate epithelial keratopathy • Systemic absorption may cause additional side effects; refer to PI if necessary
Generic Name Tafluprost **Brand Name** Zioptan	Elevated intraocular pressure	**Usual ophthalmic dose:** 0.0015% solution: instill 1 drop in the affected eye(s) once daily in the evening	• Each single-use container has adequate solution to treat both eyes (if applicable); discard immediately after use • More frequent administration may decrease the IOP-lowering effect • Monitoring: IOP and regularly examine patients who develop increased iris pigmentation • Monitor for blurred vision, burning and stinging, conjunctival hyperemia, foreign body sensation, itching, increased pigmentation of the iris, and punctate epithelial keratopathy • Systemic absorption may cause additional side effects; refer to PI if necessary
Generic Name Travoprost **Brand Name** Travatan Z	Elevated intraocular pressure	**Usual ophthalmic dose:** 0.004% solution: instill 1 drop into the affected eye(s) once daily in the evening; do not exceed once-daily dosing	• May be used with other eye drops to lower intraocular pressure • More frequent administration may decrease the IOP-lowering effect • The mean IOP reduction in African American patients appears to be greater than that in non–African American patients; the reason for this effect is unknown • Systemic absorption may cause additional side effects; refer to PI if necessary

Miscellaneous EENT Agents

Drug Name	FDA-Approved Indications	Adult Dosage Range	Precautions and Clinical Pearls
Generic Name Aflibercept **Brand Name** Eylea	**For intravitreal use only:** Diabetic retinopathy Macular degeneration Macular edema		• Intravitreal ophthalmic: for intravitreal injection only • Refer to PI for specific needle/syringe requirements

Generic Name Apraclonidine **Brand Name** Iopidine	Intraocular pressure reduction	**Usual ophthalmic dose:** 0.5% solution: instill to 2 drops in the affected eye(s) 3 times per day	• After topical instillation, finger pressure should be applied to the lacrimal sac to decrease drainage into the nose and throat and minimize possible systemic absorption • 1% solution is also available; use a separate container for each single-drop dose; discard the container after each use • Closely monitor patients who develop exaggerated reductions in intraocular pressure and monitor visual fields • Monitor cardiovascular parameters closely
Generic Name Cysteamine **Brand Name** Cystaran	Ocular cystinosis	**Usual ophthalmic dose:** 0.44% solution: instill 1 drop in each eye every hour while awake	• For topical ophthalmic use only • Available as oral formulation; refer to PI for systemic side effects as required • Monitoring: ophthalmic examination (periodic) • Ensure bottle has been thawed 24 hours prior to use; see PI for specific storage details prior to use • Record a discard date of 7 days from the day the bottle is thawed on the bottle label; do not refreeze
Generic Name Ocriplasmin **Brand Name** Jetrea	**For intravitreal use only:** Vitreomacular adhesion	Refer to PI for dosage	• For intravitreal injection only • Refer to PI for specific needle/syringe requirements
Generic Name Pegaptanib **Brand Name** Macugen	**For intravitreous use only:** Age-related macular degeneration	Refer to PI for dosage	• For intravitreal injection only • Refer to PI for specific needle/syringe requirements
Generic Name Ranibizumab **Brand Name** Lucentis	**For intravitreal use only:** Diabetic retinopathy Macular degeneration Macular edema	Refer to PI for dosage	• For ophthalmic intravitreal injection only • Refer to PI for specific needle/syringe requirements

Drug Name	FDA-Approved Indications	Adult Dosage Range	Precautions and Clinical Pearls
Generic Name Unoprostone **Brand Name** Rescula	Open-angle glaucoma Ocular hypertension	**Usual ophthalmic dose:** 0.15% solution: instill 1 drop into the affected eye(s) twice daily	• May be used with other eye drops to lower intraocular pressure • Use caution in patients with corneal abrasion • Photophobia has been reported
Generic Name Verteporfin **Brand Name** Visudyne	Subfoveal choroidal neovascularization	**Usual parenteral dose:** IV: 6 mg/m^2 body surface area; may repeat at 3-month intervals (if evidence of choroidal neovascular leakage)	• Therapy is a two-step process with specific infusion recommendations; refer to PI • Stability and compatibility information is available in the PI • Ethanol may decrease the efficacy of verteporfin; avoid use of ethanol during therapy • Monitor the intravenous site during infusion, to avoid extravasation • Not recommended for patients with hepatic impairment • Perform fluorescein angiography as recommended by manufacturer to monitor for choroidal neovascular leakage; if detected, repeat therapy Contraindications: • Patients with porphyria

Chapter 11

Gastrointestinal Agents

Author: **Kirsten Butterfoss, PharmD, CGP**

Editor: **Michelle Lewis, PharmD, MHA**

Learning Objectives

- Identify current pharmacologic agents that are appropriate for each condition/diagnosis.
- Recommend optimal pharmacologic interventions based on patient-specific characteristics.
- Provide appropriate patient-specific counseling points and optimal overall medication management.

Key Terms: Antacids and adsorbents, antidiarrheal agents, antiflatulence agents, cathartics and laxatives, cholelitholytic agents, digestants, antiemetic agents, antihistamine agents, $5HT_3$ receptor antagonists, antiulcer agents and acid suppressants, histamine H_2 antagonists, prostaglandins, protectants, proton-pump inhibitors, prokinetic agents, anti-inflammatory agents

Overview of Gastrointestinal Agents

The gastrointestinal (GI) tract is a hollow tube that extends from the mouth to the anus; its primary functions are to provide nutrition to the body and eliminate waste. The salivary glands, pancreas, liver, and gallbladder complete the GI system; they store and secrete enzymes and bile that aid in the digestive process. The liver also produces hormones and blood clotting factors, detoxifies harmful substances, and metabolizes drugs.

The GI system is innervated by the enteric nervous system (ENS), often described as the body's "second brain," as well as by the central nervous system (CNS). The CNS communicates to the ENS via the parasympathetic and sympathetic nervous systems, controlling food transit time and secretion of acid and intestinal mucus. The hypothalamic-pituitary-adrenal axis (HPA) aids in digestion by controlling hormonal release. Acetylcholine, dopamine, and serotonin as well as many of the other neurotransmitters secreted by the ENS are similar to the corresponding substances present in the CNS. These neurotransmitters are unlikely to enter the CNS; however, nerve signals sent from the GI tract to the brain may affect mood and play a role in disorders of gut-brain interactions such as irritable bowel syndrome.

Nearly everyone will experience a GI symptom—ranging from abdominal pain or heartburn to constipation or diarrhea—in his or her lifetime. The Rome IV criteria define functional GI disorders (FGIDs) as clinical indications involving GI symptoms related to a combination of hypersensitive viscera, disturbed motility, abnormal immune function, and/or altered gut microbiota, mucosal function, and CNS processing. Medications are used to control signs and symptoms of GI disorders through various mechanisms such as reducing acid secretion, replacing deficient enzymes, altering muscle tone, or increasing or decreasing gastric emptying time.

Gastric Acid Production

The two most common acid-peptic disorders are gastroesophageal reflux disease (GERD) and peptic ulcers. In these conditions, defense mechanisms (bicarbonate and mucus production, blood flow, prostaglandins) are overwhelmed by luminal aggressors (acid and pepsin production, and external factors such as nonsteroidal anti-inflammatory drugs [NSAIDs]). Additionally, the lower esophageal sphincter (LES) may not function properly to keep stomach contents from traveling back into the esophagus, leading to acid exposure in the esophagus leading to symptoms such as heartburn.

Neuronal (acetylcholine [ACh]), paracrine (histamine), and endocrine (gastrin) factors regulate parietal cell acid secretion via the M_3, H_2, and CCK-B receptors, respectively. Through cell signaling pathways, H^+/K^+ ATPase (the proton pump) is activated and exchanges hydrogen and potassium ions to maintain the pH in the stomach lumen between 1.5 and 3.5. Drug therapy can neutralize acid (antacids) or inhibit acid secretion (histamine-2 receptor antagonists [H2RAs] and proton-pump inhibitors [PPIs]).

Drug therapy can enhance or supplement the body's own mucosal defenses. Prostaglandin E_2 and prostacyclin (PGI_2) have been shown to decrease mucosal injury by stimulating mucus and bicarbonate production and increasing blood flow. Misoprostol, a prostaglandin analogue, can prevent NSAID-induced mucosal injury. Sucralfate, a sucrose sulfate-aluminum compound, selectively binds to ulcers or erosions, forming a viscous paste that creates a physical barrier to reduce further damage.

Gastrointestinal Motility

Luminal contents move through the digestive tract at various rates to allow for mixing, digestion and absorption, and temporary storage. The movement of material is coordinated by ENS and CNS signaling and hormonal control. The neurons of the ENS are organized into two types: the submucosal and myenteric ganglia. The submucosal ganglia, or *Meissner's plexus*, controls local secretion, absorption, and vascular flow. The myenteric ganglia, or *Auerbach's plexus*, increases muscle tone and controls the velocity and intensity of contractions.

More than 30 neurotransmitters have been identified in the ENS, including acetylcholine, norepinephrine, serotonin, gamma-aminobutyric acid (GABA), adenosine triphosphate (ATP), and nitric oxide. Medications that modulate the release or amount of these neurotransmitters within the GI system may alter GI motility and provide a clinical benefit for patients with FGIDs.

Stool consistency is determined by a balance of internal secretions into the lumen and absorption processes back into the blood. On average, 9 L of fluid enters the intestine daily—most of which is reabsorbed in the small intestine, leaving 100 mL to be excreted through defecation. Changes in ion secretion and luminal osmolality, intestinal motility, or tissue hydrostatic pressure can cause the stool consistency to be altered, leading to symptoms such as constipation or diarrhea. These changes can be influenced by external factors, including dietary fiber and medications, and internal processes, such as inflammatory diseases.

Nausea and Vomiting

Nausea and vomiting are symptoms caused by acute disorders and irritants or by other underlying conditions such as cancer. The three phases of these symptoms are (1) nausea—the subjective feeling of a need to vomit; (2) retching—involuntary rhythmic diaphragmatic and abdominal contractions; and (3) vomiting—rapid, forceful expulsion of contents from the GI tract.

The chemoreceptor trigger zone (CTZ), cerebral cortex, vestibular system, and GI visceral afferents send signals to the vomiting center located in the medulla oblongata. The vomiting center stimulates salivation and GI and abdominal muscle contractions leading to nausea and emesis. Neurotransmitters associated with nausea and vomiting include serotonin ($5HT_3$), neurokinin-1 (NK1), dopamine, acetylcholine, histamine, cannabinoid, opiate, and corticosteroid receptors; all of these receptors are drug therapy targets.

Inflammatory Bowel Disease

Ulcerative colitis and Crohn's disease are the two types of idiopathic inflammatory bowel disease (IBD). Although the etiology of these autoimmune disorders is unknown: genetics, infectious, environmental, and immunologic factors likely play a role in their development. Anti-inflammatory agents and sulfasalazine were the primary therapy for IBD for many years, but newer agents such as immunomodulators and biologics have since been utilized to treat exacerbations and maintain remission of the disease.

Probiotics

In recent years, the number of probiotic products on the market—as well as the number of advertisements for these agents—has increased dramatically. Traditionally, probiotics were used for digestive health maintenance purposes, but some products are now claimed to relieve allergic symptoms, reduce systemic inflammation and cholesterol, and aid in weight loss.

Probiotics are microorganisms (including bacteria and yeast) that have beneficial properties for the host. Most of these products contain lactic acid-producing bacteria, such as *Lactobacillus* or *Bifidobacterium* strains. Proposed mechanisms by which a probiotic may benefit the host include restoration of the normal balance between beneficial and pathogenic bacteria, modulation of the immune system, strengthening of the epithelial barrier, and improvement of digestion and absorption of nutrients.

Probiotics have been studied in many GI disorders, including infectious and antibiotic-associated diarrhea, irritable bowel syndrome (IBS), IBD, constipation, lactose intolerance, celiac disease, hepatic encephalopathy, and pancreatitis. Clinical research studies have been limited by small sample sizes, and many studies have not concluded that probiotics offer any clinical or statistical benefit. The most promising studies have shown that probiotics are effective in limiting antibiotic-associated diarrhea in adults. The World Gastroenterology Organization guidelines suggest that *Lactobacillus casei*, *Saccharomyces boulardii*, and *Streptococcus thermophilus* (commercially available in the product DanActive®) are modestly effective for the prevention of *Clostridium difficile*-associated disease (CDAD).

The decision to use a probiotic should consider anticipated benefits, evidence for use, cost, and patient preference. If taken to reduce antibiotic-induced diarrhea, a probiotic should be taken 2 hours before or after the antibiotic to ensure the probiotic is not adversely affected by the antibiotic.

11.1 Antacids and Adsorbents

Antacid medications are used for symptomatic relief of mild or intermittent dyspepsia and acid-peptic disorders; they work by neutralizing gastric acid and increasing gastric pH. Adverse effects related to antacid therapy are dose dependent and dependent on the particular cation of the ingested antacid. While magnesium-containing antacids can cause diarrhea, aluminum-containing products may lead to constipation, and calcium carbonate products can cause bloating, flatulence, and belching. Systemic absorption of aluminum and magnesium can occur in patients with renal impairment or renal failure. With frequent and prolonged use, aluminum hydroxide binds to phosphate in the GI tract and can lead to hypophosphatemia. Excessive ingestion of calcium carbonate can lead to hypercalcemia, alkalosis, and renal impairment. Antacids may also contain a considerable amount of sodium (sodium bicarbonate), as such volume overload can occur in susceptible patients.

When taken at the same time as other oral medications, antacids may potentially reduce the absorption of the other agent. This effect may occur as a result of the antacid's binding to or chelation of the other drugs present or by the antacid altering their absorption by increasing intragastric pH. Antibiotics including tetracyclines, azithromycin, and fluoroquinolones bind to divalent and trivalent cations, leading to decreased absorption and efficacy of these medications. Levothyroxine absorption may be reduced when taken with an antacid; to avoid this effect, it is recommended to separate doses by 4 hours.

Activated charcoal adsorbs (binds) a variety of organic compounds. It is used as an antidote to poisonings with chemicals or drugs when gastric decontamination is indicated. However, this therapy is not effective in cases of lead, lithium, cyanide, iron, ethanol, or methanol poisoning. The principal adverse reactions associated with activated charcoal administration include vomiting, constipation, diarrhea, and tongue and stool discoloration. Such side effects are more likely to occur with multiple doses and chronic administration. Adverse events are usually negligible when charcoal is administered acutely for GI decontamination in overdose. Although all these active ingredients are listed within the antacids and adsorbents category, some are not commercially available in the United States (refer to the companion drug grid for information on products containing these ingredients).

Antacids and Adsorbents

Aluminum (carbonate, hydroxide and phosphate)
Calcium carbonate
Charcoal, activated
Magnesium (carbonate, citrate, hydroxide, oxide, and trisilicate)
Sodium bicarbonate

Case Studies and Conclusions

FR is a 25-year-old female who sometimes has "mild burning" after eating spicy foods. She has no other complaints or symptoms, and reports that the burning goes away after an hour. She would like to take something to help with her symptoms.

1. Why would an antacid product be appropriate for this patient?
   a. Antacids have a long duration of action.
   b. Antacids neutralize gastric acid.
   c. Antacids are absorbed systemically before being activated.
   d. Antacids are first-line therapy for GERD.

Answer B is correct. Antacids are widely used as over-the-counter agents to relieve mild and infrequent GERD symptoms. By neutralizing gastric acid, these agents are able to increase gastric pH for a duration of 30 minutes when taken on an empty stomach to 3 hours with food.

2. When selecting an antacid product, which side effect may FR experience?
   a. Magnesium-containing antacids may cause dose-related constipation.
   b. Aluminum-containing antacids may cause dose-related diarrhea.
   c. Calcium carbonate-containing antacids may cause belching and flatulence.
   d. Calcium carbonate-containing antacids may cause dose-related diarrhea.

Answer C is correct. Antacids are generally well tolerated and minimally absorbed into the systemic circulation. Dose-related diarrhea can occur with magnesium-containing products, and dose-related constipation may occur with aluminum-containing products. Carbon dioxide gas produced by calcium carbonate products may cause belching and flatulence.

FR mentions that she is taking levothyroxine for her thyroid disorder; she would like to know if it is safe to take an antacid at the same time as her levothyroxine.

3. Which information do you provide to FR?
   a. Antacids may cause a reduced absorption of levothyroxine; separate administration of these drugs by 4 hours
   b. Antacids may cause an increase in absorption of levothyroxine; separate administration of these drugs by 4 hours
   c. Antacids do not interact with levothyroxine; both medications may be taken at the same time
   d. Levothyroxine reduces the efficacy of antacids; separate administration of these drugs by 4 hours

Answer A is correct. When taken at the same time as other oral medications, antacids may potentially increase or decrease the absorption of the other medications. This may occur by binding to or chelation of the other drugs or by altering their absorption by increasing intragastric pH.

YP is an 83-year-old female who has been experiencing "stomach pain" after eating and occasionally at bedtime. She is a nursing home resident and remains mostly in her wheelchair or bed. She has a history of congestive heart failure, osteoarthritis, and renal insufficiency.

1. Which of the following statements is true regarding antacid use in the elderly?
   a. Magnesium-containing antacids should be used cautiously in patients with renal insufficiency due to the risk of hypomagnesemia.
   b. Magnesium levels should be monitored in all patients taking antacids.
   c. Sodium bicarbonate antacids should be used cautiously in patients with renal failure.
   d. Antacid products are contraindicated for use in the elderly.

Answer C is correct. Magnesium-containing antacids may cause hypomagnesemia in patients with renal insufficiency. Sodium bicarbonate may increase fluid retention and should be used cautiously in patients with heart failure, edema, cirrhosis, and renal impairment.

2. Which of the following are nonpharmacologic options to help reduce symptoms in YP?
   a. Eat small meals throughout the day
   b. Remain upright for at least 2 hours after eating
   c. Avoid trigger foods such as carbonated beverages, caffeine, and spicy foods
   d. All of the above are correct.

Answer D is correct. Treating symptoms of heartburn may require both nonpharmacologic and pharmacologic approaches. All of the options given in this question may reduce symptoms for patients with heartburn.

YP's daughter is turning 50 years old and would like to take an antacid to prevent osteoporosis during the postmenopausal period and to help with occasional heartburn.

3. Which of the following do you recommend?
   a. A magnesium-containing antacid when needed for heartburn symptoms
   b. A calcium-containing antacid when needed for heartburn symptoms
   c. A calcium-containing antacid daily, with vitamin D
   d. A magnesium-containing antacid daily, with vitamin D

Answer C is correct. A product containing calcium should be taken daily to a target intake of 1200 mg per day of elemental calcium orally in postmenopausal women. Vitamin D can increase absorption of calcium.

11.2 Antidiarrheal and Antiflatulence Agents

Bismuth subsalicylate produces its effects through antisecretory, antibacterial, and anti-inflammatory mechanisms and is the only over-the-counter (OTC) stomach product effective in the relief of both upper and lower gastrointestinal symptoms. The salicylate in bismuth subsalicylate contributes to serum levels of this compound and may cause salicylate toxicity. Combination of bismuth subsalicylate with other salicylate products should therefore be avoided; in addition, this product should not be used in children less than 12 years of age. A temporary, harmless darkening of the stool and tongue may occur in individuals who are treated with bismuth salts.

Some antidiarrheal medications are natural opiates (morphine) or synthetic opiate agonists (diphenoxylate) that work to decrease smooth muscle contraction in the GI tract, thereby decreasing GI motility to relieve diarrhea symptoms. Diphenoxylate with atropine is indicated as adjunct therapy in the treatment of diarrhea. Infectious causes of diarrhea are usually self-limited, with hydration and management of diet being the primary treatments. If diarrhea lasts more than 48 hours, if it is bloody, if abdominal pain is present, or if the patient is experiencing a fever, further evaluation may be required. Antidiarrheal agents can be utilized to control chronic diarrhea caused by functional GI disorders such as IBS or IBD.

Another option for treating diarrhea—specifically, antibiotic-associated diarrhea (AAD)—is *Lactobacillus acidophilus*. This bacterium is a normal bowel inhabitant and is the most commonly used *Lactobacillus* species in the United States. *Lactobacillus* preparations have shown efficacy in treating and preventing AAD, but appear to be ineffective in preventing traveler's diarrhea. While the mechanism for the benefits of probiotics is not fully understood, a common theory is that the "good bacteria" suppress the growth or epithelial binding/invasion by pathogenic bacteria.

Simethicone is a mixture of inert silicon polymers that may relieve flatulence after intestinal gas has formed. This agent reduces the surface tension of gas bubbles and allows for an easier passage via belching or through the rectum. This product is safe for use in children and during pregnancy.

Antidiarrheal Agents

Bismuth salts
Diphenoxylate
Lactobacillus acidophilus
Loperamide
Opium preparations

Antiflatulence Agents

Simethicone

Case Studies and Conclusions

DB is a 55-year-old female who complains of GI symptoms.

1. Which of the following symptoms would not be appropriate to treat with bismuth subsalicylate?
   a. Diarrhea
   b. Dyspepsia
   c. Constipation
   d. Upset stomach

Answer C is correct. Bismuth subsalicylate is indicated for diarrhea to control the number of bowel movements and can relieve dyspepsia, upset stomach, and nausea. It is not indicated for constipation.

2. Which of the following adverse reactions should be discussed with DB when she is taking bismuth subsalicylate?
   a. "If you experience darkening of the tongue, you should discontinue the medication."
   b. "If you experience darkening of the stool, it indicates GI bleeding and you should discontinue the medication."
   c. "If you experience darkening of the tongue, it is temporary and not harmful."
   d. "If you experience darkening of the tongue, it is permanent."

Answer C is correct. Temporary darkening of the stool or tongue may occur when a patient is taking bismuth subsalicylate.

3. What is the mechanism of action for bismuth subsalicylate therapy to reduce DB's symptoms?
   a. Anti-inflammatory
   b. Antimicrobial
   c. Antisecretory
   d. All of the above are correct.

Answer D is correct. Bismuth is an antimicrobial agent that is effective against diarrheal pathogens, and salicylate is an antisecretory agent that reduces fluid and electrolyte losses. The antisecretory effects associated with bismuth subsalicylate may be mediated by several mechanisms, including inhibition of prostaglandin synthesis, which decreases inflammation.

AZ is a 47-year-old female who began to experience diarrhea approximately 1 day ago. She has experienced about 5 episodes per day and is afebrile.

1. Which of the following products would you recommend to manage AZ's symptoms?
   a. Loperamide
   b. Simethicone
   c. Lactobacillus acidophilus
   d. Opium preparations

Answer A is correct. Loperamide is an antidiarrheal agent that is commonly used for acute diarrhea. If the patient was experiencing a fever or other signs of infectious process, slowing down the GI tract processes may not be the most appropriate option.

When you are talking to AZ, she tells you that she is on a blood thinner, warfarin.

2. Which of the following can cause an increased risk of bleeding if taken with warfarin?
   a. Loperamide
   b. Bismuth subsalicylate
   c. Simethicone
   d. Lactobacillus acidophilus

Answer B is correct. Patients on warfarin who take salicylate-containing medication may have an increased risk of bleeding.

3. Which worsening symptoms should AZ be warned about that would make the recommended therapy inappropriate?
   a. Fever
   b. Bloody diarrhea
   c. Stomachache
   d. Both A and B are correct.

Answer D is correct. Fever and bloody diarrhea can be signs of an infectious process, and antidiarrheal agents may be inappropriate.

11.3 Cathartics and Laxatives

Constipation is characterized by its symptoms including difficult, infrequent, or seemingly incomplete defecation. The major goal when treating constipation is prevention, but for acute constipation the goal is to relieve symptoms and restore normal bowel function. Treatment for functional constipation should begin with nonpharmacologic therapy, including maintaining an adequate amount of fiber and fluid in the diet, scheduling routine time for bowel evacuation, and maintaining proper positioning when attempting a bowel movement. Reviewing the patient's medications, including both prescription and over-the-counter products, and changing or discontinuing therapy that increases the risk of constipation may provide benefit as well. Following implementation of nonpharmacologic therapy, the addition of fiber supplements, or bulk-forming agents, up to a total daily intake of 20 to 30 grams per day is recommended. Patients should be counseled that dose-dependent bloating, distension, and flatulence may occur when such agents are used.

Osmotic laxatives (i.e., lactulose, sorbitol, and polyethylene glycol [PEG]) are poorly absorbed or are nonabsorbable sugars that cause intestinal water secretion, thereby increasing fecal biomass, with secondary effects on peristalsis in the GI tract. Lactulose is an effective laxative, however, it is primarily categorized as an ammonia detoxicant and thus is covered in the companion drug grid found in the Electrolytic, Caloric, and Water Balance Agents chapter. Osmotic laxatives may cause abdominal cramping, bloating, and flatulence.

Saline laxatives such as magnesium hydroxide (milk of magnesia), magnesium citrate, and water containing high amounts of magnesium sulfate are poorly absorbed and act as hyperosmolar solutions. Hypermagnesemia, which is seen primarily in patients with renal impairment, may limit the use of these agents.

"Stool softeners," or surfactant agents such as docusate salts, lower the surface tension by reducing the oil-water interface of the stool. This results in a lower surface tension and enhanced incorporation of water and fat for stool softening. Although these agents have few adverse effects, they are less effective than other laxatives and there is little evidence to support their use in patients with chronic constipation.

Stimulant laxatives (e.g., bisacodyl, sennosides, cascara sagrada) primarily exert their effects via alteration of electrolyte transport by the intestinal mucosa. They stimulate intestinal motor activity and decrease water absorption. Diarrhea and abdominal pain are common adverse effects with the use of these agents. Evidence has not shown that stimulant laxatives cause functional impairment of the colon or increased risk of colorectal cancer, which has been a historical concern when using these agents. Adverse effects include abdominal pain, nausea and vomiting, and diarrhea.

Castor oil is another stimulant laxative used to relieve constipation and for bowel preparation prior to surgery or diagnostic procedures. The use is limited by its adverse effects such as GI irritation, rectal bleeding, and severe diarrhea. It is contraindicated for use in pregnancy and has been replaced by safer and more effective alternative FDA-approved agents for use in the United States.

Glycerin is a sweetener that is commonly used in commercial preparations of OTC and prescription medications, as well as medicinally as a rectally administered laxative. As a laxative, glycerin has an onset of action of 15 to 30 minutes and is acceptable to use intermittently for constipation or fecal impaction, including pediatrics. Adverse effects include diarrhea, nausea and vomiting, and perianal irritation.

Mineral oil is an oral and rectal lubricant laxative that retards colonic absorption of fecal water and softens the stool. This agent has been largely replaced by osmotic laxatives due to the latter's better palatability and similar efficacy. If aspirated, mineral oil can cause lipoid pneumonia; its use should be avoided in infants and the elderly.

Anthraquinone Laxatives

Bisacodyl
Senna

Stool Softeners, Lubricant Laxatives, and Others

Docusate (calcium and sodium)

Bulk-Forming Laxatives

Malt soup extract
Methylcellulose
Psyllium

Hyperosmotic Laxatives

Glycerin
Magnesium (citrate, hydroxide)
Mineral oil
Polyethylene glycol
Saline laxatives
Sodium phosphates
Sorbitol

Case Studies and Conclusions

CD is a 45-year-old female who is now complaining of constipation. She has not had a bowel movement in 4 days and normally has one bowel movement about every other day.

1. What is the initial treatment that CD should try to manage her constipation?
   a. Sorbitol
   b. Docusate
   c. Psyllium
   d. Increase the amount of fiber in the diet

Answer D is correct. The first step in the treatment of constipation is to ensure that the diet includes enough fiber. Approximately 20 to 25 g of fiber is recommended in normal diet. Adequate hydration is also vital to maintain normal bowel function.

CD returns 2 days later and has had only one small bowel movement. She does not have any other GI symptoms.

2. What should she try next?
   a. Magnesium citrate
   b. Mineral oil
   c. Docusate
   d. Polyethylene glycol

Answer D is correct. The next step in therapy would be a laxative. Mineral oil is not recommended due to its side effects. Polyethylene glycol would be the best option as an osmotic laxative. Docusate has limited efficacy in treating constipation.

3. After how many days of laxative use should CD be seen again for reevaluation of constipation and other possible causes?
   a. 2 days
   b. 7 days
   c. 10 days
   d. 14 days

Answer B is correct. Laxative treatment should not be used for more than 1 week without consulting with a medical provider.

EF is a 26-year-old female who comes in complaining of constipation for approximately 2 days.

1. Which treatment should be used?
   a. Not enough information is provided to make a decision.
   b. Increase the amount of dietary fiber
   c. Start docusate
   d. Start mineral oil

Answer A is correct. There is not enough information to make an informed decision. More information regarding EF's normal bowel habits would be needed before recommending a therapy.

EF normally has a bowel movement approximately every 1 to 2 days.

2. Which therapy would you recommend?
   a. Increased fiber
   b. Increased water
   c. Wait and see
   d. All of the above are correct.

Answer D is correct. Increased water and fiber can help with acute constipation in its early stages. It has been less than 3 days since EF's last bowel movement, which may be normal for her.

EF has a friend whom she thinks might be abusing laxatives.

3. Which of the following are signs and symptoms that a patient may experience if he or she is abusing laxatives?
   a. Chronic constipation, and excessive salivation
   b. Diarrhea, weight loss, vomiting, and abdominal pain
   c. Constipation and weight loss
   d. All of these are signs and symptoms of laxative abuse.

Answer B is correct. Laxative abusers often present with diarrhea, weight loss, vomiting, abdominal pain, thirst, edema, bone pain, and fluid and electrolyte imbalances.

11.4 Antiemetic Agents

Nausea and vomiting are associated with a variety of conditions, including GI, cardiovascular, infectious, neurologic, and metabolic diseases. These symptoms are also commonly associated with surgery, chemotherapeutic agents, radiation, and pregnancy. Several classes of drugs are available to treat nausea and vomiting that work by targeting five neurotransmitter receptor sites: muscarinic (M_1), dopamine (D_2), histamine (H_1), serotonin (5-hydroxytryptamine 3 [$5HT_3$]), and substance P (neurokinin 1 [NK1]). The choice of antiemetic agent should be based on patient-specific factors including the suspected cause for symptoms; the frequency, duration, and severity of the episodes. Additionally the ability of the patient to use oral, rectal, injectable, or transdermal medications; and the success of previous treatments should be considered.

For simple nausea and vomiting associated with motion sickness, antihistamine and anticholinergic agents are generally used. Sedation, drowsiness, dry mouth, and urinary retention are common adverse effects of these medications.

Dopamine receptor antagonists (prochlorperazine, chlorpromazine, promethazine) are effective for treatment of motion sickness, vertigo, gastroenteritis, nausea and vomiting in pregnancy (NVP), postoperative nausea and vomiting (PONV), and chemotherapy-induced nausea and vomiting (CINV). These agents may cause sedation and orthostatic hypotension; long-term use may increase the risk of extrapyramidal symptoms such as dystonia and tardive dyskinesia. Metoclopramide carries a black box warning related to its risks of producing tardive dyskinesia and increased risk associated with long-term use.

Serotonin ($5HT_3$) receptor antagonists (ondansetron, granisetron, dolasetron, and palonosetron) have replaced the dopamine antagonists as the primary treatment for multiple indications including CINV, PONV, and radiation-induced nausea and vomiting (RINV). These agents are generally well tolerated, with the most common adverse events being mild headache, asthenia, constipation, and dizziness. Electrocardiogram (ECG) alterations are a class effect of the first-generation $5HT_3$ antagonists (ondansetron, granisetron, and dolasetron). Changes are most prominent in the first 1 to 2 hours after administration and return to baseline within 24 hours; nevertheless, potentially fatal cardiac arrhythmias, including torsades de pointes, have been reported with the use of these medications. ECG monitoring is recommended in patients with electrolyte abnormalities, heart failure, or bradyarrhythmias, and in patients who are taking concomitant therapy that can cause QTc prolongation.

Substance P/neurokinin 1 receptor antagonists (aprepitant, fosaprepitant, netupitant, rolapitant) are used to prevent acute and delayed emesis in patients who are treated with highly emetogenic chemotherapy. Aprepitant has the potential to engage in many drug interactions because it is a substrate, moderate inhibitor, an inducer of specific hepatic isoenzymes. Notably, aprepitant may decrease the efficacy of oral contraceptives and may decrease the international normalized ratio (INR) for patients taking warfarin.

Cannabinoids have complex effects on the CNS and can be used alone or in combination with other antiemetic therapy. They are generally not first-line agents, but rather are an option for treatment-resistant CINV. Euphoria, drowsiness, sedation, somnolence, dysphoria, depression, hallucinations, and paranoia can occur with the use of cannabinoids.

Antihistamine Agents

Dimenhydrinate
Meclizine
Trimethobenzamide
Prochlorperazine *(see also the Psychotherapeutic Agents section in the Central Nervous System Agents chapter)*

$5HT_3$ Receptor Antagonists

Dolasetron
Granisetron
Ondansetron
Palonosetron

Miscellaneous Antiemetic Agents

Aprepitant/fosaprepitant
Dronabinol
Nabilone
Phenothiazines *(see also the Psychotherapeutic Agents section in the Central Nervous System Agents chapter)*
Promethazine *(see also the Anxiolytic, Sedative, and Hypnotic Agents section in the Central Nervous System Agents chapter)*
Scopolamine *(see also the Autonomic-Anticholinergic Agents section in the Autonomic Agents chapter)*

Case Studies and Conclusions

HJ is a 68-year-old male who was recently diagnosed with acute myeloid leukemia (AML). He is receiving treatment with cytarabine/daunorubicin. HJ needs an antiemetic for prevention of nausea and vomiting associated with chemotherapy.

1. Which treatment option is the best choice for this indication?
   a. Scopolamine patch
   b. Metoclopramide
   c. Dimenhydrinate
   d. Ondansetron

Answer D is correct. $5HT_3$ receptor antagonists are effective for prevention of CINV. An agent such as ondansetron is typically administered with a glucocorticoid such as dexamethasone.

2. Which of the following past medical history diagnoses for HJ would be concerning when prescribing a $5HT_3$ antagonist?

   a. Diabetes
   b. Heart failure
   c. Acute myeloid leukemia
   d. Hyperlipidemia

Answer B is correct. Patients with electrolyte imbalances (hypokalemia, hypomagnesemia), heart failure, or bradyarrhythmias, and those taking other medications that prolong the QT interval may require ECG monitoring.

3. What are the most common side effects that HJ may experience from a $5HT_3$ antagonist?

   a. Mild headache, constipation, low energy, and dizziness
   b. Confusion, dry mouth, and urinary retention
   c. GI symptoms including acid reflux, cramping, and diarrhea
   d. Sedation, dysphoria, and hallucinations

Answer A is correct. $5HT_3$ receptor antagonists are generally well tolerated, with mild headache being the most frequently reported adverse event, occurring in approximately 9% to 27% of patients. Constipation may occur in 5% to 10% of patients and dizziness in 7% of patients.

JS is a 35-year-old female who is planning to go on a road trip with her friends. She knows that long car rides give her motion sickness and have caused her to experience nausea and vomiting in the past.

1. Which option is best for JS to prevent motion sickness?

   a. Dimenhydrinate
   b. Haloperidol
   c. Dronabinol
   d. Ondansetron

Answer A is correct. Antihistamine agents can be used to prevent motion sickness. Dimenhydrinate 50 to 100 mg should be taken 30 to 60 minutes prior to motion. It can be taken every 4 to 6 hours, with the maximum daily dose being 400 mg.

JS has never taken dimenhydrinate before.

2. Which of the following is an important counseling point to discuss with her prior to taking this medication?

   a. "Dimenhydrinate may cause dizziness and drowsiness. Do not drive until you know how this medication will affect you."
   b. "Dimenhydrinate may cause dizziness and drowsiness, but will not impair your ability to drive."
   c. "Dimenhydrinate does not cause dizziness or drowsiness, so it will not impair your ability to drive."
   d. These are all relevant counseling points.

Answer A is correct. Dimenhydrinate may cause CNS depression. Patients should be instructed to see how this medication affects them prior to operating a motor vehicle or machinery.

JS got back from her trip and did not get car sick while taking dimenhydrinate. She now thinks it may help prevent motion sickness for her grandmother when she drives as well.

3. Which of the following statements is true regarding dimenhydrinate use for treating motion sickness in a geriatric patient?

   a. An increased dose will be necessary to achieve the same effect.
   b. The dose should be reduced if the patient has renal impairment.
   c. The medication is listed in the Beers criteria as potentially inappropriate due to its anticholinergic properties.
   d. These statements are all true.

Answer C is correct. First-generation antihistamines such as dimenhydrinate have anticholinergic properties that can result in increased risk of confusion, dry mouth, constipation, and urinary retention. Their use should be avoided in older adults due to reduced clearance with advanced age.

11.5 Antiulcer Agents and Suppressants

The treatment of peptic ulcers and GERD has been dramatically improved by the introduction of therapies that inhibit acid secretion, including histamine-2 receptor antagonists (H2RAs) and proton-pump inhibitors (PPIs). PPIs inhibitors are able to block acid secretion by inhibiting hydrogen-potassium ATPase and are considered to be more effective than H2RAs in healing duodenal and gastric ulcers as well as NSAID-induced ulcers in patients in whom treatment with NSAIDs is still required.

Proton-pump inhibitors decrease gastric acid secretion by inhibiting the H^+/K^+ ATP pump in the gastric parietal cells. The degree of acid suppression increases over the first 3 to 4 days of therapy as more proton pumps are inhibited. PPIs inhibit only those proton pumps that are actively secreting acid. They are more effective when taken 30 to 60 minutes before meals. These agents are generally well tolerated, with the most common adverse effects from their use including headache, somnolence, and dizziness. Omeprazole and esomeprazole may decrease the elimination of phenytoin, warfarin, diazepam, and carbamazepine. Patients should consult their provider before taking a PPI if they are concurrently taking clopidogrel. Use of gastric acid inhibitors has been associated with an increased risk for development of acute gastroenteritis and community-acquired pneumonia in pediatric patients. Enteric infections, vitamin B_{12} deficiency, hypomagnesemia, iron malabsorption, and bone fractures are potential adverse effects in patients taking PPIs on a long-term basis (usually more than one year). In February 2016, a study published in *JAMA Neurology* concluded that PPI use is associated with an increased risk for dementia.

Because H2RAs can cross the blood-brain barrier, dosage adjustments of these agents in patients with renal insufficiency are recommended to reduce adverse effects such as CNS symptoms. H2RA use may be limited due to tolerance that develops to gastric antisecretory effects. Taking these medications only as needed, rather than on a daily basis, may improve their efficacy.

Misoprostol is a synthetic prostaglandin analogue that acts to inhibit acid secretion and enhance mucosal defense; it is indicated for reducing the risk of NSAID-induced gastric ulcers. Its use is limited by its GI side effects and the need for frequent administration of this medication. Misoprostol is contraindicated in pregnancy due to potential abortifacient effects.

Sucralfate forms a complex by binding with positively charged proteins in exudates, thereby forming a viscous, paste-like, adhesive substance. A protective coating is formed and acts locally to protect the gastric lining against peptic acid, pepsin, and bile salts, and to promote the healing of gastrointestinal ulcers caused by *Helicobacter pylori (H. pylori)* infection. Sucralfate heals chronic ulcers without altering gastric acid or pepsin secretion. The most common side effect from its use is constipation, most likely due to the aluminum content of this medication. As with aluminum-containing antacids, long-term use of sucralfate in patients with renal insufficiency should be avoided. Sucralfate may bind and reduce the bioavailability of medications with a narrow therapeutic window, such as warfarin, phenytoin, levothyroxine, and theophylline. It is recommended to administer sucralfate at least 2 hours after these medications.

Antiulcer Agents and Acid Suppressants

Amoxicillin *(see also the Antibacterial Agents section in the Anti-infective Agents chapter)*
Antacids *(see also the Antacids and Adsorbents section)*
Clarithromycin *(see also the Antibacterial Agents section in the Anti-infective Agents chapter)*
Metronidazole *(see also the Antiprotozoal Agents section in the Anti-infective Agents chapter)*
Tetracycline *(see also the Antibacterial Agents section in the Anti-infective Agents chapter)*

Histamine (H_2) Antagonists

Cimetidine
Famotidine
Nizatidine
Ranitidine

Prostaglandins

Misoprostol

Protectants

Sucralfate

Proton-Pump Inhibitors

Dexlansoprazole
Esomeprazole
Lansoprazole
Omeprazole
Pantoprazole
Rabeprazole

Case Studies and Conclusions

BR is a 67-year-old female with complaints of episodic epigastric pain for the past 6 weeks. The pain is nonradiating and is aggravated by ingestion of food. BR has been experiencing occasional nausea, bloating, and heartburn. She denies any changes in color or frequency of bowel movements. Prior to experiencing her pain, BR was prescribed ibuprofen 600 mg three times daily for headaches.

1. Which of the following treatment options would be an appropriate recommendation for BR?
   a. Change ibuprofen to naproxen
   b. Addition of misoprostol to reduce mucosal irritation
   c. Addition of a PPI daily, and reevaluate NSAID therapy for continued use
   d. Addition of a H2RA twice daily, and reevaluate NSAID therapy for continued use

Answer C is correct. BR's symptoms are consistent with a gastric ulcer—epigastric pain, aggravated by food ingestion, and the recent start of an NSAID. PPIs have been shown to be superior in healing gastric ulcers compared to H2RAs. It is recommended that BR start a PPI and that the provider determine if an alternative therapy for her headaches would be a better option.

BR continues the prescribed therapy described in Question 1 and no longer experiences pain. Several years later, BR experiences GI symptoms including pyrosis, hypersalivation, and regurgitation consistent with GERD that occurs daily and is moderate to severe in pain intensity.

2. Which of the following therapies would you recommend for this patient?
   a. Daily PPI
   b. Daily H2RA
   c. Sucralfate
   d. Antacid

Answer A is correct. Due to her frequency and severity of symptoms, a daily PPI would be most appropriate to use. Antacids are best for mild, intermittent heartburn, while H2RAs can be utilized for mild to moderate symptoms. Tolerance is a concern with routine use of a H2RA.

3. Which adverse effects are associated with use of acid suppression therapy in a patient such as BR?
   a. Hypermagnesemia
   b. Hypercalcemia
   c. Vitamin B_{12} deficiency
   d. Vitamin D deficiency

Answer C is correct. Long-term acid suppression therapy may cause malabsorption of calcium, magnesium, and vitamin B_{12}. Periodic monitoring of these vitamins and minerals is recommended for individuals who are taking a PPI for long-term acid suppression therapy.

CR is a 75-year-old male who was diagnosed with a duodenal ulcer and started on sucralfate 1 g 4 times daily for 8 weeks.

1. Which side effect is CR likely to experience while taking sucralfate?
   a. Diarrhea
   b. Upset stomach
   c. Constipation
   d. Rash

Answer C is correct. Sucralfate contains aluminum, and the most common side effect of this medication is constipation, most likely due to its aluminum content.

CR has a history of atrial fibrillation and hypertension; he takes lisinopril, warfarin, metoprolol, and hydrochlorothiazide.

2. Which of his medications should be administered separate from sucralfate?
   a. Lisinopril
   b. Warfarin
   c. Metoprolol
   d. Hydrochlorothiazide

Answer B is correct. Sucralfate may decrease the anticoagulant effect of warfarin. It is recommended to separate the medications by administering warfarin 2 hours before or 6 hours after sucralfate.

CR completes his course of therapy for the treatment of his duodenal ulcer but continues a prophylaxis dose of 1 g twice daily. He presents to the emergency room (ER) with muscle weakness, bone pain, and altered mental status. Serum creatinine is 3.7 mg/dL and complete blood count (CBC) within normal limits (WNL) on admission.

3. Which of the following would you recommend?
   a. CR is likely experiencing a GI bleed: increase the dose of sucralfate.
   b. CR is likely experiencing a GI bleed: continue the same dose of sucralfate.
   c. CR is likely experiencing aluminum toxicity due to impaired renal function: reduce the dose of sucralfate.
   d. CR is likely experiencing aluminum toxicity due to impaired renal function: discontinue sucralfate,

Answer C is correct. CR is likely experiencing aluminum toxicity due to impaired renal function. Signs of aluminum toxicity include proximal muscle weakness, bone pain, and alterations in mental status; such toxicity may also increase the risk of fractures. The recommended dose of sucralfate for duodenal ulcer prophylaxis is 1 g twice daily, so reducing the dose may not be effective. Discontinuing sucralfate would be the best option. Alternative therapies for prophylaxis of a duodenal ulcer might include proton-pump inhibitors or histamine-2 receptor antagonists.

11.6 Miscellaneous Gastrointestinal Agents

Inflammatory bowel disease presents as two forms: ulcerative colitis (UC) and Crohn's disease (CD). Ulcerative colitis is a mucosal inflammatory condition confined to the rectum and colon, whereas Crohn's disease may cause inflammation in any part of the GI tract. Treatment of UC and CD aims to manage the inflammatory processes. Aminosalicylates, corticosteroids, antimicrobials, immunosuppressants, and biologic agents are utilized to treat active disease and to induce and maintain disease remission. Medication formulations of sulfasalazine include enemas and suppositories for the treatment of proctitis and oral agents in slow-release formulations that deliver drug to the small intestine and colon. Steroids should be reserved for induction of remission, not for maintenance treatment.

Irritable bowel syndrome is a functional GI disorder associated with recurrent abdominal pain with defecation or a change in bowel habits. IBS is classified into three main subtypes based on the predominant bowel disorder: IBS with predominant constipation (IBS-C), IBS with predominant diarrhea (IBS-D), and IBS with mixed bowel habits (IBS-M). Those individuals who do not meet the diagnostic criteria for the three main subtypes should be categorized as having IBS—unclassified (IBS-U). When managing constipation associated with IBS, after a patient fails a trial of soluble fiber and polyethylene glycol, lubiprostone or linaclotide may be tried. Lubiprostone and linaclotide increase the amount of fluid that is drawn into the intestine but can cause nausea, diarrhea, and abdominal pain. Tegaserod was approved for IBS-C but was withdrawn from the market due to cardiovascular side effects. For diarrhea symptoms associated with IBS, loperamide is suggested before meals as needed. Alosetron is a $5HT_3$ antagonist approved for the treatment of severe diarrhea associated with predominant IBS in female patients whose symptoms have lasted for at least 6 months and who have failed other treatments.

Opioid-induced constipation (OIC) has become a growing problem as the use of opioids has increased drastically. Opioid antagonists are useful to treat refractory constipation but should be avoided in the presence of bowel obstruction. Methylnaltrexone is a peripherally acting opioid antagonist that does not cross the brain-blood barrier and does not induce symptoms of opioid withdrawal. It is available as a subcutaneous injection only. Naloxegol and lubiprostone are oral opioid antagonists approved for OIC.

Cholelitholytic agents treat cholesterol gallstones by reducing biliary cholesterol secretion, reducing intestinal absorption of cholesterol, increasing hepatic bile secretion, and improving gallbladder emptying. Bile acid therapy should be used in patients with small stones and mild symptoms with mild calcification. The main side effect of these drugs is diarrhea, which occurs more frequently with chenodiol compared with ursodiol. Chenodiol can also cause hypercholesterolemia and increased serum aminotransferases. Ursodiol does not cause these side effects and is the drug of choice for gallstones.

Patients with chronic pancreatitis and severe pancreatic exocrine dysfunction cannot properly digest complex foods or absorb digestive breakdown products. This condition usually results in loose, greasy, foul-smelling stools and malabsorption of the fat-soluble vitamins (A, D, E, and K) and vitamin B_{12}. Creon is an enteric-coated formulation of lipase, amylase, and protease that is used to help break down fats, protein, and starch. It is well tolerated with minimal side effects, with the most frequent being abdominal pain and dyspepsia.

Gastroparesis can cause nausea, early satiety, bloating, and upper abdominal pain and is commonly managed with dietary modification and the use of prokinetic agents to increase the rate of gastric emptying. Metoclopramide can be utilized for diabetic gastroparesis, prevention of nausea and vomiting associated with chemotherapy, postoperatively, or for symptoms associated with GERD. Metoclopramide should be administered 10 to 15 minutes prior to meals, with an additional dose before bedtime if needed. Chronic use for longer than 12 weeks should be evaluated carefully due to the risk of tardive dyskinesia. Periodic drug holidays or dose reductions should be attempted if clinically possible. Metoclopramide is better tolerated than cisapride. The use of cisapride has been associated with drug interactions resulting in cardiac arrhythmias and death. Cisapride prescriptions can be filled only through an investigational limited-access program from the manufacturer.

Orlistat alters fat digestion by inhibiting pancreatic lipases, preventing fat from being completely hydrolyzed and increasing fecal fat excretion.

Short bowel syndrome (SBS) is a malabsorptive state caused by massive resection of the small intestine or, rarely, by congenital defect or disease associated with loss of absorption. Teduglutide is a GLP-2 analogue that has modest benefits in the treatment of SBS. It initiates and maintains the small bowel's adaptive response to resection.

Anti-inflammatory Agents

Balsalazide
Mesalamine
Olsalazine
Sulfasalazine *(see also the Antibacterial Agents section in the Anti-infective Agents chapter)*

Cholelitholytic Agents

Chenodiol
Ursodiol

Digestants

Pancrelipase

Prokinetic Agents

Cisapride
Metoclopramide

Miscellaneous Gastrointestinal Agents

Alosetron
Alvimopan
Linaclotide
Lubiprostone
Methylnaltrexone
Naloxegol
Orlistat
Teduglutide
Tegaserod
Vedolizumab
Adalimumab (also considered disease-modifying antirheumatic drugs [DMARDs])
Certolizumab (also considered disease-modifying antirheumatic drugs [DMARDs])
Infliximab (also considered disease-modifying antirheumatic drugs [DMARDs])
Octreotide *(see also the Pituitary Agents section in the Hormones and Synthetic Substitutes chapter)*

Case Studies and Conclusions

JJ is a 52-year-old woman with complaints of nausea, slight abdominal pain, early satiety, fullness, and bloating. She was recently diagnosed with gastroparesis and has tried modifying her diet and increasing hydration, but she continues to have symptoms.

1. Which of the following agents would be an appropriate treatment option for JJ?

   a. Metoclopramide
   b. Lubiprostone
   c. Mesalamine
   d. None of these.

Answer A is correct. Metoclopramide is first-line therapy for gastroparesis. It improves gastric emptying by enhancing gastric contractions and increasing postprandial fundus relaxation.

JJ's physician has prescribed metoclopramide.

2. What is the maximum amount of time that metoclopramide should be used according to the FDA?

   a. 7 days
   b. 12 weeks
   c. 2 months
   d. There is no time limit on its use.

Answer B is correct. Metoclopramide is approved by the FDA for treatment of gastroparesis for no longer than 12 weeks unless the patient's benefits outweigh the risks. Metoclopramide is associated with a risk of tardive dyskinesia that increases with longer duration of therapy and total cumulative dose.

3. JJ should be advised to contact her physician if she experiences which of the following symptoms?

   a. Any involuntary movement, especially of the tongue
   b. Any headache or dizziness
   c. Any changes in appetite, constipation, or diarrhea
   d. Any signs of infection, such as fever, chills, or body aches

Answer A is correct. Tardive dyskinesia is a serious side effect and may be irreversible. It is important to educate the patient about the risks associated with this drug. Extrapyramidal side effects, including dystonia and tardive dyskinesia, occur in 0.2% and 1% of patients, respectively.

PR is a 27-year-old female who experienced a back injury at work and is currently being treated with opioid therapy. She has been experiencing constipation and has already tried increasing her fiber intake and polyethylene glycol with no success. PR does not like needles and prefers an oral agent to manage her symptoms.

1. Which of the following therapies would be the best choice to treat PR's OIC?
   a. Naloxegol
   b. Methylnaltrexone
   c. Probiotics
   d. Increase fluid intake

Answer A is correct. Methylnatrexone is an injection and would not be a preferred agent based on this patient's preferences. Probiotics and increasing fluid intake may provide benefit for some patients for functional constipation, but these options will likely not provide enough relief for OIC. Naloxegol is an oral opioid antagonist approved for OIC.

PR has since recovered and is going to stop her opioid therapy.

2. For how long should PR continue taking naloxegol after discontinuing the opioid therapy?
   a. She should discontinue use of naloxegol as soon as she stops taking her opioid therapy
   b. For 1 week following discontinuation of her opioid therapy
   c. Until she no longer has constipation
   d. She should remain on naloxegol indefinitely

Answer A is correct. Patients should discontinue use of naloxegol when their opioid medications are discontinued.

One year later, PR is diagnosed with irritable bowel syndrome with predominant constipation. She reinjured her back at work last week and again requires opioid therapy. PR is concerned that she will experience similar changes to her bowel habits as the last time she was on opioid therapy.

3. Which of the following agents is approved to treat irritable bowel syndrome with constipation and OIC?
   a. Lubiprostone
   b. Methylnaltrexone
   c. Naloxegol
   d. All of the above are correct.

Answer A is correct. Lubiprostone is approved for chronic idiopathic constipation (dose: 24 mcg twice daily), irritable bowel syndrome with constipation in females 18 years or older (dose: 8 mcg twice daily), and OIC with chronic noncancer pain (dose: 24 mcg twice daily). Methylnaltrexone and naloxegol are not approved for IBS-C.

Tips from the Field

Using Enemas

Not everyone knows how to properly use an enema, and sometimes it is even harder to describe the process:

1. The best approach is to instruct the patient to lie on their left side with top knee bent and arms resting comfortably or the patient may kneel, then lower their head and chest forward until the left side of the face is resting on a surface with arms folded comfortably.

2. Open tube by twisting off and removing tip. A dry tip can be uncomfortable, so advise the patient to moisten the shaft/tip of the enema tube with some water or a few drops of the medication.

3. Applying an appropriate lubricant to the anal area is recommended before inserting enema.

4. With steady pressure, carefully insert the tube shaft into the rectum.
5. Squeeze tube to empty contents and keep the tube squeezed until completely removed from the rectum.
6. Often, the directions will include "retaining" the enema for a certain period of time. The patient should be prepared and plan for the evacuation of the medication contents from the bowel once the retention period is over.
7. Most patients can prepare for and are most comfortable with the evacuation of the residual contents of a rectal enema over the toilet.

Who May Be at Risk for Mechanical GI Obstruction?

1. When GI drugs are contraindicated in patients with a history of mechanical GI obstruction, clinicians may be wondering who is at risk or what symptoms might be suggestive of such blockage.
   - Patients with current symptoms of abdominal pain which may be suggestive of mechanical GI obstruction should be medically evaluated before using gastrointestinal agents.
   - Common causes of mechanical obstruction include hernias, abdominal adhesions, tumors, gastric cancer, disseminated intraperitoneal cancers, gallstones foreign bodies, diverticulitis, inflammatory bowel disease (such as Crohn's disease), and patients experiencing fecal impaction for unknown reasons.

Novel Agents Now Available for OIC with Chronic Noncancer Pain (CNCP)

1. Methylnaltrexone and naloxegol are relatively new agents for use in OIC; however, their use is contraindicated in patients with known or suspected GI obstruction and in patients at increased risk of recurrent obstruction, due to the potential for GI perforation.
2. Patients with a GI disease that may be associated with localized or diffuse reduction of structural integrity in the wall of the GI tract such as peptic ulcer disease, diverticulitis, peritoneal metastases, etc., are at higher risk for GI perforation.

Tammie Lee and Jacque

Bibliography

American Geriatrics Society. 2015 updated Beers criteria for potentially inappropriate medication use in older adults. *J Am Geriatr Soc.* 2015;63:2227-2246.

Aziz Q, Fass R, Gyawali CP, Miwa H, Pandolfino JE, Zerbib F. Esophageal disorders. *Gastroenterology.* 2016;150(6):1368-1379.

Barbara G, Feinle-Bisset C, Ghoshal UC, et al. The intestinal microenvironment and functional gastrointestinal disorders. *Gastroenterology.* 2016;150(6):1305-1318.

Boeckxstaens G, Camilleri M, Sifrim D, et al. Fundamentals of neurogastroenterology: physiology/motility—sensation. *Gastroenterology.* 2016;150(6):1292-1304.

Brandt LJ, Chey WD, Foxx-Orenstein AE, et al.; American College of Gastroenterology Task Force on Irritable Bowel Syndrome. An evidence-based position statement on the management of irritable bowel syndrome. *Am J Gastroenterol.* 2009;104(suppl 1):S1-S35.

Camilleri M, Buéno L, Andresen V, Lembo A. Pharmacologic, pharmacokinetic, and pharmacogenomic aspects of functional gastrointestinal disorders. *Gastroenterology.* 2016;150(6):1319-1331.

Canani RB, Cirillo P, Roggero P, et al.; Working Group on Intestinal Infections of the Italian Society of Pediatric Gastroenterology, Hepatology and Nutrition (SIGENP). Therapy with gastric acidity inhibitors increases the risk of acute gastroenteritis and community-acquired pneumonia in children. *Pediatrics.* 2006;117(5):e817-e820.

Cotton PB, Elta GH, Carter CR, Pasricha PJ, Corazziari ES. Gallbladder and sphincter of Oddi disorders. *Gastroenterology.* 2016;150(6):1420-1429.

Drossman DA. Functional gastrointestinal disorders: history, pathophysiology, clinical features, and Rome IV. *Gastroenterology.* 2016;150(6):1262-1279.

Drossman DA, Hasler WL. Rome IV—functional GI disorders: disorders of gut-brain interaction. *Gastroenterology.* 2016;150(6):1257-1261.

Fass R. Therapeutic options for refractory gastroesophageal reflux disease. *J Gastroenterol Hepatol.* 2012;27(suppl 3):3-7.

Fedorak RN, Dieleman LA. Probiotics in the treatment of human inflammatory bowel diseases: update 2008. *J Clin Gastroenterol.* 2008;42(suppl 2):S97-S103.

Ford AC, Moayyedi P, Lacy BE, et al. American College of Gastroenterology monograph on the management of irritable bowel syndrome and chronic idiopathic constipation. *Am J Gastroenterol.* 2014;109(suppl 1):S2-S26.

Francisconi CF, Sperber AD, Fang X, et al. Multicultural aspects in functional gastrointestinal disorders (FGIDs). *Gastroenterology.* 2016;150(6):1344-1354.

Keefer L, Drossman DA, Guthrie E, et al. Centrally mediated disorders of gastrointestinal pain. *Gastroenterology.* 2016;150(6):1408-1419.

Kostic AD, Xavier RJ, Gevers D. The microbiome in inflammatory bowel disease: current status and the future ahead. *Gastroenterology.* 2014;146(6):1489-1499.

Lacy BE, Mearin F, Chang L, et al. Bowel disorders. *Gastroenterology.* 2016;150(6);1393- 1407.

Lembo A, Camilleri M. Chronic constipation. *N Engl J Med.* 2003;349:1360-1368.

Lexicomp. *Drug Information Handbook.* 24th ed. Hudson, OH; Author: 2015.

Locke GR III, Pemberton JH, Phillips SF. American Gastroenterological Association medical position statement: guidelines on constipation. *Gastroenterology.* 2013;119(6):1761-1766.

McEvoy GK, ed. *AHFS: Drug Information.* Bethesda, MD: American Society of Health-System Pharmacists; 2016.

Müller-Lissner SA, Kamm MA, Scarpignato C, Wald A. Myths and misconceptions about chronic constipation. *Am J Gastroenterol.* 2005;100:232-242.

North American Menopause Society. Position statement: the role of calcium in peri- and postmenopausal women: 2006 position statement of the North American Menopause Society. *Menopause.* 2006;13:862-877.

Olsen KM, Hutchins GF. Evaluation of the gastrointestinal tract. In: DiPiro JT, Talbert RL, Yee GC, Matzke GR, Wells BG, Posey LM, eds. *Pharmacotherapy: A Pathophysiologic Approach.* 9th ed. New York, NY: McGraw-Hill Medical; 2014.

Sartor RB. Microbial influences in inflammatory bowel diseases. *Gastroenterology.* 2008;134(2):577-592.

Sharkey KA, Wallace JL. Treatment of disorders of bowel motility and water flux; anti-emetics; agents used in biliary and pancreatic disease. In: Brunton LL, Chabner BA, Knollmann BC, eds. *Goodman & Gilman's The Pharmacological Basis of Therapeutics.* 12th ed. New York, NY: McGraw-Hill; 2011: 1309-1322.

Stanghellini V, Chan FK, Hasler WL, et al. Gastroduodenal disorders. *Gastroenterology.* 2016;150(6):1380-1392.

Thielman NM, Guerrant RL. Clinical practice: acute infectious diarrhea. *N Engl J Med.* 2004;350:38-47.

Wald A. Is chronic use of stimulant laxatives harmful to the colon? *J Clin Gastroenterol.* 2003;36:386-389.

Wallace JL, Sharkey KA. Pharmacotherapy of gastric acidity, peptic ulcers, and gastroesophageal reflux disease. In: Brunton LL, Chabner BA, Knollmann BC, eds. *Goodman & Gilman's The Pharmacological Basis of Therapeutics.* 12th ed. New York, NY: McGraw-Hill; 2011: 1309-1322.

Wallace JL, Sharkey KA. Pharmacotherapy of inflammatory bowel disease. In: Brunton LL, Chabner BA, Knollmann BC, eds. *Goodman & Gilman's The Pharmacological Basis of Therapeutics.* 12th ed. New York, NY: McGraw-Hill; 2011: 1351-1362.

Weinberg DS, Smalley W, Heidelbaugh JJ, Sultan S; American Gastroenterological Association Institute guideline on the pharmacological management of irritable bowel syndrome. *Gastroenterology.* 2014;147(5):1146-1148.

Symbols

Symbol	Meaning	Symbol	Meaning
▲	Renal impairment: Dose adjustment is recommended.	BL	Beers list criteria (avoid in elderly).
☐	Hepatic impairment: Dose adjustment is recommended.	PD	FDA-approved pediatric doses are available.
■	Black box warning exists for this drug.	GD	FDA-approved geriatric doses are available.
QT	QTc prolongation effects have been reported.	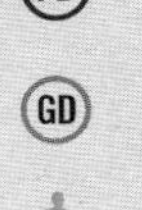	See primary body system.

Gastrointestinal Agents

Universal prescribing alerts:

- Known serious hypersensitivity to the specific drug or any other component of the product/formulation selected warrants a contraindication to its use.
- Adverse reactions associated with the use of some **gastrointestinal agents** include dizziness, drowsiness, vertigo, and fatigue; these agents may also impair the ability to perform tasks requiring mental alertness. Caution should always be recommended when using any new drug for the first time, when there is a dose change, and for continued use of known offending agents.
- Doses expressed are for usual adult dosage ranges only. "Geriatric doses" are assumed to be the same as adult doses unless otherwise noted with a symbol. Where pediatric dosing is available, a symbol will guide the reader to additional prescribing references. Refer to real-time prescribing references for these age-specific doses.
- Use of gastrointestinal agents in pregnancy is based on weighing clinical risk versus benefit; safety concerns are not represented in this grid. Refer to the package insert (PI) for more information. Clinicians should continue to provide education about the reproductive risks of any medication and offer risk-reduction strategies (which may include contraceptive use) to women of childbearing age and understand that these reproductive risks may also extend to males. Other medications may decrease the effectiveness of oral contraceptives. Where necessary, an alternative means of birth control should be explored.
- Brand names are provided for those agents still available on the market. Due to ever-changing product availability, refer to Food and Drug Administration (FDA) resources to confirm the actual brands available. This drug summary is for educational purposes only. Prescribing decisions should be based on real-time comprehensive drug databases that are updated on a regular basis.

Antacids and Adsorbents

Drug Name	FDA-Approved Indications	Adult Dosage Range	Precautions and Clinical Pearls
Generic Name Aluminum hydroxide **Brand Name** Alternagel Amphojel	**Common indications for use:** Antacid	**Usual oral OTC dose:** 640 mg (10 mL) 5 to 6 times per day, after meals and at bedtime.	• Use with caution in patients with chronic diarrhea; may lead to hypophosphatemia • Use with caution in patients with increased constipation and those at risk of this condition (e.g., geriatric patients, patients taking anticholinergics, patients with gastrointestinal [GI] obstruction, patients with undiagnosed GI/rectal bleeding) • Monitor and treat for constipation appropriately • Use with caution in patients with renal impairment; may result in aluminum toxicity • Monitor serum calcium and serum phosphate • Do not take for more than 2 weeks without doctor instruction

			• Avoid use in patients with hypophosphatemia • Avoid use in patients with colostomy, diverticulitis, or ileostomy (increases risk of electrolyte imbalance)
Generic Name Calcium carbonate **Brand Name** Maalox Rolaids Tums Many formulations with varying names (PD) (GD) ▲	Dyspepsia Chronic hypocalcemia Hyperphosphatemia (with chronic renal failure) Osteoporosis prophylaxis Pyrosis (heartburn) Nutritional supplementation	Doses vary with indication for use, formulation selected, and patient's clinical status/response **Usual OTC dose for heartburn:** Chew 1 to 2 tablets (340 to 680 mg of elemental calcium) every 2 hours not exceed 9 tablets (3060 mg of elemental calcium) per 24 hours. **Illustrative oral dosing for osteoporosis prophylaxis:** 1 to 1.5 g elemental calcium daily	• Precautions: may cause nephrolithiasis or hypercalciuria • Use with caution in patients with milk-alkali syndrome (from hypercalcemia, renal disease, or dehydration) • Use with caution in patients with increased constipation and those at risk of this condition (e.g., geriatric patients, patients with GI obstruction or ileus, patients with GI bleeding, patients with decreased gastric motility) • The amount of elemental calcium varies with the product and calcium formulation selected (i.e., elemental calcium varies based on product) • Monitor serum calcium and serum phosphate • Increased monitoring is necessary if used in patients with nephrolithiasis or hypercalciuria • Recommend administering with vitamin D to increase calcium absorption • Administer with food to increase absorption • Separate from iron to avoid lowered iron absorption Contraindications: • Hypercalcemia (hyperparathyroidism, hypercalcemia of malignancy, sarcoidosis)
Generic Name Charcoal, activated **Brand Name** Actidose-Aqua Char-Flo EZ Char Kerr Insta-Char (PD)	Digestive aid (capsules and tablets only) Poison ingestion management when gastrointestinal decontamination is recommended Effective with chemicals weighing 100 to 1000 daltons	**Usual oral dose:** 5 to 10 times the estimated weight of the drug or chemical ingested or 50 to 100 g per dose; dosages can be repeated, as needed, every 4 to 6 hours until symptoms of toxicity subside and/or serum drug concentrations have returned to a nontoxic level 25 to 100 g as a single dose, or followed by 25 to 50 g every 4 hours	• Contact poison control prior to use (to verify the appropriateness for the chemical involved in the poisoning and recommended dose of charcoal) • May cause nausea and vomiting: can give an IV antiemetic to reduce this risk • May give via nasogastric (NG) tube • Use with caution in patients with decreased bowel peristalsis: ensure bowel sounds are present • Co-administration with cathartics (i.e., sorbitol, mannitol, magnesium sulfate) is not recommended; may increase risk of fluid/electrolyte abnormalities • Ensure entire amount in container is given; agitate the container before use, rinse with water, and give the entire dose to the patient • Mix 1 g of charcoal with at least 8 mL of water • Store in a closed container • Most effective when given within 30 to 60 minutes of ingestion of poison • Monitor bowel sounds

Drug Name	FDA-Approved Indications	Adult Dosage Range	Precautions and Clinical Pearls
Generic Name Magnesium carbonate/ aluminum hydroxide **Brand Name** Acid Gone Alenic Alka Gaviscon Genaton (PD)	Symptomatic relief of dyspepsia, pyrosis (heartburn), or symptoms associated with gastroesophageal reflux disease (GERD)	**Usual oral dose:** Oral liquid: 15 to 30 mL up to 4 times per day 1 to 3 hours after meals and at bedtime (MDD: 120 mL per day) Chewable tablets: Chew 2 to 4 tablets up to 4 times per day (MDD: 16 tablets per day)	• Use with caution in patients with sodium-restricted diets such as those with heart failure; ulcerative colitis, colostomy, diverticulitis, or ileostomy; fecal impaction or GI obstruction; or chronic diarrhea • Can increase or decrease the rate and extent of absorption of other medications; refer to PI for specific drug interactions • Monitor magnesium Contraindications: • Renal disease (renal failure and severe renal impairment)
Generic Name Magnesium citrate **Brand Name** Citroma (PD)	Bowel preparation prior to surgery Intermittent use as a laxative to treat acute constipation	**Usual oral dose:** 150 to 300 mL once or in divided doses	• Use with caution in patients with renal impairment due to hypermagnesemia • Should not be used to treat chronic constipation due to the potential to create electrolyte imbalances • Use with caution in patients with myasthenia gravis or other neuromuscular diseases and in elderly patients • To improve taste, chill just before use; refer to PI for storage recommendations • Administer with 8 ounces of water • Some products contain potassium and/or sodium • Discard the remainder of solution in 24 hours Contraindications: • Presence of rectal GI bleeding
Generic Name Magnesium hydroxide **Brand Name** Dulcolax Milk of Magnesia Pedia-Lax Phillips (PD)	Occasional constipation Symptoms of hyperacidity	Dose based on indication for use and patient's clinical response **Illustrative oral dose for antacid:** 400 mg/5 mL: 5 to 15 mL as needed up to 4 times per day 311 mg/tablet: 2 to 4 tablets every 4 hours, up to 4 times per day	• Use with caution in patients with renal impairment, especially creatinine clearance (CrCl) less than 30 mL/min, due to risk of hypermagnesemia • Use with caution in patients with myasthenia gravis or other neuromuscular diseases and in elderly patients • Dilute with water before giving to the patient; follow administration with 8 ounces of water • May contain sodium

Generic Name Magnesium oxide **Brand Name** Mag-200 Mag Ox Uro-Mag (PD)	Dietary supplement Symptoms of acid indigestion and upset stomach Occasional constipation	Dose based on indication for use and patient's clinical response **Illustrative oral dose for laxative in elemental magnesium:** 2 to 4 caplets at bedtime or in divided doses (1000 to 2000 mg)	• Use with caution in patients with renal impairment due to hypermagnesemia • Use with caution in patients with myasthenia gravis or other neuromuscular diseases and in elderly patients • Take with food and 8 ounces of water • 400 mg magnesium oxide = 24 mg elemental magnesium = 19.9 mEq magnesium
Generic Name Magnesium trisilicate/ aluminum hydroxide **Brand Name** Alenic Alka Gaviscon Genaton	Symptomatic relief of dyspepsia, pyrosis (heartburn), or symptoms associated with GERD	**Usual oral dose:** Chew and swallow 2 to 4 tablets up to 4 times per day after meals or at bedtime (MDD:16 tablets per day)	• Use with caution in patients with sodium-restricted diets such as those with heart failure; ulcerative colitis, colostomy, diverticulitis, or ileostomy; fecal impaction or GI obstruction; or chronic diarrhea • Use with caution in elderly patients • Administer with a glass of water • Can increase or decrease the rate and extent of absorption of other medications; refer to PI for specific drug interactions • Monitor magnesium Contraindications: • Renal disease, including renal failure and severe renal impairment
Generic Name Sodium bicarbonate **Brand Name** Alka-Seltzer Heartburn Relief (PD)	Management of metabolic acidosis Gastric hyperacidity Overdose of certain medications, such as antidepressants and aspirin As an alkalizing agent for urine Hyperkalemia	Dose based on indication for use and patient's clinical response **Illustrative oral dose as an antacid:** 325 mg to 2 g 1 to 4 times per day	• Use with caution in patients with cirrhosis, edema, heart failure, or renal impairment • Administer oral preparations 1 to 3 hours after meals • Not the antacid of choice in elderly patients due to its sodium content • Available for parenteral administration for other acute care indications; refer to PI • Monitor: IV infusion site and for signs and symptoms of fluid retention Contraindications: • Hypocalcemia • Metabolic alkalosis

Antidiarrheal and Antiflatulence Agents

Antidiarrheal Agents

Drug Name	FDA-Approved Indications	Adult Dosage Range	Precautions and Clinical Pearls
Generic Name Bismuth salts **Brand Name** Bismatrol Diotame Kaopectate Kao-Tin Pepto-Bismol Multiple formulations are available for use (chewables, caplets, suspension)	Nonspecific diarrhea Gastric distress of the upper stomach (dyspepsia, pyrosis, nausea)	**Usual oral dose for dyspepsia:** 525 mg every 30 to 60 minutes *or* 1050 mg every hour as needed for up to 2 days for diarrhea (MDD: 4200 mg per day)	• May contain potassium, sodium, or phenylalanine; use with caution in patients with certain diet restrictions • Counsel patients that a temporary darkening of stool or the tongue can occur • Increased risk of bleeding (see universal prescribing alerts for salicylate NSAID in the Central Nervous System Agents chapter) • May increase uric acid level • Drug interactions may require dose adjustment or avoidance of certain drug combinations • Monitor serum salicylate concentration • Age-specific avoidance is required due to the potential for Reye's syndrome; refer to PI Contraindications: • GI bleeding • Hematologic disease • Salicylate hypersensitivity • Hearing impairment; tinnitus may result from toxicity
Generic Name Diphenoxylate/atropine **Brand Name** Lomotil (BL) (PD)	Adjunctive medication in the management of diarrhea	**Usual oral dose:** 5 mg 3 to 4 times per day; reduce to 2.5 mg 2 to 3 times per day, if needed; discontinue as soon as possible If no improvement after 2 days for acute diarrhea or 10 days for chronic diarrhea at the maximum dose, therapy is likely to be ineffective	• Use with caution in patients with advanced hepatorenal disease, abnormal hepatic function, renal or hepatic impairment, or acute ulcerative colitis; may cause dehydration or electrolyte imbalance • Caution patients about driving or operating heavy machinery due to central nervous system (CNS) depression • Overdose can result in severe CNS depression, including respiratory depression, coma, and death • DEA-controlled substance (synthetic opiate agonist) • Monitor: signs of severe anticholinergic effects, number and consistency of stools, fluid and electrolyte loss, hypotension, respiratory depression Contraindications: • Obstructive jaundice • Diarrhea associated with pseudomembranous enterocolitis or enterotoxin-producing bacteria

Generic Name Lactobacillus acidophilus **Brand Name** Bacid Lactinex Floranex Florajen Many others	Dietary supplement Probiotic that may be beneficial for a variety of ailments/disease states that affect the gut's normal flora; promotes normal gut flora	Dose based on indication for use and product selected; refer to the manufacturer's product label	• Do not use if the patient has an infection or intestinal damage or is immunocompromised • Discontinue if high fever develops • Usually stored in the refrigerator: check the manufacturer's recommendations • Dietary supplement: lacks rigorous trial data
Generic Name Loperamide **Brand Name** Anti-Diarrheal Diamode Imodium A-D QT PD	OTC labeling: control of symptoms of diarrhea, including traveler's diarrhea Control and symptomatic relief of chronic diarrhea associated with inflammatory bowel disease and acute nonspecific diarrhea; reduce volume of ileostomy discharge	**Usual oral dose:** 4 mg once, then 2 mg after each loose stool (MDD: 16 mg per day) Titrate maintenance dose down if used for chronic diarrhea	• Avoid use as primary therapy for acute dysentery (bloody stools with high fever), acute ulcerative colitis, bacterial enterocolitis, and pseudomembranous colitis due to broad-spectrum antibiotic use • Discontinue if the following occur: constipation, abdominal pain or distension (especially in AIDS), bloody stool, ileus, inhibition of peristalsis • Use with caution in patients with hepatic impairment • Use with caution in patients predisposed to dehydration (i.e., elderly); may contain sodium; monitor for signs and symptoms of dehydration • CNS effects: caution patients about driving or operating heavy machinery due to potential dizziness and drowsiness
Generic Name Opium preparations **Brand Name** Paregoric Opium tincture ■ PD	Treatment of diarrhea	Dose based on indication for use and patient's clinical response **Illustrative oral dose:** Paregoric (0.4 mg/mL anhydrous morphine): 2 to 4 mg 1 to 4 times per day	• Use with caution in patients with asthma, severe prostatic hypertrophy, hepatic disease, or history of opiate dependence • Morphine is an opioid agonist and has abuse potential; toxicity may result in CNS depression and respiratory depression • Dependence may develop with extended use • DEA-controlled substance Associated with: • All of the universal prescribing alerts associated with opiate agonists; refer to the Central Nervous System Agents chapter
Antiflatulence Agents			
Drug Name	**FDA-Approved Indications**	**Adult Dosage Range**	**Precautions and Clinical Pearls**
Generic Name Simethicone **Brand Name** Equalizer Gas Relief	Relief of pressure, bloating, fullness, and discomfort of gastrointestinal gas	**Usual oral dose:** 40 to 125 mg 4 times per day after meals and at bedtime as needed (MDD: 500 mg per day)	• Products contain calcium; use with caution in patients with hypercalcemia or hypercalciuria • Shake suspension before use; may mix with 30 mL of liquid, such as water • Let the strips dissolve on the tongue • To help reduce symptoms of gastrointestinal gas, avoid carbonated drinks and gas-forming foods

Drug Name	FDA-Approved Indications	Adult Dosage Range	Precautions and Clinical Pearls
Gas-X GasAid Mytab Gas Phazyme Others (PD)			

Cathartics and Laxatives

Anthraquinone Laxatives

Universal prescribing alerts:

- A group of laxatives that includes the plant-derived compounds aloe, cascara sagrada, frangula, and senna.
- See individual components for detail.

Drug Name	FDA-Approved Indications	Adult Dosage Range	Precautions and Clinical Pearls
Generic Name Bisacodyl **Brand Name** Dulcolax Fleet Bisacodyl Others	Relief of occasional constipation To prepare patients for radiologic examination or preoperative bowel preparation	**Usual oral dose:** 5 to 15 mg per day **Rectal dose:** 10 mg suppository or enema once daily	• Precautions: GI pain/obstruction/perforation, appendicitis, toxic megacolon or colitis, diverticulitis, nausea or vomiting • Stimulant laxatives are the most likely laxative agents to cause GI irritation or fluid/electrolyte loss • Discontinue if diarrhea develops • Do not administer within 1 hour of antacids, milk, or dairy products • Take the evening before desired bowel movement • More rapid results will result if taken on an empty stomach • Avoid use for longer than 1 week without physician recommendations (suppository and/or oral tablet may be used up to three times per week) • Unwrap and moisten suppository before use Absolute contraindications: • Dysphagia • GI bleeding
Generic Name Senna Sennosides	Short-term treatment of constipation Evacuation of the colon for bowel or rectal examinations	**Usual oral dose for constipation:** Sennosides 15 mg once or twice daily (MDD:34.4mg senna)	• Not recommended for use in patients experiencing stomach pain, nausea, vomiting, or a sudden change in bowel movements that lasts longer than 2 weeks • Avoid chronic use in elderly patients • Administer at bedtime with a full glass of water for bowel evacuation 6 to 12 hours later

Brand Name Senexon SennaGen SenoSol Senokot (PD)			• For more rapid results, administer on an empty stomach • Monitor: fluid/electrolyte imbalance, hypotension Contraindications: • Diarrhea or loose stools • Abdominal pain • GI obstruction or bleeding • Hemorrhoids

Stool Softeners, Lubricant Laxatives, and Others

Drug Name	FDA-Approved Indications	Adult Dosage Range	Precautions and Clinical Pearls
Generic Name Docusate calcium **Brand Name** Colace Many more (PD)	Prevention of straining during defecation and constipation Relief of occasional constipation	**Usual oral dose:** 50 to 240 mg per day (MDD: 240 mg per day)	• Ensure adequate fluid intake; mix oral liquid with milk or fruit juice to prevent throat irritation • Monitor: occasional rectal exams with impaired rectal function Contraindications: • When used for self-medication, do not use for longer than 7 days • When abdominal pain, nausea, or vomiting is present • Concomitantly with oral mineral oil
Generic Name Docusate sodium **Brand Name** Surfac Many more (PD)	See docusate calcium	**Usual oral dose:** 50 to 360 mg once daily or in divided doses **Rectal administration:** 283 mg (one enema) inserted 1 to 3 times per day	• Ensure adequate fluid intake; mix oral liquid with milk or fruit juice to prevent throat irritation • Discontinue rectal use if rash develops around the anus or if there is resistance upon insertion • Monitor: occasional rectal exams with impaired rectal function

Bulk-Forming Laxatives

Drug Name	FDA-Approved Indications	Adult Dosage Range	Precautions and Clinical Pearls
Generic Name Malt soup extract **Brand Name** Maltsupex (PD)	Bulk-forming laxative to treat constipation	**Usual oral dose:** 4 tablets 4 times per day, with liquid	• Not recommended for use in appendicitis, acute surgical abdomen, fecal impaction, intestinal obstruction, and unexplained abdominal pain • Dilute powder and oral liquid in 8 ounces of water before taking

Drug Name	FDA-Approved Indications	Adult Dosage Range	Precautions and Clinical Pearls
Generic Name Methylcellulose **Brand Name** Citrucel Soluble Fiber Therapy (PD)	Used as an adjunct in treating constipation	**Usual oral dose:** 2 caplets up to 6 times per day 2 g powder (1 tablespoon) dissolved in 8 ounces of cold water up to 3 times per day	• Some products contain phenylalanine, potassium, and/or sodium • Take with 8 ounces of water Contraindications: • Appendicitis • Esophageal stricture or perforation • Dysphagia • GI obstruction or ileus • Unexplained abdominal pain
Generic Name Psyllium **Brand Name** Evac Geri-Mucil Konsyl MetaFiber Metamucil MultiHealth Fiber Reguloid Sorbulax Others (PD)	Occasional constipation Reduce risk of coronary heart disease	**Usual oral dose:** 1 teaspoonful, 1 tablespoonful or 1 premeasured packet per day dissolved in 8 ounces of liquid and consumed 1 to 3 times per day (maximum per day 7.2 g soluble dietary fiber)	• Use with caution in patients with esophageal strictures, ulcers, stenosis, difficulty swallowing, or intestinal adhesions • Elderly patients are more likely to have inadequate fluid intake, which increases the risk of fecal impaction • Mix powder with at least 8 ounces of water or juice • When used to decrease risk of coronary heart disease, soluble fiber intake should be 7 g or more per day. along with a low-cholesterol and low-fat diet • Inhaling dust may cause runny nose, watery eyes, and wheezing • Some products may contain potassium, calcium, soy lecithin, or sodium • Per the manufacturer, administration of other prescribed oral drugs should be separated from the administration of psyllium by at least 2 hours • 3.4 g psyllium hydrophilic mucilloid = 2 g soluble fiber Contraindications: • Fecal impaction • GI obstruction

Hyperosmotic Laxatives

Universal prescribing alerts:

- A laxative class that includes sorbitol, polyethylene glycol, saline, and glycerin.
- See individual drugs for more information.

Drug Name	FDA-Approved Indications	Adult Dosage Range	Precautions and Clinical Pearls
Generic Name Glycerin **Brand Name** Fleet Liquid Glycerin Supp	Relief of occasional constipation Relief of mild mouth/throat irritation and protection of irritated areas	**Usual rectal dose for constipation:** 1 suppository inserted rectally once daily as needed or as directed	• May cause burning sensation in the rectum with use of a suppository • Do not swallow excessive amounts of oral products • Retain suppository high in the rectum for 15 minutes • Protect suppositories from heat to prevent melting

Pedia-Lax Sani-Supp Others (PD)			Contraindications: • When used for self-medication, do not use for longer than 7 days • When abdominal pain, nausea, or vomiting is present • Concomitantly with oral mineral oil
Generic Name Magnesium citrate **Brand Name** Citroma (PD)	For intermittent use to treat acute constipation For use as a bowel preparation prior to surgery or radiologic procedure	**Usual oral dose:** 195 to 300 mL once or in divided doses	• Saline cathartics should not be used in patients with history of acute abdominal pain, appendicitis, colitis, diabetes, diverticulitis, fecal impaction, GI obstruction, GI perforation, toxic megacolon, or vomiting • Use with caution in patients with renal impairment (hypermagnesemia) • Use with caution in patients with myasthenia gravis or other neuromuscular diseases and in elderly patients • Chill solution just prior to administration to increase palatability; administer each dose with 8 ounces of water; refer to PI for storage recommendations • Some products contain potassium and/or sodium • Discard the remainder of the solution within 24 hours of opening • 1 g magnesium citrate = 160 mg elemental magnesium = 13 mEq magnesium Contraindications: • For self-medication if on a low-salt diet • GI bleeding
Generic Name Magnesium hydroxide **Brand Name** Dulcolax Milk of Magnesia (PD)	Occasional constipation Dyspepsia or pyrosis	Dose based on indication for use and patient's clinical response **Illustrative oral doses:** Laxative: 400 mg/5 mL: 15 to 60 mL per day once daily at bedtime or in divided doses	• Use with caution in patients with renal impairment, especially CrCl less than 30 mL/min, due to risk of hypermagnesemia • Use with caution in patients with myasthenia gravis or other neuromuscular diseases and in elderly patients • Dilute with water before giving this medication; follow administration with 8 ounces of water • Some products contain sodium • Monitor magnesium levels
Generic Name Mineral oil **Brand Name** Fleet Oil (BL) (PD)	Relief of occasional constipation Rectal: additional indications for relief of fecal impaction and removal of barium sulfate residues following barium use	**Usual oral dose:** 30 to 90 mL in 24 hours at bedtime or in divided doses **Rectal:** 120 mL as a single dose; do not use more than one enema per day	• With extended use, may decrease the absorption of fat-soluble vitamins • Administer on an empty stomach • Shake the suspension before use; may administer with water, milk, or cocoa • Avoid use: bedridden patients and the elderly (has potential to be aspirated) • Use for longer than 1 week or if difficulty swallowing

Drug Name	FDA-Approved Indications	Adult Dosage Range	Precautions and Clinical Pearls
Generic Name Polyethylene glycol 3350 **Brand Name** Gavilax Glycolax Healthylax Miralax Pegylax (PD)	Occasional constipation	**Usual oral dose:** 17 g (1 heaping tablespoon) dissolved in 4 to 8 ounces of beverage once daily	• Can cause electrolyte imbalance with extended use or frequent dosing • Use with caution in patients with renal impairment • Do not use for longer than 1 to 2 weeks unless directed by the healthcare provider • Can dissolve in water, juice, soda, coffee, or tea • Discontinue if severe diarrhea or bleeding develops • Avoid use in patients predisposed to aspiration (those with impaired gag reflex or dysphagia) Contraindications: • Bowel obstruction • Renal disease if self-medicating
Generic Name Saline laxatives **Brand Name** Ceo-Two Fleet Enema Fleet Enema Extra OsmoPrep Others ■	Constipation Bowel cleansing Poisonings	**Illustrative oral dose as laxative:** 15 mL as a single dose; maximum single daily dose: 45 mL	• Use with caution with in patients with heart failure, electrolyte disturbance, chronic constipation, inflammatory bowel disease, renal impairment, or seizure disorder • Oral formulation: take on an empty stomach; dilute dose with 8 oz of water and follow dose with 8 oz of water; do not repeat dose within 24 hours Associated with: • Risk of acute phosphate nephropathy may be increased in patients with increased age (older than 55 years), hypovolemia, increased bowel transit time (e.g., bowel obstruction), active colitis, baseline renal disease, or known or suspected electrolyte disturbances (e.g., dehydration) • Drug interactions may require dose adjustments or avoidance of certain drug combinations (i.e., drugs that affect renal perfusion or function (e.g., diuretics, angiotensin-converting enzyme [ACE] inhibitors, angiotensin II receptor antagonists, possibly NSAIDs)
Generic Name Sodium phosphates **Brand Name** Fleet Enema Fleet Enema Extra LaCrosse Complete OsmoPrep ■ (QT) (PD)	Oral solution: short-term constipation Oral tablets: bowel cleansing before colonoscopy IV: phosphate source in parenteral nutrition or in large-volume IVs; treatment and prevention of hypophosphatemia	Dose based on indication for use, product formulation selected, and patient's clinical response **Illustrative oral dose for constipation:** Solution: 15 mL as a single dose (maximum single daily dose: 45 mL) **Laxative rectal dose:** 4.5 oz enema as a single dose	• Prolongation of QT interval has been reported (associated with hypokalemia and hypocalcemia) • Use with caution in patients with heart failure, electrolyte disturbances, GI disorders including inflammatory bowel disease, renal impairment, or seizure disorder • May precipitate if mixed with calcium; ensure compatibility before using with calcium • Parenteral product may contain aluminum; may become toxic at high doses and can cause CNS and bone toxicity (do not administer IV push). Specific monitoring required for parenteral administration • Take on an empty stomach

			• Monitor: electrolytes, calcium, phosphorus, blood urea nitrogen (BUN), creatinine if at risk for renal nephropathy, seizure, or history of electrolyte abnormalities; ECG if at risk for QTc prolongation Associated with: • Risk of acute phosphate nephropathy may be increased in patients with increased age (older than 55 years), hypovolemia, increased bowel transit time (e.g., bowel obstruction), active colitis, baseline renal disease, or known or suspected electrolyte disturbances (e.g., dehydration) • Patients receiving drugs that affect renal perfusion or function (e.g., diuretics, ACE inhibitors, angiotensin II receptor antagonists, possibly NSAIDs) may also be at increased risk
Generic Name Sorbitol	For urologic irrigation during transurethral surgery Constipation	**Usual oral dose for constipation:** 30 to 45 mL (as 70% solution) once daily **Rectal enema:** 120 mL (as 25% to 30% solution)	• Use with caution in patients with severe cardiopulmonary disease, renal impairment, or inability to metabolize sorbitol • Monitor for fluid overload and/or serum electrolyte disturbances following large volumes Contraindications • A urologic irrigation solution is available; however, is contraindicated in patients with anuria (use with caution in patients with severe renal disease/dysfunction)

Antiemetic Agents

Antihistamine Agents

Drug Name	FDA-Approved Indications	Adult Dosage Range	Precautions and Clinical Pearls
Generic Name Dimenhydrinate **Brand Name** Dramamine Driminate Motion Sickness (BL) (PD)	Prevention and treatment of motion sickness	**Usual oral dose for motion sickness:** 50 to 100 mg every 4 to 6 hours (MDD: 400 mg per day) **IM or IV dose:** 50 mg every 4 hours; maximum 100 mg every 4 hours For prevention, administer 30 to 60 minutes before exposure	• Caution patients about driving or operating heavy machinery due to CNS depression; may also increase risk of seizure • Universal prescribing alerts for anticholinergic medications (i.e., use with caution in patients with asthma, cardiovascular disease, increased intraocular pressure, prostatic hyperplasia/urinary obstruction; refer to the Autonomic Agents chapter for additional details) • Use caution in patients with pyloroduodenal obstruction, thyroid dysfunction, seizures, or hepatic impairment • Can cause increased drowsiness when combined with other sedative medications or ethanol use

Drug Name	FDA-Approved Indications	Adult Dosage Range	Precautions and Clinical Pearls
Generic Name Meclizine **Brand Name** Antivert Dramamine Less Drowsy Motion-Time Travel Sickness UniVert BL PD	Prevention and treatment of motion sickness Management of vertigo due to vestibular system dysfunction	**Usual oral dose for motion sickness:** 25 to 50 mg 1 hour before travel; can repeat in 24 hours **Usual oral dose for vertigo:** 25 to 100 mg daily in divided doses MDD: 100 mg	• Caution patients about driving or operating heavy machinery due to CNS depression • Universal prescribing alerts for anticholinergic medications (i.e., use with caution in patients with asthma, cardiovascular disease, increased intraocular pressure, prostatic hyperplasia/urinary obstruction; refer to the Autonomic Agents chapter for additional details) • Use caution in patients with pyloric/duodenal obstruction, hepatic impairment, or renal impairment • Use with caution in elderly patients • Discontinue if no response occurs in 1 to 2 weeks when used for vertigo
Generic Name Trimethobenzamide **Brand Name** Tigan PD	PONV Nausea due to gastroenteritis	**Usual oral dose:** 300 mg 3 to 4 times per day **IM dose:** 200 mg 3 to 4 times per day	• May cause adverse CNS effects such as drowsiness, seizures or coma, extrapyramidal symptoms, and skin reactions • Monitor: renal function at baseline and use with caution in patients with renal impairment; reduced dose may be necessary • Use caution in patients who are dehydrated and/ or have electrolyte imbalance • Inject IM injection into upper outer quadrant of the gluteal muscle • Not recommended for use in patients with Reye's syndrome, appendicitis, or encephalopathy due to masking of condition Contraindications: • In patients with blood dyscrasia or evidence of sensitization or jaundice with past use • Specific age-related contraindications; refer to PI
Prochlorperazine	Refer to the Central Nervous System Agents chapter.		

$5HT_3$ Receptor Antagonists			
Drug Name	**FDA-Approved Indications**	**Adult Dosage Range**	**Precautions and Clinical Pearls**
Generic Name Dolasetron **Brand Name** Anzemet QT PD	Oral: prevention of nausea and vomiting with moderately emetogenic cancer chemotherapy IV: prevention and treatment of PONV	Dose based on indication for use, product formulation selected, and patient's clinical response	• May cause serotonin syndrome, usually when used with other serotonergic agents • Injection may be diluted in apple or apple–grape juice and taken orally if the tablet cannot be swallowed • If oral prophylaxis dose has failed, do not repeat dose

		Illustrative oral dose: 100 mg within 1 hour of chemotherapy **Illustrative parenteral dose postoperative N/V:** IV: 12.5 mg as a single dose	• Efficacy for chemotherapy treatment is increased when given with dexamethasone 20 mg • Monitor: ECG and QT (in patients with renal impairment, patients with cardiovascular disease, elderly patients, those at risk of developing hypokalemia or hypomagnesemia); potassium; magnesium
Generic Name Granisetron **Brand Name** Sancuso Patch Sustol ER injection ▲ QT PD	CINV and CINV prophylaxis Prevention of radiation-associated nausea and vomiting	**Usual oral dose:** 2 mg once daily 1 hour before chemotherapy/radiation therapy *or* 1 mg twice daily, with the second dose given 12 hours later **Illustrative parenteral dose for CINV:** IV: 10 mcg/kg 30 minutes before chemotherapy **Usual transdermal dose:** Apply patch 24 to 48 hours before chemotherapy; may be worn up to 7 days	• Can cause a dose-dependent increase in ECG intervals that rarely leads to arrhythmia; avoid use in patients already at risk for QTc prolongation • Drug interactions may require dose adjustments or avoidance of certain drug combinations • Use with caution in patients at risk for cardiac conduction abnormalities • May mask progressive ileus or gastric distension • Extended release formulation may release drug for 5 to 7 days, monitor bowel sounds and consider optimizing bowel regimens in high-risk patients • May cause serotonin syndrome, usually when used with other serotonergic agents • Apply patch to clean, dry, intact skin on the upper outer arm • Do not cut the patch; protect the site from sunlight during use and 10 days after; do not apply heat • SQ doses are also available, refer to PI
Generic Name Ondansetron **Brand Name** Zofran Zofran ODT Zuplenz ■ QT PD	CINV Radiotherapy-associated nausea and vomiting Prevention of PONV	Dose based on indication for use, product formulation selected, and patient's clinical response **Illustrative oral dose for prevention of PONV:** 16 mg administered 1 hour prior to induction of anesthesia **Illustrative parenteral dose for PONV:** IM: 4 mg as single dose	• Monitor: ECG in high-risk patients, potassium, magnesium. Can cause a dose-dependent increase in ECG intervals that rarely leads to arrhythmia; avoid use in patients already at risk for QTc prolongation • Rarely causes serotonin syndrome, usually when used with other serotonergic agents • Use with caution in patients with hepatic impairment • Do not remove orally disintegrating tablets from the blister package or films from the pouch until ready for use • May mask progressive ileus or gastric distension • Do not give as needed—give prophylactically • Drug interactions may require dose adjustments or avoidance of certain drug combinations; consult the PI or drug interaction database

Drug Name	FDA-Approved Indications	Adult Dosage Range	Precautions and Clinical Pearls
Generic Name Palonosetron **Brand Name** Aloxi QT PD	CINV prophylaxis Prevention of PONV for up to 24 hours after surgery	**Usual parenteral dose for CINV:** IV: 0.25 mg 30 minutes before chemotherapy	• Does not significantly increase QTc prolongation unlike other $5HT_3$ antagonists; can decrease heart rate • Use with caution in the presence of or potential for cardiac conduction abnormalities (i.e., QTc prolongation, electrolyte abnormalities) • May cause serotonin syndrome, usually when used with other serotonergic agents • Flush the IV line with normal saline prior to and following administration • Use prophylactically only
Miscellaneous Antiemetic Agents			
Drug Name	**FDA-Approved Indications**	**Dosage Range**	**Precautions and Clinical Pearls**
Generic Name Aprepitant (oral) Fosaprepitant (IV) **Brand Name** Emend PD	Prevention of CINV Prevention of PONV	Dose based on indication for use, route of administration, and patient's clinical response **Illustrative oral dose for prevention of PONV:** 40 mg within 3 hours prior to anesthesia induction	• Monitor LFTs: has not been evaluated in patients with severe hepatic impairment or insufficiency; use with caution in this patient population • Infusion reactions have been reported. • Drug interactions may require a dose adjustment or avoidance of the combination; avoid grapefruit juice (including with the aprepitant concentration)
Generic Name Dronabinol **Brand Name** Marinol	Promotes appetite stimulation in patients with AIDS suffering from anorexia Treatment of nausea and vomiting associated with cancer chemotherapy when other agents have failed	**Usual oral dose for appetite stimulation:** 2.5 mg twice daily initially, increase to maximum of 20 mg per day Administer twice-daily dosing before lunch and dinner; administer single doses in the evening or at bedtime	• Monitor: CNS adverse effects, heart rate, blood pressure, behavioral changes • Can cause hypertension, hypotension, syncope, or tachycardia • Can exacerbate preexisting psychiatric disorders or lower the seizure threshold • DEA Schedule controlled substance • Dependence and tolerance may occur with extended use; use with caution in patients with a history of substance abuse • Caution patients about driving or operating heavy machinery due to CNS depression • Do not abruptly discontinue the medication due to potential withdrawal symptoms
Generic Name Nabilone **Brand Name** Cesamet PD	Treatment of refractory nausea and vomiting due to cancer chemotherapy	**Usual oral dose:** 1 to 2 mg twice daily (maximum: 6 mg divided in 3 doses daily)	• Monitor: blood pressure, heart rate, signs and symptoms of abuse or misuse • Use with caution in patients with cardiovascular disease due to the potential for tachycardia or orthostatic hypotension • Caution patients about driving or operating heavy machinery due to CNS depression • DEA Schedule controlled substance

			• Use with caution in patients with history of substance abuse due to the potential for tolerance and dependence • Give 1 to 3 hours before chemotherapy • Adverse psychotic reactions may develop as long as 3 days after discontinuation • Can administer a dose the night before chemotherapy and continue for 48 hours after chemotherapy • Use caution in renal and hepatic impairment
Phenothiazines	Refer to the Central Nervous System Agents chapter.		
Promethazine	Refer to the Central Nervous System Agents chapter.		
Scopolamine	Refer to the Autonomic Agents chapter.		
Antiulcer Agents and Acid Suppressants			
Amoxicillin	Refer to the Anti-infective Agents chapter.		
Antacids	Refer to the Antacids and Adsorbents section.		
Clarithromycin	Refer to the Anti-infective Agents chapter.		
Metronidazole	Refer to the Anti-infective Agents chapter.		
Tetracycline	Refer to the Anti-infective Agents chapter.		

Histamine H_2 Antagonists			
Drug Name	**FDA-Approved Indications**	**Adult Dosage Range**	**Precautions and Clinical Pearls**
Generic Name Cimetidine **Brand Name** Tagamet BL PD	**Common indications for use:** Duodenal ulcer Gastric ulcer GERD Pathological hypersecretory conditions Heartburn	Dosage depends on indication and clinical response **Illustrative oral dose for prevention of heartburn:** 200 to 400 mg per day	• Do not use if patient has trouble swallowing, vomiting with blood, or bloody stools • Can cause reversible confusion, especially in elderly patients and patients with renal or hepatic impairment • May cause vitamin B_{12} deficiency with prolonged use • Drug interactions may require dose adjustments or avoidance of certain drug combinations; consult the PI or drug interaction database • Caution in patients with renal or hepatic impairment
Generic Name Famotidine **Brand Name** Pepcid QT BL PD	**Common indications for use:** Maintenance and treatment of duodenal ulcer Treatment of GERD Active benign gastric ulcer Pathological hypersecretory conditions	Dosage depends on indication and clinical response **Illustrative dose for heartburn, indigestion, sour stomach:** Heartburn, indigestion, sour stomach: 10 to 20 mg every 12 hours; dose may be taken 15 to 60 minutes before meals	• Reversible confusion has been noted, especially with elderly patients and patients with renal or hepatic impairment • Prolonged QTc interval has been reported • May cause vitamin B_{12} deficiency with prolonged use • Use with caution in patients with moderate to severe renal impairment (CrCl less than 50 mL per minute)
Generic Name Nizatidine **Brand Name** Axid BL PD	**Common indications for use:** Treatment and maintenance therapy of duodenal ulcer Treatment of benign gastric ulcer Treatment of GERD	Dosage depends on indication and clinical response **Illustrative dose for GERD:** 150 mg twice daily	• Use with caution in patients with hepatic or renal impairment • Prolonged use may cause vitamin B_{12} deficiency
Generic Name Ranitidine **Brand Name** Zantac Others BL PD	**Common indications for use:** Duodenal ulcer Erosive esophagitis Gastric ulcer GERD Pathological hypersecretory conditions Heartburn	Dosage depends on indication and clinical response **Illustrative dose for GERD:** 150 mg twice daily	• Do not use if the patient has trouble or pain when swallowing food, vomiting with blood, or bloody or dark stools • Rare cases of reversible confusion have occurred (usually in elderly patients, severely ill patients, or patients with hepatic or renal impairment) • Elevation in ALT has occurred at higher doses or prolonged therapy • Prolonged use may lead to vitamin B_{12} deficiency

Prostaglandins

Drug Name	FDA-Approved Indications	Adult Dosage Range	Precautions and Clinical Pearls
Generic Name Misoprostol **Brand Name** Cytotec ■	Prevention of NSAID-induced gastric ulcers	**Usual oral dose:** 200 mcg 4 times daily with food	• For use only in patients at high risk of complications from gastric ulcers or at high risk of developing gastric ulcers while taking NSAIDs • Adverse cardiovascular events have been reported • May exacerbate intestinal inflammation Associated with: • Review boxed warning before considering use in females

Protectants

Drug Name	FDA-Approved Indications	Adult Dosage Range	Precautions and Clinical Pearls
Generic Name Sucralfate **Brand Name** Carafate	Short-term management of duodenal ulcers (less than 8 weeks) Maintenance therapy for duodenal ulcers	**Usual oral dose:** 1 g 4 times per day before meals and at bedtime	• Use with caution in patients with renal impairment: sucralfate is an aluminum complex and can accumulate (caution in patients undergoing dialysis) • Use with caution in patients with cardiovascular disease • Hyperglycemia has been reported with use • Use with caution in patients with conditions that impair swallowing and in patients with altered gag/cough reflex; aspiration has been reported

Proton-Pump Inhibitors

Universal prescribing alerts:

- May increase osteoporosis-related fractures, especially when used long term.
- May increase risk of *C. difficile*–associated diarrhea.
- May increase risk of pneumonia in hospitalized patients.
- Hypomagnesemia and vitamin B_{12} deficiency may occur with long-term use.
- Common FDA-approved indications for use for all PPI agents: Gastroesophageal reflux disease (GERD), *H. pylori* eradication, Zollinger-Ellison syndrome, pyrosis (heartburn).
- Use PPIs with caution and, if possible, avoid long-term (more than 14 days) use in patients with congenital long QT syndrome, as they may be at higher risk for arrhythmias.

Drug Name	FDA-Approved Indications	Adult Dosage Range	Precautions and Clinical Pearls
Generic Name Dexlansoprazole **Brand Name** Dexilant ■ (BL) (PD)	Erosive esophagitis	Dose and duration are based on indication for use and patient's clinical response **Usual oral dose:** 30 to 60 mg per day	• Can be administered without regard to meals • Monitor: LFTs and serum magnesium

Drug Name	FDA-Approved Indications	Adult Dosage Range	Precautions and Clinical Pearls
Generic Name Esomeprazole **Brand Name** Nexium ■ (BL) (PD)	**Common indications for use:** Duodenal ulcer Dyspepsia Esophagitis GERD NSAID-induced ulcer prophylaxis Upper GI rebleeding prophylaxis	Dose and duration are based on indication for use and patient's clinical response **Usual oral dose for GERD:** 20 to 40 mg per day	• Administer on an empty stomach at least 60 minutes before meals; if taken once daily, administer before the first meal of the day • Monitor: LFTs and serum magnesium • Parenteral regimens are available
Generic Name Lansoprazole **Brand Name** Prevacid (BL)	**Common indications for use:** Duodenal ulcer Dyspepsia Esophagitis GERD Gastric ulcer NSAID-induced ulcer prophylaxis Upper GI rebleeding prophylaxis	Dose and duration are based on indication for use and patient's clinical response **Usual oral dose for GERD:** 15 to 30 mg per day	• Administer on an empty stomach 30 to 60 minutes before meals; if taken once daily, administer before the first meal of the day • Monitor: LFTs and serum magnesium
Generic Name Omeprazole **Brand Name** Prilosec (BL) (PD)	**Common indications for use:** Duodenal ulcer Dyspepsia Esophagitis GERD Gastric ulcer Multiple endocrine adenoma syndrome Systemic mastocytosis	Dose and duration are based on indication for use and patient's clinical response **Usual oral dose for GERD:** 20 to 40 mg per day	• Administer on an empty stomach 30 to 60 minutes before meals; if taken once daily, administer before the first meal of the day • Monitor: LFTs and serum magnesium • Asian patients may experience higher serum concentrations

Generic Name Pantoprazole **Brand Name** Protonix QT BL PD	Esophagitis Zollinger-Ellison syndrome	Dose and duration are based on indication for use and patient's clinical response **Illustrative oral dose for esophagitis:** 40 mg per day	• Administer on an empty stomach 30 to 60 minutes before meals; if taken once daily, administer before the first meal of the day • Available as oral tablet and IV • Monitor: LFTs and serum magnesium
Generic Name Rabeprazole **Brand Name** AcipHex AcipHex Sprinkle BL PD	**Common indications for use:** Duodenal ulcer Esophagitis	Dose and duration are based on indication for use and patient's clinical response **Usual dosage range:** 20 to 40 mg per day	• Administer on an empty stomach 30 to 60 minutes before meals; if taken once daily, administer before the first meal of the day • Monitor: LFTs and serum magnesium

Miscellaneous Gastrointestinal Agents

Anti-inflammatory Agents

Drug Name	FDA-Approved Indications	Adult Dosage Range	Precautions and Clinical Pearls
Generic Name Balsalazide **Brand Name** Colazal Giazo	Ulcerative colitis	Dose varies based on indication for use and formulation selected **Usual oral dose (capsule):** 2.25 g 3 times per day for up to 8 to 12 weeks	• Use with caution in patients with hepatic dysfunction • Use with caution in patients with pyloric stenosis • Use with caution in patients with renal impairment: renal toxicity has been observed • May worsen colitis symptoms following initiation of treatment • Blood dyscrasia has been reported with use • May cause an acute intolerance syndrome (cramping, acute abdominal pain, bloody diarrhea) • May cause staining of the teeth and tongue if the capsule is opened and sprinkled on food; swallow whole

Drug Name	FDA-Approved Indications	Adult Dosage Range	Precautions and Clinical Pearls
Generic Name Mesalamine **Brand Name** Apriso Asacol Canasa Delzicol Lialda Pentasa Rowasa PD	Ulcerative colitis	Dose varies based on indication for use and formulation selected **Illustrative oral dose for treatment with Pentasa:** 1 g 4 times per day	• Cardiac hypersensitivity effects have been reported • May cause an acute intolerance syndrome (cramping, abdominal pain, bloody diarrhea) • Renal impairment has been reported • Drug interactions may require dose adjustment or avoidance of certain drug combinations • Use with caution in elderly patients: postmarketing reports suggest an increase in blood dyscrasias in patients older than 65 years • Hepatic failure has been reported • Rowasa may stain contact surfaces
Generic Name Olsalazine **Brand Name** Dipentum PD	Ulcerative colitis	**Usual oral dose:** 1 g per day in 2 divided doses	• Use with caution in patients with severe allergies or asthma • Use with caution in patients with hepatic impairment • Use with caution in patients with renal impairment • May exacerbate symptoms of colitis • Diarrhea is a common adverse effect
Sulfasalazine	Refer to the Anti-infective Agents chapter.		

Cholelitholytic Agents

Drug Name	FDA-Approved Indications	Adult Dosage Range	Precautions and Clinical Pearls
Generic Name Chenodiol **Brand Name** Chenodal	Cholelithiasis (monotherapy for gallstone dissolution)	**Usual oral dose for gallstone dissolution:** Initial: 250 mg twice daily for the first 2 weeks, increasing by 250 mg daily each week thereafter until the recommended or maximum tolerated dose is achieved Maintenance: 13 to 16 mg/kg per day in 2 divided doses	• Drug-induced liver toxicity may occur (dose related): monitor serum aminotransferase levels recommended during therapy; avoid use in patients with preexisting hepatic impairment or elevated liver enzymes • Dose-related diarrhea may occur • Bile acids may increase the risk of colon cancer (conflicting evidence) • Potentially significant drug interactions may exist; consult the PI or drug interaction database • Monitor: cholecystogram or gallbladder ultrasound; liver function tests (LFTs); serum cholesterol Contraindications: • Known hepatocyte dysfunction • Bile ductal abnormalities (i.e., cirrhosis, obstruction, disease) • Cholangitis, cholestasis, gallbladder disease, biliary-GI fistula, and pancreatitis

Generic Name Ursodiol **Brand Name** Actigall Urso 250 Urso Forte	Tablets: Primary biliary cirrhosis Capsules (Actigall): Prevention of gallstone formation in obese patients who are undergoing rapid weight loss Dissolution of gallstone in patients with radiolucent, noncalcified stones less than 20 mm in diameter, in whom cholecystectomy is not optimal	Dose based on indication for use, product formulation selected, and patient's clinical response **Usual oral dose:** Actigall: 8 to 10 mg/kg per day in 2 to 3 divided doses (dissolution) or 300 mg twice daily (prevention) **Usual oral dose primary biliary cirrhosis:** Urso: 13 to 15 mg/kg per day in 2 to 4 divided doses (with food)	• To prevent biliary obstruction, maintain bile flow during treatment • Use with caution in patients with hepatic impairment • Safety for use is not established beyond 24 months • Administer aluminum-based antacids 2 hours after taking ursodiol • Administer ursodiol 5 hours after taking bile acid sequestrants • Administer Urso and Urso Forte with food. Indications for use are brand specific, refer to PI • Urso Forte can be split in half if needed and stored for 28 days (split tablets have a bitter taste) • Monitor:gallstone disease: alanine aminotransferase (ALT), aspartate aminotransferase (AST), sonogram, hepatic disease: liver function tests monthly for the first 3 months, then every 6 months or as needed Contraindications: • Calcified cholesterol stones; radiopaque stones, or radiolucent bile pigment stones • Unremitting acute cholecystitis, cholangitis, biliary obstruction, gallstone pancreatitis, or biliary-gastrointestinal fistula

Digestants			
Drug Name	**FDA-Approved Indications**	**Adult Dosage Range**	**Precautions and Clinical Pearls**
Generic Name Pancrelipase **Brand Name** Creon Pancreaze Pertzye Ultresa Viokace Zenpep (PD)	Pancreatic insufficiency (exocrine)	Adjust dose based on body weight, clinical symptoms, and stool fat content **Maximum oral dose for Creon, Zenpep, Pancreaze:** 10,000 lipase units/kg per day or less *or* less than 4,000 lipase units per gram dietary fat per day	• Products are derived from porcine pancreatic glands • Administer with meals or snacks, and swallow whole with a generous amount of liquid; delayed-release capsules may be opened and contents added to a small amount of acidic food such as applesauce • Available brand pancreatic enzyme products are not interchangeable • Use caution in diabetic patients and those with renal impairment • Dosing should not exceed the recommended maximum dose

Prokinetic Agents			
Drug Name	**FDA-Approved Indications**	**Adult Dosage Range**	**Precautions and Clinical Pearls**
Generic Name Cisapride **Brand Name** Propulsid ▲ ■ ■ QT PD	GERD	**Usual oral dose:** 10 mg 4 times per day at least 15 minutes before meals and at bedtime; may increase to 20 mg	• Serious cardiac arrhythmias have been reported • Drug interactions may require dose adjustment or avoidance of the combination • In March 2000, the FDA announced the manufacturer would voluntarily withdraw its product from the U.S. market due to reports of heart rhythm abnormalities; the drug is available to patients who meet specific eligibility criteria for a limited-access protocol • Potential benefits should be weighed against risks prior to administration Associated with: • Do not use (contraindicated) in patients with GI hemorrhage, mechanical obstruction, GI perforation, or any situation where GI motility stimulation is dangerous • Do not use (contraindicated) in patients with prolonged QT (QTc intervals greater than 450 ms), history of QT prolongation or family history of long QT, any significant bradycardia, renal failure, history of ventricular arrhythmias, ischemic heart disease, congestive heart failure, electrolyte disorders, respiratory failure, or any other predisposing factors
Generic Name Metoclopramide **Brand Name** Metozolv Reglan ■ BL QT	Diabetic gastroparesis Gastroesophageal reflux (GERD) Prevention of: Nausea and vomiting associated with emetogenic chemotherapy PONV Radiation therapy–induced nausea and vomiting	**Usual oral dose for GERD:** 10 mg up to 4 times per day, 30 minutes before meals or food and at bedtime for 2 to 8 weeks **Usual parenteral dose:** IM/IV: 10 mg over 1 to 2 minutes; 10 days of IV formulation may be necessary	• Use with caution in patients with hypertension • Neuroleptic malignant syndrome is rarely associated with use • Proarrhythmic effects are known; use with caution in patients with heart failure and renal impairment due to risk of QT prolongation • Use with caution in patients at risk for fluid overload • Patients with NADH-cytochrome b5 reductase deficiency are at increased risk of methemoglobinemia and/or sulfhemoglobinemia • May exacerbate symptoms of Parkinson's disease • Use with caution in patients with renal impairment • Abrupt discontinuation may result in withdrawal symptoms (dizziness, headache, nervousness) Contraindications: • Situations where GI motility may be dangerous, including mechanical GI obstruction, perforation, hemorrhage, and pheochromocytoma • History of seizure disorder, or other factors predisposing patient to increased risk Associated with: • Tardive dyskinesia; discontinue in patients who develop signs or symptoms • May cause extrapyramidal symptoms: acute dystonic reactions with initial 24 to 48 hours of use; risk is higher with higher doses and in specific age groups • Mental depression has occurred, with symptoms ranging from mild to severe

Miscellaneous Gastrointestinal Agents			
Drug Name	**FDA-Approved Indications**	**Adult Dosage Range**	**Precautions and Clinical Pearls**
Generic Name Alosetron **Brand Name** Lotronex	Irritable bowel syndrome (women)	**Usual oral dose for females:** Initial: 0.5 mg twice daily for 4 weeks; may be increased to 1 mg twice daily	• Use with caution in patients with mild to moderate hepatic impairment • Drug interactions may require dose adjustment or avoidance of certain drug combinations • Indicated only for women with severe diarrhea-predominant IBS who have not responded to conventional therapy Contraindications: • History of (or current) chronic or severe constipation, intestinal obstruction, toxic megacolon • History of ischemic colitis • Hepatic impairment • Hypercoagulable state Associated with: • The need to discontinue the medication immediately in those who develop constipation: infrequent but serious complications have occurred • Ischemic colitis
Generic Name Alvimopan **Brand Name** Entereg ■	Postoperative ileus	**Usual oral dose:** Initial: 12 mg administered 30 minutes to 5 hours before surgery Maintenance: 12 mg twice daily beginning the day after surgery, for a maximum of 7 days	• Not recommended in patients having gastric or pancreatic anastomosis or complete bowel obstruction surgery • Use caution in patients with mild to moderate hepatic impairment and/or renal impairment • Patients of Japanese ancestry should be monitored closely for GI side effects due to possibility of greater drug exposure Contraindications: • Patients who have taken therapeutic doses of opioids for more than 7 consecutive days prior to use Associated with: • Requires experienced clinician who is knowledgeable in the use of this agent and specialized care setting. • Provided only by hospitals that have registered and met all requirements of the ENTEREG Access Support and Education (E.A.S.E.) program; refer to PI • Trend toward increasing incidence of myocardial infarction (MI) was observed

Drug Name	FDA-Approved Indications	Adult Dosage Range	Precautions and Clinical Pearls
Generic Name Linaclotide **Brand Name** Linzess ■	Chronic idiopathic constipation Irritable bowel syndrome with constipation	Dose varies based on indication for use and patient's clinical status **Usual oral dose for chronic idiopathic constipation:** 145 mcg once daily	• Take dose 30 minutes prior to first meal of the day • May cause diarrhea; patients should discontinue the medication if severe or persistent diarrhea occurs Contraindications: • Known or suspected mechanical gastrointestinal obstruction Associated with: • Not for use in populations of a certain age; refer to PI prior to use
Generic Name Lubiprostone **Brand Name** Amitiza □	Chronic idiopathic constipation (CIC) OIC with CNCP Irritable bowel syndrome with constipation in adult women	Dose varies based on indication for use and patient's clinical status **Usual oral dose for CIC:** 24 mcg twice daily IBS with constipation has a lower dose requirement; refer to PI	• Avoid use in patients with severe diarrhea • May cause dyspnea and chest tightness after the first dose, which resolve within a few hours • Nausea may occur; administer with food • Not approved for use in males with IBS with constipation Contraindications: • Known or suspected mechanical bowel obstruction; refer to the Tips from the Field to see who may be at higher risk or have suggestive symptoms
Generic Name Methylnaltrexone **Brand Name** Relistor ▲ □ (BL)	OIC with advanced illness OIC with CNCP	Dose varies based on indication for use and patient's clinical response **Illustrative parenteral dose for patients with OIC for CNCP (patients who weigh 62 to 114 kg):** SQ: 12 mg every other day as needed (max: 12 mg per day) Maximum oral dose: 450 mg per day	• Discontinue if severe or persistent diarrhea occurs • May precipitate symptoms of opioid withdrawal • Use with caution in patients with severe renal impairment (CrCl less than 30 mL per minute) • Discontinue all laxatives prior to use; if response is not optimal after 3 days, laxative therapy may be reinitiated • Use beyond 4 months has not been studied • Discontinue use if opioids are discontinued • Use caution if any suspected GI lesions or other patients at risk of GI perforation • For advanced illness (and various weights) dosing strategy, refer to PI Contraindications: • GI obstruction
Generic Name Naloxegol **Brand Name** Movantik ▲	OIC with CNCP	**Usual oral dose:** 25mg once daily	• Take on empty stomach at least 1 hour prior to the first meal of the day or 2 hours after the meal. • Discontinue all laxatives prior to use; if response is not optimal after 3 days, laxative therapy may be reinitiated • Use with caution in patients with severe renal impairment • Discontinue if severe or persistent diarrhea occurs • May precipitate symptoms of opioid withdrawal Contraindications: • GI obstruction and/or perforation

Generic Name Orlistat **Brand Name** Alli Xenical	Obesity management	**Usual oral dose:** Xenical: 120 mg 3 times per day with each main meal containing fat Alli: 60 mg 3 times per day	• Most patients experience gas with oily fecal discharge, loose and frequent stools, and an urgent need to go to the bathroom • Cases of severe liver injury with hepatocellular necrosis or acute liver injury have been reported • Increased urinary oxalate have occurred: monitor renal function in patients at risk • Monitor blood sugar closely in patients with diabetes • Drug–drug interactions may be significant; monitor and adjust doses as required • Patients should be advised to adhere to dietary guidelines (agent to be used in conjunction with a reduced-calorie diet and appropriate exercise) • Potential for misuse • Seizures have been reported Contraindications: • Chronic malabsorption syndrome • Cholestasis (a condition where bile cannot flow from the liver to the duodenum)
Generic Name Teduglutide **Brand Name** Gattex ▲	Short bowel syndrome	**Usual parenteral dose:** SQ: 0.05 mg/kg once daily	• May increase the risk of hyperplastic changes, including neoplasia. Development of colorectal polyps has occurred; perform a baseline colonoscopy with polyp removal less than 6 months before initiation of therapy • Fluid overload and congestive heart failure have occurred • Treatment discontinuation may result in fluid and electrolyte imbalance; monitor for these conditions • Pancreatitis has been reported; monitor lipase and amylase • Cholecystitis, cholangitis, and cholelithiasis have been reported • Discontinue treatment in patients with intestinal or stomach obstruction • Drug interactions may require dose adjustment or avoidance of certain drug combinations; refer to PI
Generic Name Tegaserod **Brand Name** Zelnorm	Females with: IBS with constipation Chronic idiopathic constipation	**Usual oral dose for females:** 6 mg twice daily before meals, for 4 to 6 weeks	• For emergency use only; denial for emergency use is possible for the those with exclusion criteria under emergency investigational new drug (IND) process: unstable angina, history of MI or stroke, hypertension, hyperlipidemia, age older than 55 years, smoking, obesity, depression, anxiety or suicidal ideation • Diarrhea may occur after starting therapy—usually a single episode within the first week—and may resolve with continued use • Potential benefits should be weighed against potential risks in qualifying patients • Safety has not been established in males Contraindications: • Severe renal impairment • Moderate to severe hepatic impairment • History of bowel obstruction • Symptomatic gallbladder disease

Drug Name	FDA-Approved Indications	Adult Dosage Range	Precautions and Clinical Pearls
Generic Name Adalimumab **Brand Name** Humira ■ (PD)	**Common indications for use:** Crohn's disease Ulcerative colitis	**Usual parenteral dose:** SQ: Initial: 160 mg (four 40-mg injections on day 1 or two 40-mg injections over 2 days), then 80 mg 2 weeks later Maintenance: 40 mg every other week, beginning day 29	• May cause pancytopenia (rare) • Patients should be up to date with all immunizations before initiating therapy • Cases of worsening heart failure have been reported • Use caution in patients with preexisting neurologic disease; monitor for behavioral changes Associated with: • Increased risk for serious infection • Lymphoma and other malignancies • Active tuberculosis or reactivation of latent infection
Generic Name Certolizumab **Brand Name** Cimzia ■	**Common indication for use:** Crohn's disease Arthritis	**Usual parenteral dose:** SQ: Initial: 400 mg, repeat dose 2 and 4 weeks after Maintenance: 200 mg every 2 weeks or 400 mg every 4 weeks	• May cause demyelinating CNS disease (rare) • Pancytopenia has occurred rarely • Hepatitis B reactivation has occurred • Patients should be up to date with immunizations before initiating therapy Associated with: • Increased risk for serious infection • Lymphoma and other malignancies • Active tuberculosis or reactivation of latent infection • Age-specific contraindications; refer to PI
Generic Name Infliximab **Brand Name** Remicade ■ (PD)	**Common indications for use:** Crohn's disease Ulcerative colitis	**Usual parenteral dose:** IV: 3 to 5 mg/kg at 0, 2, and 6 weeks, followed by 5 mg/kg every 6 to 8 weeks thereafter	• May cause hematologic toxicities (cytopenias) • Severe hepatic reactions have been reported • Reactivation of hepatitis B has occurred; evaluate before use • Infusion reactions may occur • Patients should be up to date with immunizations before initiating therapy • Use caution in patients with neurological disease or seizure disorders • Avoid sun exposure (increased risk of skin cancer) Contraindications: • Use in patients with moderate to severe heart failure (cardiovascular adverse events seen at doses greater than 5 mg/kg in these patients) Associated with: • Increased risk for serious infection • Lymphoma and other malignancies • Active tuberculosis or reactivation of latent infection
Octreotide	Refer to the Hormones and Synthetic Substitutes chapter.		

Chapter 12

Hormones and Synthetic Substitutes

Authors: **Michael S. Mac Evoy, PharmD, BCPS, CDE and Joseph Bellavia, PharmD**

Editor: **Katherine Frachetti, MD**

Learning Objectives

- Identify current pharmacologic agents that are appropriate for each condition/diagnosis.
- Recommend optimal pharmacologic interventions based on patient-specific characteristics.
- Provide appropriate patient-specific counseling points and optimal overall medication management.

Key Terms: glucocorticoids, mineralocorticoids, estrogens, progestins, androgens, hormones, receptor blockers, antiestrogens, antidiabetic agents, antihypoglycemic agents, insulin, thyroid and antithyroid agents

Overview of Hormones and Synthetic Substitutes

The term *hormone* is used broadly to describe chemicals used by the body to implement or regulate specific actions. These chemical messengers exert their effects by binding to specific tissue or organ receptors. It is the presence of these hormone chemical messengers and their affiliated receptors that lay the foundation for modern medicine and pharmacotherapy. Through the administration of exogenous compounds designed to manipulate the hormone-receptor relationship, current pharmacotherapy has the ability to control many aspects of body function. Endocrinology is the study of the body's chemical messenger systems, the hormones and their receptors, and the use of drugs to treat and cure disorders of the hormone-receptor systems.

Hormones regulate every aspect of physiologic function, and this introduction describes some of the most important ways hormones regulate our body functions. Other parts of the endocrine system are discussed in more detail within their specific sections. The endocrine system consists of all the hormones and the affiliated receptors that interact to maintain body function and regulation. Hormones are produced by glands: The glands are responsible for producing specific hormones and can be thought of as tissues specializing in the production and regulation of a specific hormonal chemical messenger. Thus, you might think of hormones as drugs produced by the body to control body functions, in contrast to drugs that are prescribed by healthcare providers and taken by patients in tablet, capsule, injectable, or other forms.

Many hormones and their glands are under the control of the pituitary gland, a small structure located in the brain. The relationship between the pituitary, another gland, and the hormone produced by that gland is termed an axis. As an example, the adrenal axis, comprises the pituitary, the adrenal glands, and cortisol.

While most of the hormones of the body are organized into specific axes, a few hormones with important regulatory functions are controlled by outside factors. The body's metabolism (or metabolic functioning) is both an example of this type of hormone regulation and one of the most common regulatory functions performed by the endocrine system. Metabolism—that is, the regulation of energy storage and utilization—results from multiple factors, ranging from the type of macronutrients consumed to the specific needs of the body at any particular time. The hormones responsible for regulating metabolic function are most commonly associated with the development of diabetes and diabetes management. The agents associated with the pharmacotherapy of diabetes are discussed in detail later in the chapter. In general, hormones regulating energy use are responsible for taking in energy in the form of macronutrients, storing excess nutrients for later use, and mobilizing energy stores for use by body tissues when the need for them arises.

Antidiabetic agents are broadly classified as agents that lower blood glucose, though many have numerous other actions in the body. The body requires insulin to properly manage the way blood glucose moves in and out of cells.

The adrenal glands regulate many of the body's stress responses. A common term used to describe the effects noticed when the body is exposed to stressful stimuli is the "fight or flight response"; a major component of this response is hormonal regulation by the adrenal glands. As mentioned previously, the adrenal glands are controlled by the pituitary gland and release the hormone cortisol. Cortisol is produced by a portion of the adrenal gland known as the cortex, and it acts on specific receptors to exert its observable functions. Among the functions regulated by the receptors bound by cortisol are serum glucose levels and fat metabolism. The effect on serum glucose was one of the first effects of cortisol discovered—which also explains why cortisol and similar compounds are termed glucocorticoids. Glucocorticoids do not just affect serum glucose: They also regulate many aspects of human physiology associated with stress, such as blood pressure, mood, inflammation, and appetite.

The diseases most commonly associated with the adrenal glands usually result from over- or under-production of the mineral or glucocorticoids. Humans are able to exogenously replace cortisol with glucocorticoid analogues so as to replenish shortfalls associated with adrenal insufficiency or to suppress inflammation and immune responses associated with autoimmune disorders. Multiple pharmacologic agents are available that can replace glucocorticoids, which differ in their relative glucocorticoid and mineralocorticoid potency. Likewise, agents are available that can replenish mineralocorticoid supplies or block these hormones' activity on blood pressure and fluid balance.

The coordinated influence of the hormones produced by the reproductive system results in the female ovulation cycle and fertility. Contraceptive agents influence the cyclic behavior of the ovulation cycle. Among their direct actions, they may halt or delay menses, impair fertility, and prevent pregnancy. Hormones used for contraception and hormonal regulation have varying degrees of activity at their receptor sites. Estrogens and progesterone are the two most common classes of hormones used to directly affect the female reproductive cycle; they are administered either to impair fertility (in the case of contraception) or to enhance fertility (so as to promote pregnancy). Estrogens and drugs that bind to estrogen receptors to exert their effect have clinical utility in many disease states not directly associated with fertility. Polycystic ovary syndrome (PCOS), hirsutism, osteoporosis, cancers, and some adrenal insufficiencies are a few of the conditions that can be treated with medications affecting the reproductive hormone axis.

The thyroid is an endocrine gland located in the neck below the larynx and surrounding the trachea. This gland contains both follicular and parafollicular cells. The follicular cells secrete thyroid hormones, while the parafollicular cells secrete calcitonin, which regulates bone homeostasis. The thyroid is responsible for producing hormones that exhibit their effects throughout the body. It is part of the hypothalamus-pituitary-thyroid (HPT) axis. The follicular cells within the thyroid synthesize and secrete thyroxine (T_4) and triiodothyronine (T_3).

The follicle cells iodinate the tyrosine in thyroglobulin. Iodine is needed to synthesize T_4 and T_3. Iodide is consumed in the diet and then taken up by the thyroid gland. Thyroid peroxidase facilitates the reaction of iodine with tyrosine residues on tyrosine, which forms T_4 and T_3. In a person with iodine deficiency, a defect in the iodine pump or a defect in thyroid peroxidase may impair the ability to synthesize T_4 or T_3 and lead to hypothyroidism.

The release of T_4 and T_3 is regulated by a negative feedback loop mediated by the hypothalamus-pituitary-thyroid axis. Thyrotropin-releasing hormone (TRH) is secreted from the hypothalamus and stimulates the anterior pituitary to secrete thyroid-stimulating hormone (TSH). TSH, in turn, stimulates the follicular cells to synthesize and secrete T_4 and T_3. These hormones are used by body tissues to regulate metabolism, oxygen consumption, and cellular processes, including cell growth and development. Both T_4 and T_3 work on multiple organs throughout the body.

Hypothyroidism (too little thyroid hormone) is most commonly caused by Hashimoto's disease, an autoimmune disorder in which the body creates antibodies that destroy thyroid tissue, which stops the body's production of thyroxine. Signs and symptoms of hypothyroidism include fatigue, weight gain, and cold intolerance. The treatment for hypothyroidism is to replace the missing hormones—that is, to remedy the deficiency in thyroxines.

12.1 Adrenal Agents

The adrenal glands are found atop each kidney. As mentioned previously, these glands are part of the hypothalamus-pituitary-adrenal (HPA) axis. Each adrenal gland consists of an adrenal cortex and an adrenal medulla. The cortex is the outer part of the gland that produces corticosteroid hormones such as glucocorticoids and mineralocorticoids. Glucocorticoids include hydrocortisone and corticosterone. Hydrocortisone, also known as cortisol, works in the body to convert fats, proteins, and carbohydrates into energy. Cortisol also regulates blood pressure and cardiovascular functions such as heart rate and blood pressure. Another common glucocorticoid is corticosterone, which regulates immune responses by suppressing inflammatory messengers produced by the immune system. Aldosterone is a mineralocorticoid secreted by the adrenal cortex whose primary function is regulation of blood pressure by maintaining the proper balance of salt and water in the systemic vasculature. Aldosterone is responsible for sodium conservation in the kidney and other locations in the body. As a critical part of the renin–angiotensin–aldosterone system, aldosterone affects total body fluid balance by regulating sodium and potassium concentrations via receptors in the kidney.

The adrenal medulla also secretes hormones, although these hormones act on receptors whose functions are very different from those of the receptors that bind the hormones of the adrenal cortex. The adrenal medulla regulates the fight-or-flight response that is stimulated by stress by secreting two hormones, epinephrine and norepinephrine. Epinephrine, also known as adrenaline, causes increased heart rate and increased insulin resistance. Norepinephrine works in conjunction with epinephrine when responding to stress: It causes vasoconstriction, resulting in an elevation in blood pressure.

Adrenal steroids are mainly used for management of adrenal insufficiency, and to suppress inflammation and immune responses. Multiple glucocorticoid agents are available that vary in their relative glucocorticoid and mineralocorticoid activity. Hydrocortisone (cortisol) has a relative potency of 1 in terms of both glucocorticoid and mineralocorticoid activity. Other glucocorticoids, such as prednisolone, methylprednisolone, and dexamethasone, have higher relative glucocorticoid activity but a reduced mineralocorticoid activity compared to hydrocortisone. Patients taking these medications could have significant adverse effects and possible complications, and must be closely monitored. Some adverse effects, such as gastrointestinal (GI) discomfort, can be mitigated by taking the glucocorticoid with food.

Among the numerous disease states associated with a dysfunction of the adrenal system is Cushing's syndrome which results from prolonged exposure to cortisol, either exogenously administered or intrinsically induced by cancer and/ or tumor. Patients typically report a constellation of symptoms that include elevated blood pressure, abdominal obesity (but often still have thin legs and arms), stretch marks, a round red "moon" face, a fat "buffalo hump" between the shoulders, as well as headaches, weak muscles, weak bones, acne, and fragile skin with impaired wound healing. Occasionally there may be changes in mood and complaints of chronic fatigue. Females may report excessive and unwanted hair growth as well as irregular menses. Most cases of Cushing's syndrome can be successfully treated. If the Cushing's syndrome is due to the administration of exogenous corticosteroids, these can often be gradually discontinued. Exogenously administered steroids that have been prescribed at higher doses and given for extended periods of time require a slow dose reduction to allow the body to gradually resume its natural production of steroids and to avoid withdrawal symptoms. For example, a regimen of 3 weeks of prednisone 20 mg per day or its equivalent is considered sufficient to suppress normal adrenal glucocorticoid production and would require a gradual tapering discontinuation. If the syndrome is caused by a tumor or cancer, it may be treated by a combination of surgery, chemotherapy, and/or radiation. Intrinsically, only increased pituitary production of adrenocorticotropic hormone (ACTH) has the potential to lead to glucocorticoid excess and Cushing's syndrome. Adrenal insufficiency can result in a number of complications, including aldosterone deficiency.

Fludrocortisone is a mineralocorticoid agonist that has a high mineralocorticoid effect but no glucocorticoid effect. This medication is administered to take advantage of its ability to increase the reabsorption of sodium by the kidney. That is, because of its effect on sodium and water balance, it can be used to treat some causes of orthostatic hypotension.

Adrenal Agents

- Beclomethasone
- Betamethasone
- Budesonide
- Ciclesonide
- Cortisone
- Dexamethasone
- Fludrocortisone
- Flunisolide
- Fluticasone
- Hydrocortisone
- Methylprednisolone
- Mometasone
- Prednisolone
- Prednisone
- Triamcinolone

Case Studies and Conclusions

ST is a 31-year-old female who has sought care from her primary care physician because of weakness and fatigue. ST also reports leg swelling. She has gained 50 pounds over the past 2 years. She has previously been diagnosed with depression and insomnia. The endocrinologist diagnosed Cushing's syndrome based on the lab findings.

1. High levels of cortisol can predispose ST to which other disease state?

    a. Diabetes
    b. Hyperthyroidism
    c. Gout
    d. Dyslipidemia

Answer A is correct. Glucocorticoids increase serum glucose as one of their major physiologic functions. Uncontrolled serum glucose leads to glucocorticoid-induced diabetes.

2. Which lab value would you expect to be elevated in a patient with Cushing's syndrome?

    a. LH
    b. FSH
    c. ACTH
    d. TSH

Answer C is correct. Only increased pituitary production of adrenocorticotropic hormone (ACTH) has the potential to lead to glucocorticoid excess and Cushing's syndrome.

3. Often Cushing disease can be caused by excess administration of glucocorticoids. If the patient experiences this adverse effect, how should it be approached?

    a. Slowly taper off the medication
    b. Stop the glucocorticoids immediately
    c. Switch to a different glucocorticoid
    d. Continue taking the glucocorticoid

Answer A is correct. Abrupt discontinuation of glucocorticoids without taper can lead to acute glucocorticoid insufficiency. A taper is needed to allow for the body's production of glucocorticoid to increase and to avoid insufficiency.

GW is a 20-year-old man who is brought to clinic after her mother found him disoriented and confused. She reports his emotions have been labile lately; in addition, he has been experiencing fatigue and a loss of focus. GW has a past medical history of type 1 diabetes and hypothyroidism. Due to GW's adrenal insufficiency, his aldosterone production is also lacking.

1. Which electrolyte abnormality could this deficiency cause?
   a. Hyperkalemia
   b. Hypokalemia
   c. Hyponatremia
   d. Hypocalcemia

Answer C is correct. Aldosterone increases sodium reabsorption by the kidneys.

2. Which of the following substances has the highest mineralocorticoid activity?
   a. Prednisone
   b. Dexamethasone
   c. Hydrocortisone
   d. Fludrocortisone

Answer D is correct. Fludrocortisone is the most potent mineralocorticoid.

3. GW has been taking 5 mg per day of prednisone for 2 weeks. When is the HPA axis considered fully suppressed?
   a. After 3 weeks of prednisone 20 mg per day or the equivalent dose of another glucocorticoid
   b. After 1 week of prednisone 1 mg per day
   c. After 1 week of hydrocortisone 10 mg per day
   d. After taking any single dose of glucocorticoids

Answer A is correct. A regimen of 3 weeks of prednisone 20 mg per day or its equivalent is considered sufficient to suppress normal adrenal glucocorticoid production.

12.2 Androgens, Estrogens, and Progestins

Synthetic androgens, estrogens, and progestins (progesterones) are commonly used to treat disorders of the reproductive endocrine axis.

Estrogen replacement is used to treat menopausal symptoms including hot flashes, vaginal dryness, dyspareunia, and atrophic vaginitis. Estrogen is available in formulations for oral, transdermal, intravaginal, intramuscular, and subcutaneous administration. Low doses are typically adequate for symptom control. Progesterone must be added for uterine protection (either in continuous or cycled regimens) in appropriate patients. Risks associated with use of these hormones vary based on age and comorbidities, but include stroke, thromboembolic disease, cardiovascular disease, and breast cancer.

Synthetic estrogens and progestins are effective for contraception. Multiple formulations are available, including oral pills, transdermal patches, intravaginal rings, subcutaneous implants, intrauterine devices, and intramuscular injections. Patient and provider preferences, along with comorbid medical conditions, guide the choice of therapy. Counseling the patient on proper technique and adherence with contraceptives is important to achieve high success rates. Conversely, several estrogen receptor agonists, including clomiphene, can be used to increase luteinizing hormone (LH) and follicle-stimulating hormone (FSH) levels so as to induce fertility.

Synthetic testosterone preparations are used to treat hypogonadism. The goal of such therapy is to replete levels so that they return to the mid-normal range. Available agents include parenteral and transdermal formulations. Longer-acting parenteral (intramuscular) injections are less expensive but can lead to fluctuating blood concentrations between injections. Injections can be painful or cause local reactions. Transdermal patches are applied to the back, abdomen, or upper arms (but not scrotum) and are convenient to administer. Skin irritation and problems with continued adhesion of the patch can occur. Transdermal gels are applied daily to the skin of the upper arms and chest. Both patches and gels aim to mimic a natural testosterone peak that occurs during the morning but provide consistent levels on a day-to-day basis. Adverse effects of all testosterone preparations include polycythemia (elevated hemoglobin), mood changes (irritability), acne, and increase in prostate-specific antigen (PSA) level. Cardiac complications are being investigated, although usually do not occur if serum levels do not rise above target ranges. Serum testosterone is a serum marker that provides information regarding appropriate repletion of testosterone. The administration of newer long-acting parenteral testosterone provides a consistent serum concentration without peaks and troughs seen with other dosage formulations.

Androgens

Danazol
Fluoxymesterone
Methyltestosterone
Oxandrolone
Testosterone

Estrogen Agonists and Antagonists

Estrogens

Estradiol
Estrogen
Estropipate

Estrogen Agonist-Antagonists

Bazedoxifene
Clomiphene
Ospemifene
Raloxifene
Tamoxifen *(see also the Hormone/Hormone Modifiers section in the Antineoplastic Agents chapter)*
Toremifene *(see also the Hormone/Hormone Modifiers section in the Antineoplastic Agents chapter)*

Progestins

Hydroxyprogesterone
Medroxyprogesterone
Norethindrone
Progesterone
Dienogest
Desogestrel
Drospirenone
Ethynodiol
Etonogestrel
Levonorgestrel
Norelgestromin
Norethindrone
Norgestimate
Norgestrel

Contraceptives

Estrogen-Progestin Combination Contraceptives

Estradiol valerate and dienogest
Ethinyl estradiol and desogestrel
Ethinyl estradiol and drospirenone
Ethinyl estradiol and ethynodiol
Ethinyl estradiol and etonogestrel

Ethinyl estradiol and levonorgestrel
Ethinyl estradiol and norelgestromin
Ethinyl estradiol and norethindrone
Ethinyl estradiol and norgestimate
Ethinyl estradiol and norgestrel
Mestranol and norethindrone

Progestin Contraceptives

Etonogestrel *(see also the Progestins section)*
Levonorgestrel *(see also the Progestins section)*
Norethindrone *(see also the Progestins section)*

Gonadotropins

Chorionic gonadotropin
Nafarelin
Goserelin *(see also the Hormone/Hormone Modifiers section in the Antineoplastic Agents chapter)*
Leuprolide *(see also the Hormone/Hormone Modifiers section in the Antineoplastic Agents chapter)*

Case Studies and Conclusions

ML is a 54-year-old man who has come in to his primary care physician because he has not been himself. He complains of diminished energy and libido, poor motivation, depressed mood, and irritability. These symptoms have been present for several months, but seem to be worsening. The primary care physician evaluates ML's labs and writes a prescription for Androgel.

1. Which of the following is an INCORRECT counseling point for Androgel?
   a. Apply to the abdomen, buttocks, forearms, or scrotum.
   b. Make sure to wash your hands after using the medication.
   c. Make sure to avoid any water activities for 2 hours after applying the medication.
   d. Ensure that women and children avoid contact with the area on which you applied the gel.

Answer A is correct. The application of Androgel should not occur on the scrotum.

2. Which of the following preparations of testosterone medications provides the most consistent levels of testosterone?
   a. Long-acting parenteral medications (Depo testosterone, Aveed)
   b. Transdermal patches (Androderm)
   c. Transdermal gels (Androgel)
   d. Buccal patches (Striant)

Answer A is correct. The newer long-acting testosterone preparations prevent variations in testosterone levels.

3. Testosterone patches try to mimic the natural peak of testosterone. When does this natural peak occur?
   a. In the morning
   b. After dinner
   c. Before falling asleep at night
   d. In the middle of the night

Answer A is correct. Testosterone peaks in the early morning hours.

JR is a 30-year-old male who is a new patient with suspected hypogonadism. Over the course of the past 2 months, he has taken weekly injections of 100 mg of testosterone. His dose was recently increased to 300 to 400 mg per week.

His most recent lab tests showed elevated total and free testosterone level. JR is experiencing gynecomastia and a rash around his eyes. He is also experiencing anxiety and palpitations. The exogenously administered testosterone suppressed the hormone axis responsible for producing testosterone.

1. Which part of his body produces testosterone?
   a. Hypothalamus
   b. Pituitary
   c. Testis
   d. Both A and B are correct.

Answer C is correct. The testis produce testosterone.

2. What is the usual starting dose for testosterone cypionate?
   a. 150–200 mg every 2 weeks
   b. 100–150 mg every week
   c. 100–150 mg every 4 weeks
   d. 150–200 mg every week

Answer A is correct. Starting doses of testosterone cypionate are typically 150–200 mg given intramuscularly every 2 weeks.

3. What is the most important monitoring value for testosterone replacement?
   a. Serum testosterone
   b. LH
   c. FSH
   d. GnRH

Answer A is correct. Serum testosterone is the only serum marker listed that provides information regarding appropriate repletion of testosterone.

EP is a 50-year-old woman who reports experiencing two or three hot flashes each day. Several times each week, her hot flashes are associated with insomnia. Her symptoms began 3 to 6 months ago and have progressed to the point where they are very bothersome. EP realizes her symptoms are likely due to menopause, but she is worried about the treatments for them because two of her friends have warned her of the risks of hormone replacement therapy.

1. Which of the following is NOT a disease-related concern with hormone replacement therapy?
   a. Increased risk of breast cancer
   b. Increased risk of hypothyroidism
   c. Increased risk of myocardial infarction
   d. Increased risk of thromboembolism

Answer B is correct. Hypothyroidism is not a major risk of estrogen replacement.

2. Which of the following disease states would contraindicate the use of hormone replacement therapy in patients?
   a. Thromboembolic disease
   b. Diabetes
   c. Hypertension
   d. Hyperthyroidism

Answer A is correct. Estrogen therapy is contraindicated in a patient with history of thromboembolic disease.

The doctor starts EP on an estrogen oral therapy.

3. Which of the following medications could be used?
   a. Premarin
   b. Oxandrin
   c. Estring
   d. Vagifem

Answer A is correct. Premarin is the only oral formulation of the estrogen formulations; Oxandrin is an androgen.

JK is a 25-year-old college student who presents to the women's health clinic for contraceptive counseling. She has been in a monogamous sexual relationship with her boyfriend for 3 years. Their primary method of contraception has been inconsistent use of male condoms. She is here to be evaluated for the use of hormonal contraceptives. JK has a past medical history of migraines.

1. Which medications could decrease effectiveness of oral contraceptives?
   a. Iron preparations
   b. Anticonvulsants
   c. Antihistamines
   d. Multivitamins

Answer B is correct. Anticonvulsants can increase the metabolism of contraceptives, rendering them less effective.

JK returns to the clinic 3 months later, complaining of never having a period since beginning the oral contraceptive pill.

2. What could be the cause of amenorrhea in this patient?
   a. Estrogen deficiency
   b. Estrogen excess
   c. Progestin deficiency
   d. Progestin excess

Answer D is correct. Amenorrhea is most commonly associated with excess levels of progestin.

JK calls the clinic in panic, saying she missed 2 days of oral contraceptives.

3. What should you advise her to do?
   a. Take the most recent missed pill and use a backup method for 7 days
   b. Continue taking the pills as she normally would; no backup method is needed
   c. Take two pills per day for the rest of this cycle
   d. Stop taking the pill for the rest of the cycle and use a backup method

Answer A is correct. According to established guidance, 2 missed days of missed oral contraceptives warrant an immediate dose and use of a backup contraceptive method for 7 days.

12.3 Antidiabetic and Antihypoglycemic Agents

The treatment for diabetes varies depending on the type of diabetes and the underlying risk factors specific to each patient. Patients with type 1 diabetes mellitus (insulin-dependent diabetes mellitus [IDDM])) are unable to produce insulin, and require multiple daily insulin injections (subcutaneous) or use of a continuous subcutaneous insulin infusion (insulin pump). The goal of this treatment is to mimic the body's natural insulin secretion patterns and maintain blood glucose within a narrow range. Insulin is available in various preparations with different timed-release profiles. The insulin regimen is customized for each patient to keep blood glucose under control. Refer to companion drug grid in order to review the differences in insulin products available and how selection is based on numerous patient-specific factors.

Patients with type 2 diabetes mellitus (non-insulin-dependent diabetes mellitus [NIDDM]) produce insulin but have increased insulin resistance; thus they have a relative deficit of insulin in the body, resulting in high blood glucose. There are several treatment options for type 2 diabetes. Multiple factors are considered when selecting a regimen, including concurrent medications and potential drug–drug interactions, chronic medical conditions, costs, and side-effect profiles.

Medications that treat type 2 diabetes work at a variety of sites. Some work in the pancreatic beta cells to increase insulin production, whereas other cells improve the body's sensitivity to insulin. Still others work to eliminate excess glucose from the body. Supplemental subcutaneous insulin is used when other therapeutic options fail to achieve adequate blood glucose control.

The backbone of therapy for type 2 diabetes is metformin—the only commercially available agent from the biguanide class. Metformin works to decrease hepatic glucose production while also increasing cell sensitivity to insulin. Nausea and diarrhea are common side effects when starting metformin, but may resolve within days to a few weeks. Slow titration to the desired dose helps to minimize these gastrointestinal side effects. Metformin may be used as a single agent or in combination with other medications.

Sulfonylureas work by stimulating insulin secretion from the pancreatic beta cells, while also suppressing glucose output from the liver. Meglitinides also increase insulin production by the pancreas, by blocking potassium channels in the pancreatic beta cells and allowing calcium to enter the cells, which then triggers insulin release. For both of these drug classes, hypoglycemia is the most common adverse effect and are considered to be the agents with the highest risk of inducing hypoglycemia by stimulating pancreatic beta cells to secrete insulin when compared to other antidiabetic agents with different mechanisms of action.

Thiazolidinediones lower blood glucose by improving insulin resistance in peripheral cells, which they accomplish by increasing the number of insulin receptors on the cells. These medications do not increase pancreatic insulin secretion. Side effects include weight gain, possible fluid retention, increased risk of heart failure, and other cardiac risks.

Incretin mimetics (GLP-1 agonists) are agonists of the GLP-1 receptor in the gut, which signals, and therefore increases, insulin secretion by the pancreas when food is present and blood glucose levels are elevated. These medications also delay gastric emptying and trigger satiety. They are administered as subcutaneous injections and are also associated with moderate weight loss. Nausea and other gastrointestinal symptoms are known side effects.

Dipeptidyl peptidase IV (DPP-4) inhibitors are a class of oral agents that prolong endogenous incretin release by the gut and result in greater and/or prolonged pancreatic insulin secretion—a mechanism of action similar to that used by GLP-1 agonists. These medication also decrease secretion of glucagon—another pancreatic hormone that increases blood glucose.

Sodium glucose cotransporter 2 (SGLT-2) inhibitors are the newest class of antidiabetic medications. They act in the kidneys on the SGLT2 receptor to reduce reabsorption of glucose, thereby promoting loss of glucose in the urine. This loss results in lowered blood glucose.

Alpha-glucosidase inhibitors delay glucose absorption by delaying digestion of carbohydrates. These agents work to decrease postprandial hyperglycemia.

Amylinomimetics are synthetic analogues of human amylin. They reduce postprandial blood glucose by prolonging gastric emptying time and reducing postprandial glucose secretion. In addition, they can suppress appetite.

Alpha-Glucosidase Inhibitors

Acarbose
Miglitol

Amylinomimetics

Pramlintide

Biguanides

Metformin

Dipeptidyl Peptidase IV (DPP-4) Inhibitors

Alogliptin
Linagliptin
Saxagliptin
Sitagliptin

Incretin Mimetics (GLP-1 Agonists)

Albiglutide
Dulaglutide
Exenatide
Liraglutide

Insulins

Insulin Aspart
Insulin Determir
Insulin Degludec
Insulin Glargine
Insulin Glulisine
Insulin Human
Insulin Lispro

Meglitinides

Nateglinide
Repaglinide

Sodium Glucose Cotransporter 2 (SGLT-2) Inhibitors

Canagliflozin
Dapagliflozin
Empagliflozin

Sulfonylureas

Chlorpropamide
Glimepiride
Glipizide
Glyburide
Tolazamide
Tolbutamide

Thiazolidinediones

Pioglitazone
Rosiglitazone

Antihypoglycemics; Glyconeolytic Agents

Glucagon

Miscellaneous Antihypoglycemic Agents

Diazoxide

Case Studies and Conclusions

LR is a 19-year-old female who was recently diagnosed with type 1 diabetes. She is being referred for a medication review. She is concerned about her glucose numbers and is worried about the new medication she will be starting. She is looking for advice on medication and her disease state.

1. Since LR has type 1 diabetes, which type of medication regimen would you recommend LR to start on?
   a. Metformin
   b. Metformin and Victoza
   c. Glyburide
   d. Lantus and Humalog

Answer D is correct. Lantus and Humalog are both insulin. Insulin is needed for patients with type 1 diabetes who are insulin deficient.

2. Which of the following medications is a type of insulin that provides a steady basal insulin level with no maximum peak?
   a. Lantus (Glargine)
   b. Humalog (Lispro)
   c. Novolog (Aspart)
   d. Humulin R (Human Regular)

Answer A is correct. Only Lantus provides a peakless steady supply of insulin after subcutaneous injection.

After LR becomes comfortable with injecting insulin, she is introduced to carbohydrate (carb) counting. At this point, the patient learns to adjust the bolus dose to specifically cover the mealtime carbohydrate consumption.

3. Which of the following medications would be used to cover mealtime glucose spikes?
   a. Humulin N
   b. Lantus (Glargine)
   c. Levemir (Detemir)
   d. Novolog (Aspart)

Answer D is correct. Novolog is the only rapid-acting insulin listed and would be used for mealtime coverage.

JR is a 45-year-old female with a 1-year history of type 2 diabetes. Her baseline $HgbA_{1c}$ was just measured as 9%, and she has symptoms including frequent urination, blurred vision, and fatigue. Her diabetes is currently uncontrolled, and she is not taking any medications. She is brought into the clinic for education on her disease state and a medication review.

1. If JR continues to have uncontrolled diabetes, which of the following complications could arise?
   a. Impaired wound healing
   b. Retinopathy
   c. Nerve damage
   d. All of the above are possible.

Answer D is correct. Impaired wound healing, retinopathy, and nerve damage are all potential complications of uncontrolled diabetes.

2. Which of the following medications is considered the backbone of therapy for type 2 diabetes?
   a. Glipizide
   b. Metformin
   c. Insulin
   d. Exenatide

Answer B is correct. Metformin is considered first-line therapy in all patients with type 2 diabetes who can tolerate it.

The doctor wants to add on a second medication to control the diabetes. This possibility makes JR nervous, because she does not want two medications to give her hypoglycemia.

3. Which of the following medications should be avoided if there are concerns about hypoglycemia?
   a. Glyburide (Micronase)
   b. Pioglitazone (Actos)
   c. Sitagliptin (Januvia)
   d. Liraglutide (Victoza)

Answer A is correct. Glyburide has the highest risk of inducing hypoglycemia by stimulating pancreatic beta cells to secrete insulin.

12.4 Parathyroid Hormones

Parathyroid hormone (PTH), along with calcitriol (the active form of vitamin D), regulates and maintains calcium and phosphorus levels in the blood. PTH increases serum calcium, excretion of phosphorus in urine (phosphaturia), and calcitriol synthesis. It acts on the bone to release calcium, and on the gut to increase absorption of both calcium and phosphorus.

Patients with hypoparathyroidism require vitamin D and calcium supplementation. PTH is needed to convert vitamin D to its active form. Therefore, it is necessary to administer vitamin D in its active form—calcitriol. For patients who are unable to maintain adequate levels of serum calcium and those who wish to prevent symptoms while on supplementation with calcium and calcitriol, a synthetic parathyroid hormone analogue is available and given subcutaneously. Calcium levels need to be monitored in these patients, and doses of supplemental calcium and calcitriol are typically decreased accordingly. Rare bone cancers have been reported with this therapy. Patients who lack PTH or who have impaired renal activation of vitamin D (as seen in patients with chronic renal failure) are unable to properly convert vitamin D into its active form and therefore would require supplementation with calcitriol, the active form of vitamin D. Hypocalcemia due to vitamin D deficiency will also result in concurrent hypophosphatemia because renal reabsorption of phosphate requires activated vitamin D. For patients who are vitamin D depleted, repletion should be started at a higher dose, typically 50,000 international units weekly to build up vitamin D stores.

Parathyroid Agents

Calcitonin
Parathyroid hormone
Teriparatide

Vitamins and Miscellaneous Parathyroid Analog Agents with Hormonal Influence

Calcitriol
Cinacalcet
Paricalcitol
Cholecalciferol [vitamin D_3] (refer to vitamins and supplements resource)
Doxercalciferol{synthetic vitamin D analog} (refer to vitamins and supplements resource)
Ergocalciferol [vitamin D_2] (refer to vitamins and supplements resource)

Case Studies and Conclusions

TJ is a 56-year-old male who visits your clinic. He has surgically induced hypoparathyroidism and supplementation will be necessary.

1. Which agent would you recommend for vitamin D replacement in TJ?
   a. Calcitriol 0.25 mcg daily
   b. Cholecalciferol 2000 units daily
   c. Ergocalciferol 2000 units daily
   d. Ergocalciferol 1000 units daily

Answer A is correct. The lack of PTH means TJ is unable to properly convert vitamin D into its active form.

2. How should TJ take his calcium carbonate to maximize its absorption?
   a. Once daily with food
   b. In divided daily doses with food
   c. Once daily on an empty stomach
   d. In divided daily doses on an empty stomach

Answer B is correct. Calcium requires sufficient stomach acid to be absorbed and should be separated into multiple smaller doses to increase its absorption.

TJ is suffering from nausea due to the large amounts of calcium carbonate he needs to take on a daily basis.

3. Which of the following medications could potentially help lower the amount of calcium carbonate he needs to take?
   a. Calcitriol
   b. Parathyroid hormone (PTH)
   c. Vitamin D
   d. Potassium phosphate

Answer B is correct. Recombinant PTH improves serum calcium deficiency and allows for lowering of the oral calcium dose.

MO is a 78-year-old woman who comes to your clinic with complaints of frequent urination and kidney stones. She has a past medical history of osteoporosis. Based on her lab values, she is diagnosed with hyperparathyroidism secondary to low levels of vitamin D.

1. What is the starting dose for vitamin D repletion therapy?
   a. 50,000 units daily for 2–3 weeks
   b. 50,000 units weekly for 2–3 weeks
   c. 1000 units daily for 2–3 weeks
   d. 5000 units daily for 2–3 weeks

Answer A is correct. Repletion should be started at a higher dose, typically 50,000 international units weekly to build up vitamin D stores.

2. Hypocalcemia due to vitamin D deficiency will also result in concurrent:
   a. Hypophosphatemia.
   b. Hyponatremia.
   c. Hypokalemia.
   d. Hypomagnesemia.

Answer A is correct. Renal reabsorption of phosphate requires activated vitamin D.

3. Which chronic disease state can cause low levels of vitamin D?
   a. Chronic hypertension
   b. Chronic renal failure
   c. Chronic type 2 diabetes
   d. Chronic obesity

Answer B is correct. Renal activation of vitamin D is impaired in patients with chronic renal failure.

12.5 Pituitary Agents

The pituitary gland, along with the hypothalamus, is the regulator of the endocrine system. The pituitary gland consists of two parts: the anterior and posterior pituitary. The anterior pituitary is part of the endocrine system; it releases multiple hormones that target other organs through their hormonal axis.

Among the anterior pituitary hormones, growth hormone regulates many physiological functions and promotes growth. Growth hormone deficiency can be treated by somatotropin (synthetic growth hormone), which is given subcutaneously daily. Growth hormone excess can be treated with the somatostatin analogue known as octreotide, which is injected as either a short- or longer-acting formulation.

The pituitary gland also secretes prolactin, a hormone that regulates mammary gland development and milk secretion. Hyperprolactinemia is often caused by an adenoma on the pituitary gland, or by taking medications that decrease dopamine levels (dopamine suppresses prolactin). Therapy with medications that are dopamine agonists is an effective way to return prolactin to the correct levels. Medications including bromocriptine, pergolidem, and cabergoline are dopamine agonists that reduce prolactin levels.

Gonadotropins (FSH {[folicle stimulating hormone], LH [leutinizing hormone]), ACTH (adrenocorticotropic hormone), and TSH (thyroid stimulating hormone) are other anterior pituitary hormones whose therapeutic targets are discussed separately in this chapter.

Pituitary Agents

Corticotropin
Desmopressin
Vasopressin

Somatostatin Agonists and Antagonists

Somatostatin Agonists

Lanreotide
Octreotide
Pasireotide

Somatotropin Agonists

Tesamorelin

Somatotropin Antagonists

Pegvisomant

Case Studies and Conclusions

CC is a 70-year-old female who recently went through a pituitary tumor removal. CC is diagnosed with panhypopituitarism secondary to the surgery.

1. Which of the following hormones is NOT released by the anterior pituitary?
   a. ACTH
   b. TSH
   c. FSH
   d. ADH

Answer D is correct. ADH is produced by the posterior pituitary.

2. When replacing hormones, which of the following deficiencies should be targeted first?
   a. ACTH deficiency
   b. Thyroxine deficiency
   c. Luteinizing hormone deficiency
   d. Calcitonin deficiency

Answer A is correct. ACTH deficiency is the most important deficiency to address due to the high mortality from Addisonian crisis associated with glucocorticoid insufficiency.

3. Which of the following regimens would cover the hormone loss from panhypopituitarism?
    a. Hydrocortisone, levothyroxine, testosterone injection
    b. Dexamethasone, levothyroxine, calcium, propranolol, vitamin D
    c. Prednisone, liothyroxine, calcium, Androgel, vitamin D
    d. Fludrocortisone, Synthroid, testosterone injection, calcium, vitamin D

Answer A is correct. Panhypopituitarism impairs ACTH, TSH, LH, and FSH production. Replacement of the functions of cortisol, thyroxines, and androgens is possible with this regimen.

LK is a 25-year-old male with a disability who has been wetting the bed for 6 months. He is healthy except for general colds.

1. Which hormone released by the pituitary gland is responsible for limiting the amount of urine produced overnight while sleeping?
    a. Antidiuretic hormone
    b. Prolactin
    c. Growth hormone
    d. Melanocyte-stimulating hormone

Answer A is correct. Antidiuretic hormone (ADH) is responsible for regulating fluid balance and urine production.

2. Which of the following is a medication that targets the posterior pituitary and is given for nocturnal enuresis?
    a. Desmopressin
    b. Prolactin
    c. Calcitonin
    d. Bromocriptine

Answer A is correct. Desmopressin specifically targets the production of ADH by the posterior pituitary.

12.6 Thyroid and Antithyroid Agents

Synthetic thyroxine, available as levothyroxine, is the drug of choice for treating hypothyroidism. Liothyronine, another available synthetic thyroid hormone, is not commonly prescribed or required. Levothyroxine is usually dosed on a mcg/kg basis and then titrated based on laboratory values (i.e., TSH level). This medication is taken once per day—typically 30 minutes before eating, because food can decrease its absorption from the gut. Administration of levothyroxine should be separated by 4 hours from any use of antacids, calcium, or iron supplements because these also decrease levothyroxine absorption. Compliance with medication is essential to successful therapy. Levothyroxine is normally well tolerated. There is potential for adverse effects if its dose is too high, including tachycardia, tremor, headache, and diarrhea.

Antithyroid drugs are used to minimize symptoms and eliminate excess thyroid hormones, which are seen with hyperthyroidism. Thioamides, including propylthiouracil (PTU) and methimazole, work to block formation of the T_4 and T_3 hormones in the thyroid gland. Propylthiouracil also inhibits the conversion of T_4 into the active form, T_3, in the peripheral tissue cells. Iodides are another class of medications that works to block thyroid hormone release. They are used to rapidly decrease thyroid levels, in critically ill patients or those requiring surgery.

Thyroid Agents

Levothyroxine
Liothyronine
Liotrix
Thyroid

Antithyroid Agents

Methimazole
Potassium iodide
Propylthiouracil

Case Studies and Conclusions

VG is a 31-year-old African American woman who is seen by a physician at your clinic. For the past few months she has felt increasingly fatigued, which she attributes to high levels of stress. She wonders if she is becoming depressed. VG also notes that for the past few months she has had more difficulty concentrating at work and has gained a few pounds. When her lab results come back, they show high levels of TSH and low levels of free T_4.

1. The high levels of TSH and low levels of free T_4 indicate that the problem of hypothyroidism is originating from which point in the thyroid axis?
   a. Hypothalamus
   b. Pituitary gland
   c. Thyroid
   d. Parathyroid

Answer C is correct. TSH is being produced properly but the thyroid gland is unable to meet the demand for producing thyroid hormones.

2. If a patient has optimal T_4 levels while taking levothyroxine but is still experiencing symptoms consistent with hypothyroidism, what would you recommend?
   a. Increase the levothyroxine dose
   b. Add on liothyroxine
   c. Switch to a different levothyroxine brand
   d. Switch levothyroxine dosing from once daily to twice daily

Answer B is correct. A patient adequately supplemented on levothyroxine who is experiencing symptoms may have impairment in peripheral activation of T_4 to T_3, so providing T_3 may be beneficial.

VG is on other medications including aspirin, lisinopril, cholestyramine, and birth control.

3. Which of these medications should not be taken within 4 hours of levothyroxine because it can affect the absorption?
   a. Lisinopril
   b. Cholestyramine
   c. Calcium
   d. Aspirin

Answer B is correct. Cholestyramine can bind levothyroxine and prevent its absorption.

CG is a 23-year-old woman who presents to her primary care physician with complaints of palpitations and a fine motor tremor. The palpitations started a few months ago and have come and gone until the past week, when they began to occur more frequently. A fine tremor began 3 weeks ago, and CG reports a 5-kg weight loss over the past 6 months despite an increased appetite and adequate food consumption. She complains of being hot and sweaty. CG is diagnosed with hyperthyroidism.

1. Which of the following is NOT a treatment option for hyperthyroidism?
    a. Methimazole
    b. Radioiodine
    c. Propranolol
    d. Paroxetine

Answer D is correct. Paroxetine is not approved for treatment of hyperthyroidism.

2. Which of the following is a serious adverse effect of thionamides?
    a. Hepatotoxicity
    b. Hypertension
    c. Hypoglycemia
    d. Hyperglycemia

Answer A is correct. Liver toxicity is a serious adverse effect associated with thionamides.

3. Given that CG ultimately needs to have a complete thyroidectomy, which medication will she need after the procedure?
    a. Levothyroxine
    b. Methimazole
    c. Radioiodine
    d. Propylthiouracil

Answer A is correct. Following complete thyroidectomy, the patient will be thyroxine deficient and, therefore, will require thyroid hormone replacement.

12.7 Miscellaneous Therapeutic Agents

Bone Resorption Inhibitors

Alendronate is a second-generation bisphosphonate and is also the first agent of this group that has demonstrated actual bone strengthening, as opposed to simply preventing bone loss. Alendronate is a more potent inhibitor of bone resorption than the first-generation agent etidronate; however, unlike etidronate, the effective dose of alendronate does not inhibit bone mineralization.

As we age bone strength and integrity change over time undergoing constant turnover with homeostatic balance maintained by osteoblasts that create bone and osteoclasts that destroy bone. Most people have adequate bone mass to last a lifetime; however, some patients with osteopenia or osteoporosis need medication intervention when bone destruction exceeds bone creation to the point where bone weakness jeopardizes the well-being of the affected individual. Fractures, along with the debilitating acute and chronic pain, are the most dangerous aspect of osteoporosis and can lead to further disability and early mortality. There are serious risks associated with hip fracture, such as deep vein thrombosis, pulmonary embolism, and increased mortality; thus, surgical intervention is usually required promptly. Women suffer bone loss at different rates than men, with an increased rate after menopause with the loss of estrogen. There are a number of ways to measure bone strength with bone scans (i.e., DEXA) and fracture risk calculators (i.e., FRAX) that assess the risk of fracture based upon several criteria, including bone mineral density (BMD), age, smoking, alcohol usage, weight, and gender. Current drug action inhibits the digestion of bone by encouraging clasts to undergo preprogrammed cell death (apoptosis) thereby slowing down bone loss. Bisphosphonates have demonstrated reduced risk of fracture but have serious GI side effects and potentially disfiguring bone necrosis that has been reported with use in patients receiving certain cancer treatment regimens, who receive longer duration of treatment, those undergoing dental procedures, such as tooth extraction, and patients with signs of local infection (including osteomyelitis).

The treatment and prevention of osteoporosis (and in some cases osteopenia) is driven by guideline-based recommendations. All women who are postmenopausal and also have experienced a previous vertebral or hip osteoporotic fracture, a BMD that is suggestive of osteoporosis at the lumbar spine, femoral neck, or total hip region, as well as other possible clinical-related issues, should receive drug therapy for osteoporosis. Other medication interventions used within this therapeutic area include fully human, highly specific, monoclonal antibody agents against receptor activator of nuclear factor kappa-beta ligand (RANKL). The protein is produced in genetically engineered mammalian (Chinese hamster ovary) cells. Denosumab blocks osteoclast activation, thereby resulting in decreased bone resorption (less bone breakdown).

Bone Resorption Inhibitors

Alendronate
Denosumab
Etidronate
Ibandronate
Pamidronate
Risedronate
Zoledronic acid
Calcitonin *(see also the Parathyroid Hormones section)*
Estrogens *(see also the Androgens, Estrogens, and Progestins section)*
Raloxifene *(see also the Androgens, Estrogens, and Progestins section)*

5-Alpha-Reductase Inhibitors

Selective inhibitors of either or both type I and type II 5-alpha-reductase, block the intracellular enzyme that catalyzes the conversion of testosterone to 5-alpha-dihydrotestosterone (DHT), thereby decreasing DHT concentrations by as much as 90% in 2 weeks and 93% in 2 years. Finasteride predominantly inhibits type II 5-alpha-reductase and is a more potent agent when compared to the others currently available, causing greater reductions of DHT. Lower DHT concentrations result in reduced prostate volume, improved urinary flow rate, and lower risk of acute urinary retention and surgery. These agents have been targeted for action to reverse male pattern baldness otherwise known as androgenetic alopecia.

5-Alpha-Reductase Inhibitors

Dutasteride
Finasteride

Tips from the Field

1. Compounding risk factors for bone loss with the use of corticosteroids include preexisting osteopenia, prolonged immobilization, family history of osteoporosis, tobacco smoking, malnutrition, and use of other medications that may reduce bone mass.
2. There is an increased risk of opportunistic infection that includes oropharyngeal candidiasis (thrush) with certain formulations and administration routes. Should thrush develop, treat it with appropriate local or systemic antifungal therapy while still continuing corticosteroid therapy (such as that administered via oral inhaler). Temporary interruption of an inhaler use should only be done under close medical supervision and individuals using intranasal and/or oral inhalation corticosteroids for extended periods (i.e., months) should be examined periodically for evidence of infection or other adverse effects on the nasal mucosa.

3. The following are general approximations of equivalent glucocorticoid dosages and may not apply to all diseases or routes of administration.

Approximately Equivalent Glucocorticoid Dosages	
Cortisone 25 mg	Methylprednisolone 4 mg
Hydrocortisone 20 mg	Triamcinolone 4 mg
Prednisolone 5 mg	Dexamethasone 0.75 mg
Prednisone 5 mg	Betamethasone 0.6 mg

4. The following is an approximate representation of general comparative topical corticosteroid potency. Check specific product formulations prior to making potency decisions.

Very High Potency	High Potency	Medium Potency	Low Potency
Betamethasone (dipropionate augmented) Clobetasol Diflorasone (diacetate ointment) Halobetasol	Amcinonide Betamethasone (dipropionate) Desoximetasone (gel, ointment, or cream 0.25% or higher) Diflorasone (diacetate cream) Fluocinolone (cream 0.2% or higher) Fluocinonide Halcinonide Triamcinolone (0.5% or greater)	Beclomethasone Betamethasone (benzoate & valerate) Clobetasone Desoximetasone (cream 0.25% or greater) Diflucortolone Fluocinolone (ointment or topical solution or cream less than 0.2%) Flurandrenolide (0.025% or greater) Fluticasone Hydrocortisone (butyrate & valerate) Mometasone Prednicarbate Triamcinolone (less than 0.5%)	Alclometasone Clocortolone Desonide Dexamethasone Flumethasone Flurandrenolide (less than 0.025%) Hydrocortisone (base & acetate)

5. Metered-dose inhalers require proper cleaning and maintenance. Some have dose counters and check of lists, expiration dates that are established based on first use, which may require initial priming and repriming if not used within a specific period of time. Refer to each PI for detailed instructions prior to using any inhaler, whether nasal or oral.

6. Estrogens, including estradiol, are available in many topical dosage forms, such as emulsions, gels, sprays, and transdermal systems. Patients should be advised to carefully read and follow administration directions to avoid accidental exposure of estradiol hormone to others, including children and pets.

7. Patients with diabetes must follow a regular, prescribed diet and exercise schedule to avoid either hypoglycemia or hyperglycemia. Conditions that predispose patients to significant fluctuations in blood glucose include fever, thyroid disease, infection, recent trauma or surgery, vomiting, diarrhea secondary to malabsorption, and certain medications can also affect insulin and oral antihypoglycemic requirements, requiring dosage adjustments. Additional consideration must always be given whenever a change in either nicotine intake or tobacco smoking status occurs. Nicotine increases circulating

cortisol and catecholamine levels, which may increase plasma glucose and tobacco smoking is known to aggravate insulin resistance. The cessation of nicotine therapy or tobacco smoking may result in a decrease in blood glucose. Conditions that predispose patients to developing hypoglycemia may alter antidiabetic agent efficacy and require more frequent blood glucose monitoring include debilitated physical condition, drug interactions, malnutrition, uncontrolled adrenal insufficiency, hypothyroidism or pituitary insufficiency. Conditions that exacerbate hyperglycemia include fever, drug interactions, female hormonal changes, severe stress, and uncontrolled hyperthyroidism and/or hypercortisolism. More frequent blood glucose monitoring may be necessary in patients with any of these conditions.

8. Patients with diabetes subjected to extreme physiologic stress such as infection, burns, or fever may require insulin in place of other antidiabetic therapy. Conditions associated with dehydration, sepsis, and hypoxemia temporarily preclude the use of biguanides such as metformin. This temporary hold on treatment also extends to surgical procedures that are associated with fluid and food restrictions and can be resumed when renal function is confirmed to be normal and when normal fluid and nutrient intake has been resumed.

9. Insulin is available in numerous dose formulations and administration devices. Read PI prior to administration. The following are a few specific tips:
   - Vials are generally recognized to have a beyond use date (BUD) of 28 days per the United States Pharmacopeial Convention (USP)
   - Vials should be stored in refrigerator prior to use; however, may be either refrigerated or kept at room temperature after first use
   - Pens are generally required to be stored in refrigerator but at room temperature once opened

Tammie Lee and Jacque

Bibliography

American Association of Clinical Endocrinologists/American College of Endocrinology. Comprehensive diabetes management algorithm. *Endocr Pract.* 2015;21(4). doi: 10.4158/EP15693.CS

American Diabetes Association. *Standards of Medical Care in Diabetes.* 2016;39(1). http://care.diabetesjournals.org/content/suppl/2015/12/21/39.Supplement_1.DC2/2016-Standards-of-Care.pdf

American Geriatrics Society. 2015 updated Beers criteria for potentially inappropriate medication use in older adults. *J Am Geriatr Soc.* 2015;63:2227–2246.

Brunton LL, Chabner B, Knollmann BC, eds. *Goodman's and Gilman's The Pharmacological Basis of Therapeutics.* 12th ed. New York, NY: McGraw-Hill; 2011.

McEvoy GK, ed. *AHFS: Drug Information.* Bethesda, MD: American Society of Health-System Pharmacists; 2016.

Melmed S, Polonsky KS, Larsen PR, Kronenberg HM, eds. *Williams Textbook of Endocrinology.* 13th ed. Philadelphia, PA: Elsevier; 2016.

PDR. Metformin hydrochloride: drug summary. http://www.pdr.net/drug-summary/Glumetza-metformin-hydrochloride-843. Accessed January 20, 2017.

PDR. Zoledronic acid: drug summary. http://www.pdr.net/drug-summary/Reclast-zoledronic-acid-437. Accessed January 20, 2017.

Symbols

- ▲ Renal impairment: Dose adjustment is recommended.
- ▢ Hepatic impairment: Dose adjustment is recommended.
- ■ Black box warning exists for this drug.
- (QT) QTc prolongation effects have been reported.
- (BL) Beers list criteria (avoid in elderly).
- (PD) FDA-approved pediatric doses are available.
- (GD) FDA-approved geriatric doses are available.
- 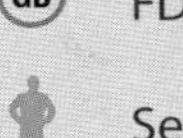 See primary body system.

Hormones and Synthetic Substitutes

Universal prescribing alerts:

- Known serious hypersensitivity to the specific drug or any other component of the product/formulation selected warrants a contraindication for its use.
- Adverse reactions associated with the use of some **hormone and synthetic substitute agents** include dizziness, drowsiness, vertigo, and fatigue; these agents may also impair the ability to perform tasks requiring mental alertness. Caution should always be recommended when using any new drug for the first time, when there is a dose change, and for continued use of known offending agents.
- Doses expressed are for usual adult dosage ranges only. "Geriatric doses" are assumed to be the same as adult doses unless otherwise noted with a symbol. Where FDA-approved pediatric dosing is available, a symbol will guide the reader to additional prescribing references. Refer to real-time prescribing references for these age-specific doses.
- Use of hormone and synthetic substitute agents in pregnancy is based on clinical risk versus benefit and safety concerns are not represented in this grid. Refer to the package insert (PI) for more information. Clinicians should continue to provide education about the reproductive risks of any medication and offer risk-reduction strategies (which may include contraceptive use) to women of childbearing age and understand that these reproductive risks may also extend to males. Other medications may decrease the effectiveness of oral contraceptives. Where necessary, an alternative means of birth control should be explored.
- Brand names provided for those products still available on the market. Due to the ever-changing product availability, refer to Food and Drug Administration (FDA) resources to confirm the actual brands available. This drug summary is intended for educational purposes only. Prescribing decisions should be based on real-time comprehensive drug databases that are updated on a regular basis.

Adrenal Agents

Universal prescribing alerts:

- These agents are associated with immunosuppressant effects and the development of localized infections including those of the nose and pharynx with *Candida albicans* as well as impaired wound healing. Patients with decreased immunity may be at higher risk of opportunistic infection and steroidal therapy may need to be interrupted during some active infections. The use of corticosteroids during the course of infection (specifically active or latent tuberculosis, certain fungal, parasitic, bacterial, or viral infections) should be cautiously initiated or continued, if medically necessary to administer to the patient. The use of nasal or orally inhaled steroids may result in localized fungal infection of the nose, mouth, and pharynx with *Candida albicans* (thrush). Patients should rinse mouth and expectorate after each use of orally inhaled steroids to decrease risk (refer to Tips from the Field to learn what to do if thrush develops).
- Reversible hyperglycemia and glucosuria has been reported in some patients receiving systemic corticosteroid therapy. Although the risk is less with inhaled corticosteroids, all steroids should generally be used with caution in those patients with diabetes mellitus because an exacerbation of diabetes may occur with significant systemic absorption of an inhaled corticosteroid.

- Psychiatric events and behavioral changes such as aggression, depression, sleep disorders, psychomotor hyperactivity, and suicidal ideation have been reported with the use of corticosteroids, and thus these agents are deemed to meet Beers criteria to avoid use in older adults with or at high risk of delirium because of the potential to induce or worsen delirium. Psychiatric events occur more commonly in patients receiving 80 mg per day of oral prednisone or equivalent. See Tips from the Field for approximate steroid dose equivalents.
- Adverse effects on bone metabolism (including decreased bone formation, increased resorption, and decreased bone integrity such as that seen in osteoporosis) have been reported with systemically administered corticosteroids. The risks of these effects are expected to be much lower with inhaled corticosteroids, however the risk is higher with high-dose inhaled formulations and in patients receiving long-term therapy of inhaled corticosteroids. See Tips from the Field for compounding risk factors.
- Glaucoma, increased intraocular pressure, and cataracts have been reported with the use of corticosteroids. Instruct patients to avoid spraying these products accidently into the eyes when using and to report any unexplained visual disturbance promptly. Prescribe with caution for patients potentially predisposed to these conditions.
- Adrenal agents are also known as glucocorticoids and are expressed in various "steroidal potencies." Prolonged use increases the likelihood of hypothalamic–pituitary–adrenal (HPA) axis suppression and the need for slow tapering. Topical products result in varying degrees of systemic absorption, so they may also share the risk of similar adverse effects as agents that are administered orally.
- Other reported adverse effects: GI irritant effects (take with food), fat distribution changes resulting in the "buffalo hump", moon face (Cushingoid appearance), striae or stretchmarks. Steroids should generally not be applied to the face or thin skin.

Drug Name	FDA-Approved Indications	Adult Dosage Range	Precautions and Clinical Pearls
Generic Name Beclomethasone dipropionate **Brand Name** (Nasal) Beconase Beconase AQ Qnasal (Oral inhalation) QVAR BL	Beconase AQ: seasonal or perennial allergic and nonallergic (vasomotor) rhinitis QVAR: maintenance treatment of asthma as prophylactic therapy	**Illustrative dose for oral inhaler (MDI) for patient not on oral steroids:** Initial dose: 1 to 2 puffs (40 mcg per puff) twice daily; the usual maximum dose is 320 mcg inhaled orally twice daily	• Dose varies with indication for use, formulation selected, and patient's clinical response • May cause mild nasopharyngeal irritation, nasal discomfort, epistaxis, nasal ulceration, and nasal septal perforation • Avoid use in patients with nasal ulcers, recent nasal surgery or trauma • MDI not for treatment of acute bronchospasms • Symptomatic relief may not occur in some patients for as long as 2 weeks • Patients should prime devices (and shake container if directed to do so) prior to use according to the manufacturer's recommendations as outlined in the PI

Drug Name	FDA-Approved Indications	Adult Dosage Range	Precautions and Clinical Pearls
Generic Name Betamethasone Dipropionate Valerate **Brand Name** Betamethasone Diprolene Diprolene AF Luxiq BL	**Common indications for use:** Relief of inflammation and pruritic manifestations of corticosteroid-responsive dermatoses Inflammatory conditions (i.e., asthma, chronic obstructive pulmonary disease [COPD])	Dose varies with indication for use, formulation selected, and patient's clinical response **Usual topical dose for eczema:** 0.05% (non-augmented) cream or ointment: apply a thin layer to the affected area(s) once or twice daily	• Treatment beyond 2 weeks is not recommended • Do not use more than 50 g topically per week • Apply a thin layer topically; use sparingly • Do not use in treatment or rosacea • Many formulations available (including augmented gel and parenteral formulations); use care when prescribing and refer to PI • For severe respiratory conditions: recommend parenteral administration initially particularly where airway obstruction is present; refer to PI
Generic Name Budesonide **Brand Name** Pulmicort Rhinocort Entocort EC Uceris BL	**Common indications for use:** Asthma Allergic rhinitis Crohn's disease Ulcerative colitis	Dose varies with indication for use, formulation selected, and patient's clinical response **Illustrative oral (inhaled) dose:** Pulmicort oral inhalation powder: 360 mcg twice daily (MDD: 720 mcg twice daily) **Illustrative oral dose for Crohn's disease:** 9 mg once daily in the morning for up to 8 weeks	• Many formulations available: systemic (oral), inhaled, intranasal and rectal • One actuation of the 180 mcg oral inhaler strength delivers 160 mcg of budesonide from the mouthpiece; one actuation of the 90 mcg strength delivers 80 mcg of budesonide from the mouthpiece • Avoid use in patients with severe hepatic impairment
Generic Name Ciclesonide **Brand Name** Alvesco (Oral MDI) Omnaris (Intranasal) Zetonna (Intranasal) BL	Maintenance treatment of asthma as prophylactic therapy Allergic rhinitis	Dose varies with indication for use, formulation selected, and patient's clinical response **Illustrative oral (inhaled) dose for asthma:** Initial: 80 mcg inhaled twice daily (MDD: 160 mcg twice daily)	• May cause headache, nasopharyngitis, sinusitis, pharyngolaryngeal pain, upper respiratory infection, arthralgia, nasal congestion, pain in extremities, and back pain • For those without an adequate response after 4 weeks, higher doses may provide additional symptom control

Generic Name Cortisone acetate BL	**Common indications for use:** Addison's disease Allergic rhinitis Anaphylaxis	Dose varies with indication for use, formulation selected, and patient's clinical response **Illustrative dose for anaphylaxis:** Oral/IM: 25 to 300 mg administered once daily or on alternate days	• Available as: oral and IM • Once a satisfactory response is achieved, dosage should be reduced to the lowest possible for maintenance. Lower initial dosage may be adequate Contraindications: • Fungal infections
Generic Name Dexamethasone acetate **Brand Name** Decadron BL	**Common indications for use:** Addison's disease Anaphylaxis Asthma	Dose varies with indication for use, formulation selected, and patient's clinical response **Illustrative oral dose for asthma:** Initial: 0.75 to 9 mg per day, given in 2 to 4 divided doses	• For severe respiratory conditions: recommend parenteral administration initially particularly where airway obstruction is present (refer to PI) • Numerous dose formulations available, use care when selecting and administering (oral, parenteral, ophthalmic, etc.) Contraindications: • Refer to ophthalmic cautions in the Eye, Ear, Nose, and Throat Preparations chapter
Generic Name Fludrocortisone BL	**Common indications for use:** Addison's disease Adrenocortical insufficiency Adrenogenital syndrome	**Illustrative oral dose for Addison's disease:** 0.1 mg once daily (dose may range 0.1 mg 3 times per week to 0.2 mg once daily).	• Use as a supplement to hydrocortisone or cortisone for Addison's and other indications; refer to PI • Reduce the dose (i.e., to 0.05 mg once daily) if transient hypertension (HTN) due to therapy develops Contraindications: • Fungal infection
Generic Name Flunisolide **Brand Name** Aerospan (oral inhalation) Nasarel (intranasal) BL PD	**Common indications for use:** Allergic rhinitis Asthma Bronchospasm prophylaxis	**Illustrative oral (inhaled) dose for asthma:** Inhale 2 puffs (80 mcg per puff) via oral inhalation twice daily	• Prime prior to first use or if not used for more than 2 weeks • Use check-off chart to keep track of the amount of medicine used Contraindications: • Infection • Status asthmaticus

Drug Name	FDA-Approved Indications	Adult Dosage Range	Precautions and Clinical Pearls
Generic Name Fluticasone **Brand Name** Arnuity (oral inhalation) Flovent (oral inhalation) Veramist (nasal) Flonase (nasal) BL PD	**Common indications for use:** Addison's disease Asthma Dermatitis	**Usual oral (inhaled) dose for asthma:** 88 mcg (44 mcg per spray) via oral inhalation twice daily; not to exceed 440 mcg twice daily	• Multiple dosage forms available (including topical creams and ointments); use care when selecting and administering • Dose expressed as illustrative example for asthma is for patients previously treated with bronchodilators alone • Additional dosage regimens available for patients previously treated with oral and/or inhaled steroids; refer to PI prior to use Contraindications: • Acute bronchospasm • Status asthmaticus
Generic Name Hydrocortisone acetate cypionate sodium phosphate sodium succinate BL PD	**Common indications for use:** Addison's disease Anaphylaxis Asthma	Dose varies with indication for use, formulation selected, and patient's clinical response **Illustrative doses for asthma:** Oral: 20 to 240 mg (base) per day, given in 2 to 4 divided doses IM/IV/SQ: 15 to 240 mg (base) per day, given in divided doses every 12 hours	• Available in numerous dosage formulations including topical, rectal, EENT and oral; use care when selecting and administering • Administer parenterally (IV or IM) initially for the treatment of severe respiratory conditions or those compromising the airway Contraindications: • Fungal infection • Intrathecal administration
Generic Name Methylprednisolone acetate **Brand Name** Medrol Solu-Medrol Depo-Medrol BL	**Common indications for use:** Addison's disease Anaphylaxis Asthma	Dose varies with indication for use, formulation selected, and patient's clinical response **Illustrative oral dose for non-urgent allergic conditions:** 4 to 48 mg, depending on disease treated, per day administered in 4 divided doses **Illustrative parenteral dose for urgent intervention for anaphylaxis:** IV: 1 to 2 mg/kg per dose (maximum: 125 mg per dose)	• Available in numerous dosage formulations; use care when selecting and administering • Available in a dose pack for acute interventions for inflammatory or allergic conditions • Parenteral administration is recommended when urgent treatment is required such as necessary for severe conditions like anaphylaxis, angioedema, or urticarial transfusion-related reactions

Generic Name Mometasone **Brand Name** Asmanex Elocon Nasacort BL PD	**Common indications for use:** Asthma Dermatitis Rhinitis	Dose varies with indication for use, formulation selected, and patient's clinical response **Illustrative oral (inhalation powder) dose for asthma:** Initial: Inhale 220 mcg once daily in the evening (MDD: 440 mcg, as single or divided dose)	• Available in numerous dosage formulations (EENT, topical, and oral inhalation); use care when selecting and administering • Titrate to the lowest effective dose once asthma stability is achieved • Inhaled mometasone undergoes extensive first-pass metabolism in the liver; use caution in patients with hepatic impairment • Confirm dose counter is working properly prior to use • Digital dose counter will display the doses remaining; watch for '00' when the cap will lock and the unit must be discarded
Generic Name Prednisolone acetate sodium phosphate **Brand Name** Veripred BL PD	**Common indications for use:** Addison's disease Asthma Dermatitis	Dose varies with indication for use, formulation selected, and patient's clinical response **Illustrative oral dose for asthma exacerbation**: 40 to 80 mg per day in 1 to 2 divided doses until optimal clinical improvement is confirmed	• Available in numerous dosage forms (EENT, topical, parenteral, and oral); use care when selecting and administering • Guidelines recommend peak expiratory flow is 70% of predicted or personal best as clinical goal and therapeutic resolution for asthma exacerbation; total course of treatment is generally 3 to 10 days Contraindications: • Fungal infection • Viral infection (i.e., varicella)
Generic Name Prednisone **Brand Name** Deltasone Rayos (DR)	**Common indications for use:** Addison's disease Asthma Angioedema	Dose varies with indication for use and patient's clinical response **Illustrative oral dose for asthma exacerbation:** 40 to 80 mg per day in 1 to 2 divided doses until optimal clinical improvement is confirmed	• Pro-drug of prednisolone • Guidelines recommend peak expiratory flow is 70% of predicted or personal best as clinical goal and therapeutic resolution for asthma exacerbation; total course of treatment is generally 3 to 10 days Contraindications: • Fungal infection • Viral infection (i.e., varicella)

Drug Name	FDA-Approved Indications	Adult Dosage Range	Precautions and Clinical Pearls
Generic Name Triamcinolone acetonide hexacetonide **Brand Name** Aristospan Kenalog Trivaris (BL) (PD)	**Common indications for use:** Asthma Aphthous ulcers Dermatitis	Dose varies with indication for use, formulation selected, and patient's clinical response **Illustrative parenteral dose for severe asthma exacerbation:** IM: 60 mg; usual range is 40 to 80 mg	• Available in numerous dosage forms (EENT, topical, and parenteral); use care when selecting and administering • Specific formulations are recommended for individual indications (i.e., Trivaris is only indicated as adjunctive therapy for short-term administration of an acute episode or exacerbation); refer to PI • In some cases, use is recommended only when other treatment has failed; refer to PI • Dose titrations should be based on patient response and duration of symptom relief Contraindications: • Acute bronchospasm • Fungal infection • Status asthmaticus

Androgens, Estrogens, and Progestins

Androgens

Drug Name	FDA-Approved Indications	Adult Dosage Range	Precautions and Clinical Pearls
Generic Name Danazol **Brand Name** Cyclomen (Canada) ■	Endometriosis Fibrocystic breast disease Hereditary angioedema	Dose varies with indication for use and patient's clinical response **Illustrative oral dose for endometriosis:** 200 to 800 mg per day in 2 divided doses; continue treatment uninterrupted for 3 to 9 months	• Increased low-density lipoprotein (LDL) cholesterol, central nervous system (CNS) changes, jaundice, hematuria • Patients on hypoglycemic agents should monitor blood glucose closely • Drug interactions may require dose adjustments or avoidance of certain drug combination • Onset of action is 4 weeks • Peliosis hepatitis and benign hepatic adenoma have been reported with long-term use Contraindications: • Marked renal and/or hepatic impairment • Severe cardiac disease • Acute intermittent porphyria • Undiagnosed vaginal bleeding Associated with: • Thromboembolic events: thromboembolism, thrombotic, and thrombophlebitic events have been reported (including life-threatening or fatal strokes) • Benign increased intracranial pressure

Generic Name Fluoxymesterone **Brand Name** Androxy	Hypogonadism Delayed puberty (males) Inoperable breast carcinoma (females)	Dose varies with indication for use and patient's clinical response **Illustrative oral dose for hypogonadism:** 5 to 20 mg per day	• Risk of gynecomastia in males • Risk of menstrual irregularities • Use with caution in patients with hepatic impairment • DEA-controlled substance • Monitor females for signs of virilization Contraindications: • Males with breast or prostate carcinoma
Generic Name Methyltestosterone **Brand Name** Android Methitest Testred (BL)	Delayed puberty Hypogonadotropism Hypogonadism Primary hypogonadism Metastatic breast cancer (females)	Dose varies with indication for use and patient's clinical response **Illustrative oral dose for hypogonadism:** 10 to 50 mg once daily	• May cause gynecomastia or VTE; if either occurs, discontinue the therapy • DEA-controlled substance • Use with extreme caution in patients with hepatic, renal, or cardiovascular disease • Monitor for edema, anxiety, depression, acne, baldness, gastrointestinal (GI) irritation, leukopenia, and hepatic dysfunction • Hypoglycemia agents may have increased effects Contraindications: • Males with breast cancer or prostate cancer
Generic Name Oxandrolone **Brand Name** Oxandrin ■ (PD) (GD)	Weight gain (adjunct therapy)	**Usual oral dose:** 2.5 to 20 mg per day in 2 to 4 doses; course of treatment is 2 to 4 weeks and can be repeated periodically	• Blood lipid changes with increased risk of arteriosclerosis • DEA-controlled substance • Monitor liver function tests (LFTs), cholesterol profile, international normalized ratio (INR)/prothrombin time (PT) in patients on anticoagulant therapy • Drug interactions may require dose adjustments or avoidance of certain drug combinations Contraindications: • Nephrosis • Breast carcinoma • Prostate carcinoma • Hypercalcemia Associated with: • Peliosis hepatitis • Liver cell tumors may not be apparent until liver failure or intra-abdominal hemorrhage occur • Black box contraindication for use in renal impairment

Drug Name	FDA-Approved Indications	Adult Dosage Range	Precautions and Clinical Pearls
Generic Name Testosterone **Brand Name** Androderm Androgel Axiron Depo-Testosterone Fortesta Testopel Striant ■ (BL)	Metastatic breast cancer Delayed puberty (males) Hypogonadism, hypogonadotropic or primary	Dose varies with indication for use, formulation selected, and patient's clinical response **Illustrative parenteral dose for males with hypogonadism:** IM: 50 to 400 mg once every 2 to 4 weeks **Illustrative topical dose for males with hypogonadism:** Transdermal patch: Apply 2 to 7.5 mg for 24 hours	• Multiple formulations available; use care when selecting and administering • Starting dose of testosterone cypionate is typically 150 to 200 mg • DEA-controlled substance • Apply the medication to clean, dry skin; do not apply to scrotum • Patch may contain metal; remove it prior to undergoing magnetic resonance imaging (MRI) Contraindications: • Breast cancer (males) • Prostate cancer • Cardiac, renal, or hepatic disease (certain formulations) Associated with: • Risk of secondary exposure (transdermal gel/solution); refer to PI for strategies to prevent transfer to other people • Pulmonary oil microembolism (testosterone undecanoate) • Risk of serious reactions to oil injections even in patients who have tolerated previous doses

Estrogen Agonists and Antagonists

Estrogens

Universal prescribing alerts:

- Cancer risk: Estrogen and estrogen/progestin therapy in postmenopausal women has been associated with an increased risk of breast cancer and, thus, is contraindicated in patients with known, suspected, or history of breast cancer. Additionally, estrogens have been associated with endometrial cancer in women with an intact uterus. Estrogens are also contraindicated in the presence of hepatocellular cancer, hepatic adenoma (or in severe hepatic disease of any type).
- Cerebrovascular risk: Estrogens have been associated with an increased risk of cerebrovascular disease (i.e., stroke), venous thrombosis (venous thromboembolism or VTE) and pulmonary embolism (PE) and are therefore contraindicated in patients with an active or past history of MI, stroke, and/or thromboembolic disease as well as for patients with known protein C deficiency, protein S deficiency, or antithrombin deficiency or other known thrombophilic disorders associated with increased risk of venous thrombosis. The addition of a progestin to an estrogen regimen adds an even greater risk of cardiovascular events (i.e., MI).
- Dementia: Estrogen and estrogen/progestin therapy increases the risk of dementia in geriatric women 65 years and older.
- These agents are associated with danger of accidental exposure. See Tips from the Field for strategies to reduce risk.

Drug Name	FDA-Approved Indications	Adult Dosage Range	Precautions and Clinical Pearls
Generic Name Estradiol **Brand Name** Alora Climara Delestrogen Depo-Estradiol Divigel Estrace Evamist Femring Vivelle-Dot ■ (BL)	Metastatic breast cancer Hypoestrogenism (female) Osteoporosis prevention (female) Advanced prostate cancer Vasomotor symptoms associated with menopause Vulvar and vaginal atrophy associated with menopause	**Illustrative doses for ovarian failure:** Oral: 0.5 to 2 mg daily Parenteral: IM (cypionate in oil): 1.5 to 2 mg every 4 weeks Topical: apply 1 patch (0.025 to 0.05 mg per patch) once or twice weekly depending on brand and clinical need	• Available in numerous dosage forms; use care when selecting and administering (i.e., oral, patches, gels, emulsions, vaginal inserts, etc.) • Precautions: transdermal patch may contain metal; remove it prior to undergoing MRI • Estrogens should be used for the shortest duration possible (risk versus benefit considered) • Avoid alcohol: routine use increases estrogen levels and risk of breast cancer; recommend frequent breast and OBGYN exams • Monitor for VTE, edema, HTN, and CNS changes throughout therapy • May cause impaired glucose intolerance Associated with: • All universal prescribing alerts for estrogens
Generic Name Estrogen, conjugated **Brand Name** Premarin ■ (BL)	Abnormal uterine bleeding (injection only) Metastatic breast cancer Hypoestrogenism (female) Osteoporosis prevention (female) Advanced prostate cancer Vasomotor symptoms associated with menopause Vulvar and vaginal atrophy associated with menopause	Dose varies with indication for use, formulation selected, and patient's clinical response **Illustrative doses for hormone replacement for symptoms of menopause:** Oral: 0.3 mg daily in continuous or cyclic administration Intravaginal: 0.5 to 2 g per day cyclically; 0.5 g twice weekly **Illustrative parenteral dose abnormal uterine bleeding:** IV/IM: 25 mg and repeat in 6 to 12 hours if needed	• Estrogens should be used at the lowest dose and for the shortest duration possible • Consider overall risk versus benefit • Avoid alcohol; routine use increases estrogen levels and risk of breast cancer and osteoporosis • Monitor for VTE, edema, HTN, and CNS changes throughout therapy • Recommend frequent breast & OBGYN exams • Patients with diabetes should monitor their blood glucose due to impaired glucose intolerance • Cyclic administration: 3 weeks on with 1 week off, or 25 days on with 5 days off Associated with: • All universal prescribing alerts for estrogens

Drug Name	FDA-Approved Indications	Adult Dosage Range	Precautions and Clinical Pearls
Generic Name Estropipate Esterified estrogen **Brand Name** Menest Ogen ■ (BL)	Hypoestrogenism Osteoporosis prevention Vasomotor symptoms associated with menopause Vulval and vaginal atrophy associated with menopause	Dose varies with indication for use, formulation selected, and patient's clinical response **Illustrative oral dose for esterified estrogens for primary ovarian failure:** 0.3 to 1.25 mg daily or cyclically **Usual oral dose for estropipate for vasomotor symptoms of menopause:** 0.75 to 6 mg per day, cyclical administration	• Before and during use, consider risk versus benefit Associated with: • All universal prescribing alerts for estrogens

Estrogen Agonist-Antagonists

Universal prescribing alerts:
- Beers criteria due to potential to exacerbate incontinence.

Drug Name	FDA-Approved Indications	Adult Dosage Range	Precautions and Clinical Pearls
Generic Name Bazedoxifene **Brand Name** Duavee ■ (BL)	**Common indications for use:** Postmenopausal osteoporosis prophylaxis Vasomotor symptoms For women with an intact uterus	**Usual oral dose:** Take 1 tablet daily (contains 20 mg bazedoxifene in combination with 0.45 mg conjugated estrogens)	• Do not use with additional estrogens • Use is not recommended in patients with renal impairment • Keep tablets in the original packaging; do not place them in a pill box • Swallow tablets whole • Stop therapy 4 to 6 weeks before surgery • Monitor for edema, blood pressure, and VTE/deep vein thrombosis (DVT) • Perform yearly breast exams; perform mammograms based on patient age and previous exams Contraindications: • Hepatic impairment • Estrogen-dependent neoplasia and undiagnosed abnormal uterine bleeding Associated with: • All universal prescribing alerts for estrogens

Generic Name Clomiphene citrate	Infertility	**Illustrative oral dose for premenopausal females:** Initial: 50 mg once daily for 5 days	• Patients with polycystic ovarian syndrome (PCOS) may need lower initial doses (i.e., 25 mg once daily for 5 days). • In women with recent menstrual bleeding or progestin-induced bleeding, therapy should be initiated on or about the fifth day of the cycle following the first day of withdrawal or menstrual bleeding • Therapy may be started at any time in women who have not had recent uterine bleeding. • Only effective for women with intact hypothalamic-pituitary tract/ovarian response
Generic Name Ospemifene **Brand Name** Osphena ■	Treatment of moderate to severe dyspareunia (symptom of vulvar and vaginal atrophy, due to menopause)	**Usual oral dose:** 60 mg daily with food	• Do not use estrogens or an estrogen agonist/antagonist concomitantly with this medication • Drug interactions may require dose adjustments or avoidance of certain drug combinations • May increase the risk of cancer of the lining of the uterus Contraindications: • Undiagnosed abnormal genital bleeding • Known or suspected estrogen-dependent neoplasia • Active DVT, pulmonary embolism (PE), or a history of these conditions • Active arterial thromboembolic disease (e.g., stroke and myocardial infarction [MI]), or a history of these conditions • Known, suspected, or history of breast cancer • Severe hepatic impairment Associated with: • All universal prescribing alerts for estrogens
Generic Name Raloxifene **Brand Name** Evista ■	**Common indication for use:** Prevention or treatment of osteoporosis in postmenopausal women	**Usual oral dose:** 60 mg once daily	Contraindications: • DVT, VTE Associated with • An increased risk of fatal stroke was observed
Tamoxifen	Refer to the Antineoplastic Agents chapter.		
Toremifene	Refer to the Antineoplastic Agents chapter.		

Progestins			

Universal prescribing alerts:
• Contraindications for use:
  • Patients with current or history of thrombosis or thromboembolic disease and undiagnosed abnormal vaginal bleeding
  • Patients with known or suspected breast cancer, cervical cancer, uterine cancer, vaginal cancer or other hormone-sensitive cancer
  • Patients with uncontrolled HTN
• May cause decreased glucose tolerance, may exacerbate psychiatric conditions and may cause fluid retention; use care in high-risk patients or in those with conditions that may be influenced by these effects.
• Progesterone should be used cautiously in patients with hyperlipidemia. Although hyperlipidemia is associated with estrogen-progestin combinations, the effects of progestin-only oral contraceptives on serum lipids have not been studied. Serum lipoproteins (HDL and LDL) should be monitored during therapy with progesterone.
• Estrogen/progestin combination therapy does not prevent mild cognitive impairment (memory loss) and has been found to increase the risk of dementia in women 65 years and older.			

Drug Name	**FDA-Approved Indications**	**Adult Dosage Range**	**Precautions and Clinical Pearls**
Generic Name Hydroxyprogesterone caproate **Brand Name** Makena	Preterm labor prophylaxis of singleton pregnancy	**Usual parenteral dose:** IM: 250 mg once weekly	• Administer in upper outer quadrant of gluteus maximus; apply pressure to the injection site • Not for IV use • Specific cyclic administration is required; refer to PI Contraindications: • All universal prescribing alerts for progestins
Generic Name Medroxyprogesterone **Brand Name** Depo-Provera Provera	Abnormal uterine bleeding Secondary amenorrhea Contraception Endometrial hyperplasia Endometrial carcinoma Endometriosis	**Usual oral dose for secondary amenorrhea:** 5 mg or 10 mg per day for 5 to 10 days **Usual parenteral dose for routine contraception:** IM: 150 mg every 3 months SQ: 104 mg every 3 months	• Prescribe at the lowest dose and for the shortest duration possible • Administer the first dose during the first 5 days of the menstrual period • Verify appropriate calcium and vitamin D levels • Monitor for vision changes, migraines, and BMD • Various formulations available for use (some require shaking before use) Contraindications: • Angioedema • Thrombophlebitis • Thromboembolic disorders • Significant hepatic impairment Associated with: • Loss of BMD • Dementia • Breast cancer • Increased cardiovascular risk

Generic Name Norethindrone **Brand Name** Aygestin Camila Errin Heather Ortho Micronor	Abnormal uterine bleeding Secondary amenorrhea Contraception Endometriosis	**Usual oral dose for secondary amenorrhea:** Acetate tablets: 2.5 to 10 mg once daily for 5 to 10 days	• Do not miss the daily dose if used for contraception; take at the same time each day • Backup contraception is required if the dose is administered 3 or more hours late and at the start of use • Monitor for vision changes, migraines, BMD, pregnancy status, weight, depression, and lipid profiles • Products are not interchangeable; refer to PI for selection and administration Contraindications: • Liver tumors • Thromboembolic disorders • All universal prescribing alerts for progestins
Generic Name Progesterone **Brand Name** Crinone Endometrin Prometrium	Amenorrhea Dysfunctional uterine bleeding Estrogen replacement Infertility	**Usual dose for amenorrhea:** Oral: 400 mg single dose in the evening for 10 days Intravaginal gel (4% or 8%): Administer every other day up to a total of 6 doses Parenteral: IM: 5 to 10 mg once daily for 6 to 8 days	• For amenorrhea, therapy usually starts 8 to 10 days prior to the anticipated first day of menstruation Associated with: • All universal prescribing alerts for progestins
Dienogest Desogestrel Drospirenone Ethynodiol diacetate Etonogestrel Levonorgestrel Norelgestromin Norethindrone Norgestimate Norgestrel	**Common indications for use:** Contraception and other indications based on specific products FDA approval	Refer to product labeling for directions for use	• Universal prescribing cautions for contraceptives and progestins (refer to specific sections)

Contraceptives

Universal prescribing alerts:

- A backup method of contraception is required for no less than 7 days at the start of therapy; refer to specific product PI for further information.
- Refer to product-specific PI for recommendations if any of the following situations apply: If the contraceptive ring is removed for at least 3 hours, if the patch is detached for more than 24 hours, or if 2 consecutive oral doses are missed (or 1 dose is missed in the extended cycle).

- Dose varies with indication for use, formulation selected, and patient's clinical response (common indications for use can include contraception, acne vulgaris premenstrual dysphoric disorder and hormonal regulation).
- Immediately rinse with cool/lukewarm water and reinsert the contraceptive ring if accidental removal occurs.
- Oral contraceptives are classified as monophasic, biphasic, triphasic, or estrophasic.
- Oral contraceptive regimens can be a conventional cycle, extended cycle, or continuous.
- Estrogen in combination products: ethinyl estradiol.
- Progestins in combination products: norgestrel, norgestimate, levonorgestrel, etonogestrel, drospirenone, desogestrel.
- Drug interactions may require dose adjustment and use of a backup method of birth control; refer to the PI.

Drug Name	FDA-Approved Indications	Adult Dosage Range	Precautions and Clinical Pearls
Estrogen–Progestin Combinations			
See associated letter for brand containing: **Estradiol valerate and:** Dienogest (A) **Ethinyl estradiol and:** Desogestrel (B) Drospirenone (C) Ethynodiol diacetate(D) Etonogestrel (E) Levonorgestrel(F) Norelgestromin (G) Norethindrone (H) Norgestimate (I) Norgestrel (J) **Mestranol and:** Norethindrone (K) ■ (BL)	**Common indications for use:** Contraception and other indications based on specific products: Natazia (A) Apri (B & others) Beyaz/Yaz (C & others) Kelnor/Zovia (D) Nuvaring (E) Seasonale/Seasonique(F) Xulane (G) Loestrin (H) Ortho-Tricylen (I & others) Ogestrel (J) Necon 1/50 (K)	**Illustrative oral dose:** Should be taken around the same time daily **Illustrative intravaginal dose:** Insert a ring for 3 weeks, then remove for 1 week **Illustrative transdermal dose:** Apply a patch once weekly for 3 weeks, then remove for 1 week	Contraindications: • Undiagnosed abnormal bleeding • Classic migraine • Active liver disease • Severe HTN • Thromboembolism • Coronary artery disease (CAD) • Breast cancer Associated with: • Increased risk of cardiovascular events with cigarette smoking and use of oral contraceptives
Progestin Contraceptives			
Etonogestrel	Refer to the Progestins section.		
Levonorgestrel	Refer to the Progestins section.		
Norethindrone	Refer to the Progestins section.		

Gonadotropins

Drug Name	FDA-Approved Indications	Adult Dosage Range	Precautions and Clinical Pearls
Generic Name Chorionic gonadotropin **Brand Name** Ovidrel Novarel Pregnyl	Assisted reproductive technologies (ART) and ovulation induction in females Hypogonadotropic hypogonadism in adult and adolescent males	**Usual parenteral dose:** Ovidrel SQ: 250 mcg administered 1 day after the last dose of a follicle-stimulating agent	• Risk of ovarian enlargement and ovarian hyperstimulation syndrome • Educate patients on self-administration, including reconstitution, injection technique, storage, and disposal of needles/syringes • Monitor for enlarged abdomen, cardiorespiratory status, urine output, and vital signs • Preferred route for certain formulations (urine-derived products) is IM administration • Ovidrel (recombinant Human Chorionic Gonadotropin [HCG]) is only for SQ administration Contraindications: • Uncontrolled thyroid or adrenal dysfunction • Uncontrolled organic intracranial lesion • Abnormal uterine bleeding • Ovarian cysts • Sex hormone–dependent tumors
Generic Name Nafarelin **Brand Name** Synarel	**Common indications for use:** Endometriosis	**Usual intranasal dose for endometriosis:** 1 spray (200 mcg per spray) into one nostril in the morning and 1 spray into the other nostril in the evening	• Treatment should start between days 2 and 4 of the menstrual cycle • If amenorrhea is not achieved after 2 months, the dose may be increased to 1 spray (200 mcg) in both nostrils every morning and every evening • Monitor bone density should be established prior to treatment and verified to be within normal limits and reevaluated as recommended; refer to PI • Bone density values should be within normal limits prior to retreatment Contraindications: • Undiagnosed abnormal uterine bleeding
Goserelin	Refer to the Antineoplastic Agents chapter.		
Leuprolide	Refer to the Antineoplastic Agents chapter.		

Antidiabetic and Antihypoglycemic Agents

Alpha-Glucosidase Inhibitors

Universal prescribing alerts:

- The terms Insulin-dependent diabetes mellitus (IDDM) and non-insulin-dependent diabetes mellitus (NIDDM) are used instead of type 1 diabetes and type 2 diabetes, respectively, in this grid.

- Conditions that predispose patients to developing hypoglycemia may alter antidiabetic agent efficacy; refer to Tips from the Field for a review of which patients may be at higher risk of developing hypoglycemia.
- When these agents are administered concomitantly with sulfonylureas, they will cause further lowering of blood glucose.
- These agents do not reverse any of the pathophysiologic dysfunction associated with insulin-dependent diabetes mellitus (IDDM) and therefore should not be used as monotherapy in IDDM.
- The hydrolysis of sucrose (cane sugar) to fructose and glucose is inhibited by alpha glucosidase inhibitors and thus products containing sucrose are unsuitable for the rapid correction of hypoglycemia. Patients should be aware of the need to have a readily available source of glucose (such as dextrose, d-glucose) to treat hypoglycemic episodes. In severe hypoglycemia, intravenous dextrose or glucagon injections may be needed.

Drug Name	FDA-Approved Indications	Adult Dosage Range	Precautions and Clinical Pearls
Generic Name Acarbose **Brand Name** Precose	Management of NIDDM	**Usual oral dose:** Initial: 25 mg 3 times per day Maintenance: 50 to 100 mg 3 times per day	• Administer with the first bite of each main meal • May cause flatulence and diarrhea • Will reduce postprandial blood glucose • Monitor blood glucose and $HgbA_{1c}$: may reduce $HgbA_{1c}$ by as much as 0.5% to 1% • One-hour postprandial glucose levels throughout treatment and a glycosylated hemoglobin (HgbA1c) level at 3 months should be used to determine response to therapy Contraindications: • Diabetic ketoacidosis or cirrhosis inflammatory bowel disease • Partial intestinal obstruction or predisposition to intestinal obstruction and colonic ulceration • Chronic intestinal diseases associated with marked disorders of digestion or absorption
Generic Name Miglitol **Brand Name** Glyset	Management of NIDDM	**Usual oral dose:** Initial: 25 mg 3 times per day Maintenance: 50 to 100 mg 3 times per day	• Administer with the first bite of each main meal • May cause flatulence and diarrhea • Monitor blood glucose and $HgbA_{1c}$; may reduce $HgbA_{1c}$ by as much as 0.5% to 0.8% • One-hour postprandial glucose levels throughout treatment and a glycosylated hemoglobin (HgbA1c) level at 3 months should be used to determine response to therapy • Not recommended in patients with severe renal impairment Contraindications: • Diabetic ketoacidosis or cirrhosis inflammatory bowel disease • Partial intestinal obstruction or predisposition to intestinal obstruction and colonic ulceration • Chronic intestinal diseases associated with marked disorders of digestion or absorption

Amylinomimetics

Drug Name	FDA-Approved Indications	Adult Dosage Range	Precautions and Clinical Pearls
Generic Name Pramlintide **Brand Name** Symlin ■	Adjunctive treatment with mealtime insulin in IDDM Management of NIDDM	**Usual parenteral dose:** SQ: Initial 15 mcg with gradual dose increases of 15 mcg no sooner than every 3 days to target of 60 mcg prior to each major meal	• May cause nausea, vomiting, and weight loss; if nausea persists, decrease dose • Major meal should be at least 250 kcal or 30 g of carbohydrates • Increases the feeling of fullness after a meal Associated with: • Hypoglycemia if the patient is on insulin and the insulin dose is not reduced • Should only be used in patients that have failed to achieve adequate glycemic control despite individual insulin management and are receiving ongoing care under the guidance of a healthcare provider skilled in the use of insulin

Biguanides

Universal prescribing alerts:

- Use of these agents is contraindicated in patients with metabolic acidosis. Metformin is associated with a risk for lactic acidosis and therefore should not be used in patients with lactic acidosis, a form of metabolic acidosis.
- Conditions that predispose patients to developing hypoglycemia may alter antidiabetic agent efficacy. Refer to Tips from the Field for a review of which patients may be at higher risk of developing hypoglycemia.
- Delayed stomach emptying may alter blood glucose control; monitor patients with diarrhea, gastroparesis, GI obstruction, ileus, or vomiting carefully. Conditions that predispose patients to developing hypoglycemia or hyperglycemia may alter antidiabetic agent efficacy. Refer to Tips from the Field to see who may be at higher risk.

Drug Name	FDA-Approved Indications	Adult Dosage Range	Precautions and Clinical Pearls
Generic Name Metformin **Brand Name** Fortamet Glucophage Glucophage XR Glumetza ■ (PD) (GD)	Adjunct to diet and exercise to improve glycemic control in adults with NIDDM	**Usual oral dose:** Initial IR: 500 mg twice per day; increase dose gradually by 500 mg weekly up to 2000 mg daily (in divided doses) Glucophage XR: 500 mg once daily; may increase up to 2000 mg once daily	• Warn against excessive alcohol intake • Not recommended in patients with hepatic impairment • Ensure normal renal function before initiating and at least annually thereafter • Temporarily discontinue in patients undergoing radiologic studies with intravascular administration of iodinated contrast materials or any surgical procedures necessitating restricted intake of food and fluids • May cause vitamin B_{12} deficiency and may lower vitamin B_{12} levels; monitor hematologic parameters annually Contraindications: • Patients with renal impairment Associated with: • May cause lactic acidosis in patients with cardiovascular, renal, or hepatic dysfunction

Dipeptidyl Peptidase IV (DPP-4) Inhibitors			
Universal prescribing alerts: • May cause hypoglycemia: When an insulin secretagogue (i.e., sulfonylurea) or insulin is used in combination with these agents, a lower dose of the insulin secretagogue or insulin may be required to minimize the risk of this adverse effect. • These agents are not substitutes for insulin in patients who require insulin and should not be used in patients with type 1 diabetes mellitus or for the treatment of diabetic ketoacidosis. • Conditions that predispose patients to developing hypoglycemia may alter antidiabetic agent efficacy. Refer to Tips from the Field for a review of patients who may be at higher risk of developing hypoglycemia.			
Drug Name	**FDA-Approved Indications**	**Adult Dosage Range**	**Precautions and Clinical Pearls**
Generic Name Alogliptin **Brand Name** Nesina ▲	Adjunct to diet and exercise to improve glycemic control in adults with NIDDM	**Usual oral dose:** 25 mg once daily	• May cause serious hypersensitivity reactions including anaphylaxis, angioedema, and exfoliative skin conditions • Well tolerated and may contribute to a 0.5 to 1% decrease in A1c • Acute (sometimes fatal) cases of pancreatitis and hepatic failure have been reported; do not restart if liver injury is confirmed and no alternative etiology can be found • Specific recommendations for patients undergoing dialysis; refer to PI
Generic Name Linagliptin **Brand Name** Tradjenta	Adjunct to diet and exercise to improve glycemic control in adults with NIDDM	**Usual oral dose:** 5 mg once daily	• Acute pancreatitis has been reported • May cause serious hypersensitivity reactions including anaphylaxis, angioedema, and exfoliative skin conditions • May cause severe and disabling arthralgia
Generic Name Saxagliptin **Brand Name** Onglyza	Adjunct to diet and exercise to improve glycemic control in adults with NIDDM	**Usual oral dose:** 2.5 mg or 5 mg once daily, taken regardless of meals	• May cause serious allergic reactions: exfoliative skin conditions (Stevens-Johnson syndrome), anaphylaxis, and angioedema • May cause hypoglycemia when added to sulfonylureas, insulin, or metformin • Drug interactions may require dose adjustments or avoidance of certain drug combinations • Acute pancreatitis has been reported • Arthralgia has been reported • No hypoglycemia occurs when saxagliptin is used as monotherapy • Weight neutral • Specific recommendations for patients undergoing dialysis; refer to PI

Generic Name Sitagliptin **Brand Name** Januvia ▲	Adjunct to diet and exercise to improve glycemic control in adults with NIDDM	**Usual oral dose:** 100 mg once daily	• May cause serious allergic reactions: exfoliative skin conditions (Stevens-Johnson syndrome), anaphylaxis, and angioedema • Arthralgia has been reported • Acute pancreatitis has been reported • Specific recommendations for patients undergoing dialysis; refer to PI

Incretin Mimetics (GLP-1 Agonists)

Universal prescribing alerts:

- Pancreatitis has been reported. Consider other therapies in patients with a history of pancreatitis.
- Discontinue promptly if pancreatitis is suspected and do not restart if pancreatitis is confirmed.
- Conditions that predispose patients to developing hypoglycemia may alter antidiabetic agent efficacy; refer to Tips from the Field for a review of which patients may be at higher risk of developing hypoglycemia.
- Associated with thyroid C-cell tumors in animals; the human relevance is unknown (dose dependent and treatment duration dependent).
- These agents have specific storage (and some require reconstitution); refer to PI.
- When administering concomitantly with insulin, administer as separate injections (never mix together). The two injections may be injected in the same body region, but the injections should not be adjacent to each other.

Drug Name	FDA-Approved Indications	Adult Dosage Range	Precautions and Clinical Pearls
Generic Name Albiglutide **Brand Name** Tanzeum ■	Adjunct to diet and exercise to improve glycemic control in adults with NIDDM	**Usual parenteral dose:** SQ initial: 30 mg once weekly. Dose can be increased to 50 mg once weekly	• May be given without regard to food • If a dose is missed, administer it as soon as noticed, as long as the next regularly scheduled dose is due at least 3 days later • May cause GI side effects and reduced weight • Refer to PI for reconstitution directions Associated with: • Contraindication for use in patients with history of specific cancers; refer to PI
Generic Name Dulaglutide **Brand Name** Trulicity ■	Adjunct to diet and exercise to improve glycemic control in adults with NIDDM	**Usual parenteral dose:** Initial SQ: 0.75 mg once weekly; dose can be increased to 1.5 mg once weekly for additional glycemic control	• May be given without regard to food • May cause hypoglycemia • Hypersensitivity reactions have been reported; discontinue if suspected • Requires reconstitution prior to use Associated with: • Contraindication for use in patients with history of specific cancers; refer to PI

Drug Name	FDA-Approved Indications	Adult Dosage Range	Precautions and Clinical Pearls
Generic Name Exenatide **Brand Name** Bydureon Byetta ■	Adjunct to diet and exercise to improve glycemic control in adults with NIDDM	Dose varies with indication for use, formulation selected, and patient's clinical response: **Usual parenteral dose Bydureon:** Initial SQ: 2 mg once weekly **Usual parenteral dose Byetta:** Initial SQ: 5 mcg twice daily	• Requires reconstitution prior to use • Use care when selecting and administering different formulations (i.e., Bydureon is an extended release product) • Should not be administered after a meal • Administer Byetta at any time within the 60-minute period **before** the morning and evening meals • Dose can be increased to 10 mcg twice daily after 1 month of Byetta therapy Associated with: • Contraindication for use in patients with history of specific cancers; refer to PI
Generic Name Liraglutide **Brand Name** Saxenda Victoza ■	Saxenda: Adjunct to a reduced-calorie diet and increased physical activity for chronic weight management in adult patients Victoza: Adjunct to diet and exercise to improve glycemic control in adults with NIDDM	**Usual parenteral dose for Saxenda:** Initial SQ: 0.6 mg per day for 1 week; increase by 0.6 mg per day in weekly intervals until a maximum dose of 3 mg per day is achieved **Usual parenteral dose for Victoza:** Initial SQ: 0.6 mg per day for 1 week, then increase the dose to 1.2 mg	• If the 1.2-mg dose does not result in acceptable glycemic control, the dose can be increased to 1.8 mg • Indicated for use for obesity with an initial body mass index (BMI) of 30 kg/m^2 or greater or 27 kg/m^2 or greater (overweight) with at least 1 weight-related comorbid condition (e.g., HTN, NIDDM) • Administer subcutaneously in the abdomen, thigh, or upper arm and rotate injection sites • Administer daily at any time, independent of meals • If a dose is missed, resume the once-daily regimen with the next scheduled dose; do not give an extra dose or a higher dose • If doses are missed for more than 3 days, initiate therapy at 0.6 mg per day to avoid GI symptoms Associated with: • Contraindication for use in patients with history of specific cancers; refer to PI
Insulins			
Universal prescribing alerts: • May cause weight gain. • May cause hypoglycemia. • Considered to be effective in all patients. • Consider starting insulin, in combination with metformin therapy with or without other non-insulin therapies, when the blood glucose is greater than 300 mg/dL to 350 mg/dL and/or the $HgbA_{1c}$ is 10% or greater.			

- Insulin may be more effective than other therapies when hyperglycemia is severe, especially if the patient is symptomatic or has any catabolic features (e.g., weight loss, ketosis).
- May reduce $HgbA_{1c}$ by as much as 1.5% to 3.5%.
- Changes in insulin regimen should be managed under close medical supervision and increase the frequency of blood glucose monitoring.
- May cause potentially life-threatening hypoglycemia.
- Monitor blood glucose, and increase monitoring frequency with changes in insulin dosage, use of glucose-lowering medications, meal pattern, or physical activity; in patients with renal or hepatic impairment; and in patients with hypoglycemia unawareness.
- Hypoglycemia due to medication errors: Accidental mix-ups between insulin products can occur.
- Hypokalemia may be life-threatening. Monitor potassium levels in patients at risk of hypokalemia; if indicated, treat for fluid retention and heart failure.
- Observe for signs and symptoms of heart failure; consider dosage reduction or discontinuation if heart failure occurs.
- Certain insulin formulations are appropriate for insulin pump use. Hyperglycemia and ketoacidosis due to insulin pump device malfunction have been reported. Monitor glucose and administer by subcutaneous injection if pump malfunction occurs.
- Beers list criteria when used as "sliding scale" insulin due to the potential for a higher risk of hypoglycemia without improvement in hyperglycemia management regardless of care setting (i.e., exclusive use of rapid or short acting insulins to manage hyperglycemia without an established basal or long-acting insulin).
- Products have specific storage requirements that change based on continuum of use and product type; refer to Tips from the Field.

Drug Name	FDA-Approved Indications	Adult Dosage Range	Precautions and Clinical Pearls
Generic Name Insulin Aspart **Brand Name** Novolog	To improve glycemic control in patients with diabetes mellitus	Dosage varies and is individualized depending on previous regimen, concurrent medications, and other factors (i.e., lifestyle) IV/SQ Continuous Intermittent	• Onset/Peak and duration **are approximate** and values can vary among individuals • Onset of action: 10 to 20 minutes • Peak: 40 to 50 minutes • Duration of effect: 3 to 5 hours • Continuous SQ may be used with insulin pump • Earlier peak glucose lowering effect when compared to regular insulin • Shorter than the duration of regular insulin
Generic Name Insulin Detemir **Brand Name** Levemir	To improve glycemic control in patients with diabetes mellitus	Dosage varies and is individualized depending on previous regimen, concurrent medications, and other factors (i.e., lifestyle) Intermittent SQ injection only	• Onset/Peak and duration **are approximate** and values can vary among individuals • Onset of action: 1.1 to 2 hours • Peak: none • Duration of effect: 7.6 to 24 hours (dose dependent) • IDDM, the average initial dose is 0.5 to 0.6 units/kg per day (NIDDM often requires lower initial doses); most patients require at least 3 injections per day

Drug Name	FDA-Approved Indications	Adult Dosage Range	Precautions and Clinical Pearls
Generic Name Insulin Degludec **Brand Name** Tresiba	To improve glycemic control in patients with diabetes mellitus	Dosage varies and is individualized depending on previous regimen, concurrent medications, and other factors (i.e., lifestyle) SQ dosing regimen	• Ultralong-acting basal insulin analogue; initial dose range for IDDM-insulin naive patients is 0.2 to 0.4 units/kg per day • Insulin degludec may be given at any time of day; however, doses must be given at least 8 hours apart. • May administer one-third to one-half of the total daily insulin requirement once daily; the remaining total daily insulin dose should be short-acting insulin (divided between each daily meal)
Generic Name Insulin Glargine **Brand Name** Lantus Toujeo Basaglar	To improve glycemic control in patients with diabetes mellitus	Dosage varies and is individualized depending on previous regimen, concurrent medications, and other factors (i.e., lifestyle) Intermittent SQ injection	• Onset/Peak and duration **are approximate** and values can vary among individuals and with brand selected • Onset of action for Lantus: 1.1 hours • Onset of action for Toujeo: 6 hours • Peak: none • Median duration of action: 24 hours • IDDM, the average initial dose is 0.5 to 0.6 units/kg per day (NIDDM often requires lower initial doses); most patients require at least 3 injections per day • Use care when selecting and administering (products are not interchangeable); available in two concentrations as a prefilled Solostar pen: 100 units/mL and 300 units/mL • Basaglar available only in KwikPen
Generic Name Insulin Glulisine **Brand Name** Apidra	To improve glycemic control in patients with diabetes mellitus	Dosage varies and is individualized depending on previous regimen, concurrent medications, and other factors (i.e., lifestyle) IV/SQ Continuous Intermittent	• Onset/Peak and duration **are approximate** and values can vary among individuals • Onset of action: approximately 20 minutes • Peak: approximately 55 minutes • Duration of effect: approximately 4 to 5.3 hours • Continuous SQ may be used with insulin pump • IDDM, the average initial dose is 0.5 to 0.6 units/kg per day (NIDDM often requires lower initial doses); most patients require at least 3 injections per day • More rapid than the onset of regular insulin • Earlier peak glucose lowering effect when compared to regular insulin • Exhibits a shorter duration of action compared to regular insulin • Should be given within 15 minutes before to 20 minutes after starting a meal because of its rapid onset (compared to regular insulin)

Generic Name Insulin human regular **Brand Name** Humulin R Novolin R	To improve glycemic control in patients with diabetes mellitus	Dosage varies and is individualized depending on previous regimen, concurrent medications, and other factors (i.e., lifestyle) Based on specific product selected (buffered versus unbuffered): IV/SQ Continuous Intermittent	• Onset/Peak and duration **are approximate** and values can vary among individuals and with brand selected • Take 30 minutes before meals • Onset of action: 30 minutes • Peak: 1 to 3.5 hours • Duration of effect: 8 hours • IDDM, the average initial dose is 0.5 to 0.6 units/kg per day (NIDDM often requires lower initial doses); most patients require at least 3 injections per day • Can mix with NPH insulin • Unbuffered regular insulin (500 units/mL) is considerably longer (mean 21 hours, range: 13 to 24 hours) • Only regular (unbuffered) insulin (100 units/mL) may be administered intravenously. • Do NOT use Humulin R U-500 intravenously
Generic Name Insuline human isophane (NPH) **Brand Name** Humulin N Novolin N	To improve glycemic control in patients with diabetes mellitus	Dosage varies and is individualized depending on previous regimen, concurrent medications, and other factors (i.e., lifestyle) SQ	• Onset/Peak and duration **are approximate** and values can vary among individuals and with brand name products selected • Can mix with aspart, glulisine, lispro, and regular insulin • Onset of action: 1 to 2 hours • Peak: 2.8 to 13 hours • Duration of effect: 16 to 24 hours
Generic Name Insulin human inhaled **Brand Name** Afrezza Exubera	To improve glycemic control in patients with diabetes mellitus	Inhaled oral: single-inhalation cartridge (4 to 8 units) before meals Afrezza 4 units (one 4-unit cartridge) is approximately equal to SQ prandial insulin up to 4 units	• Onset/Peak and duration **are approximate** and values can vary among individuals and with brand selected • IDDM, the average initial dose is 0.5 to 0.6 units/kg per day (NIDDM often requires lower initial doses); most patients require at least 3 injections per day • May increase risks of adverse effects in patients with lung cancer, ketoacidosis hypokalemia, fluid retention, and heart failure associated with thiazolidinediones (TZDs)

Drug Name	FDA-Approved Indications	Adult Dosage Range	Precautions and Clinical Pearls
			• The metabolism and elimination of inhaled human insulin are comparable to regular human insulin • Onset of action: 15 to 30 minutes • Peak: 53 minutes • Duration of effect: 160 minutes • Administer at the beginning of a meal Associated with: • Acute bronchospasm therefore contraindicated in patients with chronic pulmonary disease, such as asthma or COPD • Use during periods of hypoglycemia
Generic Name Insulin Lispro **Brand Name** Humalog	To improve glycemic control in patients with diabetes mellitus	Dosage varies and is individualized depending on previous regimen, concurrent medications, and other factors (i.e., lifestyle) Based on specific product selected (refer to PI) IV/SQ Continuous Intermittent	• Onset/Peak and duration **are approximate** and values can vary among individuals • Onset of action: 15 to 30 minutes • Peak: 30 minutes to 2.5 hours • Duration of effect: 3 to 6.5 hours • IDDM, the average initial dose is 0.5 to 0.6 units/kg per day (NIDDM often requires lower initial doses); most patients require at least 3 injections per day

Meglitinides

Drug Name	FDA-Approved Indications	Adult Dosage Range	Precautions and Clinical Pearls
Generic Name Nateglinide **Brand Name** Starlix	Adjunct to diet and exercise to improve glycemic control in adults with NIDDM	**Usual oral dose:** 60 mg 3 times per day; may increase to 120 mg per dose if needed	• May be used in addition to, but not as a substitute for, metformin or a thiazolidinedione when glucose control cannot be maintained with monotherapy • Dosage for combination therapy is identical to monotherapy; hypoglycemic symptoms should be monitored closely • Use with oral sulfonylureas is not justified nor recommended • Use caution in hepatic impairment Contraindications: • IDDM • Ketoacidosis

Drug Name	FDA-Approved Indications	Adult Dosage Range	Precautions and Clinical Pearls
Generic Name Repaglinide **Brand Name** Prandin	Adjunct to diet and exercise to improve glycemic control in adults with NIDDM	**Usual oral dose:** 0.5 to 4 mg 15 to 30 minutes before meals up to 4 times per day	• If patient skips a meal they should skip the associated dose • Combination therapy of repaglinide with metformin, or a thiazolidinedione is indicated if glucose control cannot be maintained with monotherapy Contraindications: • IDDM • Ketoacidosis
Sodium Glucose Cotransporter 2 (SGLT-2) Inhibitors			
Universal prescribing alerts: • May cause hypoglycemia, genital mycotic infections, increased LDL cholesterol levels, hypotension, and renal function impairment.			
Drug Name	**FDA-Approved Indications**	**Adult Dosage Range**	**Precautions and Clinical Pearls**
Generic Name Canagliflozin **Brand Name** Invokana ▲	Adjunct to diet and exercise to improve glycemic control in adults with NIDDM	**Usual oral dose:** 100 mg once daily in the morning with first main meal of the day; may gradually increase to 300 mg daily if needed	• Correct any volume depletion prior to initiation of treatment (hyperkalemia has been reported) • Use care where there is increased risk of hypoglycemia; refer to Tips from the Field for conditions that put patients at higher risk • Dose-related increased LDL has been reported • Not recommended in hepatic impairment • Monitor patients for tissue necrosis and/or infection of the legs and feet • May be associated with increased risk of stroke • Fractures (rare, in susceptible patients) and decreases in BMD reported Contraindications: • Renal failure • Dialysis
Generic Name Dapagliflozin **Brand Name** Farxiga	Adjunct to diet and exercise to improve glycemic control in adults with NIDDM	**Usual oral dose:** 5 to 10 mg per day	• May be associated with increased risk of bladder cancer • Dose-related increased LDL has been reported • Use care where there is increased risk of hypoglycemia; refer to Tips from the Field for conditions that put patients at higher risk • Do not initiate if creatinine clearance (CrCl) less than 60 mL per minute Contraindications: • Renal failure • Dialysis

Drug Name	FDA-Approved Indications	Adult Dosage Range	Precautions and Clinical Pearls
Generic Name Empagliflozin **Brand Name** Jardiance	Adjunct to diet and exercise to improve glycemic control in adults with NIDDM	**Usual oral dose:** 10 to 25 mg per day	• Take without regard to food • Do not initiate if CrCl less than 45ml/minute • May cause renal function impairment • Dose-related increased LDL has been reported • Use care where there is increased risk of hypoglycemia; refer to Tips from the Field for conditions that put patients at higher risk Contraindications: • Renal failure • Dialysis
Sulfonylureas			
Universal prescribing alerts: • Avoid use in patients with glucose-6-phosphate dehydrogenase deficiency (G6PD deficiency); anemia has been reported. • Contraindications include IDDM and ketoacidosis. • Recommended to give once daily dose with breakfast.			
Drug Name	**FDA-Approved Indications**	**Adult Dosage Range**	**Precautions and Clinical Pearls**
Generic Name Chlorpropamide **Brand Name** Diabinese ▲ (BL)	NIDDM	**Usual oral dose:** Initial: 100 to 250 mg once daily; may increase gradually up to a maximum of 750 mg per day	• Classified as a first-generation sulfonylurea • Hypoglycemia is more common compared with second-generation sulfonylureas • May cause weight gain • Avoid in patients with renal dysfunction and hepatic disease (i.e., hepatic porphyria or cirrhosis); may cause edema due to antidiuretic properties
Generic Name Glimepiride **Brand Name** Amaryl	NIDDM	**Usual oral dose:** Initial: 1 mg once daily; may gradually increase up to a maximum 8 mg per day if needed	• Classified as a third-generation sulfonylurea • For elderly patients and patients with hepatic or renal dysfunction, start with low doses and titrate up
Generic Name Glipizide **Brand Name** Glucotrol Glucotrol XL ■	NIDDM	**Usual oral dose:** Initial: 5 mg once daily May gradually increase up to usual range of 10 to 15 mg per day	• Classified as a second-generation sulfonylurea

Generic Name Glyburide **Brand Name** Diabeta Micronase Glynase ▲ (BL)	NIDDM	**Usual oral dose:** 2.5 mg once daily; may gradually increase up to maximum 20 mg per day if needed.	• Classified as a second-generation sulfonylurea • Micronized and conventional formulations of glyburide are not bioequivalent
Generic Name Tolazamide **Brand Name** Tolinase	NIDDM	**Usual oral dose:** Initial: 100 to 250 mg once daily; may increase dose gradually up to 500 mg twice daily before meals	• Classified as a first-generation sulfonylurea • Doses over 500 mg should be divided and given twice daily
Generic Name Tolbutamide **Brand Name** Orinase	NIDDM	**Usual oral dose:** 1 to 2 g daily once daily (or may be given in divided doses); may increase dose up to maximum 3 g per day	• Classified as a first-generation sulfonylurea • Relatively short half-life and is metabolized to inactive metabolites, it may have a safety advantage (versus longer-acting agents) for the treatment of elderly patients • Use caution in patients with uremia, renal failure, or severe renal impairment
Thiazolidinediones			
Drug Name	**FDA-Approved Indications**	**Adult Dosage Range**	**Precautions and Clinical Pearls**
Generic Name Pioglitazone **Brand Name** Actos	NIDDM	**Usual oral dose:** 15 mg once daily	• May cause weight gain (retention of fluid) • May cause volume retention and congestive heart failure: do not initiate in patients with New York Heart Association (NYHA) Class III/IV heart failure • May possibly increase the risk of bladder cancer; do not use in patients with active bladder cancer • Increased fracture risk • Reduces triglyceride level • Improves HDL cholesterol • Drug interactions may require dose adjustment • May reduce $HgbA_{1c}$ by as much as 0.5% to 1.4% • Little, if any, hypoglycemia occurs when pioglitazone is used as monotherapy • May reduce cardiovascular disease (CVD) risk

Drug Name	FDA-Approved Indications	Adult Dosage Range	Precautions and Clinical Pearls
Generic Name Rosiglitazone **Brand Name** Avandia	NIDDM	**Usual oral dose:** Initial: 4 mg once daily	• Increases LDL cholesterol

Antihypoglycemics; Glycogenolytic Agents

Drug Name	FDA-Approved Indications	Adult Dosage Range	Precautions and Clinical Pearls
Generic Name Glucagon **Brand Name** GlucaGen	Hypoglycemia Diagnostic aid in radiologic examinations to temporarily inhibit GI tract movement	**Usual parenteral dose:** IM/IV/SQ: 1 mg; may repeat in 15 minutes as needed	• Use with caution in patients with prolonged fasting, starvation, or chronic hypoglycemia • Supplemental carbohydrates should be given to patients who respond to glucagon for severe hypoglycemia, so as to prevent secondary hypoglycemia • Monitor blood glucose levels closely Contraindications: • Insulinoma and/or pheochromocytoma

Miscellaneous Antihypoglycemic Agents

Drug Name	FDA-Approved Indications	Adult Dosage Range	Precautions and Clinical Pearls
Generic Name Diazoxide **Brand Name** Proglycem (BL) (PD)	Hypoglycemia	**Usual oral dose:** 3 to 8 mg/kg per day in divided doses every 8 to 12 hours	• Use caution in patients in whom sodium and water retention could be detrimental (i.e., uncompensated CHF and cardiac disease) • Prolonged hypoglycemia can exacerbate renal failure • Use caution in uremia • Parenteral formulations are available for alternative indications; refer to PI prior to use (for non-glycemic indications) Contraindications: • Aortic coarctation • Arteriovenous shunt

Parathyroid Agents

Drug Name	FDA-Approved Indications	Adult Dosage Range	Precautions and Clinical Pearls
Generic Name Calcitonin **Brand Name** Miacalcin	**Common indications for use:** Hypercalcemia Osteoporosis Paget's disease	**Illustrative parenteral dose for osteoporosis treatment:** IM/SQ: 100 iu once daily, once every other day, or 3 times per week	• Reserved for use in osteoporosis for use in women who are more than 5 years past menopause and in whom estrogens cannot be used (more effective therapies are available) • Give with supplemental calcium and vitamin D • Calcitonin-salmon nasal spray has not been shown to increase spinal BMD in early postmenopausal women

		Illustrative intranasal dose: 200 iu (1 activation) intranasally in one nostril once daily; alternate nostril used daily	• Serious reactions (anaphylactic) have been reported with use; refer to PI prior to use • Hypocalcemia and increased risk of secondary malignancy has been reported with use • Avoid intranasal dose if there is nasal trauma
Generic Name Parathyroid hormone **Brand Name** Natpara	Hypocalcemia Hypoparathyroidism	**Illustrative parenteral maximum dose:** SQ: 100 mcg per day Actual dose based on baseline evaluation of essential labs	• Prior to starting therapy must establish a baseline of essential labs (including but not limited to 25-hydroxyvitamin D and serum calcium), must collect and evaluate during treatment and upon discontinuation; refer to PI for specific details • Severe hypercalcemia has been reported Associated with: • Osteosarcoma
Generic Name Teriparatide **Brand Name** Forteo ■	Treatment of osteoporosis	**Usual parenteral dose:** SQ: 20 mcg once daily	• Recommended for the treatment of osteoporosis in postmenopausal women with osteoporosis who are at a high risk of fracture or in men with primary osteoporosis or hypogonadal osteoporosis who are at a high risk of fracture • Use for more than 2 years with a lifetime is not recommended • Has actions similar to parathyroid hormone thus use in patients with hyperparathyroidism should be avoided Associated with: • Rare cases of secondary malignancy (osteosarcoma)
Vitamins and Miscellaneous Parathyroid Analog Agents with Hormonal Influence			
Generic Name Calcitriol **Brand Name** Rocaltrol	**Common indications for use:** Hyperparathyroidism Hypocalcemia Hypoparathyroidism Psoriasis Renal osteodystrophy	**Illustrative oral dose for hyperparathyroidism:** Initial: 0.25 mcg per day; may increase dosage to 0.5 mcg per day if necessary	• Serum calcium, phosphorus, alkaline phosphatase, and creatinine concentrations should be determined initially, monthly for 6 months, then periodically (dosage adjustments are based on these values); refer to PI • Hypercalcemia and/or cardiac arrhythmias have been reported • Use caution in patients with hyperphosphatemia due to the risk of metastatic calcification • Encourage hydration and maintain adequate fluid intake • Avoid sun exposure may increase risk of skin tumor formation; use appropriate precautions • Avoid other photosensitizing agents Contraindications: • Hypercalcemia • Hypervitaminosis D • Ocular exposure (topical agents) • Accidental exposure to unintended skin (do not occlude with dressing)

Drug Name	FDA-Approved Indications	Adult Dosage Range	Precautions and Clinical Pearls
Generic Name Cinacalcet **Brand Name** Sensipar	**Common indications for use:** Hypercalcemia in patients with parathyroid carcinoma Hyperparathyroidism	**Usual dose for hyperparathyroidism** Initial: 30 mg twice daily May gradually increase dose to 90 mg twice daily	• Dosage should be titrated every 2 to 4 weeks through sequential doses • Higher doses may be needed to normalize serum calcium concentrations • Measure serum calcium within 1 week of initiation or dose adjustment • Once maintenance dose has been established, measure serum calcium no less than every 2 months; use caution in hepatic impairment • Hypotension, worsening heart failure, and/or arrhythmia have been reported with use • Seizures have been reported with use Contraindications: • Hypocalcemia
Generic Name Paricalcitol **Brand Name** Zemplar (PD)	**Common indications for use:** Prevention and treatment of secondary hyperparathyroidism	**Illustrative oral dose for hyperparathyroidism:** Initial: 1 mcg once daily or 2 mcg 3 times per week	• Serum intact parathyroid hormone (iPTH) concentration, calcium, phosphorus, alkaline phosphatase, and creatinine concentrations should be determined initially, at least every 2 weeks for 3 months, monthly for 3 months, and then every 3 months thereafter • Dosage adjustments are based on these values; refer to PI **Contraindications:** • Hypercalcemia • Hypervitaminosis D
Cholecalciferol [vitamin D_3]	Refer to vitamins and supplements resource.		
Doxercalciferol [synthetic vitamin D analog]	Refer to vitamins and supplements resource.		
Ergocalciferol [vitamin D_2]	Refer to vitamins and supplements resource.		

Pituitary Agents

Drug Name	FDA-Approved Indications	Adult Dosage Range	Precautions and Clinical Pearls
Generic Name Corticotropin **Brand Name** HP Acthar (PD)	**Common indications for use:** Collagen diseases Dermatologic diseases Diuresis in nephrotic syndrome	Dose varies with indication for use, formulation selected, and patient's clinical status **Illustrative parenteral dose:** IM/SQ: 80 to 120 units per day for 2 to 3 weeks	• May increase risk of electrolyte disturbances, hypersensitivity reactions, and immunosuppression • Use with caution in patients with history of cardiovascular disease, GI disease, liver and renal impairment, or myasthenia gravis • Administer at room temperature • Check the patient's vaccination record; if necessary, administer vaccines prior to initiation of therapy

	Multiple sclerosis Ophthalmic diseases Rheumatic disorders Serum sickness Symptomatic sarcoidosis	Discontinue with gradual tapering of the dose if prolonged therapy was used	• Monitor for infection, HTN, behavioral mood disturbances, cataracts, and glaucoma • Hypothyroidism may worsen • Long-term therapy may require osteoporosis prophylaxis Contraindications: • Scleroderma • Osteoporosis • Systemic fungal infections • Ocular herpes simplex • Peptic ulcer • Recent surgery • Congestive heart failure (CHF) • Uncontrolled HTN • Primary adrenocortical insufficiency • Adrenocortical hyperfunction • Co-administration of live vaccines • IV administration
Generic Name Desmopressin **Brand Name** DDAVP DDAVP Rhinal Tube Stimate ▲ (PD)	Diabetes insipidus Hemophilia A Von Willebrand disease (type 1) Primary nocturnal enuresis	Dose varies with indication for use, formulation selected, and patient's clinical status **Usual parenteral dose:** IV/SQ: 2 to 4 mcg per day in 2 doses or 1/10 of maintenance intranasal dose **Usual intranasal dose:** 10 to 40 mcg per day as a single dose or divided into 2 doses **Usual oral dose:** 0.05 mg twice daily	• Risk of severe hypersensitivity reactions, hyponatremia, and thrombotic events • Use with caution in patients with history of polydipsia, coronary artery insufficiency, or hypertensive cardiovascular disease • Should not be used in patients with type 2B von Willebrand disease requiring hemostasis due to risk of platelet aggregation, thrombocytopenia, and thrombosis • Evaluate the patient's risk of renal impairment and hyponatremia before beginning therapy • Limit fluids to amounts sufficient to reduce the risk of water intoxication (fluid restriction should be observed 1 hour before to 8 hours after administration of tablets) • Interrupt treatment if a condition develops requiring increased water consumption (e.g., vomiting, fever, vigorous exercise) • Monitor for VTE, hyponatremia, and water intoxication during therapy • Monitor pulse and blood pressure for IV infusions Contraindications: • Hyponatremia • Moderate to severe renal impairment (CrCl less than 50 mL per minute)

Drug Name	FDA-Approved Indications	Adult Dosage Range	Precautions and Clinical Pearls
Generic Name Vasopressin **Brand Name** Pitressin Synthetic Vasostrict (PD)	Diabetes insipidus (Pitressin Synthetic only) Vasodilatory shock (Vasostrict only)	Dose varies with indication for use, formulation selected, and patient's clinical status **Illustrative parenteral dose for central diabetes insipidus:** IM/SQ: 5 to 10 units 2 to 4 times per day as needed	• May increase risk of water intoxication • Use with caution in patients with history of asthma, cardiovascular disease, goiter, migraine, renal impairment, seizures, or vascular disease • Titrate to lowest dose possible to maintain blood pressure • Ensure proper needle and catheter placement; monitor to avoid extravasation • If extravasation occurs, stop the infusion and refer to the guidance in the PI for management • Monitor cardiac status, blood pressure, CNS status, fluid balance, and signs or symptoms of water intoxication Contraindications: • Uncorrected chronic nephritis with nitrogen retention (Pitressin Synthetic only)
Somatostatin Agonists and Antagonists			
Somatostatin Agonists			
Drug Name	FDA-Approved Indications	Adult Dosage Range	Precautions and Clinical Pearls
Generic Name Lanreotide **Brand Name** Somatuline	**Common indications for use:** Acromegaly Neuroendocrine tumor (NET)	**Illustrative parenteral dose for acromegaly using (Somatuline depot):** SQ: Initial: 90 mg every 4 weeks for 3 months	• Designated orphan drug by FDA for acromegaly • After 3 months, adjust dose based on growth hormone (GH) concentration, insulin growth factor-1 (IGF-1), and clinical symptoms • Administer via deep subcutaneous injection • May cause bradycardia; use care in patients with cardiac disease • Inhibit the secretion of insulin and glucagon; may cause hyper or hypoglycemia • Use caution in hepatic impairment
Generic Name Octreotide **Brand Name** Sandostatin (QT)	**Common indications for use:** Acromegaly Vasoactive intestinal peptide tumors (VIPoma)	**Illustrative parenteral dose for acromegaly:** Initial SQ: 50 mcg 3 times daily (usual range 100 to 200 mcg per dose)	• Designated orphan drug by FDA for acromegaly • Some patients require doses up to 500 mcg 3 times daily • IM regimens are available for those who cannot tolerate SQ • May increase risk of developing acute cholecystitis, ascending cholangitis, biliary obstruction, and cholestatic hepatitis • May cause hypo or hyperglycemia; use caution in patients with diabetes • Specific recommendations for patients with renal disease and undergoing dialysis • Use caution in patients with hepatic disease • May cause hypothyroidism and/or goiter • May cause B12 deficiency

Drug Name	FDA-Approved Indications	Adult Dosage Range	Precautions and Clinical Pearls
Generic Name Pasireotide **Brand Name** Signifor Signifor LAR ■ QT	Acromegaly Cushing's disease	Dose varies with indication for use, formulation selected, and patient's clinical status **Illustrative parenteral dose for acromegaly:** IM: 40 to 60 mg once every 28 days SQ: 0.6 or 0.9 mg twice daily	• Risk of cholelithiasis, bradycardia, QT prolongation, hepatic complications, diabetes, hypocortisolism, and hypothyroidism • Allow to reach room temperature for at least 30 minutes before reconstitution • Give intramuscular injection into the gluteus • Monitor at baseline (and periodically during treatment): $HgbA_{1c}$, EKG/ECG, thyroid/adrenal/gonadal function, liver function tests, potassium, magnesium Contraindications: • IV administration
Somatotropin Agonists			
Drug Name	**FDA-Approved Indications**	**Adult Dosage Range**	**Precautions and Clinical Pearls**
Generic Name Tesamorelin **Brand Name** Egrifta BL	HIV-associated lipodystrophy	**Usual parenteral dose:** SQ: 2 mg once daily	• Risk of fluid retention, injection-site reactions, diabetes, malignancy, and mortality in acute critical illness • Administer preferably in the abdomen, while rotating sites • Monitor for fluid retention and blood glucose: diabetes mellitus and retinopathy have been reported • Check serum insulin-like growth factor (IGF-1) levels at baseline and during therapy for risk of malignancy • For SQ use only; not for IV or IM use Contraindications: • Disruption of hypothalamic–pituitary axis due to hypophysectomy, hypopituitarism, pituitary tumor/surgery, head irradiation or head trauma, or active malignancy
Somatotropin Antagonists			
Drug Name	**FDA-Approved Indications**	**Adult Dosage Range**	**Precautions and Clinical Pearls**
Generic Name Pegvisomant **Brand Name** Somavert ■ BL	Acromegaly	**Usual parenteral dose:** SQ: 40 mg once as a loading dose; 10 mg once daily as a maintenance dose; MDD: 30 mg per day; titrate by dose increments of 5 mg based on serum IGF levels	• Increased risk of elevated hepatic enzymes more than 10 times the upper limit of normal (ULN) has been reported. Perform LFTs at baseline and monthly or weekly depending on levels • Risk of lipohypertrophy • Second-line therapy • Initial dose should be administered under prescriber supervision • Rotate the injection site daily; do not rub the injection site (for SQ use only)

Thyroid and Antithyroid Agents

Thyroid Agents

Drug Name	FDA-Approved Indications	Adult Dosage Range	Precautions and Clinical Pearls
Generic Name Levothyroxine (T_4) **Brand Name** Levothyroid Levoxyl Synthroid ■	Hypothyroidism	**Usual dose:** Oral/IV: 25 to 300 mcg per day IV: Oral ratio = 1:2	• Use with caution and reduce dosage in patients with cardiovascular disease • Overdosing levothyroxine in elderly patients may lead to atrial fibrillation and increased risk of fracture • Take on an empty stomach at least 30 minutes before breakfast, with a full glass of water • Thyroid-stimulating hormone (TSH) levels should be measured 6 to 8 weeks after therapy is initiated, every 6 to 8 weeks until normal, and then every 6 months • Slight reduction in symptoms is noted within 1 to 2 weeks; the full effect occurs 1 to 2 months after initiation of therapy • Drug interactions may require dose adjustments or the avoidance of certain drug combinations • Separate from the levothyroxine dose by at least 4 hours from other agents (i.e., aluminum [antacids], calcium, cholestyramine, iron, magnesium, multivitamins with fat-soluble vitamins [A, D, E, and K], folate, orlistat, sevelamer, sodium kayexalate, etc); refer to PI for additional details Contraindications: • Acute MI • Thyrotoxicosis • Uncorrected adrenal insufficiency Associated with: • The need to not use for the treatment of obesity
Generic Name Liothyronine (T_3) **Brand Name** Cytomel ■	Hypothyroidism	**Usual oral dose:** 25 to 75 mcg per day	• Use caution in patients with acute MI and preexisting cardiac disease • Symptoms of other endocrine disorders, such as diabetes mellitus, can be unmasked or exacerbated with use; use care • Parenteral administration is available for patients unable to take oral (IV use only) Contraindications: • Thyrotoxicosis • Uncorrected adrenal insufficiency Associated with: • The need to not use for the treatment of obesity

Generic Name Liotrix (T_3 and T_4) (1:4) **Brand Name** Thyrolar ■	Hypothyroidism	**Usual oral dose:** Initial: 1 tablet of Thyrolar-1/2 (contains 25 mcg T_4 with 6.25 mcg T_3) once daily **Usual oral maintenance dose:** 50 to 100 mcg T_4 with 12.5 to 25 mcg T_3 per daily	• Use care when selecting and administering Thyrolar-1/4, 1/2, 1, 2, or 3 (designates how much T4 and T3 each tablet contains) Contraindications: • Thyrotoxicosis • Uncorrected adrenal insufficiency Associated with: • The need to not use for the treatment of obesity
Generic Name Thyroid, dessicated **Brand Name** Armour Thyroid ■	Hypothyroidism	**Usual oral dose:** Initial: 30 mg once daily for most patients May increase to usual range for most patients between 60 to 120 mg daily	• Use caution in patients with acute MI and preexisting cardiac disease • Symptoms of other endocrine disorders, such as diabetes mellitus, can be unmasked or exacerbated with use; use care Contraindications: • Thyrotoxicosis • Uncorrected adrenal insufficiency Associated with: • The need to not use for the treatment of obesity
Antithyroid Agents			
Drug Name	FDA-Approved Indications	Adult Dosage Range	Precautions and Clinical Pearls
Generic Name Methimazole **Brand Name** Tapazole	Graves' disease Hyperthyroidism Thyrotoxicosis	**Usual oral dose for mild hyperthyroidism:** Initial: 15 mg per day given in 1 to 3 divided doses	• Doses are usually given in 3 equally divided doses at 8-hour intervals • Do not use in patients who have experienced drug induced agranulocytosis • Leukopenia has been reported • Use caution in hepatic impairment

Drug Name	FDA-Approved Indications	Adult Dosage Range	Precautions and Clinical Pearls
Generic Name Potassium iodide **Brand Name** SSKI Thyroshield	Only the case of radioactive emergency for thyroid protection to prevent radioactive iodide uptake	**Usual oral dose:** 1 to 2 drops every 8 hours	• Monitor: thyroid function test, signs and symptoms of hyperthyroidism • Dilute in a glass of water, juice, or milk; take with food or milk to reduce stomach upset Contraindications: • Dermatitis herpetiforms • Hypocomplementemic vasculitis • Nodular thyroid condition with heart disease
Generic Name Propylthiouracil	Graves' disease with hyperthyroidism or toxic multinodular goiter Symptoms of hyperthyroidism in preparation for thyroidectomy or radioactive iodine therapy in patients who are intolerant of methimazole	**Usual oral dose:** Initial: 300 mg per day, divided and given every 8 hours Maintenance: 100 to 150 mg per day divided	• Temporary hypothyroidism, agranulocytosis, or hyperplastic thyroid • Intolerance of methimazole and when surgery or radioactive iodine therapy is not an appropriate treatment option • May cause GI upset, constipation, dysgeusia • Monitor: LFTs, complete blood count (CBC), PT, thyroid function tests (TSH, free T_4, total T_3; every 4 to 6 weeks until euthyroid) • Patients with severe hyperthyroidism, very large goiters, or both: initial dose may be increased to 400 mg daily Associated with: • Severe liver injury and acute liver failure

Miscellaneous Therapeutic Agents

Bone Resorption Inhibitors

Universal prescribing alerts:

- Supplement calcium and vitamin D if dietary intake is inadequate.
- Severe, potentially life-threatening, hypocalcemia has been reported with the use of some of these agents; refer to PI.
- Contraindications for bisphosphonate use: esophageal stricture, achalasia or increased risk of aspiration, preexisting hypocalcemia and/ or the inability stand or to sit upright for no less than 30 minutes after taking a dose. All agents have been associated with osteonecrosis of the jaw; refer to PI for additional details and refer to chapter reading to see who may be at higher risk.

Drug Name	FDA-Approved Indications	Adult Dosage Range	Precautions and Clinical Pearls
Generic Name Alendronate **Brand Name** Fosamax Binosto	Treatment of osteoporosis Prophylaxis of postmenopausal osteoporosis Paget's disease	**Illustrative oral dose for adult postmenopausal females for osteoporosis prevention:** 5 mg once daily or 35 mg once weekly	• Osteonecrosis of the jaw has been reported; have dental evaluation and corrective interventions done prior to starting this agent • May cause rash that is worsened with sun exposure; use appropriate precautions • Avoid effervescent tablets in patients who are on a sodium restriction • Avoid in severe renal impairment Contraindications: • Universal prescribing alerts for bisphosphonates

Generic Name Denosumab **Brand Name** Prolia Xgeva	**Common indications for use:** Osteoporosis treatment and prophylaxis	**Illustrative parenteral dose for the treatment of postmenopausal women at high risk for fracture:** **Prolia:** SQ: 60 mg once every 6 months	• Monoclonal antibody; may impair immunity and increase the risk of infection; use caution • Osteonecrosis of the jaw has been reported; have dental evaluation and corrective interventions done prior to starting this agent • Severe injection reactions have been reported • Different products are indicated for different treatments; use caution when selecting and administering • All patients should receive 1000 mg of calcium and at least 400 international units of vitamin D daily • If a dose is missed, administer the dose as soon as possible and schedule future injections every 6 months from that date Contraindications: • Severe (sometimes fatal) hypocalcemia; use extra care in patients with renal impairment who may be predisposed • Review PI with women of childbearing age prior to use
Generic Name Etidronate ▲	**Common indications for use:** Heterotopic ossification Hypercalcemia Paget's disease	**Usual oral dose for Paget's disease:** Initial: 5 to 10 mg/kg per day for no longer than 6 months	• Higher dose regimens for shorter duration are available for urgent or more intense treatment; refer to PI • Osteonecrosis of the jaw has been reported; have dental evaluation and corrective interventions done prior to starting this agent • Retreatment after initial treatment requires specific criteria and caution; refer to PI Contraindications: • Universal prescribing alerts for bisphosphonates
Generic Name Ibandronate **Brand Name** Boniva	Osteoporosis treatment and prophylaxis	**Usual oral dose for prevention for postmenopausal females:** 2.5 mg once daily Alternatively may give: 150 mg once monthly on the same date each month	• Parenteral formulations and regimens are available; refer to PI • Osteonecrosis of the jaw has been reported; have dental evaluation and corrective interventions done prior to starting this agent • Supplement calcium and vitamin D if dietary intake is inadequate Contraindications: • Universal prescribing alerts for bisphosphonates

Drug Name	FDA-Approved Indications	Adult Dosage Range	Precautions and Clinical Pearls
Generic Name Pamidronate	**Common indications for use:** Hypercalcemia Paget's disease	**Usual parenteral dose for Paget's disease:** IV: 30 mg once daily for 3 days (total dose: 90 mg); administer each dose over 4 hours. If clinically indicated, patient may be retreated with the same dose.	• Osteonecrosis of the jaw has been reported; have dental evaluation and corrective interventions done prior to starting this agent • Correct electrolyte imbalances prior to use or when detected during use • May cause acute deterioration in renal function, including acute renal failure; patients with underlying kidney disease may be at higher risk • Universal prescribing alerts for bisphosphonates
Generic Name Risedronate **Brand Name** Actonel Atelvia	**Common indications for use:** Osteoporosis treatment and prevention Paget's disease	**Illustrative oral doses for prevention in postmenopausal women:** IR: 5 mg once daily before breakfast Alternatively may give: IR: 35 mg once weekly before breakfast	• Twice monthly and monthly regimens are also available; refer to PI for specific formulations and indication for use • Osteonecrosis of the jaw has been reported; have dental evaluation and corrective interventions done prior to starting this agent • Use care when selecting and administering these agents; multiple formulations that may not be interchangeable (i.e., Atelvia is delayed release) Contraindications: • Universal prescribing alerts for bisphosphonates
Generic Name Zoledronic acid **Brand Name** Reclast Zometa ▲	**Common indications for use:** Hypercalcemia Osteoporosis treatment and prevention Paget's disease	**Illustrative parenteral dose for prevention in postmenopausal females:** IV: 5 mg once every other year	• Administer over no less than 15 minutes at a constant rate of infusion • If dietary intake is not sufficient, patients also should be supplemented with no less than 1200 mg calcium and 800 to 1000 international units of vitamin daily • Indications and cautions are product specific; refer to PI prior to selecting or administering • Severe, potentially life-threatening, hypocalcemia has been reported. Correct imbalances prior to use and throughout the course therapy Contraindications: • Use patients with evidence of acute renal impairment and in those with a creatinine clearance of less than 35 ml/min or renal failure
Calcitonin	Refer to the Parathyroid Hormones section.		
Estrogens	Refer to the Androgens, Estrogens, and Progestins section.		
Raloxifene	Refer to the Androgens, Estrogens, and Progestins section.		

5-Alpha-Reductase Inhibitors

Universal prescribing alerts:

- Patients with a large residual urinary volume and/or severely diminished urinary flow may not be good candidates for 5-alpha-reductase inhibitor therapy and should be carefully monitored for urinary tract obstruction.

Drug Name	FDA-Approved Indications	Adult Dosage Range	Precautions and Clinical Pearls
Generic Name Dutasteride **Brand Name** Avodart	BPH	**Usual oral dose for adult males with BPH:** 0.5 mg once daily	• For adult males only • Capsule contents may cause irritation of the oropharyngeal mucosa; swallow whole • Avoid blood donation • PSA concentrations are expected to decrease even with diagnosis of prostate cancer • Can be used in combination with tamsulosin for greater efficacy Contraindications: • Refer to PI for women who are within childbearing age
Generic Name Finasteride **Brand Name** Propecia Proscar	Alopecia (Propecia) BPH (Proscar)	**Usual oral dose for adult males with BPH:** 5 mg daily	• Delayed results expected; may take 6 to 12 months to see therapeutic results • For adult males only • Avoid blood donation • PSA concentrations are expected to decrease even with diagnosis of prostate cancer • Caution in hepatic impairment • Women should not touch tablets with bare skin Contraindications: • Refer to PI for women who are within childbearing age

Chapter 13

Skin and Mucous Membrane Agents

Authors: **Tammie Lee Demler, PharmD, BS Pharm, MBA, RPh, BCPP and Charlene Meyer, PharmD**

Editor: **Claudia Lee, RPh, MD**

Learning Objectives

- Identify current pharmacologic agents that are appropriate for each condition/diagnosis.
- Recommend optimal pharmacologic interventions based on patient-specific characteristics.
- Provide appropriate patient-specific counseling points and optimal overall medication management.

Key Terms: Skin, mucous membranes, anti-infective agents, antibacterial agents, antiviral agents, antifungal agents, allylamines, azoles, benzylamines, hydroxypyridones, oxaboroles, polyenes, thiocarbamates, scabicides, pediculicides, anti-inflammatory agents, antipruritics, local anesthetic agents, astringents, cell stimulants, cell proliferants, detergents, emollients, demulcents, protectants, keratolytic agents, keratoplastic agents, depigmenting agents, pigmenting agents, sunscreen agents

Overview of Skin and Mucous Membrane Agents

Skin

The skin is the largest organ of the human body and makes up approximately 15% of the total body weight. As a key component of the integumentary system, the skin has many functions. It represents the first line of defense of the immune system, preventing pathogens and chemicals from entering the body by providing a strong physical barrier that contains infection-fighting macrophages and enzymes that break down foreign substances and metabolize medications. In addition, the skin helps regulate temperature, maintains hydration, and has receptors for touch and pain.

The skin comprises three distinct layers: the epidermis, the dermis, and the hypodermis. The epidermis is the outer layer that contains squamous cells, whose tight junctions protect the body from foreign invasions by creating a barrier against pathogens' entry. The epidermis continuously produces more skin cells to repair and replace the skin cells as they die and are sloughed off. The epidermis is also home to melanocytes, the cells that create melanin, the substance that produces the pigmentation of the skin. The greater the amount of melanin, the darker the skin, and the more efficient its blocking potential against harmful ultraviolet radiation.

The middle layer of the skin, the dermis, is highly vascular; it also contains connective tissues, nerves, hair follicles, and glands. Macrophages in this layer help defend the body and also serve a critical role in healing damaged skin.

The deepest layer of the skin is the hypodermis, or subcutaneous tissue. Here, more blood vessels are found, in addition to a protective layer of adipose cells. Adipose cells, along with sweat glands, play a crucial role in regulating the body's temperature. The hypodermis differs in thickness depending on its location on the body and on the specific person. As people age, this layer of skin becomes thinner—a factor that can lead to differences in medication delivery as well as less effective protection against foreign invaders. Pediatric patients are also at risk of infections and injuries due to the immaturity of this protective tissue in children.

Damage to the skin can result in either superficial or deep wounds. Superficial wounds that affect only the epidermis are more likely to heal without a scar or changes in skin structure. By comparison, wounds that extend farther into the dermis or hypodermis can cause scarring and potential loss of function for nerves or other structures if damage is severe enough. During the process of healing, a wound becomes highly vascularized to provide more oxygen to the tissues; oxygen is a key input that supports rapid cell proliferation. The healing skin may appear reddened and irritated. The new tissue created during wound healing consists of collagen, which is highly fibrous and the source of the uneven appearance of the regrowth. Over time, the number of blood vessels decreases as the structure of the skin becomes secure once again.

For pharmacologic therapy, the skin and mucous membranes provide a viable alternative administration route, albeit one that also presents a new set of barriers to drug delivery. For example, the skin varies in thickness; thus, a more potent medication may need to be applied to achieve suitable results in the thicker regions, such as the palms of the hands and the soles of the feet. Hairy areas may also require a different vehicle of administration—to cover the whole surface of the scalp, for example. The target of the medication is also important to consider. Are we treating an ailment of the skin, in which case a local effect is desired, or are we using this route as another entry point into the systemic circulation? To achieve systemic circulation, the medication needs to bypass the continuous skin layers that are meant to keep foreign invaders out. In contrast, other medications are meant to stay on the skin, thereby avoiding systemic adverse effects.

Disease and medical illness may influence the rate of absorption of medications through the skin. Certain skin conditions, such as eczema, psoriasis, and cold sores, interrupt the integrity of the skin, breaking down the skin's natural protective barrier. This can lead to the potential introduction of pathogens and an unintended increase of medication side effects. When the skin is healed, the normal rate of absorption resumes.

Creams, lotions, ointments, gels, foams, shampoos, sprays, and patches all can be used to help achieve the desired therapeutic effects. Nevertheless, each of these formulations also comes with vehicle-specific limitations. Lotions are aqueous based and are meant to hydrate, but are generally not very effective, leaving the skin susceptible to dryness due to evaporation. Ointments are oil based, which can cause staining of clothing and a greasy residue. The oily property of ointments, however, provides a physical barrier that reduces water loss through the skin; as a result, ointments have a greater hydrating potential than creams or lotions. By comparison, creams have a greater hydrating potential than lotions, are less greasy than ointments, and offer a middle-of-the-road moisturizing base. Foams and shampoos are often used on hairy areas of the body, especially the scalp. Patches allow for a continuous release of medication through the skin for either a local or systemic effect.

Mucosal Membranes

Mucosal membranes, also called mucosa, are moist linings that are adapted to specific functions of the body. Both the mucosa and the skin are continuous protective layers that guard against the entry of pathogens. Mucosal membranes are found in the oral cavity, nasopharynx, gastrointestinal tract, and urogenital area. Similar in structure to the skin, these structures have an epithelial layer that sits above connective tissue. The thickness and the type of epithelium vary depending on the location. Mucosa is often surrounded by smooth muscle, whereas in the gastrointestinal tract the smooth muscle lies between the epithelium and connective tissue.

Mucosa is also adapted to handle mechanical stress, such as the chewing and swallowing of food. Antibacterial enzymes are produced within these tissues to provide additional protection. As suggested by its pink appearance, mucosa is highly vascularized, which allows for a quick onset of action for systemic medication delivery. Age has little effect on mucosa, unlike with the skin. Diseases that cause dryness or breaks in the mucosal surface can increase the risk of infection or lead to unintended increased absorption (and effects) of medications.

13.1 Anti-infective Agents

Topical anti-infective agents offer an administration option that provides treatment directly to the infected location without risking significant systemic side effects. For example, this localized benefit is seen with the use of antifungal agents. Since many of these agents are known to cause hepatic dysfunction and require careful monitoring when used systemically, topical antifungal agents offer therapeutic benefits but with minimal systemic absorption, which reduces this unnecessary risk.

The ability to penetrate the skin is a key factor to consider during anti-infective treatment. Nail beds are difficult to penetrate, so the failure rate when treating nail fungus (onychomycosis) with topical medications is high. Topical antiviral agents can be used to treat cold sores, help with pain, and reduce the number of days with symptoms. Topical antibacterials can be used for various reasons, including prophylaxis against infection and the treatment of acne, rosacea, and other superficial infections. As with all antibacterial agents, repeated use may cause resistance. It is recommended to wash one's hands before and after applying treatment to prevent the spread of infection. Despite the generally low systemic absorption of these topical agents, patients should not use a topical anti-infective therapy if they have a true allergy to the medication.

Antibacterial Agents

Bacitracin
Clindamycin
Erythromycin
Gentamycin
Metronidazole
Mupirocin
Neomycin
Retapamulin
Dapsone (*see also the Antimycobacterial Agents section in the Anti-infective Agents chapter*)
Tetracycline (*see also the Antibacterial Agents section in the Anti-infective Agents chapter*)

Antiviral Agents

Acyclovir
Docosanol
Penciclovir

Antifungal Agents

Allylamines

Naftifine
Terbinafine

Azoles

Butoconazole
Clotrimazole
Econazole
Efinaconazole
Ketoconazole
Luliconazole
Miconazole
Oxiconazole
Sertaconazole
Sulconazole
Terconazole
Tioconazole

Benzylamines

Butenafine

Hydroxypyridones

Ciclopirox

Oxaboroles

Tavaborole

Polyenes

Nystatin

Thiocarbamates

Tolnaftate

Miscellaneous Antifungal Agents

Clioquinol
Gentian violet
Undecylenic acid

Scabicides and Pediculicides

Benzyl alcohol
Crotamiton
Ivermectin
Lindane
Malathion
Permethrin
Pyrethrins with piperonyl butoxide
Spinosad
Sulfur *(see also the Other Skin and Mucous Membrane Agents section)*

Miscellaneous Local Anti-infectives Agents

Benzalkonium chloride
Iodine
Mafenide
Selenium sulfide
Silver sulfadiazine
Boric acid (*see also the Anti-infective Agents section in the Eye, Ear, Nose, and Throat Preparations chapter*)
Chlorhexidine (*see also the Anti-infective Agents section in the Eye, Ear, Nose, and Throat Preparations chapter*)

Case Studies and Conclusions

Patient AJ is a 50-year-old female with severe hepatic disease, hypercholesterolemia, hypertension, and hepatitis B. Today she comes to your clinic with complaints of itchy feet. Upon closer examination, the doctor determines that AJ has tinea pedis and onychomycosis. AJ is really concerned because it is almost sandal season and she is embarrassed by her diagnosis.

1. What do you recommend to treat her tinea pedis?
   a. Ciclopirox solution
   b. Nystatin suspension
   c. Fluconazole tablets
   d. Econazole cream

Answer D is correct. Ciclopirox solution, fluconazole tablets, and nystatin oral suspension are not indicated for tinea pedis. Ciclopirox solution is indicated only for onychomycosis.

2. Which regimen do you recommend to treat this patient's onychomycosis?

   a. Efinaconazole solution weekly for 48 weeks
   b. Terbinafine 250-mg tablet daily for 12 weeks
   c. Clotrimazole cream twice daily for 12 weeks
   d. Nystatin solution swish and swallow 4 times daily for 12 weeks

Answer A is correct. Clotrimazole cream is not indicated for onychomycosis, and treatment would need to continue for at least 6 months. Nystatin solution is used only to treat oral thrush. Although terbinafine would treat onychomycosis, AJ has severe hepatic impairment so its use is not recommended in this patient.

You remember reading that onychomycosis is difficult to treat topically due to medications' inefficient penetration of the nail bed. To ensure greater success, you want to recommend an additional agent to use with the patient's currently prescribed efinaconazole solution.

3. Which added medication do you choose?

   a. Econazole cream
   b. Tolnaftate cream
   c. Urea cream
   d. Nystatin cream

Answer C is correct. Urea cream will help thin the nail bed and provide for better penetration by the topical agent. Adding another antifungal medication will not increase the ability to penetrate the nail bed.

Wilbert is an 18-year-old male with a history of type 1 diabetes (IDDM). He comes to you asking for help for his itching. His arm itches so much that he accidently scratched himself and now has a superficial wound. You notice a familiar rash pattern that is often associated with burrows under the skin and realize that his itchiness may be caused by scabies.

1. Which therapy do you recommend to treat scabies?

   a. Permethrin shampoo
   b. Permethrin cream
   c. Ivermectin lotion
   d. Lindane lotion

Answer B is correct. Permethrin shampoo and ivermectin lotion are indicated for lice only. Lindane lotion should be used only after first-line therapy has failed, due to its severe side effects of neurotoxicity.

It has been a few days since Wilbert's wound started. Knowing that he has diabetes, you want to make sure the wound heals properly.

2. Which topical antibiotic do you recommend to help this patient avoid infection?

   a. Metronidazole
   b. Dapsone
   c. Clindamycin
   d. Mupirocin

Answer D is correct. Mupirocin is considered a first-line therapy due to its excellent degree of tissue penetration and low rate of skin irritation. Metronidazole topical therapy is indicated for rosacea. Clindamycin and dapsone topical formulations are indicated for treatment of acne vulgaris.

Wilbert is also interested in an over-the-counter remedy for his cold sore. His prom is coming up soon, and he wants something to make the cold sore go away quickly.

3. Which therapy do you recommend?
   a. Docosanol
   b. Benzocaine gel
   c. Menthol cream
   d. Mupirocin

Answer A is correct. While benzocaine and menthol will help relieve the pain, they do not shorten the length of symptoms in the same way that docosanol does. Mupirocin is an antibiotic and will not treat cold sores, which are caused by a viral infection.

13.2 Anti-inflammatory Agents

Steroids are the first-line agents to treat local inflammation caused by immune reactions or skin diseases such as eczema, as they help with inflammation and itching. If applicable, topical steroid agents are preferred due to the adverse effects associated with systemic use of steroids. When used on a long-term basis, topical steroids can potentially cause thinning of the skin.

Steroids vary in potency depending on the medication and the strength used. Potent steroids should not be used on thinner skin areas such as the face and groin; they should also be limited in both duration of use and amount of product applied at each application. It is important that patients wash their hands before and after use of these medications to reduce unnecessary steroid exposure to other areas. Many of these products are also cross-referenced for systemic use in the Hormones and Synthetic Substitutes chapter and for use in the Eye, Ear, Nose, and Throat Preparations chapter.

Anti-inflammatory Agents

Alclometasone
Amcinonide
Betamethasone
Clobetasol
Clocortolone
Desonide
Desoximetasone
Diflorasone
Fluocinolone
Flurandrenolide
Halcinonide
Hydrocortisone
Mometasone
Prednicarbate
Triamcinolone

Case Studies and Conclusions

JD is a 25-year-old male hand model who expresses significant concern when diagnosed with eczema. He says, "Please give me the strongest medication that you have; I tried the OTC products and they don't do anything for my condition." The eczema appears only on his hands as a red rash and pustules. It is extremely itchy and unsightly.

1. Which steroid would you recommend to JD to clear his skin?
   a. Prednisone 5-mg tablets daily
   b. Hydrocortisone 1% cream twice daily
   c. Fluocinolone 0.1% cream twice daily
   d. Fluorouracil 5% cream twice daily

Answer C is correct. A systemic agent such as prednisone is not needed to treat this topical problem, and it can cause undesired side effects if used on a long-term basis. Hydrocortisone is a low-potency steroid that JD has already tried in over-the-counter (OTC) products, but that failed to relieve his problem. Fluorouracil is used to treat certain types of skin cancer and is not indicated for eczema.

2. Given that JD's profession is hand modeling, which information is important for him to know when using topical steroids?
   a. Topical steroids may cause striae, which are often not reversible.
   b. Topical steroids have a high risk of causing hyperglycemia.
   c. Topical steroids can cause skin atrophy, which is always irreversible.
   d. Topical steroids can suppress growth with long-term use.

Answer A is correct. Topical steroids can cause hyperglycemia, but this is not common. Skin atrophy is generally reversible with the discontinuation of the medication. Systemic steroids can suppress growth in pediatric patients only.

JD returns 2 weeks later and happily shows you that his eczema has improved. Unfortunately, he went to a masquerade ball, and the mask he wore has caused him to develop an itchy rash on his cheek. There are no comedones or scratch marks. You decide to recommend a topical steroid to relieve the itchiness and redness.

3. Which topical steroid would you recommend for JD?
   a. Hydrocortisone 2.5%
   b. Fluocinolone 0.1%
   c. Clobetasol 0.05%
   d. Mometasone 0.1%

Answer A is correct. Only low-potency steroids are recommended for use on the face and genital regions due to the increased sensitivity and absorption that occurs in these areas. Of the choices presented here, only hydrocortisone is considered a low-potency medication.

13.3 Antipruritic and Local Anesthetic Agents

Local anesthetics can be used to numb an area, either to treat pain or in preparation for minor surgery. Their topical application allows the patient to avoid side effects of strong systemic pain medication or the risks that come with complete anesthesia. The effects of topical anesthetics usually do not last more than a few hours, so these medications may be reapplied frequently.

Antipruritic medications can help treat rashes and itching due to a number of causes, including immune responses. Patients should wash their hands before and after use of these agents. These agents work through various pathways and clinicians should be familiar with the mechanism of action and potential concerns with systemic absorption (i.e., doxepin is an antidepressant that should not be combined with MAO inhibitors). While systemic absorption is generally minimal, the degree of absorption and potential adverse effects—if any—should be evaluated prior to use.

Antipruritic and Local Anesthetic Agents

Benzocaine
Dibucaine
Doxepin
Ethyl chloride
Phenazopyridine
Pramoxine
Diphenhydramine (*see also the First-Generation Antihistamine Agents section in the Antihistamine Agents chapter*)

Case Studies and Conclusions

MB is a 36-year-old African American male who recently went camping deep in the woods. He received a bug bite that is now itchy and painful and he would like to get relief from these symptoms. He also reports that he just finished his linezolid regimen for pneumonia 7 days ago. He is tired of taking pills. After his visit with you, MB needs to drive to his parents' house which is 4 hours away.

1. Which therapy would you recommend to help stop the itchiness?
   a. Diphenhydramine capsule
   b. Diphenhydramine cream
   c. Clean the area with green soap
   d. Doxepin cream

Answer B is correct. Diphenhydramine capsules will cause drowsiness, and MB needs to stay awake for the drive to his parents' house. Green soap will not help because the itchiness is not caused by an allergen immediately on his skin. Doxepin cream should not be used in patients with glaucoma or urinary retention, or within 14 days of using monoamine oxidase (MAO) inhibitors such as linezolid. It should be noted that diphenhydramine cream may not work well for everyone; if it does not, you would recommend OTC hydrocortisone cream.

MB has benzocaine spray at home. He asks if he can use it for the pain of the bug bite.

2. What would you tell him?
   a. Pramoxine works faster than benzocaine but can only be applied 3 times daily.
   b. Benzocaine is not used for bites, but rather is used only in the mouth or throat.
   c. Benzocaine cannot be used within 14 days of using linezolid.
   d. Benzocaine spray wears off in 1 to 2 hours and can be applied no more than 4 times daily.

Answer D is correct. Benzocaine wears off quickly and the total applications per day are limited. Pramoxine works as quickly as benzocaine and can be applied more often than 3 times per day. Benzocaine does not interact with MAO inhibitors and can be used for any minor pain topically; however, its use must be limited. The FDA has warned that caution is required when using benzocaine because oral benzocaine liquid, spray, lozenge, and topical gel products include a serious methemoglobinemia warning. This warning states that use of a product containing benzocaine may cause methemoglobinemia, a rare but serious condition that must be treated promptly because it reduces the amount of oxygen carried in blood.

MB calls your office a week later and says he received a severe burn while cooking dumplings. The burn is blistering and covers the skin from the back of his hand all the way to his elbow. He asks if he can use the benzocaine spray for his burn to help stop the pain.

3. What do you recommend?
   a. Yes, the benzocaine will act quickly and will numb the area.
   b. Use benzocaine on the area, then bandage the burn.
   c. This is too large of an area to treat with benzocaine; MB should go to the ER for proper care.
   d. Use ibuprofen instead of benzocaine, because its relief will last longer than that with benzocaine.

Answer C is correct. If the wound is deep or large, then benzocaine is not recommended due to the potential for systemic absorption and adverse effects. Since the burn covers a large area, MB should be instructed to seek medical attention to receive proper wound care.

13.4 Other Skin and Mucous Membrane Agents

Various medications are used for superficial conditions, and some can be used for cosmetic alterations. Depigmenting agents, for example, help acne scars to fade and are used to treat other abnormal hyperpigmentation of the skin. Because these are lightening agents, they may stain clothing.

Astringents are used to remove dead skin on the face, giving it a healthy glow. Cell stimulants promote cell turnover; they are used to treat acne vulgaris and have the added benefit of lightening acne scars. Keratolytic agents are used to thin thickened areas of skin or to treat acne vulgaris. Coal tar can be used for a variety of purposes, including treating psoriasis and dandruff, although it tends to be smelly and greasy, and can stain clothing. Patients should wash hands before and after using these products.

Sunscreens are topical products that help to protect the skin from the sun's ultraviolet (UV) radiation. Sunscreen agents absorb or block the harmful UV rays. Two types of UV radiation—UVA and UVB—damage the skin and increase the risk of skin cancer. Sunscreens vary in their ability to protect against UVA and UVB. Numerous reports questioning the safety of several sunscreen products have arisen since the 2000s. One ingredient in particular—oxybenzone—is a synthetic estrogen that was thought to cause hormonal adverse effects. Multiple studies thereafter came to the conclusion that oxybenzone is not absorbed into the body sufficiently to cause any of the suspected adverse effects. Titanium dioxide is another UV blocker that had concerns due to the danger of toxicity if the dry powder is inhaled. Both of these products maintain their status of FDA-approved sunblock, but it is always important to use any sunblock as directed and to read the caution label on the product before use. The minimum sun protection factor (SPF) rating needed for a product to properly protect the skin is SPF15, although products are also available at much higher SPF values (and contain an even greater amount of chemicals). Regardless of what SPF is used, sunscreens should be reapplied every few hours. There are a number of sunscreen ingredients approved by the FDA for OTC use. There are numerous brand names associated with these ingredients; refer to the specific product's ingredients prior to selection and use.

Astringents

Aluminum acetate
Aluminum chloride hexahydrate

Cell Stimulants and Proliferants

Palifermin
Tretinoin

Detergents

Green soap

Emollients, Demulcents, and Protectants

Vitamins A and D

Keratolytic Agents

Salicylic acid
Sulfur
Urea

Keratoplastic Agents

Coal tar

Depigmenting Agents

Hydroquinone

Pigmenting Agents

Methoxsalen

Sunscreen Agents

Sunscreens

Case Studies and Conclusions

TA is a 17-year-old Caucasian female who is at your clinic asking for treatment for her acne. She has a few comedones on her nose and forehead. Currently, TA uses benzoyl peroxide for acne twice daily on her skin. She has no significant past history. She does enjoy tanning on a regular basis and playing outside sports during the summer.

1. Which medication do you recommend to treat TA's acne?
   a. Aluminum acetate
   b. Tretinoin
   c. Salicylic acid
   d. Hydroquinone

Answer C is correct. Tretinoin and hydroquinone cause sun sensitivity and should not be used when sun tanning. Hydroquinone is not indicated for acne, but rather for dark-pigmented spots on skin caused by acne, age, and other reasons. Aluminum acetate is not indicated for acne.

TA also asks about sunscreen.

2. Which of the following statements is correct?
   a. When selecting sunscreen, it should be at least SPF 10.
   b. Sunscreen should be reapplied at least every 2 hours.
   c. Sunscreen does not need to be a broad-spectrum product to provide adequate protection.
   d. SPF 70 protects the skin 100% from harmful UV rays.

Answer B is correct. The minimum-rated sunscreen that should be used is SPF 15. Broad-spectrum products protect against both UVA and UVB radiation and are recommended. No sunscreen protects 100% from the sun, and protection increases by very small increments with products rated beyond SPF 45.

13.5 Miscellaneous Skin and Mucous Membrane Agents

The remaining topical agents are used for an even larger variety of disease states. Most are used to treat acne vulgaris, such as dapsone and doxycycline. These agents may irritate the skin and cause dryness. Diclofenac is a member of the nonsteroidal anti-inflammatory drugs (NSAID) family and is available as a gel for local pain relief. Collagenase is used for debridement of wounds, such as ulcers or burns.

Fluorouracil is a chemotherapy agent used to treat certain types of skin cancer. Patients and healthcare providers should wear gloves while administering this agent and wash hands after its use. Irritation to the skin is expected during treatment. Please refer to the companion drug grid for a review of all of these miscellaneous agents.

Miscellaneous Skin and Mucous Membrane Agents

Acitretin
Adapalene
Alitretinoin
Aminolevulinic acid
Azelaic acid
Bexarotene
Brimonidine
Calcipotriene
Collagenase
Eflornithine
Fluorouracil
Imiquimod
Ingenol
Isotretinoin
Mechlorethamine
Minoxidil
Pimecrolimus
Podofilox
Podophyllum resin
Secukinumab
Sinecatechins
Tacrolimus
Tazarotene
Ustekinumab
Diclofenac *(see also the Analgesic and Antipyretic Agents section in the Central Nervous System Agents chapter)*
Doxycycline *(see also the Antibacterial Agents section in the Anti-infective Agents chapter)*
Finasteride *(see also the Miscellaneous Therapeutic Agents section in the Hormones and Synthetic Substitutes chapter)*

Case Studies and Conclusions

PJ is a 55-year-old female with a past history of hypertension, diabetes, chronic obstructive pulmonary disease (COPD), and psoriasis. Her current medications include lisinopril 10 mg daily, amlodipine 5 mg daily, Advair 250/50 twice daily, metformin 1000 mg twice daily, and triamcinolone 0.1% cream twice daily. Lately, her psoriasis has been acting up and she has asked your advice about its treatment.

1. What would you recommend for PJ's psoriasis?
   a. Add calcipotriene cream to triamcinolone
   b. Discontinue triamcinolone and start calcipotriene
   c. Add diclofenac cream to triamcinolone
   d. Discontinue triamcinolone and start diclofenac cream

Answer A is correct. Calcipotriene cream is a vitamin D analogue that is more effective when used with a steroid. Using both medications together will improve the efficacy of treatment compared to either agent alone. Diclofenac cream is used to treat pain and will not help to reduce symptoms of psoriasis.

PJ also asked about minoxidil cream for her husband. Over the last few years, he has lost more and more hair and now has a bald patch in the middle of his head.

2. Which of the following statements about minoxidil is correct?
   a. Minoxidil treatment shows results within 4 weeks.
   b. Minoxidil has a 50% chance of curing baldness.
   c. Minoxidil is most effective in people older than 65 years.
   d. Stopping minoxidil use will cause noticeable hair loss.

Answer D is correct. Minoxidil takes 4 months to 1 year to show results and cannot cure baldness. Minoxidil is best used in people younger than 40 years, when hair loss first starts.

WJ is a 33-year-old Caucasian female who arrives at the clinic for her annual health visit. Upon examining her skin, you notice an abnormal spot with discoloration. It is diagnosed as superficial basal cell carcinoma. WJ is worried about using chemotherapy agents because she is a very busy mother with three young children. She often forgets to eat breakfast in the morning because she is busy putting the children on the bus.

1. Which medication do you recommend?
   a. Imiquimod
   b. Fluorouracil
   c. Ingenol
   d. Bexarotene

Answer A is correct. Bexarotene is indicated for cutaneous T-cell lymphoma only and ingenol is used to treat actinic keratosis. Fluorouracil is used twice daily, whereas imiquimod can be used 5 times a week at bedtime, which is a better dosing for this patient given her busy schedule, and she will not have to handle her children while the cream soaks in overnight.

2. Given that WJ wants to know more about imiquimod, which side effect should you counsel this patient about?
   a. Use imiquimod daily at bedtime for 5 days; wash hands before and after use.
   b. This medication does not affect the immune system.
   c. Imiquimod may cause premature aging, so the patient should use a supplemental "beauty cream."
   d. Local inflammation, chest pain, and influenza-like symptoms are common reactions with imiquimod use.

Answer D is correct. With any chemotherapy agent, the immune system can be compromised by its systemic absorption. Use of imiquimod for 5 days is indicated in antiviral-resistant genital herpes. For carcinoma treatment, the imiquimod regimen should last for 6 weeks.

Tips from the Field

1. Reducing systemic absorption of topical skin and mucous membrane agents should always be part of the overall treatment plan. Absorption is increased by the use of occlusive dressings, application to broken skin and to large surface areas. Do not apply to broken skin, do not apply heat (i.e., heating blanket, use sauna, etc.), and do not apply excessive amounts of the product. Use guidelines of limits of topical steroids based on potency and do not overuse. Gel formulations are generally more potent than creams and therefore should not be used on the underarm or groin areas where absorption may be greater.

2. For vaginal cream, only those dosage formulations specified for vaginal use should be used intravaginally. Topical products differ in pH from vaginal products; therefore, topical cream, gel, and lotion are for topical application to the skin only.

3. For topical cream, a thin layer should be rubbed into the affected areas. Cosmetics, sunscreens, and/or moisturizers often may be used after applying cream or lotion, if needed. Refer to PI prior to use for the product you have selected. Allow lotion to dry and wait until approximately 5 minutes have passed.

4. For the proper treatment of lice, nits (eggs) should be removed with a nit comb. Proper disinfection of the environment is also critical for success. This includes machine washing of all personal effects such as scarfs, coats, and linens for no less than 20 minutes. Those articles that cannot be washed should be either sent for drycleaning, sprayed with appropriate disinfecting products, or sealed in a plastic bag for 4 weeks. Combs and hairbrushes should be soaked in hot water that is at least 130°F for 10 minutes. Encourage parents to remind children not to share personal grooming articles with others to decrease the transmission of lice and other infections.

5. Even though sunscreen can help protect us from the sun's damaging rays, there are other actions we can take to keep us even safer such as avoiding the sun during the high intensity times in the middle of the day and finding shade whenever possible.

6. Wearing protective clothing (including hats) and polarized sunglasses that wrap around the eyes are both ways to keep oneself protected from sun exposure.

7. Self-tanning products are not the same as sunscreens; however, some tanning products also contain sunscreens (read labels carefully prior to use).

8. The American Cancer Society and other agencies recommend the use of broad-spectrum UV radiation blockers with SPF of 30 or greater during sun exposure, with periodic reapplication of sunscreen to ensure continuous protection.

9. Use good products responsibly and apply enough—experts suggest a "shot glass" (1 fluid ounce) volume for a total body application.

10. To reduce absorption, avoid applying to broken or irritated skin and be sure to apply regularly according to instructions. This includes reapplying after swimming and sweating. Water-resistant products should include instructions on how frequently to reapply.

11. Be sure to read and follow instructions and do not use expired products.

12. Apply sunscreen to all areas of the skin that are exposed and include areas often forgotten like bottom of feet and bald spots of head.

13. The higher the SPF, the greater the concentration of chemicals contained in the sunscreen product. The FDA 2001 guidelines recommend that SPF of no greater than 50 is necessary because there is inadequate data demonstrating that higher SPF products offer greater protection than the lower products.

Tammie Lee and Jacque

Bibliography

American Geriatrics Society. 2015 updated Beers criteria for potentially inappropriate medication use in older adults. *J Am Geriatr Soc.* 2015;63:2227–2246.

Bensen HAE, Watkinson AC, eds. *Topical and Transdermal Drug Delivery: Principles and Practice.* Hoboken, NJ: Wiley; 2011.

Demler TL. Is sunscreen really toxic? These studies might shock you. https://www.consumerhealthdigest.com/beauty-skin-care/is-sunscreen-really-toxic-study-revealed.html. Accessed January 20, 2017.

McEvoy GK, ed. *AHFS: Drug Information.* Bethesda, MD: American Society of Health-System Pharmacists; 2016.

Peate I, Nair M. *Anatomy and Physiology for Nurses at a Glance.* Chichester, West Sussex, UK: John Wiley & Sons; 2015.

Skin Cancer Foundation. The Skin Cancer Foundation's guide to sunscreens. http://www.skincancer.org/prevention/sun-protection/sunscreen/the-skin-cancer-foundations-guide-to-sunscreens. Accessed November 28, 2016.

Skin Cancer Foundation. Sunscreens explained. May 12, 2002. http://www.skincancer.org/prevention/sun-protection/sunscreen/sunscreens-explained. Accessed November 28, 2016.

Squier C, Brogden K. *Human Oral Mucosa: Development, Structure and Function.* Chichester, West Sussex, UK: John Wiley & Sons; 2010.

U.S. Food and Drug Administration. Code of Federal Regulations Title 21. April 1, 2016. http://www.accessdata.fda.gov/scripts/cdrh/cfdocs/cfcfr/CFRSearch.cfm?fr=358.650. Accessed January 20, 2017.

U.S. Food and Drug Administration. FDA permits manufacturers of oral health care benzocaine products to include a methemoglobinemia warning. May 12, 2014. http://www.fda.gov/downloads/Drugs/DrugSafety/UCM396988.pdf. Accessed May 15, 2016.

Symbols

▲	Renal impairment: Dose adjustment is recommended.	(BL)	Beers list criteria (avoid in elderly).
■ (gray)	Hepatic impairment: Dose adjustment is recommended.	(PD)	FDA-approved pediatric doses are available.
■	Black box warning exists for this drug.	(GD)	FDA-approved geriatric doses are available.
(QT)	QTc prolongation effects have been reported.		See primary body system.

Skin and Mucous Membrane Agents

Universal precautions:

- Known serious hypersensitivity to the specific drug or any other component of product/formulation selected warrants a contraindication for its use.
- Adverse reactions associated with the use of **some skin and mucous membrane agents** include dizziness, drowsiness, vertigo, and fatigue; these agents may also impair the ability to perform tasks requiring mental alertness. Caution should always be recommended when using any new drug for the first time, when there is a dose change, and for continued use of known offending agents.
- Do not use polyethylene glycol–based ointments in conditions where absorption of large quantities is possible (e.g., extensive burns or open wounds), especially in the presence of moderate or severe renal impairment. It is generally advised that topical antibiotic preparations should be avoided with IV cannula or at central IV sites because of the potential to promote fungal infections and antimicrobial resistance. Refer and confirm information available in the PI and within current anti-infective guidelines prior to selection and use of these products relative to this type of administration.
- Doses expressed are for usual adult dosage ranges only. "Geriatric doses" are assumed to be the same as adult doses unless otherwise noted with a symbol. Where FDA-approved pediatric dosing is available, a symbol will guide the reader to additional prescribing references. Refer to real-time prescribing references for these age-specific doses.
- Use of skin and mucous membrane agents in pregnancy is based on weighing clinical risk versus benefit and safety concerns are not represented in this grid. Refer to the package insert (PI) for more information. Clinicians should continue to provide education about the reproductive risks of any medication and offer risk-reduction strategies (which may include contraceptive use) to women of childbearing age and understand that these reproductive risks may also extend to males. Other medications may decrease the effectiveness of oral contraceptives. Where necessary, an alternative means of birth control should be explored.
- Brand names are provided for those products still available on the market. Due to the ever-changing product availability, refer to Food and Drug Administration (FDA) resources to confirm the actual brands available. This drug summary is intended for educational purposes only. Prescribing decisions should be based on real-time comprehensive drug databases that are updated on a regular basis.

Anti-infective Agents

Antibacterial Agents

- Prolonged use may result in fungal or bacterial superinfections including, but not limited to, *Clostridium difficile*–associated diarrhea (CDAD).
- Refer to universal prescribing alerts (including black box warnings) for the systemic use of anti-infective agents in the Anti-infective Agents chapter.

Drug Name	FDA-Approved Indications	Adult Dosage Range	Precautions and Clinical Pearls
Generic Name Bacitracin	Topical infection prevention	**Usual topical dose**: Apply a thin film 2 to 3 times daily, depending upon the severity of the infection	• Over-the-counter (OTC) use: use for more than 1 week is not recommended (do not exceed 5 applications per day) • Apply to clean skin and limit application to affected area only (avoid covering large areas of the body to limit systemic absorption) • Apply a small amount equal to the surface area of the fingertip • May cover the treated area with a sterile bandage
Generic Name Clindamycin **Brand Name** Cleocin Clindagel Evoclin	Severe acne Bacterial vaginosis	**Usual topical dose for acne:** 1% gel/pledget/lotion/solution: apply a thin film twice daily Alternatively may use: 1% foam: apply once daily	• Use with caution in patients with a history of gastrointestinal (GI) disease • Use care when selecting and administering; many dosage forms are available and may not be interchangeable • The topical solution (including pledgets) contains alcohol • Foam: dispense directly into cap or onto a cool surface; do not dispense directly into the hands or on the face (foam will melt on contact with warm skin) • Lotion: shake well immediately before use • Do not use skin products near the eyes, nose, or mouth • Wash hands before and after use. Wash affected area and gently pat dry • Only use those dosage formulations specified for intravaginal use. Intravaginal dosage forms are not for topical therapy and topical therapy is not for intravaginal use • Where applicable, use only the applicator(s) supplied by the manufacturer
Generic Name Erythromycin **Brand Name** Emcin Ery pad	Treatment of superficial infections of the skin Acne	**Illustrative topical dose for acne:** 2% pledget/gel/ointment/solution: apply a thin layer to the affected area 2 times per day	• Do not use topical preparations near the eyes, nose, mouth, or other mucous membranes • Cleanse and pat dry the affected area prior to application. • Wear gloves during application; refer to PI for when this precaution is appropriate • Gently rub pledgets over affected skin; several pledgets may be required per application
Generic Name Gentamicin	Treatment of superficial infections of the skin	**Usual topical dose:** 0.1% cream/ointment: apply a thin film to the affected area 3 to 4 times per day	• Apply gently to clean skin and avoid further contamination of the infected skin • May be covered with sterile gauze • Remove crusts from impetigo prior to fresh application to optimize exposure of infection to the antibiotic

Generic Name Metronidazole **Brand Name** MetroCream Metrogel	Topical infection	**Illustrative topical dose for acne rosacea:** 0.75% gel/cream/lotion: apply to affected area 2 times per day; reevaluate after 3 to 5 days if no clinical response	• Avoid contact with the eyes • Use with caution in patients with renal impairment • Do not use topical products orally or vaginally • Prior to administration, cleanse area with a mild, nonirritating cleanser • To minimize local irritation, wait 20 minutes after cleansing before applying cream, gel, or lotion • Topical cream and ointment: may cover treated areas with gauze dressing • Topical cream and ointment: components may be absorbed systemically and may cause drying and irritation
Generic Name Mupirocin **Brand Name** Bactroban Centany	Topical infection	**Usual topical dose for impetigo:** 2% cream/ointment: apply to affected area 3 times per day; reevaluate after 3 to 5 days if no clinical response **Illustrative intranasal dose for the elimination of Methicillin-resistant *Staphylococcus aureus* (MRSA) colonization:** Apply approximately one-half of ointment from the single-use tube into one nostril and the other half into the other nostril twice daily (morning and evening) for 5 days	• Topical ointment and intranasal: use with caution in patients with renal impairment • Intranasal ointment: after application, press sides of the nose together and gently massage to spread ointment throughout for approximately 1 minute; discard tube after use • Do not use concurrently with other nasal products • Do not apply topical ointment to the eye and only intranasal formulations should be used in the nose • May cover treated areas with gauze dressing
Generic Name Neomycin **Brand Name** Neosporin	Skin infections	**Usual topical dose:** 0.5% cream/ointment: apply a thin layer to the affected area 1 to 4 times per day Usually used in combination with other anti-infectives	• Sensitivity, especially in prolonged use, has been reported • Burn patients require special care; refer to PI for additional details • Care should be taken to avoid further contamination of the infected skin • Treated area may be covered with sterile gauze

Drug Name	FDA-Approved Indications	Adult Dosage Range	Precautions and Clinical Pearls
Generic Name Retapamulin **Brand Name** Altabax (PD)	Impetigo	**Usual topical dose**: 1% ointment: apply a thin layer to the affected area twice daily for 5 days	• May cover the treatment area with a sterile bandage or gauze dressing if needed • Refer to PI for specific body surface area (BSA) limits • For external use only; not for ophthalmic administration, oral, intranasal, or vaginal administration
Dapsone	Refer to the Anti-infective Agents chapter.		
Tetracycline	Refer to the Anti-infective Agents chapter.		
Antiviral Agents			
Drug Name	FDA-Approved Indications	Adult Dosage Range	Precautions and Clinical Pearls
Generic Name Acyclovir **Brand Name** Sitavig Zovirax	Herpes virus infections	Dose based on indication for use, formulation selected, and patient's clinical response **Illustrative topical dose for genital herpes simplex virus:** 5% ointment (initial episode): ½-inch ribbon of ointment for a 4-inch square surface area every 3 hours (6 times per day) for 7 days	• Herpes labialis: treatment should begin with the first signs or symptoms • Available in many dose formulations including buccal tablets, which are also available for application to the area of the upper gum above the incisor tooth on the same side as the symptoms; do not apply to the inside of the lip or cheek; refer to PI for additional details • Once adhered, the tablet will gradually dissolve. Do not crush, chew, suck, or swallow the tablet • If the tablet is swallowed within the first 6 hours, instruct the patient to drink a glass of water and apply a new tablet (no action is needed if this occurs after 6 hours)
Generic Name Docosanol **Brand Name** Abreva	Cold sores Fever blisters	**Usual topical dose for herpes labialis (cold sores):** 10% cream: apply 5 times per day to the affected area of the face or lips	• Available as an OTC product • Avoid applying directly inside the mouth • Apply to affected area only; rub in gently and completely • Start at first sign of cold sore or fever blister (tingle) and continue until healed; early treatment ensures best results • If not healed within 10 days, discontinue use and contact the healthcare provider

Drug Name	FDA-Approved Indications	Adult Dosage Range	Precautions and Clinical Pearls
Generic Name Penciclovir **Brand Name** Denavir (PD) (GD)	Recurrent herpes simplex labialis (cold sores)	**Usual topical dose for herpes labialis (cold sores):** 1% cream: apply cream at the first sign of symptom of cold sore (e.g., tingling, swelling) and every 2 hours during waking hours for 4 days	• Application to mucous membranes is not recommended • Apply only to herpes labialis on the lips and face • Apply a sufficient amount to cover lesions; gently rub into the affected area • Monitoring: reduction in virus shedding, negative cultures for herpes virus; resolution of pain and healing of cold sore lesion
Antifungal Agents			
Allylamines			
Drug Name	FDA-Approved Indications	Adult Dosage Range	Precautions and Clinical Pearls
Generic Name Naftifine **Brand Name** Naftin (PD)	**Common indications for use:** Tinea infections Tinea pedis	**Illustrative topical dose for tinea pedis:** 1% cream: apply a thin layer once daily to the affected area and surrounding skin for up to 4 weeks 1% gel: apply a thin layer twice daily to the affected area and surrounding skin for up to 4 weeks	• Avoid occlusive dressings • Monitoring parameters: culture and KOH exam; reevaluate if no improvement after 4 weeks of therapy • Monitor for signs of application site exfoliation, erythema, and dermatitis • Teach patient proper administration or application and necessity of completing full therapy • Apply to affected area and healthy surrounding skin (½-inch margin)
Generic Name Terbinafine **Brand Name** Lamisil (PD)	**Common indications for use:** Tinea pedis Tinea cruris Tinea corporis	**Usual topical dose for tinea pedis:** 1% gel: apply a thin layer to the affected area once daily for at least 1 week 1% cream: apply a thin layer on the bottom or sides of the feet twice daily for 2 weeks	• Some formulations are available OTC • Avoid occlusive dressing of the affected areas unless otherwise directed by the prescriber • Improvements may continue for the 2 to 6 weeks after terbinafine therapy is discontinued (manufacturer recommends that patients not be designated as therapeutic failures until 2 to 6 weeks off therapy have passed and patient is re-evaluated)
Azoles			
Drug Name	FDA-Approved Indications	Adult Dosage Range	Precautions and Clinical Pearls
Generic Name Butoconazole **Brand Name** Gynazole-1	**Common indications for use:** Vulvovaginal candidiasis	**Usual intravaginal dose:** 2% sustained release cream: insert 1 applicatorful intravaginally as a single dose	• Contains mineral oil, which may weaken latex or rubber (condoms or diaphragms); use of these products within 72 hours of treatment is not recommended • Associated with less leakage, so can be applied at any time during the day or night • May be used during menstruation; however, patient should not use tampons during treatment • Abdominal pain, fever greater than 100°F, or foul-smelling vaginal discharge may be symptoms of another vaginal infection or pelvic inflammatory disease requiring urgent reevaluation and intervention

Drug Name	FDA-Approved Indications	Adult Dosage Range	Precautions and Clinical Pearls
Generic Name Clotrimazole **Brand Name** Alevazol Gyne-Lotrimin	**Common indications for use:** Treatment of susceptible fungal infections Cutaneous candidiasis Vulvovaginal candidiasis	**Usual topical dose for cutaneous candidiasis:** 1% cream/solution: apply a thin layer twice daily; if no improvement occurs after 4 weeks, reevaluate diagnosis **Usual intravaginal dose for vulvovaginal candidiasis:** 1% cream: insert 1 applicatorful daily (preferably at bedtime) for 7 consecutive days or alternatively 2% cream for 3 days	• Apply sparingly • Some formulations available as OTC • Protect hands with latex gloves • Do not use occlusive dressings • Use the brand/formulation specific to the indication; vaginal creams are formulated specifically for this use • Transmucosal (troche) dosage available for oral candidiasis; refer to PI
Generic Name Econazole **Brand Name** Ecoza	Fungal infection	Dose based on indication for use, formulation selected, and patient's clinical response **Illustrative topical dose for tinea pedis:** 1% cream/foam: apply a thin (but sufficient) layer to the affected area(s) once daily for 4 weeks	• Avoid heat, flame, and smoking during and immediately following application of the foam; topical foam is flammable • Occasionally, longer treatment periods may be required • Reassess diagnosis if no clinical improvement after 2 weeks • For topical external use only
Generic Name Efinaconazole **Brand Name** Jublia	Onychomycosis	**Usual topical dose:** Apply to affected toenail(s) once daily for 48 weeks	• Wait at least 10 minutes after showering, bathing, or washing the area prior to application • Squeeze the bottle and apply one drop onto the toenail • If the great toe is affected, apply a second drop to the end of the toenail • Monitor for site dermatitis or vesicles and pain at application site; assess for ingrown toenails

Generic Name Ketoconazole **Brand Name** Extina Ketodan Nizoral Nizoral A-D Xolegel (PD)	Fungal infections (i.e., tinea) Cutaneous candidiasis Seborrheic dermatitis Dandruff	Dose based on indication for use, formulation selected, and patient's clinical response **Illustrative topical dose for fungal infections:** 2% cream: rub gently into the affected area once daily Shampoo: apply to damp skin, lather, leave on 5 minutes, and rinse	• Use care when selecting or administering product; various formulations have specific indications for use • Foam/gel: do not expose to open flame or smoking during or immediately after application • Foam: formulation contains alcohol and propane/butane; do not puncture or incinerate container • Shampoo: may remove curl from permanently wavy hair, cause hair discoloration, and change hair texture • Do not apply directly to hands • Treatment duration varies based on the specific fungal infection
Generic Name Luliconazole **Brand Name** Luzu	Tinea pedis Tinea cruris Tinea corporis	**Usual topical dose:** 1% cream: apply to the affected area and roughly 1 inch of the immediate surrounding area(s) once daily for 2 weeks	• Monitor for localized dermatitis and cellulitis during use • For topical external use only; not for ophthalmic, oral, or intravaginal use
Generic Name Miconazole **Brand Name** Desenex Vagistat Zeasorb-AF	Vulvovaginal candidiasis Skin and mucous membrane fungal infections	**Illustrative topical dose for tinea corporis/pedis:** 2% cream: apply a thin layer twice daily for 4 weeks **Usual intravaginal dose for vulvovaginal candidiasis:** 2% cream: insert 1 applicatorful at bedtime for 7 days; 4% cream can be used for 3 days Alternatively may use: 100 mg suppository: insert 1 suppository vaginally at bedtime for 7 days; 200 mg dose can be used for 3 days 1200 mg suppository: 1 suppository (one-time dose), without regard to time of day	• Many formulations are available; use care when selecting and administering. Specific for fungoid tincture: patients with diabetes, circulatory problems, and renal or hepatic dysfunction should contact prescriber before use • Products are specifically formulated for indications (and locations) for use and are not interchangeable • Vaginal products are petrolatum based and may damage rubber or latex condoms or diaphragms; separate use by 3 days • Consult with the prescriber prior to OTC use if there is vaginal itching/discomfort, pain, chills, nausea and vomiting, foul-smelling discharge, or experiencing first vaginal yeast infection • Contact prescriber if no symptom improvement occurs after 3 days or the infection lasts more than 7 days

Drug Name	FDA-Approved Indications	Adult Dosage Range	Precautions and Clinical Pearls
Generic Name Oxiconazole **Brand Name** Oxistat	Tinea infections	**Usual topical dose for tinea pedis:** 1% cream/lotion: apply a thin layer to the affected areas 1 to 2 times per day for 2 weeks	• Avoid occlusive dressings • For hairy areas, use lotion • Shake lotion prior to use
Generic Name Sertaconazole **Brand Name** Ertaczo	Tinea pedis	**Usual topical dose for tinea pedis:** 2% cream: apply a thin layer between toes and to surrounding healthy skin twice daily for 4 weeks	• Make sure skin is dry before applying • Avoid use of occlusive dressings • Reevaluate use if no response occurs within 2 weeks
Generic Name Sulconazole **Brand Name** Exelderm	Fungal infections	Dose based on indication for use, formulation selected, and patient's clinical response **Illustrative topical dose for tinea pedis:** 1% cream/solution: apply a thin layer to the affected area twice daily for 4 weeks	• Wash hands before and after use and use universal infection prevention precautions (i.e., gloves) for application, as appropriate • Apply to skin that is clean and dry • Occlusive dressings should be avoided, since these dressings provide favorable conditions for yeast growth
Generic Name Terconazole **Brand Name** Terazol Zazole	Vulvovaginal candidiasis	**Illustrative intravaginal dose for vulvovaginal candidiasis:** 0.4%: vaginal cream: insert 1 applicatorful at bedtime for 7 consecutive days; 0.8% cream may be used for 3 consecutive days 80 mg vaginal suppository: insert 1 suppository intravaginally at bedtime for 3 consecutive days	• Petrolatum-based vaginal products may damage rubber or latex condoms or diaphragms; concurrent use is not recommended • Lack of response: repeat microbiological studies (KOH smear and/or cultures) in patients who do not respond to terconazole to confirm the diagnosis and rule out other pathogens • Vaginal cream: use the applicator provided by the manufacturer; wash the applicator after each use
Generic Name Tioconazole **Brand Name** Vagistat	Vulvovaginal candidiasis	**Illustrative intravaginal dose:** 6.5% ointment: insert 1 applicatorful intravaginally just prior to bedtime, as a single dose	• Available OTC • Petrolatum-based vaginal products may damage rubber or latex condoms or diaphragms; separate use by 3 days • Most patients will experience relief of symptoms within 7 days. If symptoms do not improve in 3 days or remain after 7 days, patient should be reevaluated

Benzylamines

Drug Name	FDA-Approved Indications	Adult Dosage Range	Precautions and Clinical Pearls
Generic Name Butenafine **Brand Name** Lotrimin Ultra Mentax	**Common indications for use:** Topical tinea infections	Dose based on indication for use, formulation selected, and patient's clinical response **Illustrative topical dose for tinea corporis/cruris infection:** Apply a thin layer once daily to the affected area for 2 weeks	• For topical external use on the skin only (not for ophthalmic, oral or intravaginal use) • When used for self-medication (OTC), do not use on nails or scalp or for vaginal yeast infections • Avoid occlusive dressings • Apply to skin that is clean and dry • Culture and KOH exam, clinical signs of tinea pedis • Wash hands before and after use and use universal infection prevention precautions (i.e., gloves) for application, as appropriate

Hydroxypyridones

Drug Name	FDA-Approved Indications	Adult Dosage Range	Precautions and Clinical Pearls
Generic Name Ciclopirox **Brand Name** Ciclodan CNL8 Nail Loprox Penlac (PD)	**Common indications for use:** Tinea infections Cutaneous candidiasis Seborrheic scalp dermatitis Onychomycosis	Dose based on indication for use, formulation selected, and patient's clinical response **Illustrative topical dose for tinea pedis:** 0.77% cream/lotion/gel or suspension: apply a thin layer to affected area twice daily; gently massage into affected areas	• Avoid use of occlusive dressings or wrappings • For topical use only as directed; not for ophthalmic, oral, or intravaginal use • Available in many dosage formulations and may be applied to the skin as a lotion or cream, to the scalp as a shampoo, and to the nails as a nail lacquer solution; use care when selecting and administering products • Lacquer (solution): apply evenly over nail and surrounding skin at bedtime (or allow 8 hours before washing); apply daily over previous coat for 7 days; after 7 days, may remove with alcohol and continue cycle • Gently massage into affected areas and surrounding skin • Shampoo: apply roughly 5 mL (1 teaspoonful) to wet hair, lather, leave in place for approximately 3 minutes, and then rinse; may use up to 10 mL for longer hair • If no improvement occurs after 4 weeks of treatment, reevaluate diagnosis

Oxaboroles

Drug Name	FDA-Approved Indications	Adult Dosage Range	Precautions and Clinical Pearls
Generic Name Tavaborole **Brand Name** Kerydin	Onychomycosis	**Usual topical dose:** 5% solution: apply to affected toenail(s) once daily for 48 weeks	• Apply to completely cover affected toenail surface using the provided dropper; apply under the tip of each affected toenail as well • Monitor for signs of application site exfoliation, erythema, dermatitis, and ingrown toenail • Avoid pedicures, and use of nail polish or cosmetic nail products during treatment • Keep away from heat or flame

Polyenes			
Drug Name	**FDA-Approved Indications**	**Adult Dosage Range**	**Precautions and Clinical Pearls**
Generic Name Nystatin **Brand Name** Nyamyc Nyata Nystop Pediaderm AF Complete (PD)	Fungal infections (cutaneous and mucocutaneous)	**Usual topical dose for cutaneous candidiasis:** Cream/ointment (100,000 units/g): apply to the affected areas twice daily or as indicated until healing is complete. Alternatively may use: Powder: apply 2 to 3 times per day **Usual dose for oral candidiasis (thrush):** Swish 4 to 6 mL in the mouth 4 times per day; continue treatment for at least 48 hours after symptoms are resolved	• Cream is usually preferred to ointment for intertriginous areas; very moist lesions are best treated with topical powder • Apply liberally • For fungal infection of the feet, the powder should be dusted in all footwear (in addition to application to the feet) • Divide dose of oral suspension so that one-half is placed in each side of the mouth (cheek pouch) • Treatment usually requires 7 to 14 days

Thiocarbamates			
Drug Name	**FDA-Approved Indications**	**Adult Dosage Range**	**Precautions and Clinical Pearls**
Generic Name Tolnaftate **Brand Name** Fungi-Guard Tinactin	Tinea pedis Tinea cruris Tinea corporis	**Usual topical dose for tinea infection:** 1% cream/solution/powder: apply a thin layer twice daily to the affected area for 2 to 4 weeks	• When used for self-medication (OTC use), contact the healthcare provider if the condition does not improve within 4 weeks • Duration of use is based on the indication; may use for up to 4 weeks for tinea pedis or tinea corporis, and up to 2 weeks for tinea cruris • Not recommended in the treatment of deeper skin infections or infection of the nail beds • Wash and dry the affected area; do not use occlusive bandage

Miscellaneous Antifungal Agents			
Drug Name	**FDA-Approved Indications**	**Adult Dosage Range**	**Precautions and Clinical Pearls**
Generic Name Clioquinol **Brand Name** Ala-Quin Dermasorb AF kit	Tinea and other skin infections	**Usual topical dose:** 3% cream (with hydrocortisone 0.5%): apply 3 to 4 times per day	• Apply between the toes; wear well-fitting, ventilated shoes and change shoes/socks at least once daily • Treatment duration is based on infection and indication for use • Discontinue if aggravation of the lesions or surrounding skin occurs • If there is no improvement, discontinue and reevaluate • Products can stain the skin, fabric, hair, and nails

			• Avoid prolonged use; can result in overgrowth of nonsusceptible organisms • May interfere with certain thyroid function tests; manufacturer recommends that at least 1 month elapse between discontinuing topical therapy and performing such tests • May produce false-positive results in the ferric chloride test for phenylketonuria when the drug is present in urine • Not effective for fungal infections of the scalp or nails Contraindications: • Viral and TB skin lesions
Generic Name Gentian violet	Topical infection	**Usual topical dose for infection:** Apply to the affected area once to twice daily	• May stain skin and clothing • Safer and more effective topical anti-infective agents are now available • Apply directly to the wound or with a cotton applicator • Do not cover a with bandage Contraindications: • When used for self-medication, do not use on ulcerative lesions
Generic Name Undecylenic acid	Tinea pedis Ringworm (except nails and scalp)	**Usual topical dose for tinea pedis:** 25% ointment/solution: apply twice daily to the affected area for 4 weeks	• With OTC use, contact the prescriber if the condition does not improve within 4 weeks • Clean the affected area and dry thoroughly • Apply a thin layer over affected area • For tinea pedis (athlete's foot), pay special attention to the spaces between the toes; wear well-fitting, ventilated shoes; and change shoes and socks at least once daily • For topical external use only (do not use on scalp or nails) and avoid contact with the eyes

Scabicides and Pediculicides

Universal prescribing alerts:

- Environmental planning is required to eliminate reinfection. Contaminated clothing and bed linens should be washed on hot cycle or dry-cleaned, and all clothing and bedding should be changed the day after application when these products are used.
- These products are poisonous if ingested; take appropriate precautions to avoid accidental exposure.

Drug Name	FDA-Approved Indications	Adult Dosage Range	Precautions and Clinical Pearls
Generic Name Benzyl alcohol **Brand Name** Ulesfia	Head lice	**Usual topical dose for head lice:** 5% lotion: apply appropriate volume for the patient's hair length to dry hair and completely saturate the scalp; leave on for 10 minutes, then rinse thoroughly with water; repeat in 7 days	• With self-medication (OTC use), discontinue use and notify the prescriber if the condition worsens or does not improve within 7 days, or if swelling, rash, or fever develops; do not use for more than 7 days unless so instructed by the healthcare professional • Lotion: apply to dry hair until completely saturated; leave on for 10 minutes, followed by a thorough water rinse; wash hands after application • Use in conjunction with an overall lice management program: dry-clean or wash all clothing, hats, bedding, and towels in hot water; wash all personal care items (e.g., combs, brushes, hair clips) in hot water • May use a fine-tooth or special nit comb to remove nits and dead lice
Generic Name Crotamiton **Brand Name** Eurax	Scabies Symptomatic treatment of pruritus	**Usual topical dose for scabies:** 10% cream/lotion: apply a thin layer and massage the drug onto the skin of the entire body from the neck to the toes (with special attention to skin folds, creases, and interdigital spaces); repeat application in 24 hours; may retreat if new lesions appear or itching persists more than 2 to 4 weeks after initial treatment	• Although approved by FDA for use, the Centers for Disease Control and Prevention (CDC) does not recommend crotamiton for use in scabies • Do not apply to acutely inflamed, raw, or weeping skin • Shake lotion well before use • Take a bath or shower prior to application and take a cleansing bath 48 hours after the final application • Trim fingernails and apply under nails (can use toothbrush—dispose after use) • Contaminated clothing and bed linens should be washed on hot cycle or dry-cleaned; all clothing and bedding should be changed the day after application
Generic Name Ivermectin **Brand Name** Sklice Soolantra (PD) (GD)	Head lice Rosacea	**Usual topical dose for head lice:** 0.5% lotion: apply sufficient amount (up to 1 tube) to completely cover dry scalp and hair; for single-dose use only (discard any remaining); leave on for 10 minutes (start timing after complete coverage is achieved); rinse hair thoroughly with warm water	• Ivermectin cream is administered topically for rosacea; use care when selecting and administering products • Avoid contact with eyes and lips (and wash hands) • Topical lotion: for use on scalp and scalp hair only • Apply lotion to dry scalp and hair closest to the scalp first, then apply outward toward ends of hair; completely cover scalp and hair. Nit combing is not required • Should be a portion of a whole lice removal program, including washing or dry-cleaning all clothing, hats, bedding, and towels recently worn or used by the patient, and washing combs, brushes, and hair accessories in hot soapy water; monitor scalp for live lice

Generic Name Lindane ■ (PD)	Lice infestation Scabies	**Usual topical dose for scabies:** 1% lotion: apply a thin layer of lotion and massage it on the skin from the neck to the toes; after 8 to 12 hours, bathe and remove the drug Do not retreat; do not leave on for more than 8 hours **Illustrative topical dose for head lice (based on hair length):** 1% shampoo: apply 30 ml to dry hair without adding water, leave in place for 4 minutes only then add small quantities of water to hair until a good lather forms; immediately rinse all lather away and avoid unnecessary contact of lather with other body surfaces Apply only 1 time and do not retreat	• Use with caution in patients with hepatic impairment • Do not use on open wounds or sores; do not apply occlusive dressings • Hazardous: use appropriate precautions for handling and disposal; caregivers should apply with gloves (avoid natural latex) • For treatment only; not to be used to prevent infestation • Shake well prior to use • Most patients will require 30 mL (1 ounce); larger adults may require up to 60 mL • Skin should be free of any other topical preparations prior to application; wait at least 1 hour after bathing or showering to apply lotion • Oil-based hair dressing may increase toxic potential • Shampoo: Wait at least 1 hour after washing hair before applying. Hair should be washed with a shampoo not containing a conditioner; hair and skin of head and neck should be free of any topical preparations prior to application. Do not cover with shower cap or towel. • Itching may occur as a result of killing lice; it does not necessarily indicate treatment failure or need for retreatment Contraindications: • Uncontrolled seizure disorders • Crusted (Norwegian) scabies or other skin conditions (e.g., atopic dermatitis, psoriasis) that may increase systemic absorption Associated with: • Severe neurologic toxicities: seizures and death have been reported with use; use with caution in patients weighing less than 50 kg, with head trauma, or with HIV infection • Not a drug of first choice; use only in patients who have failed or cannot tolerate first-line agents
Generic Name Malathion **Brand Name** Ovide	Head lice infection	**Usual topical dose for head lice:** 0.5% lotion: apply a sufficient amount to cover and thoroughly moisten dry hair and scalp; allow hair to dry naturally; leave uncovered and after 8 to 12 hours wash hair with non-medicated shampoo; rinse and use a fine-toothed (nit) comb to remove dead lice and eggs	• Leave hair uncovered after application • Lotion is flammable; do not expose lotion or hair wetted with malathion to open flames or electric heat sources (e.g., hair dryer, curling iron, flat iron) • Apply to dry hair and scalp; rub gently until thoroughly moistened • If required, administer a second application in 7 to 9 days; further treatment is generally not necessary

Drug Name	FDA-Approved Indications	Adult Dosage Range	Precautions and Clinical Pearls
Generic Name Permethrin **Brand Name** Elimite Nix (PD)	Head lice Scabies	**Usual topical dose for head lice:** 1% lotion: apply a sufficient amount to saturate the hair and scalp (especially behind ears and nape of neck); leave on hair for no longer than 10 minutes, then rinse off with warm water; use nit comb remove remaining nits **Usual topical dose for scabies:** 5% cream: apply to skin from the head to the soles of the feet (rinse after 8 to 14 hours); 1 application is generally curative but retreatment is appropriate if living mites persist after 7 to 14 days of initial treatment	• Treatment may temporarily exacerbate the symptoms of itching, redness, and swelling • Wear gloves when applying • Shake cream rinse/lotion well before using • Prior to application, wash hair with conditioner-free shampoo; rinse with water and towel dry • A single application is generally sufficient, but may repeat 7 days after first treatment if lice or nits are still present • Mites rarely infect the scalp of adults, although the hairline, neck, temple, and forehead may be infested in infants and geriatric patients; 30 g is sufficient for the average adult • External topical use only (not nose, ears, mouth, etc.)
Generic Name Pyrethrins with piperonyl butoxide **Brand Name** Rid complete (PD)	Lice infestation	**Usual topical dose:** Gel or liquid: shake well before use; apply the undiluted liquid to dry hair and scalp or to any infested area until entirely wet and then wash off after 10 minutes; do not use on eyelashes or eyebrows	• Not effective for treatment of scabies (mite infestation) • Also available as a shampoo • Repeat treatment in 7 to 10 days to assure eradication of unhatched nits; two consecutive applications should not be administered within 24 hours

Generic Name Spinosad **Brand Name** Natroba (PD)	Head lice	**Usual topical dose:** 0.9% suspension: apply a sufficient amount of spinosad suspension to cover dry scalp and hair; leave on for 10 minutes and then rinse thoroughly with warm water (if live lice are still seen 7 days after the first treatment, apply a second treatment)	• Shake well prior to use • Wash hands after application • Shampoo may be used immediately after the product is completely rinsed off • Application amount depends on the amount of hair; up to one full bottle (120 ml) may be required depending on the length of hair • Scalp and hair should be dry prior to application • Do not ingest and avoid accidental exposure with eyes, mouth, or any mucus membrane
Sulfur	Refer to the Other Skin and Mucous Membrane Agents section.		
Miscellaneous Local Anti-infective Agents			
Drug Name	**FDA-Approved Indications**	**Adult Dosage Range**	**Precautions and Clinical Pearls**
Generic Name Benzalkonium chloride **Brand Name** Revitaderm	**Common indications for use:** Prophylactic disinfection of the intact skin Treatment of superficial injuries and infected wounds	Drug is diluted in various concentrations depending on the indication **Illustrative topical dose for abrasions and wounds:** 0.13% topical foam: apply a thin layer of foam 1 to 3 times daily	• Rapidly germicidal for many pathogenic bacteria and fungi • Use care when selecting and administering; multiple formulations available for use (not interchangeable) • Wipe away any dirt or debris with a sterile gauze prior to use • Inactivated by anionic compounds (e.g., soap): before applying quaternary ammonium compounds to the skin for preoperative disinfection, all traces of soap should be removed prior to use • Allow the foam to dissipate into the wound and wipe away any excess with a sterile gauze; the foam should be allowed to dry before covering the wound with a sterile bandage • Gel may become discolored when in contact with tissue fluids
Generic Name Iodine (povidone) Iodine (cadexomer) **Brand Name** Betadine Iodoflex Iodosorb	Topical: antiseptic for the management of minor, superficial skin wounds; preoperative disinfection of skin	**Usual topical dose as antiseptic for minor cuts, scrapes, and burns:** Apply small amount to the affected area 1 to 3 times per day	• Use with caution in patients with renal impairment • Iodosorb is also available in a Cadexomer matrix dressing that provides sustained release of iodine (Iodosorb and Iodoflex) • Some products have guidelines for maximum application amounts; refer to PI prior to use • Not for application to large areas of the body or for use with tight or air-excluding bandages; improper use may lead to product contamination • When used for self-medication (OTC), do not use on deep wounds, puncture wounds, animal bites, or serious burns without consulting with the prescriber • Notify the prescriber if condition does not improve within 7 days Contraindications for Iodosorb and Iodoflex: • Hashimoto's thyroiditis • Graves' disease • Nontoxic nodular goiter

Drug Name	FDA-Approved Indications	Adult Dosage Range	Precautions and Clinical Pearls
Generic Name Mafenide **Brand Name** Sulfamylon	Burn treatment	**Illustrative topical dose:** 8.5% cream: apply 1 to 2 times per day with a sterile-gloved hand; apply to a thickness of approximately 1/16 inch The burned area should be covered with cream at all times	• Prolonged use may result in fungal or bacterial superinfection • Use with caution in patients with glucose-6-phosphate dehydrogenase (G6PD) deficiency • Use with caution in patients with burns and acute renal impairment; may cause metabolic acidosis • Cream: dressings are typically not required, but if necessary only a thin layer of dressings should be used; apply to the debrided area with a sterile gloved hand • Powder for solution: cover graft area with 1 layer of fine mesh gauze; secure the irrigation dressing with a bolster dressing and wrap as appropriate • Continue treatment until healing is progressing well or the burn site is ready for grafting • Teach patient appropriate application
Generic Name Selenium sulfide **Brand Name** Anti-Dandruff Dandrex Tersi	Itching and flaking of the scalp associated with dandruff Control of scalp seborrheic dermatitis Tinea versicolor	**Usual topical dose for tinea versicolor:** 2.5% lotion: apply to the affected area and lather with small amounts of water; leave on skin for 10 minutes, then rinse thoroughly; apply every day for 7 days	• Due to the risk of systemic toxicity, do not use on damaged skin or mucous membranes • Shake the bottle well before using • May damage jewelry; remove before treatment • Invert canister to administer foam • Available as a shampoo; refer to PI for use and guidance • Avoid accidental exposure to genitals, eyes, mouth, and other mucous membranes
Generic Name Silver sulfadiazine **Brand Name** Silvadene SSD	Prevention and treatment of infection in second- and third-degree burns	**Usual topical dose for antiseptic, burns:** 1% cream: apply once or twice daily (to a thickness of approximately 1/16 inch)	• Prolonged use may result in fungal or bacterial superinfection, • Systemic absorption may be significant; adverse reactions may occur; dressings are not required but may be used • Use with caution in patients with G6PD deficiency; hemolysis may occur • Use with caution in patients with renal or hepatic impairment • Apply with a sterile-gloved hand • Burned area should be covered with cream at all times • Monitoring: serum electrolytes, urinalysis, renal function tests, complete blood count (CBC) in patients with extensive burns on long-term treatment • Monitor for development of granulation, rash, or irritation of unburned areas.
Boric acid	Refer to the Eye, Ear, Nose, and Throat Preparations chapter.		
Chlorhexidine	Refer to the Eye, Ear, Nose, and Throat Preparations chapter.		

Anti-inflammatory Agents

Universal prescribing alerts:

- Topical steroids may cause hypercorticism or suppression of the hypothalamic–pituitary–adrenal (HPA) axis, particularly in patients receiving high doses for prolonged periods. Refer to universal prescribing alerts in the Hormones and Synthetic Substitutes chapter for systemic side effects of corticosteroids.
- Topical corticosteroids may be absorbed percutaneously, which may cause manifestations of Cushing's syndrome, hyperglycemia, or glycosuria. Absorption is increased by occlusive dressings and application to denuded skin or large surface areas.
- Prolonged use may result in fungal or bacterial superinfection; discontinue if dermatologic infection persists.
- Monitor for HPA axis suppression (adrenocorticotropic hormone [ACTH] stimulation test, morning plasma cortisol test, urinary free cortisol test), signs of bacterial or fungal infection, and response to treatment.
- Local adverse reactions may occur (e.g., skin atrophy, burning, irritation, dryness, hypopigmentation, allergic contact dermatitis) and may be irreversible. They are more likely to occur with occlusive and prolonged use.
- Use of occlusive dressings is not recommended.
- The foams and sprays are flammable.
- These agents are generally not for routine use on the face, underarms, or groin area. Avoid the use of high-potency steroids on the face. Refer to Tips from the Field in the Hormones and Synthetic Substitutes chapter for steroidal potencies and relative equivalency between steroidal products.
- Discontinue these medications when control achieved; if improvement is not seen within 2 weeks, reassessment of the diagnosis may be necessary.
- Topical corticosteroids should not be used to treat acne vulgaris, acne rosacea or perioral dermatitis as they may aggravate these conditions.
- Topical corticosteroids may delay the healing of non-infected wounds, such as venous stasis ulcers and may mask the normal inflammatory response to local infections
- Psychiatric events and behavioral changes such as aggression, depression, sleep disorders, psychomotor hyperactivity, and suicidal ideation have been reported with the use of corticosteroids, and thus these agents are deemed to meet Beers criteria to avoid in older adults with or at high risk of delirium because of the potential of inducing or worsening delirium. Psychiatric events occur more commonly in patients receiving 80 mg per day of oral prednisone or equivalent. See Tips from the Field for steroid dose equivalents in the Hormones and Synthetic Substitutes chapter.
- Universal prescribing alerts for potential corticosteroidal systemic absorption; refer to Tips from the Field to reduce chance of absorbing topical products systemically.

Drug Name	FDA-Approved Indications	Adult Dosage Range	Precautions and Clinical Pearls
Generic Name Alclometasone **Brand Name** Aclovate	**Common indications for use:** Treatment of inflammation of corticosteroid-responsive dermatosis	**Usual topical dose for dermatitis:** 0.05% cream/ointment: apply a thin layer to the affected area 2 to 3 times per day	• Avoid use of topical preparations on weeping or exudative lesions
Generic Name Amcinonide	**Common indications for use:** Relief of the inflammatory and pruritic manifestations of corticosteroid-responsive dermatoses (high-potency corticosteroid)	**Usual topical dose for dermatitis:** 0.1% cream/ointment/lotion: apply a thin layer to affected area 2 to 3 times per day	• Absorption is increased by the use of occlusive dressings, application to denuded skin, and application to large surface areas

Drug Name	FDA-Approved Indications	Adult Dosage Range	Precautions and Clinical Pearls
Generic Name Betamethasone **Brand Name** Diprolene Diprolene AF Luxiq PD	**Common indications for use:** Dermatoses Dermatoses of the scalp (foam only)	Dose based on indication for use, formulation selected, and patient's clinical response **Illustrative topical dose for dermatoses of the scalp:** 0.12% foam: apply to the scalp twice daily, in the morning and at night	• Specific guidelines exist for the amount to be used (i.e., grams) over time; refer to PI • Avoid concurrent use of other corticosteroids • Withdraw therapy with gradual tapering of dose by reducing the frequency of application or substituting a less potent steroid • Apply cream, ointment, and lotion formulations sparingly to affected areas; not for use on broken skin or in areas of infection • Do not apply to wet skin unless so directed • Do not cover with an occlusive dressing • Foam: Invert the can and dispense a small amount onto a saucer or other cool surface; do not dispense directly into hands. Pick up small amounts of foam and gently massage into affected areas until the foam disappears. Repeat until entire affected scalp area is treated
Generic Name Clobetasol **Brand Name** Clobex Clodan Olux Temovate PD	**Common indications for use:** Steroid-responsive dermatoses	Dose based on indication for use, formulation selected, and patient's clinical response **Illustrative topical dose for contact dermatitis:** 0.05% gel/foam/ointment: apply twice daily for up to 2 weeks (maximum dose: 50 g per week or 50 mL per week)	• Specific guidelines exist for the amount to be used (i.e., grams) over time; refer to PI • Use care when selecting and administering products (not interchangeable, i.e., emollient vs non-emollient creams) • Do not use if there is atrophy at the treatment site • Minimize contact to non-affected areas of the body • Shampoo: Use on dry hair. Do not use a shower cap or bathing cap while shampoo is on the scalp. Leave in place for 15 minutes, then wet hair, lather, and rinse hair and scalp completely • Spray: spray directly onto affected area of skin; gently and completely rub into skin after spraying • Primary infections: initiate or continue only if the appropriate anti-infective treatment is instituted
Generic Name Clocortolone **Brand Name** Cloderm	**Common indications for use:** Steroid-responsive dermatoses	**Usual topical dose for dermatitis:** 0.1% cream: apply a thin layer gently; rub into affected area 3 times per day	• Primary infections: initiate or continue only if the appropriate anti-infective treatment is instituted • Specific guidelines exist for the amount to be used (i.e., grams) over time; refer to PI

Generic Name Desonide **Brand Name** Desonate DesOwen LoKara Verdeso (PD)	**Common indications for use:** Atopic dermatitis Corticosteroid-responsive dermatoses	**Usual topical dose for atopic dermatitis:** 0.05% cream/ointment: apply a thin layer 2 to 4 times per day daily	• Primary infections: initiate or continue only if the appropriate anti-infective treatment is instituted • Do not use on open wounds • Apply sparingly, using the smallest amount needed to adequately cover the affected area • Specific guidelines exist for the amount to be used (i.e., grams) over time; refer to PI • Foam, lotion: shake well before use
Generic Name Desoximetasone **Brand Name** Topicort	**Common indications for use:** Relief of inflammation and pruritic symptoms of corticosteroid-responsive dermatosis Plaque psoriasis	**Usual topical dose for plaque psoriasis treatment:** 0.25% spray: apply a thin film to affected area twice daily	• Use care when selecting and administering products; formulations are indication specific and not interchangeable • Primary infections: initiate or continue only if the appropriate anti-infective treatment is instituted • Specific guidelines exist for the amount to be used (i.e., grams) over time; refer to PI
Generic Name Diflorasone **Brand Name** ApexiCon Psorcon (PD)	Dermatoses	**Usual topical dose for dermatitis:** 0.05% cream/ointment (non-emollient): apply a thin layer 1 to 3 times per day	• Primary infections: initiate or continue only if the appropriate anti-infective treatment is instituted • Apply the smallest amount that will cover the affected area • Do not use if there is atrophy at the treatment site • Minimize contact to non-affected areas of the body • Specific guidelines exist for the amount to be used (i.e., grams) over time; refer to PI
Generic Name Fluocinolone **Brand Name** Capex Derma-Smoothe/FS Body Synalar (PD) (GD)	**Common indications for use:** Dermatitis or psoriasis of the scalp Atopic dermatitis	Dose based on indication for use, formulation selected, and patient's clinical response **Illustrative topical dose for atopic dermatitis:** 0.01% Derma-Smoothe/FS body oil: apply a thin layer to affected area 3 times per day	• Not for oral, ophthalmic, or intravaginal use • Do not apply to the face, axillae, or groin unless directed by the healthcare provider • Primary infections: initiate or continue only if the appropriate anti-infective treatment is instituted • Capex: prior to dispensing, empty the contents of the capsule into the liquid shampoo and shake well; discard after 3 months

Drug Name	FDA-Approved Indications	Adult Dosage Range	Precautions and Clinical Pearls
Generic Name Flurandrenolide **Brand Name** Cordran	**Common indications for use:** Corticosteroid-responsive dermatoses	**Usual topical dose for dermatitis:** 0.05% cream/lotion/ointment: apply a thin layer to the affected area 2 to 3 times per day	• Use appropriate antibacterial or antifungal agents to treat concomitant skin infections; discontinue treatment if the infection does not resolve promptly • Shake lotion well before use • Available in many dosage formulations including a medicated tape, which is most effective for dry, scaling, localized lesions; tape is not recommended for intertriginous lesions • Shave or clip hair in the treatment area to promote adherence and easy removal • Replacement of tape every 12 hours is best tolerated, but tape may be left in place for 24 hours if well tolerated; allow skin to dry 1 hour before applying new tape • May be used just at night and removed during the day • Do not tear medicated tape; always cut
Generic Name Halcinonide **Brand Name** Halog	**Common indications for use:** Relief of inflammatory and pruritic effects of corticosteroid-responsive dermatoses (high-potency topical corticosteroid)	**Usual topical dose for dermatitis:** 0.01% cream/ointment/solution: apply sparingly 2 to 3 times per day	• Primary infections: initiate or continue only if the appropriate anti-infective treatment is instituted • Avoid use of topical preparations on weeping or exudative lesions • Specific instructions provided if an occlusive dressing is needed for severe conditions; refer to PI for details • A thin film is effective; avoid excessive application • Specific guidelines exist for the amount to be used (i.e., grams) over time; refer to PI
Generic Name Hydrocortisone **Brand Name** Anusol-HC Preparation H PD	**Common indications for use:** Anal and genital itching (external) Dermatoses	Dose based on indication for use, formulation selected, and patient's clinical response **Usual topical dose for dermatosis:** 0.1% cream/gel/ointments/sprays: apply a thin film to the affected area 3 to 4 times per day	• Primary infections: initiate or continue only if the appropriate anti-infective treatment is instituted • Formulations vary (hydrocortisone butyrate, hydrocortisone valerate); refer to PI for specific guidance on selections • With self-medication (OTC), contact the prescriber if the condition worsens, symptoms persist for more than 7 days, or rectal bleeding occurs • Shake lotion well before use • Rectal foam and suspensions are also available for use
Generic Name Mometasone **Brand Name** Elocon PD	**Common indications for use:** Corticosteroid-responsive dermatoses	**Usual topical dose for dermatoses:** Apply sparingly; do not use occlusive dressings 0.1% cream/ointment/lotion: apply a thin layer to the affected area once daily	• Primary infections: initiate or continue only if the appropriate anti-infective treatment is instituted • Absorption is increased by application to broken skin or to large surface areas

Generic Name Prednicarbate **Brand Name** Dermatop	**Common indications for use:** Corticosteroid-responsive dermatoses	**Usual topical dose for dermatoses:** 0.1% cream/ointment: apply a thin film to the affected area twice daily	• For topical external use only (i.e., not for intravaginal use) • Primary infections: initiate or continue only if the appropriate anti-infective treatment is instituted
Generic Name Triamcinolone **Brand Name** Dermasorb TA Kenalog Oralone Trianex (PD)	**Common indications for use:** Dermatoses (corticosteroid-responsive) Oral inflammatory and ulcerative lesions	Dose based on indication for use, formulation selected, and patient's clinical response **Illustrative topical dose eczema:** 0.025% cream/ointment/lotion: apply thin film to the affected area 2 to 4 times per day	• Also available as a topical lotion, aerosol, and oral paste • Aerosol solution: do not inhale if spraying near face; container may be used upright or inverted; spray at a distance of 3 to 6 inches from the affected area • May be used with occlusive dressings for management of psoriasis or recalcitrant conditions; if an infection develops, discontinue dressings • Oral paste: apply a small amount to the oral cavity until a thin, smooth film develops; do not rub in, as it may result in a granular, gritty sensation and crumbling; apply at bedtime • Primary infections: initiate or continue only if the appropriate anti-infective treatment is instituted • Frequency of application is based on the severity of the condition

Antipruritic and Local Anesthetic Agents

Drug Name	FDA-Approved Indications	Adult Dosage Range	Precautions and Clinical Pearls
Generic Name Benzocaine **Brand Name** Benzodent Anbesol Americaine (PD)	Temporary pain reliever	These are general dosing guidelines; refer to the specific product labeling for dosing instructions **Illustrative topical dose for bee stings, insect bites, minor burns, and sunburn:** 20% topical spray: apply to affected area 3 to 4 times per day as needed	• Methemoglobinemia has been reported following topical use, particularly with higher-concentration (14% to 20%) spray formulations applied to the mouth or mucous membranes; alternatives such as topical lidocaine preparations should be considered for patients at higher risk of this reaction • Monitoring: cyanosis, dyspnea, weakness, tachycardia • High systemic levels and toxic effects (e.g., irregular heartbeat) • Avoid wraps/dressings to cover the skin following application and avoid large areas of broken skin • Record the number of sprays administered and the length of each spray (maximum spray duration of 2 seconds) • Use caution to prevent gagging or choking with oral formulation; avoid food or drink for 1 hour Contraindications: • Secondary bacterial infection of the affected area • Ophthalmic use

Drug Name	FDA-Approved Indications	Adult Dosage Range	Precautions and Clinical Pearls
Generic Name Dibucaine **Brand Name** Nupercainal PD GD	**Common indications for use:** Dermal pain/itching Hemorrhoids/anorectal disorders Rectal pain/itching	These are general dosing guidelines; refer to the specific product labeling for dosing instructions **Illustrative topical dose for skin abrasions/insect bites/ itching:** 1% ointment: apply to affected area up to 3 to 4 times per day (MDD: 30 g per day)	• Topical application: high systemic levels and toxic effects (i.e., methemoglobinemia, irregular heartbeats, respiratory depression, seizures, death) have been reported in patients who (without supervision of a trained professional) have applied topical anesthetics in large amounts (or to large areas of the skin), left these products on for prolonged periods of time, or used wraps/dressings to cover the skin following application • Self-medication (OTC use): for external use only • Notify the prescriber and discontinue use if the condition worsens, if it does not improve within 7 days, or if redness, irritation, swelling, bleeding, or other symptoms develop or increase • Do not use in large quantities, particularly over raw surfaces or blistered areas
Generic Name Doxepin **Brand Name** Prudoxin Zonalon PD	**Common indication for use:** Dermatitis	**Usual topical dose for atopic dermatitis:** 5% cream: apply a thin film 4 times per day with at least a 3- to 4-hour interval between applications; not recommended for use for more than 8 days	• Increased risk of renal and/or hepatic disease resulting from excessive systemic absorption may occur following prolonged exposure to this known liver and kidney toxin • Doxepin is significantly absorbed following topical administration; plasma levels may be similar to those achieved with oral administration • Avoid occlusive dressings: may increase absorption • Drowsiness has been reported; use care Contraindications: • Universal prescribing alerts for anticholinergic effects, and black box warnings for this drug when used systemically; refer to the Autonomic Agents chapter and the Central Nervous System Agents chapter for additional details
Generic Name Ethyl chloride	**Common indications for use:** Local anesthetic in minor operative procedures and injections	Dose based on indication for use, formulation selected, and patient's clinical response	• Increased risk of renal and/or hepatic disease resulting from excessive systemic absorption may occur following prolonged exposure to this known liver and kidney toxin • Formulation is flammable; avoid use near open flame or electrical cautery equipment

	Relieve pain caused by minor sports (i.e., injury, bruises)	**Usual topical dose for anesthesia prior to injections:** Spray the affected area 3 to 7 seconds when using a spray bottle (4 to 10 seconds when using a spray can) until the tissue becomes white	• Spray the area until the skin just turns white; avoid frosting the skin (use as you would ice) • If used for local freezing of tissues, apply petroleum to adjacent skin areas for protection
Generic Name Phenazopyridine **Brand Name** Azo-Gesic Pyridium	Dysuria, symptomatic relief	**Usual oral dose for dysuria, symptomatic relief:** 200 mg 3 times per day after meals for 2 days when used concomitantly with an antibacterial agent	• Use leads to reddish-orange discoloration of the urine • Discontinue the drug if skin or sclera develops a yellow color; may indicate drug accumulation due to impaired renal excretion • Use with caution in patients with G6PD deficiency • May stain contact lenses if they are handled after touching tablets; may stain fabric or clothing • Does not treat urinary infection; acts only as an analgesic • When used for self-medication, patients should be instructed to discontinue use if symptoms last for more than 2 days or if an adverse reaction occurs • Monitoring: patients with diabetes should perform serum glucose monitoring, as phenazopyridine may interfere with certain urine testing reagents Contraindications: • Renal insufficiency and impairment
Generic Name Pramoxine **Brand Name** Prax Proctofoam Sarna Sensitive PD	Temporary relief of pain and itching associated with hemorrhoids, burns, minor cuts, scrapes, or minor skin irritations	Dose based on indication for use, formulation selected, and patient's clinical response **Illustrative topical dose for minor skin irritation:** 1% lotion/cream/gel: apply to the affected area up to 3 to 4 times per day	• Available in many dosage formulations (including those for self-medication OTC use); use care when selecting and administering products • Notify the prescriber if the condition worsens or does not improve within 7 days; if it clears up and occurs again within a few days; or if it is accompanied by additional symptoms (i.e., swelling, rash, irritation) • Do not use topical products on open wounds or large areas of the body • Lotion: apply sparingly; use the minimal effective dose • Foam: shake well; dispense onto a clean tissue and apply externally; do not insert into rectum • Wipes: gently pat perianal area with wipe; discard wipe after single use
Diphenhydramine	Refer to the Antihistamine Agents chapter.		

Other Skin and Mucous Membrane Agents

Astringents

Drug Name	FDA-Approved Indications	Adult Dosage Range	Precautions and Clinical Pearls
Generic Name Aluminum acetate **Brand Name** Domeboro	Skin irritation	**Usual topical dose for soak:** Soak affected area in solution for 15 to 30 minutes as needed; may repeat 3 times per day or as directed May also use as a wet dressing or compress: soak a clean, soft, white cloth in solution and apply it loosely to the affected area for 15 to 30 minutes; may repeat as needed for 4 to 8 hours or as directed	• Discontinue use if irritation occurs, condition worsens, or symptoms persist more than 7 days • Consult the prescriber if irritation or sensitivity increases • Do not allow the dressing to dry out, but do not occlude the dressing to prevent evaporation (i.e., with plastic or other material) • Dissolve in cool or warm water prior to use; stir or shake until fully dissolved; do not strain or filter and discard solution after each use (for soak/wet dressing/compress); refer to PI for directions for preparing solution
Generic Name Aluminum chloride hexahydrate **Brand Name** Drysol Xerac AC	**Common indications for use**: Astringent in the management of hyperhidrosis Debridement	Dose based on indication for use, formulation selected, and patient's clinical response **Illustrative topical dose for hyperhidrosis:** Apply once daily at bedtime; once excessive sweating has stopped, may decrease to once or twice per week, or as needed; wash treated area in the morning	• Topical application only • Discontinue if skin irritation occurs • Do not apply to broken or recently shaved skin • May be harmful to certain metals or fabrics • Antiperspirant: apply to dry skin; cover area with plastic wrap held in place with a snug-fitting T-shirt; do not hold in place with tape

Cell Stimulants and Proliferants

Drug Name	FDA-Approved Indications	Adult Dosage Range	Precautions and Clinical Pearls
Generic Name Palifermin **Brand Name** Kepivance	**Common indications for use:** Mucositis prophylaxis in certain patients receiving myelotoxic therapy	**Usual parenteral dose:** IV: 60 mcg/kg per day for 3 consecutive days before and 3 consecutive days after myelotoxic therapy; total of 6 doses	• Edema, erythema, pruritus, rash, oral/perioral dysesthesia, taste alteration, tongue discoloration and thickening may occur; instruct patients to report mucocutaneous effects • Refer to PI for specific administration schedules for various regimens (timing relative to myelotoxic chemotherapy) • Hazardous: use appropriate precautions for handling and disposal • Refer to PI for specific administration requirements including concurrent use of heparin and filtering precautions • Allow the solution to reach room temperature prior to administration; do not use if at room temperature for more than 1 hour

Generic Name Tretinoin **Brand Name** Atralin Avita Renova Refissa Retin-A (PD) (GD)	Acne vulgaris Palliation of fine wrinkles, mottled hyperpigmentation, and facial skin roughness (Refissa/Renova)	**Usual topical dose for acne vulgaris:** Apply a thin layer once daily to acne lesions before bedtime or in the evening	• Increases susceptibility/sensitivity to UV light; avoid or minimize excessive exposure to sunlamps or sunlight (daily sunscreen use recommended) • Increased skin sensitivity to weather extremes of wind or cold; do not apply to sunburned skin • Use with caution in patients with eczema; may cause severe irritation; apply 30 minutes after washing skin • Indication-specific guidance on duration of treatment is available; refer to PI • If combination topical therapy is required, consider separating their applications (i.e., one agent in the morning and the other in the evening or before bedtime) • Avoid use of additional astringents (or alcohol bases) • Gel is flammable; do not expose to high temp or flame • Hazardous: use appropriate precautions for handling and disposal • Refer to systemic adverse effects with oral use in the Antineoplastic Agents chapter (and associated black box warnings)

Detergents

Drug Name	FDA-Approved Indications	Adult Dosage Range	Precautions and Clinical Pearls
Generic Name Green soap	**Common indications for use:** Topical detergent cleansing of skin and hair Cleansing of surgical operators and assistants	Dose based on indication for use, formulation selected, and patient's clinical response	• Germicidal agents (e.g., chlorhexidine gluconate, hexachlorophene, povidone-iodine) have generally replaced green soap for many uses • Does not have germicidal activity, but the alcohol present in green soap tincture provides an antiseptic action • Green soap prepared from green-colored oils such as green olive oil, or artificial colors; however, green soap is not necessarily green • Store in well-closed containers

Emollients, Demulcents, and Protectants

Drug Name	FDA-Approved Indications	Adult Dosage Range	Precautions and Clinical Pearls
Generic Name Vitamins A and D **Brand Name** A+D Original Baza Clear Clocream Sween Cream	Temporary relief of discomfort due to chapped skin or lips, cuts and scrapes, or minor burns	**Usual topical dose as skin protectant:** Apply to affected areas as needed	• Do not use on animal bites, severe burns, deep or puncture wounds, or lacerations

Keratolytic Agents			
Drug Name	**FDA-Approved Indications**	**Adult Dosage Range**	**Precautions and Clinical Pearls**
Generic Name Salicylic acid **Brand Name** Betasal Compound W Keralyt Salex Sebasorb	**Common indications for use:** Acne Dermatitis Hyperkeratotic skin disorders Removal of warts, calluses, or corns	**Illustrative topical OTC dose for acne:** 2% or less concentrated products: use to cleanse skin once or twice per day Products contain significant ranges of concentration strength for specific indications for use; caution when selecting and administering formulations	• Do not combine use of topical salicylic acid with use of other salicylates or drugs that can increase serum concentrations; systemic absorption following topical use may occur and lead to toxicity; refer to the Central Nervous System Agents chapter for universal prescribing alerts for salicylates • Apply to affected areas only; do not apply to broken skin or large areas of body • See products for specific instructions; use only one topical acne product at a time if irritation occurs • Use sunscreen and limit sun exposure during use and for 1 week afterward; do not use before UVB phototherapy • Discontinue use if excessive peeling or stinging occurs • Avoid inhaling vapors Contraindications are product and indication specific: • Example: corn/warts, when used for self-medication (OTC use), do not use if you have diabetes or have poor blood circulation; do not use on irritated skin, any area that is infected or reddened, moles, birthmarks, warts with hair growing from them, genital warts, or warts on the face or mucous membranes
Generic Name Sulfur **Brand Name** Avar Plexion Rosanil (PD)	Acne vulgaris Rosacea Seborrheic dermatitis	**Illustrative topical dose for acne:** 5% gel/cream/lotion: apply to the entire affected area 1 to 3 times per day	• Lotions, ointments, creams, or soaps contain 1% to 10% sulfur; at least 2% sulfur is generally necessary to produce a sufficient keratolytic effect • Many combination products include sulfacetamide; read the package labeling prior to use • If excessive skin irritation develops or increases, discontinue and consult a physician or pharmacist • Do not use sulfur with resorcinol for self-medication of large areas of the body or with broken skin • When used for self-medication of acne, topical sulfur-containing preparations generally should not be used concurrently with other topical acne medications unless otherwise directed by a prescriber Contraindications: • Kidney disease

Drug Name	FDA-Approved Indications	Adult Dosage Range	Precautions and Clinical Pearls
Generic Name Urea **Brand Name** Aluvea Carmol Kerafoam Utopic Others	Hyperkeratotic conditions	**Usual topical dose:** Apply 1 to 3 times per day Concentrations less than 45% generally for xerosis/pruritus and 40–50% for keratolytic action	• Some products may cause photosensitivity; use skin protection and limit sun exposure during therapy and for 1 week after • Urea cream may facilitate better penetration by other topical agents; refer to PI prior to use for this purpose • Discontinue if redness, discomfort, or irritation occurs • Apply to affected area; rub in until completely absorbed • May cover with adhesive bandage/gauze or plastic film • Shake the lotion, foam, and suspension vigorously before administering the dose Contraindications: • OTC labeling: when used for self-medication, do not use on irritated, infected, or open skin

Keratoplastic Agents

Drug Name	FDA-Approved Indications	Adult Dosage Range	Precautions and Clinical Pearls
Generic Name Coal tar **Brand Name** Balnetar Ionil-T Scytera Theraplex T Others	**Common indications for use:** Eczema Seborrheic dermatitis Psoriasis	Dose based on indication for use, formulation selected, and patient's clinical response **Illustrative topical dose for eczema or dermatitis:** 2% foam: apply to the affected area 1 to 4 times per day; decrease to less frequent use once controlled	• May increase photosensitivity; avoid exposure to direct sunlight for 24 hours following application and use appropriate precautions • May stain hair and clothing

Depigmenting Agents

Drug Name	FDA-Approved Indications	Adult Dosage Range	Precautions and Clinical Pearls
Generic Name Hydroquinone **Brand Name** Aclaro EpiQuin Melpaque Others	Gradual bleaching of hyperpigmented skin conditions	**Illustrative topical dose:** 4% cream/gel: apply a thin layer and rub in twice daily	• Limit application to an area no larger than the face and neck or the hands and arms • Monitor for skin irritation • Discontinue therapy if lightening effect is not noted after 2 months of treatment • May cause photosensitivity; use skin protection and limit sun exposure Contraindications: • Sunburn • Depilatory usage

Pigmenting Agents			
Drug Name	**FDA-Approved Indications**	**Adult Dosage Range**	**Precautions and Clinical Pearls**
Generic Name Methoxsalen **Brand Name** Oxsoralen ■ (PD) (GD)	**Common indications for use:** Treatment of severe, recalcitrant, disabling psoriasis Repigmentation of idiopathic vitiligo (in conjunction with UVA)	Illustrative oral doses are available based on the patient's weight and indication for use; refer to treatment protocols for UVA exposure guidelines and PI for product dosing details	• Product should *not* be dispensed to the patient • Products are not interchangeable; use caution when selecting and administering Contraindications: • Diseases associated with photosensitivity (e.g., lupus, porphyria) • Invasive skin cancer • Melanoma or history of melanoma Associated with: • Requires experienced clinician who is knowledgeable in the use of this agent • Serious burns may occur from UV radiation or sunlight (even if exposed through glass) if the recommended exposure schedule is exceeded and/or protective clothing/sunscreen is not used • Methoxsalen concentrates in the lens; shield eyes from direct and indirect sunlight for 24 hours to prevent possible formation of cataracts • Avoid sun (including sun lamp) exposure for 8 hours after methoxsalen exposure • Protective clothing, eyewear, and sunscreen (do not apply sunscreen to psoriatic areas) should be used for several days after combined methoxsalen/UVA therapy

Sunscreen Agents			
Drug Name	**FDA-Approved Indications**	**Adult Dosage Range**	**Precautions and Clinical Pearls**
Sunscreens (PD)	Photoprotection	**Illustrative topical dose for photoprotection:** Apply to all exposed areas of skin at least 15 minutes prior to sun exposure; reapply at least every 2 hours and more frequently after swimming, excessive sweating, or towel drying	• Inhaling the fumes from these preparations may be harmful; use care when administering • PABA and PABA esters may permanently stain light-colored clothing and upholstery yellow or brown; do not put clothing over the treated area until the applied product has dried • Suntanning products that do not contain sunscreen ingredients do not protect the skin from sunburn; repeated exposure of unprotected skin while tanning may increase the risk of skin aging, skin cancer, and other harmful effects to the skin even if sunburn does not occur • Apply evenly and liberally to all exposed areas of the skin, least 15 minutes prior to sun exposure; 1 ounce of sunscreen is considered to be adequate to cover all exposed areas

			• Avoid products with SPF greater than 50; the FDA's 2011 guidelines suggest that there are not adequate data demonstrating that these products provide more protection than lower-SPF products. • Note that a higher SPF requires a greater concentration of chemicals to achieve the higher number.

Miscellaneous Skin and Mucous Membrane Agents

Drug Name	FDA-Approved Indications	Adult Dosage Range	Precautions and Clinical Pearls
Generic Name Acitretin **Brand Name** Soriatane ■	Psoriasis	**Usual oral dose:** 25 to 50 mg per day, as a single dose with main meal	• May cause a decrease in night vision, visual changes and/or tolerance of contact lenses • Monitoring: lipid profile, liver function tests, renal function, blood glucose in patients with diabetes; evaluate for bone abnormalities (with long-term use); CBC and mental health (depression and suicidal thoughts); use with caution in patients with a history of mental illness • Lipid changes are common and generally reversible upon discontinuation; fatal fulminant pancreatitis has been reported • Reported conditions: capillary leak syndrome, exfoliative dermatitis, tinnitus and impaired hearing • Hazardous: use appropriate precautions for handling and disposal • May cause hepatitis (including fatalities); may occur early in treatment • May take 2 to 3 months to achieve the full benefits and most patients experience relapse of psoriasis after discontinuing the medication • Not indicated for the treatment of acne Contraindications: • Severe hepatic or renal dysfunction • Chronic abnormally elevated blood lipid levels Associated with: • Avoid alcohol ingestion and blood donation • Requires experienced clinician who is knowledgeable in the use of this agent • Pseudotumor cerebri

Drug Name	FDA-Approved Indications	Adult Dosage Range	Precautions and Clinical Pearls
Generic Name Adapalene **Brand Name** Differin	Acne vulgaris	**Usual topical dose:** 0.1 % gel/cream/lotion: apply once daily in the evening before bedtime	• Use is associated with increased susceptibility/sensitivity to UV light: avoid sunlamps or excessive sunlight exposure; daily sunscreen use and other protective measures are recommended • Erythema, dryness, scaling, stinging/burning, or pruritus may occur; most likely during first few weeks of therapy, but risk lessens with continued use • Avoid waxing as depilatory method is not recommended • Moisturizers may be used if necessary; avoid products that contain irritants (i.e., acids) • Apply lotion after washing gently with a mild or soapless cleanser and then pat dry; dispense a nickel-size amount (3 to 4 pump actuations) to cover the entire face • A mild transitory sensation of warmth or stinging has been reported with use
Generic Name Alitretinoin **Brand Name** Panretin	Topical treatment of cutaneous lesions in AIDS-related Kaposi's sarcoma	**Usual topical dose:** 0.1% gel: initially apply twice daily to lesions; may gradually increase application frequency to 3 to 4 times per day based on lesion tolerance	• May be photosensitizing (based on experience with other retinoids); minimize sun or other UV exposure of treated areas • Do not use occlusive dressings and do not use concurrently with topical products containing DEET (e.g., insect repellant) • Wait 20 minutes after a shower or bath before applying and do not swim or bathe for at least 3 hours after application • Hazardous: use appropriate precautions for handling and disposal • Apply sufficient gel to cover lesion(s) with a generous coating; allow gel to dry 3 to 5 minutes after application before covering with clothing • Avoid accidental exposure to non-affected skin and membranes • Response may be observed within 2 weeks of initiation, but typically a longer period is required
Generic Name Aminolevulinic acid **Brand Name** Levulan Kerastick	Actinic keratosis of scalp or face	**Illustrative topical dose for actinic keratosis:** 10% gel: apply as directed to lesions and cover with an appropriate occlusive dressing for 3 hours then remove dressing and excess gel and initiate illumination treatment; treatment may be repeated at a treatment site (once) after 3 months	• Recommended gel application: 1 mm thick layer of topical gel to lesions on the scalp or face, and to 5 mm of surrounding skin • Should be applied only by qualified medical personnel to avoid application to perilesional skin; not intended for application by patients • Treatment site will become photosensitive following application; instruct patients to avoid exposure to sunlight, bright indoor lights, or tanning beds during the period prior to blue light treatment • Concomitant use of other known photosensitizing agents may increase the degree of photosensitivity reaction

			• Exposure may result in lesion burning, edema, erythema, and stinging and may also occur during blue light treatment • Therapy should be applied to either scalp or face lesions, but not both simultaneously • Do not wash the application area during the time between application and photosensitization; after photosensitization, gently rinse actinic keratosis with water and pat dry • Following blue light treatment, lesions will temporarily redden, swell, and/or scale; these effects should resolve within 4 weeks after treatment • If unable to perform the blue light treatment after topical application or if treatment with blue light is interrupted or stopped, advise the patient to avoid sunlight/bright light exposure to treated lesions (and wear a wide-brimmed hat or other protective apparel) for at least 40 hours after application; burning/stinging sensation may still occur Contraindications: • Product specific (based on strength); cutaneous photosensitivity at wavelengths of 400 to 450 nm patients with photodermatoses • Porphyria
Generic Name Azelaic acid **Brand Name** Azelex Finacea	Acne vulgaris Rosacea	**Usual topical dose for acne vulgaris:** 20% cream: apply a thin layer to the affected area(s) twice daily (morning and evening)	• Asthma exacerbation has been reported with use • Herpes infection exacerbation has been reported with use • Skin irritation and hypopigmentation (e.g., pruritus, burning, stinging) may occur, usually during the first weeks of therapy • The foam contains flammable propellants; avoid fire, flame, and smoking during and immediately after use • May reduce to once daily if persistent skin irritation occurs; improvement is usually seen within 4 weeks • Reassess gel use if no improvement is seen after 12 weeks • Avoid the use of occlusive dressings and accidental exposure to non-affected areas (including mucous membranes, eyes, etc.) • Shake the foam canister well before use • Monitor for sensitivity, severe irritation, and hypopigmentation in dark-skinned patients at regular intervals during therapy

Drug Name	FDA-Approved Indications	Adult Dosage Range	Precautions and Clinical Pearls
Generic Name Bexarotene **Brand Name** Targretin ■	Cutaneous T-cell lymphoma	**Usual topical dose:** Apply to lesions once every other day for first week, then increase on a weekly basis to once daily, twice daily, 3 times per day, and finally 4 times per day, according to individual lesion tolerance	• Pancreatitis has been reported; avoid use in patients at high risk • Bone marrow suppression (i.e., neutropenia), symptoms of hypothyroidism and hypoglycemia have been reported • May cause photosensitization; minimize sunlight and artificial UV light exposure during treatment • Drug interactions may require dose adjustments or avoidance of certain drug combinations • Vitamin A intake should be limited; refer to PI • Avoid use of insect repellents containing DEET • Apply a sufficient amount to cover the lesion generously and allow the gel to dry before covering with clothing • Visual disturbances have been reported; seek appropriate care • Avoid application to normal skin; do not apply near mucosal surfaces • Use of occlusive dressings is not recommended • If applying after bathing/showering/swimming, wait 20 minutes prior to application of the therapy and for at least 3 hours following application (if possible) • Following application, wipe excess gel from the finger with a disposable tissue and wash hands with soap and water • Continue therapy as long as the patient derives a benefit from it • Response is usually observed with application at 2 to 4 times per day: may decrease frequency if local toxicity occurs; for severe irritation, temporarily withhold for a few days until symptoms subside
Generic Name Brimonidine **Brand Name** Mirvaso	Rosacea	**Usual topical dose:** 0.33% gel: apply a thin layer once daily to the 5 areas of the face: central forehead, each cheek, nose, and chin	• Apply one pea-size amount to affected area • EENT dosage formulations are available also for the treatment of elevated intraocular pressure • Avoid the eyes and lips and wash hands after application

Generic Name Calcipotriene **Brand Name** Calcitrene Dovonex Sorilux	Plaque psoriasis	**Illustrative topical dose:** 0.005% cream/solution or foam: apply a thin layer to the affected skin twice daily	• May cause transient increases in serum calcium (reversible); monitor serum calcium • Transient irritation of both lesions and surrounding uninvolved skin may occur; avoid application to unaffected areas • Foam and solution are flammable; keep away from fire • Avoid excessive exposure to sunlight or phototherapy • Foam, solution (scalp psoriasis): prior to using, comb hair to remove debris; apply only to scalp lesions, when hair is dry • Do not use concurrently with products that may alter the pH of the vehicle (e.g., topical lactic acid); if use of multiple topical agents is necessary, apply at separate times throughout the day • Combining calcipotriene with a topical corticosteroid is more effective (and may result in few adverse events) than when either treatment is used alone • When applied to large areas of skin or for extensive periods of time, monitor for adverse skin or systemic reactions Contraindications: • Demonstrated hypercalcemia or evidence of vitamin D toxicity • Use on the face (cream, ointment) • Acute psoriatic eruptions (scalp solution)
Generic Name Collagenase **Brand Name** Santyl ■	Dermal ulcers	**Usual topical dose:** Apply once daily (or more frequently if the dressing becomes soiled) until debridement of necrotic tissue is complete and granulation tissue is well established	• Debriding enzymes may increase the risk of bacteremia; monitor debilitated patients for systemic bacterial infections • Prior to application, cleanse the wound of debris and digested material using appropriate wound cleaning protocol • If infection is present, refer to PI for appropriate actions • Enzymatic activity is optimal at a pH of 6–8; take precautions to ensure optimal pH at the application site • Apply collagenase directly to the wound or to a sterile gauze pad, which is then applied to the wound and secured • Application should be carefully confined to the area of the wound; transient erythema may occur in surrounding tissues when it is not confined • When applied to large areas or for extensive periods of time, monitor for adverse reactions • Associated with: specific precautions when used parenterally for injection (not applicable for skin and mucous); refer to PI

Drug Name	FDA-Approved Indications	Adult Dosage Range	Precautions and Clinical Pearls
Generic Name Eflornithine **Brand Name** Vaniqa	Reduction of unwanted facial hair in females	**Usual topical dose:** Apply a thin layer of cream to affected areas of the face and areas under the chin twice daily, at least 8 hours apart	• Parenteral formulations are available for protozoal infections; serious adverse effects are associated with systemic exposure and include anemia, ototoxicity, seizures and caution in renal impairment; avoid exposure to EENT and mucous membranes • Hair removal techniques must still be continued; wait at least 5 minutes after removing hair to apply the cream • Do not wash area for at least 4 hours following application • Makeup and sunscreen may be used over treated area(s) after the cream has dried
Generic Name Fluorouracil **Brand Name** Carac Efudex ■	Actinic or solar keratosis Basal cell carcinoma (5%)	Dose based on indication for use, formulation selected, and patient's clinical response **Illustrative topical dose for basal cell carcinoma:** 0.5% cream/solution: apply a thin layer to lesions twice daily for up to 3 to 6 weeks, as tolerated	• Progressive percentage strengths are available with varying degrees of duration, based on the indication for use and recommended affected skin location • Application results in erythema followed by vesiculation, desquamation, erosion, and reepithelialization, which may persist for several weeks after discontinuation; may also cause bruising, burning, dryness, irritation, ulceration • Topical fluorouracil is associated with photosensitivity, including severe sunburn; avoid prolonged exposure to sunlight or UV irradiation • Complete healing may not be evident for 1 to 2 months following treatment • Hazardous: use appropriate precautions for handling and disposal • Apply 10 minutes after washing, rinsing, and drying the affected area; apply a sufficient amount to cover lesions, preferably using a nonmetal applicator or suitable glove • Do not cover the area with an occlusive dressing Contraindications: • Dihydropyrimidine dehydrogenase (DPD) enzyme deficiency: affected individuals may exhibit severe toxicity with topical fluorouracil; life-threatening systemic toxicity has been reported

Generic Name Imiquimod **Brand Name** Aldara Zyclara	Treatment of external genital and perianal warts/condyloma postulati Actinic keratosis Superficial basal cell carcinoma	Dose based on indication for use, formulation selected, and patient's clinical response **Illustrative topical dose for superficial basal cell carcinoma:** 5% Aldara cream: apply a thin layer 5 times per week on alternative days prior to bedtime; leave on for 8 hours (recommended duration of treatment is 6 weeks)	• Intense local inflammatory reactions may occur after a few applications and may be accompanied by systemic symptoms (fever, malaise, myalgia, chronic graft-versus-host disease) • May increase sunburn susceptibility; use protective measures • Not intended for oral, nasal, intravaginal, or ophthalmic use • Severe inflammation of female external genitalia following topical application may lead to severe vulvar swelling and urinary retention • Use with caution in patients with preexisting autoimmune disorders • Administration is not recommended until tissue is healed from any previous drug or surgical treatment • Treatment should not be prolonged beyond the recommended period due to missed doses or rest periods • Prime the Zyclara pump prior to first use; no further priming is required throughout therapy • Actinic keratosis: wash the treatment area and thoroughly dry it prior to application; do not occlude the application site • External genital warts: apply to external or perianal warts; not for vaginal use • Superficial basal cell carcinoma: see the PI for specific application (diameter and margins) guidance • Reduction in lesion size is indicative of a therapeutic response
Generic Name Ingenol **Brand Name** Picato (GD)	Actinic keratosis	**Usual topical dose for face or scalp:** 0.015% gel: apply once daily to the affected area for 3 consecutive days	• Refer to PI for guidance on application to contiguous affected areas of skin • Do not cover with bandages or occlusive dressings • Apply to intact and non-irritated skin only; severe reactions (e.g., erythema, vesiculation, postulation) can occur • Avoid inadvertent transfer to other individuals • Administration of gel is not recommended until the skin is healed from any previous drug or surgical treatment • Avoid washing or touching the treatment area for at least 6 hours; following this period of time, patients may wash the area with a mild soap • Avoid sun exposure and use appropriate protection • Patients not achieving clearance or who experience recurrence after achieving clearance 8 weeks or longer after the initial treatment may benefit from a second treatment course

Drug Name	FDA-Approved Indications	Adult Dosage Range	Precautions and Clinical Pearls
Generic Name Isotretinoin **Brand Name** Absorica Claravis Zenatane ■ (PD)	Severe recalcitrant nodular acne	Dose based on indication for use, formulation selected, and patient's clinical response **Usual oral dose:** 0.5 to 1 mg/kg per day in 2 divided doses for 15 to 20 weeks Dose adjustments or a second course may be required; these decisions are patient specific	• May decrease bone mineral density; osteoporosis, osteopenia, fractures, and delayed healing have been reported • May cause clinical hepatitis, elevated liver enzymes, and impaired glucose metabolism • Marked elevations of serum triglycerides may occur; use with caution in patients with hypertriglyceridemia or those who may be at high risk of that condition (e.g., patients with diabetes) • Avoid prolonged exposure to UV rays or sunlight • May cause depression, psychosis, mood disturbance, and (rarely) suicidal or violent behaviors • Monitor patients with diabetes closely and all patients for changes in CBC with differential and platelet count, baseline sedimentation rate, glucose, creatine phosphokinase (CPK), lipids, liver function tests (LFTs), and changes in vision • Avoid dermatological procedures skin resurfacing procedures (i.e., waxing, dermabrasion, laser, etc.) during and for at least 6 months after discontinuation; there is a risk of scarring • Administer with a meal (except Absorica, which may be taken without regard to meals) • Limit vitamin A intake; some formulations contain soybean oil • Monitor skin for unusual or serious reaction Contraindications: • Specific blood donation restrictions; refer to PI Associated with: • Age-specific contraindication; refer to PI prior to use
Generic Name Mechlorethamine **Brand Name** Valchlor ■	Cutaneous T-cell lymphoma	**Usual topical dose:** 0.016% gel: apply a thin layer once daily to affected areas of skin	• Wear nitrile gloves when applying; wash hands thoroughly with soap and water after handling/application • Avoid accidental skin exposure; wash area thoroughly for at least 15 minutes with soap and water; remove any contaminated clothing if inadvertent exposure occurs • Dose adjustment for toxicity/skin ulceration, blistering, or dermatitis (moderately severe to severe): withhold treatment; may reinitiate treatment with a reduced frequency once adverse effects have resolved; refer to PI for guidance • Discard any unused product 60 days after opening the packaging. • Avoid fire, flame, and smoking until dried

			• Apply to completely dry skin at least 4 hours before or 30 minutes after showering or washing; allow the treated area(s) to dry for 5 to 10 minutes after application before covering with clothing (do not use occlusive dressings over areas) • May apply emollients (moisturizers) to the treated area 2 hours before or 2 hours after application
Generic Name Minoxidil **Brand Name** Rogaine ■	Alopecia	**Illustrative topical dose for males**: 5% foam aerosol/solution: apply twice daily Continuous therapy for 4 months may be necessary for hair growth	• Changes in hair color and texture may occur • Formulations are flammable; avoid fire and flames • For use on the scalp only • Apply directly to the hair-thinning areas of the scalp; massage into the scalp with fingers; wash hands after application • Foam may melt upon contact with warm fingers; rinse the fingers in cold water and thoroughly dry prior to use Contraindications: • If the patient's degree of hair loss differs from that shown on the product labeling or with use of other agents on the scalp • If there is no family history of hair loss, if loss is sudden or patchy or is unknown • If the scalp is red, inflamed, infected, irritated, or painful • Do not use products on women that are labeled for use on men
Generic Name Pimecrolimus **Brand Name** Elidel ■	Atopic dermatitis (mild to moderate)	**Usual topical dose:** 1% cream: apply a thin layer to the affected area twice daily; limit application to the involved areas	• Should not be used in immunocompromised patients, including those on concomitant systemic immunosuppressive therapy • Therapy has been associated with an increased risk of developing herpes simplex (opportunistic infection) and warts • Hazardous: use appropriate precautions for handling and disposal • Avoid artificial or natural sunlight exposure, even when pimecrolimus is not on the skin • Burning at the application site is most common in the first few days after therapy initiation; it improves as the atopic dermatitis improves • Do not use with occlusive dressings • Discontinue use when symptoms have resolved; reevaluate if symptoms persist longer than 6 weeks • Moisturizers may be applied after use of pimecrolimus cream • Avoid use in patients with ichthyosis, specifically Netherton's syndrome (congenital ichthyosiform erythroderma) Associated with: • Topical calcineurin inhibitors (including pimecrolimus) have been associated with rare cases of lymphoma and skin malignancy • Avoid continuous long-term use and limit use to only affected area for the shortest duration possible

Drug Name	FDA-Approved Indications	Adult Dosage Range	Precautions and Clinical Pearls
Generic Name Podofilox **Brand Name** Condylox	External genital warts Perianal warts	**Usual topical dose for genital and perianal warts:** 0.5% solution/gel: apply twice daily (morning and evening) for 3 consecutive days, then withhold use for 4 consecutive days; cycle may be repeated up to 4 times until there is no visible wart tissue	• Solution must be applied with applicator; not for perianal use • Most skin reactions are mild to moderate and do not increase during the treatment period; severe skin reactions can occur and most frequently noted within the first 2 weeks of treatment • Cutaneous use only (not for warts on mucous membranes) • Flammable and poisonous; keep away from fire or flames • Apply to warts using either the applicator supplied with the drug (gel, solution) or with the finger (gel only) while minimizing exposure to surrounding normal tissues • Allow the gel or solution to dry before allowing return of the opposing skin surfaces to their normal positions; wash hands after application • Monitoring: adequate healing and tolerability of treatment • Discontinue after 4 treatment cycles if incomplete response occurs and consider alternative treatment; do not repeat use
Generic Name Podophyllum resin **Brand Name** Podocon	Topical treatment of soft external genital warts	**Usual topical dose:** Applied by physician only	• Use of large amounts of drug should be avoided • Do not use if the wart or surrounding tissue is inflamed or irritated • To be applied by a physician only Contraindications: • Application to bleeding warts, birthmarks, moles, or warts with hair growth • Diabetes or poor circulation • Concurrent use of steroids
Generic Name Secukinumab **Brand Name** Cosentyx	Ankylosing spondylitis Psoriasis Psoriatic arthritis	**Usual parenteral dose for psoriasis:** SQ (without a loading dose): 150 mg every 4 weeks	• May be administered with or without a loading dose • With a loading dose: SQ: 150 mg at weeks 0, 1, 2, 3, and 4 followed by 150 mg every 4 weeks • Exacerbations of inflammatory bowel disease have been reported; avoid use in patients at higher risk (i.e., with Crohn's disease) • Do not be administer to patients with active tuberculosis (TB) infection and evaluate patients for TB infection before treatment • Ensure appropriate immunizations prior to initiating therapy; do not administer vaccinations during therapy (live vaccines may cause infection and non-live vaccinations may not elicit ad adequate immune response to prevent disease) • Discard product if it contains particulate matter, is cloudy, or discolored and discard unused portion (not stored for later use) • Refrigerate (between 36° and 46°F), store in carton until time of use, and do not freeze

Generic Name Sinecatechins **Brand Name** Veregen	Treatment of external genital and perianal warts secondary to condylomata acuminata	**Usual topical dose:** 15% ointment: apply a thin layer (approximately 0.5-cm strand) 3 times per day to all external genital and perianal warts until all warts have been cleared (maximum duration: 16 weeks)	• Local skin reactions are common; continue treatment if possible, but severe skin reactions may require discontinuation • Not intended for treatment of human papillomavirus disease • Women should continue to undergo regular gynecologic examination including screening for cervical dysplasia • For topical use only: ointment is *not* intended for internal use; avoid topical application to open wounds • Avoid exposure of treated area to sun and UV light and do not apply an occlusive dressing • Wash hands before and after application; apply a thin layer of ointment with the fingers; do not wash the ointment off the affected area after application • Sexual contact should be avoided while ointment is on the skin • For females using tampons for menses during treatment; tampon should be inserted prior to application of the ointment • May stain clothing or bedding
Generic Name Tacrolimus **Brand Name** Protopic ■	Moderate to severe atopic dermatitis in immunocompetent patients not responsive to conventional therapy or when conventional therapy is not appropriate	**Illustrative topical dose:** 0.03% ointment: apply a thin layer to the affected area twice daily; rub in gently and completely Discontinue use when symptoms have cleared If no improvement occurs within 6 weeks, patients should be reexamined to confirm the diagnosis	• Do not apply to areas of active bacterial or viral infection (may cause further immunosuppression in already immunocompromised patients) • Monitor for signs of opportunistic infection • Not recommended for patients with skin diseases that may increase systemic absorption (e.g., Netherton's syndrome) • Hazardous: use appropriate precautions for handling and disposal • Second-line therapy for atopic dermatitis/eczema treatment; limit use to patients who have not responded to other therapies • Avoid exposure of treated area to sun and UV light and do not apply an occlusive dressing • Apply only to affected area(s) • Burning at application site is common in the first few days after therapy initiation; (decreases as condition improves) • Continue therapy as long as signs and symptoms persist; discontinue if resolution occurs • Reevaluate if symptoms persist longer than 6 weeks Associated with: • Rare cases of malignancy (including skin and lymphoma) • Limit to short-term and intermittent treatment using the minimum amount necessary for symptom control and only on involved areas

Drug Name	FDA-Approved Indications	Adult Dosage Range	Precautions and Clinical Pearls
Generic Name Tazarotene **Brand Name** Avage Fabior Tazorac	**Common indications for use:** Acne Psoriasis Wrinkling Hyper- and hypopigmentation	**Illustrative dose for acne:** 0.1% cream/gel: apply a small amount to the affected area once daily in the evening	• Causes photosensitivity; avoid exposure to sunlight and sunlamps and use in patients with personal or family history of skin cancer • Treatment can increase skin sensitivity to weather extremes • In patients experiencing excessive skin irritation (e.g., pruritus, burning), discontinue therapy or reduce to tolerable dosing interval • Avoid use of concomitant topical agents (i.e., medicated or abrasive soaps, cosmetics with a strong drying effect) due to increased skin irritation • Foam propellant is flammable; use care • Avoid application of gel to more than 20% of body surface • Do not apply to eczematous, abraded/broken/sunburned skin • Monitoring: disease severity in patients with plaque psoriasis during therapy (reduction in erythema, scaling, induration); clinical response and skin tolerance
Generic Name Ustekinumab **Brand Name** Stelara GD	Plaque psoriasis Psoriatic arthritis	Dose based on indication for use, formulation selected, and patient's clinical response **Illustrative parenteral dose for plaque psoriasis:** SQ: patients weighing 100 kg or less: 45 mg and repeat 4 weeks later, then every 12 weeks thereafter	• Antibody formation to ustekinumab has been observed; this effect has been associated with decreased serum levels and therapeutic response in some patients • May increase the risk for infection, malignancy, or activation of latent infections. Monitor closely if a new infection develops during treatment; in case of a serious infection, discontinue or withhold therapy until infection resolves • Do not initiate therapy if active infection is present and initiate treatment of latent TB before therapy begins • Live vaccines should not be given concurrently • Use with caution in combination with other immunosuppressive drugs • May decrease the protective effect of desensitization procedures and may increase the risk of an allergic reaction to a dose of allergen immunotherapy • Patients who weigh more than 100 kg may require higher doses to achieve adequate serum levels; refer to PI • Consider therapy discontinuation in any patient who fails to demonstrate a response after 12 weeks of therapy • Administer by subcutaneous injection into the top of the thigh, abdomen, upper arms, or buttocks; rotate sites • Do not inject into tender, bruised, erythematous, or indurated skin and avoid injections into areas where psoriasis is present

			• Monitoring: TB screening; CBC; ustekinumab-antibody formation; signs and symptoms of infection, reversible posterior leukoencephalopathy syndrome (RPLS), and squamous cell skin carcinoma • Following an interruption in therapy, retreatment may be initiated at the initial dosing interval • IV administration is limited to non-dermatologic indications • Single-use vial or single-use prefilled syringe do not contain preservatives; discard any unused portion
Diclofenac	Refer to the Central Nervous System Agents chapter.		
Doxycycline	Refer to the Anti-infective Agents chapter.		
Finasteride	Refer to the Hormones and Synthetic Substitutes chapter.		

Chapter 14

Smooth Muscle Relaxants

Authors: **Wayne H. Grant, PharmD, MBA and Laura Rumschik, PharmD**

Editor: **Margaret A. Huwer, PharmD**

Learning Objectives

- Identify current pharmacologic agents that are appropriate for each condition/diagnosis.
- Recommend optimal pharmacologic interventions based on patient-specific characteristics.
- Provide appropriate patient-specific counseling points and optimal overall medication management.

Key Terms: gastrointestinal agents, genitourinary smooth muscle relaxants, antimuscarinic agents, $beta_3$-adrenergic agonists, respiratory smooth muscle relaxants

Overview of Smooth Muscle Relaxants

Smooth muscle is found in the walls of hollow organs, including blood vessels, airways, the gastrointestinal (GI) tract, and bladder. The term "smooth muscle" reflects the lack of visible striation in skeletal muscle. Contractions of these muscles are primarily controlled by the autonomic nervous system, as part of involuntary daily functions such as digestion and blood pressure maintenance. Both the sympathetic (adrenergic) and parasympathetic (cholinergic) nervous systems act on smooth muscle. A wide variety of drugs are available that can affect these systems throughout the body. Like skeletal and cardiac muscle, smooth muscle is made up of thick myosin and thin actin filaments. These components act in concert, creating muscle contractions. Vasodilators work to reduce this contractility, thereby leading to smooth muscle relaxation. Further discussion of specific bronchial vasodilators is found in other chapters within this text.

14.1 Gastrointestinal and Genitourinary Smooth Muscle Relaxants

Overactive Bladder and Urinary Incontinence

Overactive bladder (OAB) syndrome is defined as urinary urgency with or without urinary incontinence. Antimuscarinics are used to treat both urinary incontinence and overactive bladder. Parasympathetic muscarinic stimulation causes detrusor muscle contraction and sphincter muscle relaxation. Drug therapy, therefore, seeks to have the opposite effects, leading to muscarinic (M_2) receptor antagonism. M_2 receptors are the most prevalent targets, but M_3 receptors have been linked to detrusor contraction as well.

Genitourinary Smooth Muscle Relaxants

Overactive bladder and urinary incontinence have historically been treated with antimuscarinic agents. Systemic inhibition of muscarinic receptors may lead to blurred vision, constipation, and dry mouth, ultimately creating adherence issues. Oxybutynin has been linked to the highest discontinuation rates, so transdermal and topical gel formulations have been developed that are designed to decrease these systemic effects. Anticholinergic effects could also worsen other disease states such as glaucoma and urinary retention. Drowsiness, dizziness, and confusion can occur with such agents; these effects are most problematic for elderly patients. This cascade of adverse events is less common with trospium, darifenacin, solifenacin, and fesoterodine.

Members of this drug class are generally metabolized by the liver; thus, they require dose reductions with concomitant use of hepatic enzyme inhibitors and should not be used with inhaled formulations such as ipratropium. Drugs within the class have been shown to have statistically significant differences in efficacies, but these small differences have not been shown to be clinically significant.

Flavoxate is considered an antispasmodic, but it also has local anesthetic effects and, at high doses, antimuscarinic effects. Mirabegron is a newer agent that offers less anticholinergic effects than the other antimuscarinics. It activates the β_3 receptor in the bladder to relax the detrusor smooth muscles while the bladder is filling, thereby allowing this organ to hold more urine for longer amounts of time. Mirabegron may be preferred over other agents due to its more tolerable side-effect profile. Tachycardia and arrhythmias are a concern with both flavoxate and mirabegron.

Antimuscarinic Agents

Darifenacin
Fesoterodine
Flavoxate
Oxybutynin
Solifenacin
Tolterodine
Trospium

Selective Beta$_3$-Adrenergic Agonists

Mirabegron

Case Studies and Conclusions

A patient is currently taking oxybutynin ER 10 mg. He complains of dry mouth and constipation, although his frequency of urination has been decreased effectively.

1. What can be changed in this patient's regimen to address the adverse effects he is experiencing?
   a. Switch to the transdermal or gel formulation
   b. Take the medication on an empty stomach
   c. Increase his daily fluid intake
   d. Switch to the immediate-release formulation

Answer A is correct. Switching to a transdermal or gel formulation of oxybutynin will address the adverse effects because these alternative administration forms essentially eliminate presystemic metabolism, thereby preventing this small, lipophilic drug and its metabolite from crossing the blood–brain barrier easily and decreasing the potential adverse effects.

2. If the patient requested a topical dosage form, how would you instruct the patient to use the new regimen?
   a. Apply the transdermal patch to rotated abdomen, hip, and gluteal sites
   b. Apply the topical gel to the gluteal region only
   c. Decrease the oral dose by half when adding a patch
   d. Warm the patch in the microwave oven prior to use

Answer A is correct. Topical administration should be rotated among sites to reduce administration-site reactions. The patch can be applied to the abdomen, hip, and gluteal region. The gel may be applied to the abdomen, thighs, and upper arms/shoulders. The patch is heat sensitive and should not be heated. Also, it should not be used concurrently with an oral formulation.

3. Which additional side effects would you expect to become more concerned about with the use of oxybutynin as the patient ages?
   a. Increased urinary tract infections
   b. Drowsiness, dizziness, and confusion
   c. Dermatologic rashes
   d. Increased sleep continuity

Answer B is correct. Drowsiness, dizziness, and confusion are common in older adults; hence, oxybutynin is on the Beers list. Increased sleep continuity is an improvement in total sleep time; this effect does not occur with anticholinergic products, although they do cause somnolence.

A 60-year-old patient is interested in starting mirabegron. She is currently taking lisinopril for hypertension, baclofen for back spasms, and sertraline for depression.

1. Which of this patient's current health problems should be closely monitored if she is started on mirabegron and why?
   a. Hypotension; blood pressure may decrease with use of mirabegron.
   b. Anemia; a decreased red blood cell count may occur with use of mirabegron.
   c. Hypertension; blood pressure may increase with use of mirabegron.
   d. Leukopenia; a decreased absolute neutrophil count may occur with use of mirabegron.

Answer C is correct. Clinicians should be aware that patients may experience an exacerbation of hypertension, as blood pressure may increase with use of mirabegron.

2. How would you explain to the patient how mirabegron works and differs from the other treatment options available?
   a. Mirabegron relaxes the bladder when it is filling by activating receptors.
   b. Mirabegron has less adverse drug reactions than the older medications that block receptors throughout the body.
   c. Mirabegron has selective receptor action, so it does not influence all receptors in the body.
   d. All of the above are correct.

Answer D is correct. All of these statements are true.

3. When would you not want to give mirabegron to a patient?
   a. If the patient cannot produce or expel urine
   b. If the patient has congenital QTc prolongation
   c. If the patient is on medications that increase the QTc interval
   d. All of these conditions are contraindications to mirabegron use.

Answer D is correct. All of these conditions are contraindications to mirabegron use.

14.2 Respiratory Smooth Muscle Relaxants

Airway smooth muscle is a vital tissue involved in the regulation of bronchomotor tone. This tissue is present in the trachea and in the bronchial tree up to the terminal bronchioles. It increases in mass with chronic airway diseases—a change that may represent either a pathologic process or an injury-repair response due to chronic inflammation. Some studies have shown that airway smooth muscle may become an "active participant" in modulating inflammation in chronic lung diseases versus existing as a "passive" contractile tissue; this role suggests that it may serve as an important potential new target for the treatment of chronic lung diseases.

Methylxanthines

Methylxanthines such as theophylline are structurally related to caffeine and act as adenosine receptor antagonists to prevent bronchoconstriction. They act similarly to β_2 agonist bronchodilators in that they prevent degradation of cyclic adenosine monophosphate (cAMP) through nonselective phosphodiesterase inhibition. The bronchodilatory effects are most apparent when plasma concentrations of theophylline are greater than 10 mcg/mL; anti-inflammatory effects are responsible for the drug's efficacy when concentrations are less than this level. Intravenous methylxanthines are generally used in acute asthma or chronic obstructive pulmonary disease (COPD) exacerbations when patients cannot tolerate nebulized sympathomimetics.

Oral sustained-release formulations can be added to maintenance therapy if maximally effective doses of first-line immediate release agents are ineffective, although their role in therapy is controversial. Plasma levels should be closely monitored in either case, as these medications have narrow therapeutic ranges.

Theophylline was the first methylxanthine designed to treat asthma and COPD and remains the standard for therapeutic drug monitoring. Theophylline's targeted concentration is 10 mcg/mL in adults (or 5 to 15 mcg/mL). Adverse drug reactions are most commonly seen with doses greater than 15 mcg/mL and are caused by phosphodiesterase type 4 inhibition, resulting in headache, nausea, and vomiting. Tachycardia, agitation, and gastric acid secretion are caused by excess adenosine receptor antagonism. While chronic theophylline toxicity is associated with minimal GI symptoms, acute toxicity is characterized by severe, repetitive vomiting. Conditions such as comorbid heart failure (HF) have also been linked to decreased clearance of theophylline.

The methylxanthines are metabolized by the liver and thus require higher doses when patients are given medications that compete for the same hepatic pathway (such as beta blockers) or in patients who are cigarette smokers. Although these agents are unique in having anti-inflammatory and bronchodilation effects, their use has declined since more efficacious drugs have become available that produce less adverse drug effects. Over the years, methylxanthines have fallen out favor; today, they are generally prescribed only when response to β_2 agonists, anticholinergics, and/or inhaled corticosteroids is insufficient.

Respiratory Smooth Muscle Relaxants

Aminophylline
Theophylline
Anticholinergic agents *(see also the Autonomic-Anticholinergic Agents section in the Autonomic Agents chapter)*
Sympathomimetic (adrenergic) agents *(see also the Autonomic-Sympathomimetic Adrenergic Agents section in the Autonomic Agents chapter)*
Vasodilating agents *(see also the Vasodilating Agents section in the Cardiovascular Agents chapter and the Phosphodiesterase Type 4 Inhibitors and Miscellaneous Respiratory Agents section in the Respiratory Tract Agents chapter)*

Case Studies and Conclusions

An elderly woman with diabetes and congestive heart failure (CHF) presents with an acute asthma exacerbation. Intravenous aminophylline is to be started to treat this condition.

1. Which theophylline plasma level range should be targeted in adults?
   a. 5 to 15 mcg/mL
   b. 50 to 150 mcg/mL
   c. 10 to 20 mcg/mL
   d. 100 to 200 mcg/mL

Answer A is correct. The target range for theophylline is 5 to 15 mcg/mL in adults.

2. Which symptom would the patient display if she experienced acute theophylline toxicity, and what may be the patient-specific risk factor contributing to the development of such toxicity?
   a. Hypoglycemia; comorbid diabetes
   b. Abdominal pain; female gender
   c. Respiratory alkalosis; intravenous administration
   d. Repetitive vomiting; comorbid congestive heart failure

Answer D is correct. While chronic theophylline toxicity is associated with minimal GI symptoms, acute toxicity is characterized by severe, repetitive vomiting. Comorbid HF has been linked to decreased clearance of theophylline. While abdominal pain is a symptom, female gender does not make this presentation more likely. Respiratory alkalosis and hypoglycemia are not symptoms of acute theophylline toxicity.

As the aminophylline is being given, you notice a visitor bring the patient coffee and a breakfast sandwich.

3. What might be a concern here?

   a. IV theophylline should be given on an empty stomach
   b. Caffeinated coffee may increase the side effects of theophylline
   c. Nothing—these foods are acceptable choices for the patient to consume
   d. Caffeinated coffee may exacerbate acute asthma symptoms

Answer B is correct. Theophylline is structurally related to caffeine, a known bronchodilator. Concomitant use can increase risk of nausea, insomnia, irregular heartbeats, or seizures.

A 27-year-old male patient with asthma is currently taking a long-acting beta-agonist and an inhaled steroid, but still requires daily use of his rescue inhaler.

1. Assuming the patient is already taking the maximum doses of his current medications, which medication and formulation would you start?

   a. Intravenous theophylline
   b. Immediate-release oral theophylline
   c. Sustained-release oral theophylline
   d. Any of these options is appropriate.

Answer C is correct. IV theophylline is reserved for acute exacerbations of asthma. Immediate-release options are no longer manufactured, having been replaced by sustained-release options that have more stable plasma levels.

2. How would you instruct the patient to take the medication to maintain consistent plasma levels?

   a. Either with or without food, as long as he is consistent with his choice
   b. With a high-fat meal
   c. With a full glass of water on an empty stomach
   d. Only on days when he feels he needs it

Answer A is correct. Food affects absorption of theophylline and, therefore, its plasma levels. The sustained-release dose can be adjusted to accommodate how the patient takes the medication, as long as he takes it the same way every day.

3. How will the patient know if this medication is effective therapy for him?

   a. The patient will be able to stop using his inhalers.
   b. The patient will be able to tolerate doses associated with a plasma level beyond 15 mcg/mL.
   c. Theophylline is a first-line therapy and should work for everyone.
   d. The patient will experience symptomatic relief and will require the rescue inhaler only 1 or 2 days per week.

Answer D is correct. Rescue inhalers should ideally be needed 2 or fewer days per week. Adequate control will be achieved if the patient reaches this point, while still taking his other medications. He has already tried first-line inhalers and, therefore, requires an adjunctive (add-on) medication.

Tips from the Field

1. Topical gels (including oxybutinin) are typically flammable; therefore, exposure to fire, flame, and tobacco-smoking should be avoided until the gel has dried.

2. Accidental exposure to other people and pets can result from numerous products, including topical gels. In order to minimize this risk of unintentional exposure, patients should wait until the gel dries after application and then cover the application (if appropriate) when skin-to-skin contact with others is possible.

3. Urinary incontinence can result from a variety of causes. Patients should be made aware that fluid restriction does not solve the problem and can result in dehydration and overly concentrated urine, which can irritate the bladder and cause increased feelings of urgency.
4. Patients should be encouraged to seek treatment for incontinence and not feel as though they just have to live with the embarrassment and reduced quality of life. Equally important are non-pharmacotherapeutic interventions such as using the restroom at regular intervals, even before the bladder feels full. Exercises specifically focused on bladder strength can be very helpful, but so can maintaining an overall healthy lifestyle that includes regular exercise, healthy diet, weight control, limited alcohol consumption, and smoking cessation.

Tammie Lee and Jacque

Bibliography

American Geriatrics Society. 2015 updated Beers criteria for potentially inappropriate medication use in older adults. *J Am Geriatr Soc.* 2015;63:2227-2246.

Amrani Y, Panettieri RA. Airway smooth muscle: contraction and beyond. *Int J Biochem Cell Biol.* 2003;35(3):272-276.

Brunton LL, Chabner BA, Knollmann BC, eds. *Goodman & Gilman's The Pharmacological Basis of Therapeutics.* 12th ed. New York, NY: McGraw-Hill; 2011.

Ferreira J, Drummond M, Pires N, Reis G, Alves C, Robalo-Cordeiro C. Optimal treatment sequence in COPD: can a consensus be found? *Rev Port Pneumol.* 2016;22:39-49.

Golan DE, ed. *Principles of Pharmacology.* 3rd ed. Philadelphia, PA: Lippincott Williams & Wilkins; 2012.

Juliato CRT, Baccaro LF, Pedro AO, Costa-Paiva L, Lui-Filho J, Pinto-Neto AM. Subjective urinary urgency in middle age women: a population-based study. *Maturitas.* 2016;85:82-87.

Lexi-Comp Online. Hudson, OH: Lexi-Comp; 2015. http://online.lexi.com/action/home

McEvoy GK, ed. *AHFS: Drug Information.* Bethesda, MD: American Society of Health-System Pharmacists; 2016.

Paulsen DF. *Histology and Cell Biology: Examination and Board Review.* 5th ed. New York, NY: McGraw-Hill; 2010.

PDR. Oxybutynin: drug summary. http://www.pdr.net/drug-summary/Oxytrol-for-Women-oxybutynin-3260. Accessed January 20, 2017.

Symbols

- ▲ Renal impairment: Dose adjustment is recommended.
- ◼ Hepatic impairment: Dose adjustment is recommended.
- ■ Black box warning exists for this drug.
- (QT) QTc prolongation effects have been reported.
- (BL) Beers list criteria (avoid in elderly).
- (PD) FDA-approved pediatric doses are available.
- (GD) FDA-approved geriatric doses are available.
-  See primary body system.

Smooth Muscle Relaxants

Universal prescribing alerts:

- Known serious hypersensitivity to the specific drug or any other component of the product/formulation selected warrants a contraindication for its use.
- Adverse reactions associated with the use of some **smooth muscle relaxant agents** include dizziness, drowsiness, vertigo, and fatigue; these agents may also impair the ability to perform tasks requiring mental alertness. Caution should always be recommended when using any new drug for the first time, when there is a dose change, and for continued use of known offending agents.
- Doses expressed are for usual adult dosage ranges only. "Geriatric doses" are assumed to be the same as adult doses unless otherwise noted with a symbol. Where FDA-approved, pediatric dosing is available, a symbol will guide the reader to additional prescribing references for these age-specific doses. Refer to real-time prescribing references for these age-specific doses.
- Use of smooth muscle relaxant agents in pregnancy is based on weighing clinical risk versus benefit and safety concerns are not represented in this grid. Refer to the package insert (PI) for more information. Clinicians should continue to provide education about the reproductive risks of any medication and offer risk-reduction strategies (which may include contraceptive use) to women of childbearing age and understand that these reproductive risks may also extend to males. Other medications may decrease the effectiveness of oral contraceptives. Where necessary, an alternative means of birth control should be explored.
- Brand names are provided for those products still available on the market. Due to the ever-changing product availability, refer to Food and Drug Administration (FDA) resources to confirm the actual brands available. This drug summary is intended for educational purposes only. Prescribing decisions should be based on real-time comprehensive drug databases that are updated on a regular basis.

Gastrointestinal and Genitourinary Smooth Muscle Relaxants

Antimuscarinic Agents

Universal prescribing alerts:

- Antimuscarinic agents are contraindicated in patients with narrow-angle glaucoma, urinary retention, paralytic ileus, gastrointestinal (GI) or genitourinary (GU) obstruction, urinary retention, or gastric retention. Consider universal prescribing alerts for anticholinergic agents (refer to Autonomic Agents chapter).
- Angioedema is possible even after just the first dose.
- Monitor for central nervous system (CNS) effects.
- Use caution in hot weather and while exercising (due to risk of heat prostration).
- Use with caution in patients with myasthenia gravis.

Drug Name	FDA-Approved Indications	Adult Dosage Range	Precautions and Clinical Pearls
Generic Name Darifenacin **Brand Name** Enablex ■ (BL)	Symptomatic management of bladder overactivity (urge incontinence, urgency, frequency)	**Usual oral dose:** 7.5 to 15 mg per day	• Take with liquid and swallow whole • Drug interactions may require dose adjustment or avoidance of certain drug combinations Contraindications: • Closed-angle glaucoma • GI obstruction, gastroparesis and pyloric stenosis • Urinary retention
Generic Name Fesoterodine **Brand Name** Toviaz ▲ (BL)	Symptomatic management of bladder overactivity (urge incontinence, urgency, frequency)	**Usual oral dose:** 4 to 8 mg per day	• Swallow whole • Drug interactions may require dose adjustments or avoidance of certain drug combinations • Not recommended for patients with hepatic impairment
Generic Name Flavoxate **Brand Name** Urispas (BL)	Symptomatic management of dysuria, nocturia, suprapubic pain, and urgency Incontinence in patients with cystitis, urethritis, or prostatitis	**Usual oral dose:** 100 to 200 mg 3 to 4 times per day	Contraindications: • GI obstruction or GI hemorrhage • Urethral stricture, obstruction and/or retention
Generic Name Oxybutynin **Brand Name** Ditropan XL Gelnique Oxytrol (BL) (PD) (GD)	Symptomatic treatment of uninhibited or reflex neurogenic bladder Symptomatic treatment of detrusor overactivity due to a neurologic condition (XL only)	**Usual oral dose:** IR: 5 mg 2 to 4 times per day ER: 5 to 30 mg per day **Usual topical dose:** Topical gel: apply 84 to 100 mg per day (three 3% pumps or contents of one 10% gel packet) Transdermal patch: apply 1 patch (3.9 mg per day patch) twice weekly	• Use with caution in patients with hyperthyroidism or Parkinson's disease • Swallow XL tablets whole • XL tablet shells may be seen in stool • Gel delivered in a device that must be "pumped" 3 times and that dose should be applied topically once daily to clean, dry, intact skin on the abdomen, upper arms/shoulders, or thighs. Rotate sites to avoid local irritation • Gel is flammable; use caution • Avoid accidental exposure; refer to Tips from the Field to limit this risk • Apply the transdermal patch to rotated abdomen, hip, and buttocks sites Contraindications: • GI obstruction or GI hemorrhage • Urethral stricture, obstruction, and/or retention
Generic Name Solifenacin **Brand Name** Vesicare ▲ ■ (QT) (BL)	Symptomatic management of bladder overactivity (urge incontinence, urgency, frequency)	**Usual oral dose:** 5 to 10 mg per day	• Swallow tablet whole with liquids • Drug interactions may require dose adjustments or avoidance of certain drug combinations Contraindications: • GI obstruction or GI hemorrhage • Urethral stricture, obstruction and/or retention

Generic Name Tolterodine **Brand Name** Detrol Detrol LA QT BL	Symptomatic management of bladder overactivity (urge incontinence, urgency, frequency)	**Usual oral dose:** IR: 1 to 2 mg twice daily ER: 2 to 4 mg per day	• Use with caution in patients with renal or hepatic impairment • Swallow the ER tablet whole Contraindications: • GI obstruction or GI hemorrhage • Urethral stricture, obstruction, and/or retention
Generic Name Trospium **Brand Name** Sanctura Sanctura XR QT BL	Symptomatic management of bladder overactivity (urge incontinence, urgency, frequency, and neurogenic bladder)	**Usual oral dose:** IR: 20 mg twice daily ER: 60 mg per day	• Use with caution in patients with renal or hepatic impairment • Take on an empty stomach • ER capsules should be taken in the morning with water, 2 hours apart from alcohol consumption Contraindications: • GI obstruction or GI hemorrhage • Urethral stricture, obstruction, and/or retention

Selective Beta$_3$-Adrenergic Agonists

Drug Name	FDA-Approved Indications	Adult Dosage Range	Precautions and Clinical Pearls
Generic Name Mirabegron **Brand Name** Myrbetriq QT	Symptomatic management of bladder overactivity (urge incontinence, urgency, frequency)	**Usual oral dose:** 25 to 50 mg per day	• Recommendation to start with 25 mg dose for 8 weeks; if there is inadequate improvement, may increase dose to improve efficacy • Angioedema is possible even after just the first dose • Not recommended in severe hepatic impairment • Dose-related increases in blood pressure can occur • Use with caution in patients with bladder flow obstruction, hepatic or renal impairment • Swallow the tablet whole • Drug interactions may require dose adjustments or avoidance of certain drug combinations

Respiratory Smooth Muscle Relaxants

Universal prescribing alerts:

- These agents can exacerbate existing cardiac arrhythmias and can increase oxygen demand and should be used with caution in patients at risk (i.e., cardiac disease and history of myocardial Infarction).
- Use caution in patients with hepatic impairment and moderate to severe hepatic disease such as cirrhosis, acute hepatitis, cholestasis, or alcoholic liver disease. These agents undergo extensive hepatic metabolism and dose adjustments may be required.
- Encouraging smoking cessation is critical, especially for individuals with respiratory illness. Because the effect of tobacco on liver enzymes is not related to the nicotine component, sudden smoking cessation may result in a reduced clearance that results in increased serum concentration of theophylline, despite the initiation of nicotine replacement. Monitor theophylline serum concentrations carefully when smoking status changes and adjust doses accordingly.
- Theophylline also should be used cautiously in patients with respiratory infection, severe hypoxemia and when fever is present. Dose adjustments may be warranted.

- These agents should be used with caution in patients with gastritis, gastroesophageal reflux disease (GERD), hiatal hernia, or active peptic ulcers. Theophylline stimulates gastric secretions and may aggravate symptoms related to these conditions.
- Use caution in patients with prostatic hypertrophy. Theophylline may cause diuretic effects and relaxation of smooth muscle resulting in increase urinary retention, so it should be used with caution in these patients.

Drug Name	FDA-Approved Indications	Adult Dosage Range	Precautions and Clinical Pearls
Generic Name: Aminophylline ■ (BL) (PD) (GD)	Symptomatic treatment of reversible airway obstruction due to chronic lung diseases	**Illustrative parenteral dose (expressed as theophylline) for asthma exacerbation:** IV: 0.4 mg/kg per hour up to a maximum of 900 mg per day in otherwise healthy nonsmokers	• Aminophylline is a compound of theophylline (has ethylenediamine added) and is less potent • Theophylline dose is 80% of aminophylline • If using a loading dose, give over 30 minutes • If extravasation occurs, immediately stop the infusion and follow the management guidelines provided in the PI • Theophylline toxicity (repetitive vomiting) is likely in patients with congestive heart failure (CHF), cor pulmonale, hepatic disease, and sepsis • Narrow therapeutic index drug; dose to target theophylline concentrations; refer to PI
Generic Name Theophylline **Brand Name** Theophylline Uniphyl Theo-24 Various others ▲ ■ (BL) (PD) (GD)	Symptomatic management or prevention of reversible obstructive airway diseases	**Illustrative parenteral dose (expressed as theophylline) for asthma exacerbation:** IV: 0.4 mg/kg per hour up to a maximum of 900 mg per day in otherwise healthy nonsmokers **Usual oral dose:** ER: initial 300 to 400mg once per day; may increase dose to 400 to 600 mg once per day if needed and tolerated	• Increase oral doses gradually (no sooner than every 3 days per manufacturer). Adjust dose to maintain therapeutic range • Evening doses are not recommended due to caffeine like effects. Monitor for CNS effects • ER tablets can be taken with or without food • ER formulations are intended only for chronic disease management; do not use in treatment of acute symptoms of asthma and reversible bronchospasm • Theophylline toxicity (repetitive vomiting) is likely in patients with CHF, cor pulmonale, hepatic disease, and sepsis • Use with caution in patients with severe cardiac disease, hyperthyroidism, peptic ulcer disease, or seizure disorders • Lower doses are recommended for patients who cannot be monitored and have risk factors for reduced theophylline clearance • Multiple formulations available, use care when selecting and administering • Narrow therapeutic index drug; dose to target theophylline concentrations; refer to PI
Anticholinergic agents		Refer to the Autonomic Agents chapter.	
Sympathomimetic (adrenergic) agents		Refer to the Autonomic Agents chapter.	
Vasodilating agents		Refer to the Cardiovascular Agents chapter and the Respiratory Tract Agents chapter.	

Index

A

B

C

D

E

F

G

N

O

P

Q

R

V

W